PROLOG

OBSTETRICS

SIXTH EDITION

CRITIQUE BOOK

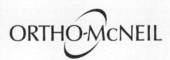

Ortho–McNeil Pharmaceutical is pleased to provide *PROLOG: Obstetrics,*
Sixth Edition, to future specialists in obstetrics and gynecology.
Recognizing the importance of high-quality education, Ortho–McNeil is
privileged to introduce this valuable educational resource.

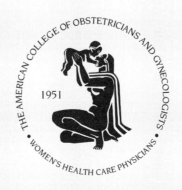

THE AMERICAN COLLEGE OF OBSTETRICIANS AND GYNECOLOGISTS

1951

WOMEN'S HEALTH CARE PHYSICIANS

ISBN 978-1-932328-43-1

12345/21098

The American College of Obstetricians and Gynecologists
409 12th Street, SW
PO Box 96920
Washington, DC 20090-6920

Contributors

PROLOG Editorial and Advisory Committee

CHAIR

Ronald T. Burkman, Jr, MD, Chair
  Chair, Department of Obstetrics and
    Gynecology
  Baystate Medical Center
  Springfield, Massachusetts
  Deputy Chair and Professor
  Department of Obstetrics and
    Gynecology
  Tufts University School of Medicine
  Boston, Massachusetts

MEMBERS

Bernard Gonik, MD
  Professor and Fann Srere Chair of
    Perinatal Medicine
  Division of Maternal–Fetal Medicine
  Department of Obstetrics and
    Gynecology
  Wayne State University School of
    Medicine
  Detroit, Michigan
Louis Weinstein, MD
  Paul A. and Eloise B. Bowers Professor
    and Chair
  Department of Obstetrics and
    Gynecology
  Thomas Jefferson University
  Philadelphia, Pennsylvania
Sterling B. Williams, MD
  Vice President, Education
  The American College of Obstetricians
    and Gynecologists
  Washington, DC

PROLOG Task Force for *Obstetrics*, Sixth Edition

COCHAIRS

George A. Macones, MD
  Professor and Chair
  Department of Obstetrics and
    Gynecology
  Washington University at St. Louis
  St. Louis, Missouri
Isabelle A. Wilkins, MD
  Professor and Director
  Division of Maternal and Fetal
    Medicine
  Department of Obstetrics and
    Gynecology
  University of Illinois at Chicago
  Chicago, Illinois

MEMBERS

David Acker, MD
  Associate Professor
  Division of Maternal–Fetal Medicine
  Dept. of Obstetrics, Gynecology, and
    Reproductive Sciences
  Harvard Medical School
  Chief of Obstetrics
  Brigham and Women's Hospital
  Boston, Massachusetts
Vincenzo Berghella, MD
  Professor and Director
  Division of Maternal–Fetal Medicine
  Director, Maternal–Fetal Medicine
    Fellowship Program
  Department of Obstetrics and
    Gynecology
  Jefferson Medical College of Thomas
    Jefferson University
  Philadelphia, Pennsylvania

Continued on next page

PROLOG Task Force for *Obstetrics,* Sixth Edition *(continued)*

Andrea D. Kemp, MD, MPH
Assistant Professor and Associate
Residency Director
Division of Maternal–Fetal Medicine
Department of Obstetrics and
Gynecology
University of Illinois at Chicago
Chicago, Illinois

Bill C. Mabie, MD
Clinical Professor of Obstetrics and
Gynecology
Division of Maternal–Fetal Medicine
Department of Obstetrics and
Gynecology
University of South Carolina,
Greenville
Greenville Hospital Systems
Greenville, South Carolina

Joan M. Mastrobattista, MD
Associate Professor
Director, Prenatal Diagnosis
Division of Maternal–Fetal Medicine
Department of Obstetrics, Gynecology,
and Reproductive Sciences
University of Texas Health Science
Center Houston
Houston, Texas

Ana Monteagudo, MD
Professor
Department of Obstetrics and
Gynecology
Associate Director, Ob–Gyn
Ultrasound Unit
New York University School of
Medicine
New York, New York

Dotun Aberdoye Ogunyemi, MD
Director, Maternal–Fetal Medicine
Division of Obstetrics
Department of Obstetrics and
Gynecology
Harbor–UCLA Medical Center
Los Angeles, California

John T. Repke, MD
Professor and Chairman
Department of Obstetrics and
Gynecology
Penn State University College of
Medicine
Obstetrician–Gynecologist-in-Chief
The Milton S. Hershey Medical Center
Hershey, Pennsylvania

Anthony C. Sciscione, DO
Director of Maternal–Fetal Medicine
and Residency Program Director
Department of Obstetrics and
Gynecology
Christiana Hospital
Newark, Delaware
Department of Obstetrics and
Gynecology
Christiana Hospital
Newark, Delaware

Sally Y. Segel, MD
Assistant Professor
Director of Maternal–Fetal Medicine
Fellowship
Division of Maternal–Fetal Medicine
Department of Obstetrics and
Gynecology
Oregon Health and Science University
Portland, Oregon

ACOG STAFF
Erica Bukevicz
Senior Manager, Educational
Development and Testing
Division of Education

Christopher T. George, MA
Editor, PROLOG

CONFLICT OF INTEREST DISCLOSURE

This PROLOG unit was developed under the direction of the PROLOG Advisory Committee and the Task Force for *Obstetrics*, Sixth Edition. PROLOG is planned and produced in accordance with the Standards for Enduring Materials of the Accreditation Council for Continuing Medical Education. Any discussion of unapproved use of products is clearly cited in the appropriate critique.

Current guidelines state that continuing medical education (CME) providers must ensure that CME activities are free from the control of any commercial interest. The task force and advisory committee members declare that neither they nor any business associate nor any member of their immediate families has material interest, financial interest, or other relationships with any company manufacturing commercial products relative to the topics included in this publication or with any provider of commercial services discussed in the unit except for **Ronald T. Burkman Jr, MD,** who is a consultant with Pfizer, Inc., and Ortho-McNeil Pharmaceutical, and has received speaker support from Ortho-McNeil Pharmaceutical, Wyeth, Inc., Berlex, Inc., and Organon, Inc. **Anthony C. Sciscione, MD,** is on the speaker's bureau of Adeza Biomedical. All potential conflicts have been resolved through multiple task force and advisory committee review of all content.

Preface

Purpose

PROLOG (Personal Review of Learning in Obstetrics and Gynecology) is a voluntary, strictly confidential, self-evaluation program. PROLOG was developed specifically as a personal study resource for the practicing obstetrician–gynecologist. It is presented as a self-assessment mechanism that, with its accompanying performance information, should assist the physician in designing a personal, self-directed life-long learning program. It may be used as a valuable study tool, reference guide, and a means of attaining up-to-date information in the specialty. The content is carefully selected and presented in multiple-choice questions that are clinically oriented. The questions are designed to stimulate and challenge physicians in areas of medical care that they confront in their practices or when they work as consultant obstetrician–gynecologists.

PROLOG also provides the American College of Obstetricians and Gynecologists (ACOG) with one mechanism to identify the educational needs of the Fellows. Individual scores are reported only to the participant; however, cumulative performance data and evaluation comments obtained for each PROLOG unit help determine the direction for future educational programs offered by the College.

Process

The PROLOG series offers the most current information available in five areas of the specialty: obstetrics, gynecology and surgery, reproductive endocrinology and infertility, gynecologic oncology and critical care, and patient management in the office. A new PROLOG unit is produced annually, addressing one of those subject areas. *Obstetrics,* Sixth Edition, is the first unit in the sixth 5-year PROLOG series.

Each unit of PROLOG represents the efforts of a special task force of subject experts under the supervision of an advisory committee. PROLOG sets forth current information as viewed by recognized authorities in the field of women's health. This educational resource does not define a standard of care, nor is it intended to dictate an exclusive course of management. It presents recognized methods and techniques of clinical practice for consideration by obstetrician–gynecologists to incorporate in their practices. Variations of practice that take into account the needs of the individual patient, resources, and the limitations that are special to the institution or type of practice may be appropriate.

Each unit of PROLOG is presented as a two-part set, with performance information and cognate credit available to those who choose to submit their answer sheets for confidential scoring. The first part of the PROLOG set is the Question Book, which contains educational objectives for the unit and multiple-choice questions, and an answer sheet with return mailing envelope. Participants can work through the book at their own pace, choosing to use PROLOG as a closed- or open-book assessment. Return of the answer sheet for scoring is encouraged but voluntary.

The second part of PROLOG is the Critique Book, which reviews the educational objectives and questions set forth in the Question Book and contains a discussion, or critique, of each question. The critique provides the rationale for correct and incorrect options. Current, accessible references are listed for each question.

Continuing Medical Education Credit

The American College of Obstetricians and Gynecologists (ACOG) is accredited by the Accreditation Council for Continuing Medical Education (ACCME) to provide continuing medical education for physicians. ACOG designates this educational activity for a maximum of *25 AMA PRA Category 1 Credits*™ or up to a maximum of 25 Category 1 ACOG cognate credits. Physicians should claim credit only commensurate with the extent of their participation in the activity.

Fellows who submit their answer sheets for scoring will be credited with the number of hours they designate in the appropriate box on the answer sheet. (Important: Unless hours are noted, CME credit cannot be awarded and the test sheet will be returned.) Participants who return their answer sheets for CME credit will receive a Performance Report that provides a comparison of their scores with the scores of a sample group of physicians who have taken the unit as an examination. An individual may request credit only once for each unit. *Please allow 1 month to process answer sheets.*

Credit for PROLOG *Obstetrics*, Sixth Edition, is initially available through December 2010. During that year, the unit will be reevaluated. If the content remains current, credit is extended for an additional 3 years, with credit for the unit automatically withdrawn after December 2013.

Conclusion

PROLOG was developed specifically as a personal study resource for the practicing obstetrician–gynecologist. It is presented as a self-assessment mechanism that, with its accompanying performance information, should assist the physician in designing a personal, self-directed learning program. The many quality resources developed by the College, as detailed each year in the ACOG *Publications and Educational Materials Catalog*, are available to help fulfill the educational interests and needs that have been identified. PROLOG is not intended as a substitute for the certification or recertification programs of the American Board of Obstetrics and Gynecology.

PROLOG CME SCHEDULE

Obstetrics, Fifth Edition (2003)	Credit through 2008
Gynecology and Surgery, Fifth Edition (2004)	Credit through 2009
Reproductive Endocrinology and Infertility, Fifth Edition (2005)	Credit through 2010
Gynecologic Oncology and Critical Care, Fifth Edition (2006)	Reevaluated in 2008– Credit through 2011
Patient Management in the Office, Fifth Edition (2007)	Reevaluated in 2009– Credit through 2012
Obstetrics, Sixth Edition (2008)	Reevaluated in 2010– Credit through 2013

PROLOG Objectives

PROLOG is a voluntary, strictly confidential, personal continuing education resource that is designed to be both stimulating and enjoyable. By participating in PROLOG, obstetrician–gynecologists will be able to do the following:

- Review and update clinical knowledge
- Recognize areas of knowledge and practice in which they excel, be stimulated to explore other areas of the specialty, and identify areas requiring further study
- Plan continuing education activities in light of identified strengths and deficiencies
- Compare and relate present knowledge and skills with those of other participants
- Obtain continuing medical education credit, if desired
- Have complete personal control of the setting and of the pace of the experience

The obstetrician–gynecologist who completes *Obstetrics*, Sixth Edition, will be able to:

- Demonstrate an understanding of maternal and fetal physiology and pathophysiology and the impact on normal and complicated pregnancies
- Identify components of antepartum care that optimize maternal and perinatal outcomes in uncomplicated pregnancies, including education regarding normal pregnancy
- Diagnose and plan efficacious and cost-effective management of medical and obstetric conditions encountered during the antepartum period
- Identify the risks and prognosis of selected complications of pregnancy and in the neonate
- Describe invasive and noninvasive methods of fetal assessment in the antepartum period and identify the risks, indications, predictive value, and the physiologic basis for the tests
- Diagnose problems and manage obstetric emergencies
- Select appropriate management strategies for intrapartum care and delivery
- Consider medical–legal principles, risk management, and office management guidelines in obstetric practice

Obstetrics, Sixth Edition, includes the following topics:

SCREENING AND DIAGNOSIS
Abruptio placentae
Acute appendicitis in pregnancy
Acute fatty liver of pregnancy
Amnionitis
Anemia
Antiphospholipid syndrome
Aspiration pneumonia
Breast mass in pregnancy
Causes of stillbirth
Cerebral palsy
Cervical insufficiency
Cervical length
Cystic fibrosis
Cytomegalovirus
Diagnostic accuracy in fetal distress
Disseminated intravascular coagulopathy
Down syndrome
Elevated maternal serum alpha-fetoprotein level
Fetal acid–base assessment
Fetal complications of maternal hypothyroidism

MEDICAL MANAGEMENT

External version
Operative complications in the obese patient
Placenta accreta
Postpartum hemorrhage
Tubal sterilization
Vaginal birth after a cesarean delivery
Vaginal breech delivery of second twin

EPIDEMIOLOGY
Cocaine use
Congenital malformations due to isotretinoin
Cytomegalovirus
Epidural complications
Labor induction
Lupus and pregnancy
Maternal and fetal side effects of tocolysis
Maternal human immunodeficiency virus
Neonatal outcomes
Preterm labor
Recurrence of gestational diabetes mellitus

COUNSELING
Advanced maternal age counseling
Counseling for a woman with a prior cesarean delivery
Elective cesarean delivery
Fetal death
Folic acid supplementation during pregnancy
Immunization in pregnancy
Influenza vaccination
Labor induction
Maternal human immunodeficiency virus
Neonatal outcomes
Perinatal survival
Peripartum cardiomyopathy
Smoking cessation
Triplets
Tubal sterilization
Use of peak flow meter in asthma

ETHICAL AND LEGAL ISSUES
Elective cesarean delivery

A subject matter index appears at the end of the Critique Book.

PROLOG

OBSTETRICS

SIXTH EDITION

1

Fetal heart effects of narcotics

A healthy 24-year-old primigravid woman at term is in active labor. She receives intravenous meperidine hydrochloride (Demerol, Mepadin) for analgesia, after which there is a decrease in heart rate variability. The most likely type of fetal heart rate change that would be expected is

      (A) increased acceleration amplitude
      (B) increased baseline fetal heart rate
      (C) sinusoidal heart rate pattern
*   (D) decreased number of accelerations

Although many patients receive regional anesthesia for analgesia during labor, opioids such as morphine sulfate, meperidine hydrochloride, and fentanyl citrate (Oralet, Sublimaze) also are used for this purpose. These agents can be administered either intravenously or intramuscularly.

It is generally believed that opioids are not as effective as regional anesthesia in providing analgesia in labor, and this is partially supported by a meta-analysis of randomized trials. In some circumstances, epidural anesthesia is contraindicated (eg, maternal thrombocytopenia or allergy to local anesthetics), and knowledge of the maternal, fetal, and neonatal effects of opiates is necessary.

Narcotics act centrally in the parturient and are associated with drowsiness, nausea, vomiting, and respiratory depression. Most narcotics also cross the placenta and can have transient fetal and neonatal effects. If used within hours of delivery, the neonate may manifest central nervous system depression, slowing of respiratory rate, and changes in muscle tone. These effects can be reversed quickly with an opioid antagonist such as naloxone hydrochloride (Narcan).

Because most narcotics freely cross the placenta, they also can affect the fetal heart rate tracing transiently. It is generally believed that maternal narcotic administration can lead to a decrease in the baseline fetal heart rate and decrease variability. However, the most common change in the fetal heart rate associated with narcotic use is a decrease in the number of fetal heart rate accelerations. Pseudosinusoidal heart rate tracings have been reported transiently with the use of butorphanol tartrate (Stadol), although the mechanism of this finding remains unclear. Narcotics are not associated with an increase in acceleration amplitude or with an increase in the baseline fetal heart rate.

The change in acceleration frequency may make interpretation of intrapartum fetal heart rate tracings more challenging. It cannot be assumed that observed alterations in acceleration frequency are caused by narcotics alone, and there may be a need for use of other methods of reassurance of fetal status. Fetal scalp stimulation and vibroacoustic stimulation are reliable tests to exclude acidosis, if accelerations are noted after stimulation.

Anim-Somuah M, Smyth R, Howell C. Epidural versus non-epidural or no analgesia in labour. Cochrane Database of Systematic Reviews 2005, Issue 4. Art. No.: CD000331. DOI: 10.1002/14651858.CD000331. pub2.

Hatjis CG, Meis PJ. Sinusoidal fetal heart rate pattern associated with butorphanol administration. Obstet Gynecol 1986;67:377–80.

Intrapartum fetal heart rate monitoring. ACOG Practice Bulletin No. 70. American College of Obstetricians and Gynecologists. Obstet Gynecol 2005;106:1453–60.

* Indicates correct answer.
Note: See Appendix A for a table of normal values for laboratory tests.

1

2

Hepatitis B virus

A 29-year-old woman, gravida 2, para 1, is positive for hepatitis B surface antigen (HBsAg) on initial prenatal screening. On further questioning, she informs you that she was HBsAg positive during her last pregnancy 2 years ago. Further evaluation yields the following test results:

Test	Abbreviation	Result
Hepatitis B surface antigen	HBsAg	Positive
Hepatitis B e antigen	HBeAg	Positive
Antibody to hepatitis B surface antigen	HBsAb	Negative
Antibody to hepatitis B core antigen	HBcAb	Negative
Antibody to hepatitis B core antigen	HBcAb	Positive
Alanine aminotransferase	ALT	88 units/L
Aspartate aminotransferase	AST	112 units/L

These findings are most consistent with

* (A) early acute hepatitis B infection
* (B) resolved hepatitis B infection
* (C) previous hepatitis B vaccination
* (D) chronic active hepatitis B infection
* (E) chronic inactive hepatitis B infection (carrier)

An estimated 2 billion people worldwide have been infected or are currently infected with hepatitis B virus (HBV). Acute hepatitis B infection occurs in 1–2 in 1,000 pregnancies, and chronic infection is present in 5–15 of 1,000 pregnancies. Of patients who become infected with HBV, 85–90% will experience complete resolution with the remaining 10–15% becoming chronically infected. These individuals are at risk of later developing chronic or persistent hepatitis and cirrhosis with significant risk of morbidities associated with chronic liver disease, including hepatocellular carcinoma. Because of the highly pathogenic and infectious nature of hepatitis B, the Centers for Disease Control and Prevention has recommended that all pregnant women be routinely tested for HBsAg during an early prenatal visit (ie, in the first trimester), even if they have been previously vaccinated or tested. Perinatal transmission of HBV can occur in up to 20% of women who are HBsAg positive, with this rate increasing to 90% if a woman is seropositive to both HBsAg and HBeAg.

Numerous different antigens and antibodies are associated with HBV infection, but at least one serologic marker is present during each of the different phases of HBV infection (Table 2-1). After a person is exposed to HBV, serum serologic markers, including HBsAg and HBeAg (a marker of active HBV replication), first appear, followed by increases in serum aspartate aminotransferase (AST) and alanine aminotransferase (ALT) levels. The first indication of acute HBV infection is the presence of HBsAg, which appears as early as 1 week after initial exposure to HBV and before the onset of symptoms or serum elevation. Typically, HBsAg becomes detectable 6–10 weeks after exposure to the virus (Fig. 2-1; see color plate).

Acute HBV infection usually presents as a subclinical, mild illness, and most patients do not report any discernible symptoms. Up to 30% of patients will develop scleral icterus, nausea and vomiting, and right upper quadrant tenderness. In an acute or recently acquired infection, hepatitis B core (HBc) antibodies will first appear, usually at the onset of acute HBV infection, with the immunoglobulin M (IgM) class appearing first and persisting for up to 6 months. Thereafter, the immunoglobulin G (IgG) HBc antibodies will appear and persist for life.

In persons who recover from HBV infection, HBsAg usually is eliminated from the blood in 3–4 months, and HBs antibodies develop during convalescence. The presence of HBs antibodies typically indicates immunity from HBV infection. In persons who are successfully immunized, only the HBs antibodies will be detected. Transient HBsAg positivity has been reported for up to 18 days after vaccination. This is a clinically insignificant finding and is not associated with elevations in liver enzymes.

Chronic active HBV infection is diagnosed by the presence of HBsAg for more than 6 months, accompanied by persistent or intermittent elevations of serum ALT or AST levels. The typical patient with chronic active HBV infection has both HBsAg and HBeAg in serum, reflecting

TABLE 2-1. Interpretation of Serologic Test Results for Hepatitis B Virus Infection

Serologic Marker				
HBsAg	IgM HBc Antibodies	IgG HBc Antibodies	IgG HBs Antibodies	Interpretation
–	–	–	–	Never infected
+	–	–	–	Early acute infection; transient + after vaccination
+	+	+	–	Acute infection
–	+	+	–	Acute resolving infection
–	+	–	+	Recovered from past infection and immune
+	+	–	–	Chronic infection
–	–	–	+	Immune after vaccination

IgG, immunoglobulin G; IgM, immunoglobulin M; HBc, hepatitis B core; HBsAg, hepatitis B surface antigen.

Modified from Mast EE, Margolis HS, Fiore AE, Brink EW, Goldstein ST, Wang SA, et al. A comprehensive immunization strategy to eliminate transmission of hepatitis B virus infection in the United States: recommendations of the Advisory Committee on Immunization Practices (ACIP) part 1: immunization of infants, children, and adolescents [published erratum appears in MMWR Morb Mortal Wkly Rep 2006;55:158–9]. MMWR Recomm Rep 2005;54(RR-16):1–31.

active viral replication, infectivity, and hepatic inflammation. In persons who become chronically infected, HBsAg and HBc antibody persist, typically for life.

In active HBV carriers, HBsAg is still detectable in serum; however, because the virus is not actively replicating, the HBeAg will be negative and these carriers will be positive for the HBe antibodies.

American College of Obstetricians and Gynecologists. Viral hepatitis in pregnancy. ACOG Educational Bulletin 248. Washington, DC: ACOG; 1998.

Gastrointestinal disorders. In: Cunningham FG, Leveno KJ, Bloom SL, Hauth JC, Gilstrap L 3rd, Wenstrom KD, editors. Williams obstetrics. 22nd ed. New York (NY): McGraw-Hill; 2005. p. 1111–23.

Mast EE, Margolis HS, Fiore AE, Brink EW, Goldstein ST, Wang SA, et al. A comprehensive immunization strategy to eliminate transmission of hepatitis B virus infection in the United States: recommendations of the Advisory Committee on Immunization Practices (ACIP) part 1: immunization of infants, children, and adolescents [published erratum appears in MMWR Morb Mortal Wkly Rep 2006;55:158–9]. MMWR Recomm Rep 2005;54(RR-16):1–31.

Servoss JC, Friedman LS. Serologic and molecular diagnosis of hepatitis B virus. Infect Dis Clin North Am 2006;20:47–61.

3

Fetal complications of maternal hypothyroidism

A 33-year-old woman, gravida 3, para 2, at 10 weeks of gestation comes to the office for her first prenatal visit. She reports that she had hypothyroidism in the distant past but was never treated. She is asymptomatic. Physical examination is normal. On bimanual examination, her uterus is 10 weeks in size and the fetal heart rate is 150 beats per minute. Her thyroid-stimulating hormone (TSH) level is 13.1 microunits/mL, free thyroxine (free T_4) level is 0.7 ng/dL, and her antithyroid peroxidase antibody level is high. The best next step in the patient's care is

* (A) begin levothyroxine
  (B) repeat serum TSH and free T_4 after 20 weeks of gestation
  (C) measure serum thyroid-stimulating immunoglobulins
  (D) perform ultrasonography of the maternal thyroid

Although the patient is asymptomatic, she has laboratory evidence of overt hypothyroidism with an elevated serum TSH level and a low free T_4 level. She also has an elevated antithyroid peroxidase antibody level, which indicates that the likely cause of her hypothyroidism is chronic autoimmune thyroiditis (Hashimoto's disease). The antithyroid peroxidase antibodies also indicate an increased risk of her developing other autoimmune diseases, such as adrenal insufficiency or type 1 diabetes mellitus.

Hypothyroidism in pregnancy has been associated with preeclampsia, gestational hypertension, abruptio placentae, preterm delivery, and neuropsychologic deficits in the child. The fetus begins to produce thyroid hormone at approximately 12 weeks of gestation, and it depends on maternal free T_4 for brain development in the first trimester. It is important to treat patients with hypothyroidism as early as possible in pregnancy. Therefore, the best next step for this patient would be to begin treatment with levothyroxine. Ideally, the hypothyroidism would be identified and treated before pregnancy. An initial dose of levothyroxine should be started in this patient, and the serum TSH should be reassessed 4–6 weeks after therapy is begun. The goal would be to achieve a serum TSH in the reference range.

The other answer choices to this question provide a diversion from the primary goal of starting treatment. The option to repeat serum TSH and free T_4 measurements after 20 weeks of gestation relates to a common problem encountered with TSH screening in early pregnancy. The finding of a suppressed TSH level raises the possibility of hyperthyroidism versus thyroid-stimulating activity of human chorionic gonadotropin (hCG). The question can be resolved by repeating the TSH and free T_4 measurements after 20 weeks of gestation when the hCG level has plateaued at a lower level for the remainder of the pregnancy. Thyroid-stimulating immunoglobulins have a pathophysiologic role in Graves disease but are not pertinent in this patient who has hypothyroidism. Performing ultrasonography of the thyroid is unnecessary in this case.

Although this is a case of overt hypothyroidism, a current widely discussed topic in the obstetric and endocrinology literature is whether all pregnant women should be screened for subclinical hypothyroidism. The diagnostic criteria for subclinical hypothyroidism are an elevated TSH level with a normal free T_4 level. In 1999, two studies showed a lower intelligence quotient (IQ) in children of mothers who had high serum TSH concentrations. These studies were retrospective and noninterventional. They included patients with overt hypothyroidism without treatment, patients with overt hypothyroidism with inadequate treatment, and patients with subclinical hypothyroidism. The authors concluded that all of these groups should be treated. The studies showed an association but not cause and effect. No studies have been performed to determine whether treating subclinical hypothyroidism can prevent the lower IQ. A large Maternal–Fetal Medicine Units Network trial is underway to determine whether early treatment of subclinical hypothyroidism during pregnancy is effective in improving children's intellectual ability at age 5 years. The importance of this problem for pregnant women and the absence of adequate research evidence have prompted recommendations by some organizations for routine screening of all pregnant women for hypothyroidism. The American College of Obstetricians and Gynecologists currently recommends screening of pregnant women with a personal history, physical examination, or symptoms of a thyroid disorder.

Gharib H, Tuttle RM, Baskin HJ, Fish LH, Singer PA, McDermott MT. Subclinical thyroid dysfunction: a joint statement on management from the American Association of Clinical Endocrinologists, the American Thyroid Association, and the Endocrine Society. J Clin Endocrinol Metab 2005;90:581–5; discussion 586–7.

Haddow JE, Palomaki GE, Allan WC, Williams JR, Knight GJ, Gagnon J, et al. Maternal thyroid deficiency during pregnancy and subsequent neuropsychological development of the child. N Engl J Med 1999; 341:549–55.

Pop VJ, Kuijpens JL, van Baar AL, Verkerk G, van Son MM, de Vijlder JJ, et al. Low maternal free thyroxine concentrations during early pregnancy are associated with impaired psychomotor development in infancy. Clin Endocrinol (Oxf) 1999;50:149–55.

Spong CY. Subclinical hypothyroidism: should all pregnant women be screened? [editorial]. Obstet Gynecol 2005;105:235–6.

Surks MI, Ortiz E, Daniels GH, Sawin CT, Col NF, Cobin RH, et al. Subclinical thyroid disease: scientific review and guidelines for diagnosis and management. JAMA 2004;291:228–38.

Thyroid disease in pregnancy. ACOG Practice Bulletin No. 37. American College of Obstetricians and Gynecologists. Obstet Gynecol 2002;100:387–96.

4

Testing strategies for fetal lung maturity

A 36-year-old multiparous woman who had a cesarean delivery 3 years ago was told not to avoid spontaneous labor in future pregnancies. She now is seen at 36 weeks of gestation for an amniocentesis to assess fetal lung maturity prior to a planned cesarean delivery. An anterior placenta is encountered, and the amniotic fluid sample is bloody. The most appropriate test to assess fetal pulmonary maturity is

    (A) lecithin–sphingomyelin ratio
* (B) phosphatidylglycerol
    (C) foam stability test
    (D) fluorescence polarization
    (E) lamellar bodies

Assessment of fetal pulmonary maturity is recommended when an elective delivery is planned before 39 weeks of gestation or in instances of uncertain gestational age. Patients with conditions precluding vaginal delivery, such as prior transfundal myomectomy, prior classical cesarean delivery, or complete placenta previa, may undergo maturity testing before a planned cesarean delivery. Additional situations where amniocentesis may be indicated are late entry into care or discrepancies between menstrual and ultrasound dating.

Respiratory distress syndrome (RDS) is one of the leading causes of death in newborn infants and results from insufficient amounts of pulmonary surfactant. As bronchial development progresses throughout pregnancy, fetal alveoli are lined with type II pneumocytes that produce a group of phospholipids known as surfactant. These intracellular stores of phospholipids are known as lamellar bodies, which are the storage form of surfactant that are released into the alveolar spaces. Surfactant reduces the surface tension within alveolar spaces, facilitating effective gas exchange after the infant is born. Premature infants deficient in surfactant are difficult to infuse with oxygen because of higher surface tension within the alveoli. The surfactant component present in greatest quantity is lecithin (phosphatidylcholine). Another component of the surfactant compound, phosphatidylglycerol, appears later in gestation, and thus its presence indicates a more advanced state of pulmonary maturity. Additional surface-active components include phosphatidylinositol, phosphatidylethanolamine, proteins, and cholesterol.

Several methods are available to assess fetal pulmonary maturity (Table 4-1). Direct tests of lung maturity are categorized into biochemical and biophysical tests. Biochemical tests, which measure the concentration of particular components of pulmonary surfactant, include the lecithin–sphingomyelin (L/S) ratio, the presence of phosphatidylglycerol, and the fluorescence polarization test. Biophysical tests, which measure the surface-active effects of phospholipids, include the foam stability index, lamellar body counts, and optical density testing of amniotic fluid at 650 nm. The tests for pulmonary maturity predict the absence of RDS with greater certainty than they predict pulmonary immaturity (presence of RDS). A "mature" test result suggests that the likelihood of delivering an infant with RDS is less than 5%.

The most significant limitation of these tests is that most are affected by the presence of contaminants in the amniotic fluid, such as blood or meconium, that can interfere with proper interpretation. The accuracy of four of the tests—the L/S ratio, foam stability index, fluorescence polarization, and measurement of optical density at 650 nm—can be compromised by the presence of either blood or meconium contamination. Lamellar body counts are marginally affected by meconium, but the presence of whole blood in the sample has a biphasic effect that leads to a lower count or falsely immature result. Only the phosphatidylglycerol analysis is affected by neither blood nor meconium contamination. Because the amniotic fluid sample in this scenario is contaminated with blood, the most appropriate test of pulmonary maturity is phosphatidylglycerol.

TABLE 4-1. Commonly Used Direct Tests of Fetal Lung Maturity

Test*	Technique	Time/Ease of Testing†	Threshold	Predictive Value (%) of Test		Relative Cost	Notes
				Mature Result	Immature Result		
Lecithin–sphingomyelin ratio	Thin-layer chromatography	4+	2.0–3.5	95–100	33–50	High	Many variations in technique; laboratory variation significantly affected by blood and meconium
Phosphatidylglycerol	Thin-layer chromatography	4+	"Present" (usually means less than 3% of total phospholipid)	95–100	23–53	High	Not affected by blood, meconium; vaginal pool samples satisfactory
	Antisera	1+	0.5 = low positive 2.0 = high positive	95–100	23–53	Commercial version—moderate	Not affected by blood, meconium; vaginal pool samples satisfactory
Foam stability index	Ethanol added to amniotic fluid, solution shaken, presence of stable bubbles at meniscus noted	2+	47 or 48 or less	95	51	Laboratory—low Commercial version—moderate	Affected by blood, meconium, vaginal pool debris, silicone-coated test tubes
Fluorescence polarization	Fluorescence polarization	1+	55 mg/g of albumin‡ or less	96–100	47–61	Moderate	Minimal intraassay and interassay variability; simple testing procedure affected by blood and meconium
Optical density at 650 nm	Spectrophotometric reading	1+	Optical density 0.15 or less	98	13	Low	Simple technique
Lamellar body counts	Counts using commercial hematology counter	2+	30,000–40,000 (still investigational)	97–98	29–35	Low	Promising technique

*Commercial versions are available for all tests except optical density and lamellar body counts.

†Range in complexity: 1+ indicates procedure is simple, is available all the time, requires only short procedure time, and personnel effort is not intensive; 4+ indicates procedure is complex or difficult, time consuming, and, therefore, frequently not available at all times.

‡The manufacturer has reformulated the product and revised the testing procedure. Currently, the threshold for maturity is 55; with the original assay, it was 70.

Modified from the American College of Obstetricians and Gynecologists. Assessment of fetal lung maturity. ACOG Technical Bulletin 230. Washington, DC: ACOG; 1996.

American College of Obstetricians and Gynecologists. Assessment of fetal lung maturity. ACOG Educational Bulletin 230. Washington, DC: ACOG; 1996.

Ashwood ER. Standards of laboratory practice: evaluation of fetal lung maturity. National Academy of Clinical Biochemistry. Clin Chem 1997;43:211–4.

Grenache DG, Parvin CA, Gronowski AM. Preanalytical factors that influence the Abbott TDx Fetal Lung Maturity II assay. Clin Chem 2003;49:935–9.

Neerhof MG, Dohnal JC, Ashwood ER, Lee IS, Anceschi MM. Lamellar body counts: a consensus on protocol. Obstet Gynecol 2001;97:318–20.

5

Parvovirus

A 31-year-old woman, gravida 4, para 3, comes to the office at 22 weeks of gestation for routine prenatal care. She states that parvovirus infection (fifth disease) recently was diagnosed in her youngest child. The woman feels well and her vital signs are normal, including a temperature of 37°C (98.6°F). A review of systems and physical examination are normal. The best method to diagnose acute maternal parvovirus B19 infection is

    (A) viral culture
    (B) maternal rash
*   (C) maternal immunoglobulin G (IgG) and immunoglobulin M (IgM) antibody titers to parvovirus B19
    (D) polymerase chain reaction testing for parvovirus B19 in maternal serum

Human parvovirus infection, also known as *erythema infectiosum* or *fifth disease*, is a common, self-limited, usually benign infection associated with childhood. The parvovirus subtype most often associated with human infection is B19, although the A6/K71 and V9 subtypes are present is some populations.

Parvovirus B19 is communicated from person to person by the respiratory route and is very contagious. Viremia usually develops 7 days after inoculation and persists for 4 days after the initial viremia. A facial rash, often having a "slapped cheek" appearance, follows approximately 2 weeks after inoculation. The rash then spreads to the trunk and extremities. Other common symptoms are low-grade fever, flulike symptoms, and symmetric arthralgias. Although this is a common constellation of signs and symptoms in children, the presentation in adults can be varied. Parvovirus B19 is an *Erythrovirus* and is replicated in erythroid progenitor cells. In its late stages, infection results in aplastic anemia and red cell hemolysis.

Because of the effect of parvovirus B19 on red blood cell precursors, the classic laboratory finding is anemia with a normal reticulocyte count. This stage lasts approximately 7–10 days, with a full recovery of the bone marrow in approximately 3 weeks. Healthy adults are rarely significantly affected by the anemia, and 20% of women infected by parvovirus B19 are unaware of their infection. Despite the lack of maternal symptoms, their fetuses may still be adversely affected. In patients with diseases characterized by fast erythrocyte turnover, the anemia can be severe and life threatening.

Maternal diagnosis is based on symptoms consistent with infection, but these are not universally present. In pregnancy, it is worthwhile to test for parvovirus B19 in any woman who has symptoms or who has been exposed to a sick contact. The most common method to differentiate between an acute and a past infection is with IgG and IgM parvovirus B19 antibody titers. Women who have been exposed to infection recently but have an isolated elevation in IgG have been infected in the past and are immune. However, if IgM alone or IgM and IgG are elevated, serial titers are warranted to establish the presence of an acute infection.

Among women infected with parvovirus B19, the associated rate of fetal infection has not been established. Recently, polymerase chain reaction (PCR) testing for parvovirus B19 has become available and can be performed on maternal blood, fetal blood, or amniotic fluid. This test directly detects the presence of the virus particle and is very reliable when performed by a reputable laboratory. However, PCR should not be used as a primary test because of its expense and limited availability and the potential to miss the short period of maternal viremia.

The effects of maternal parvovirus B19 infection on the fetus are most often benign, and the majority of pregnancies progress without incident. However, women who have an infection in the first trimester have an increased risk of spontaneous abortion, and infections in the second and third trimesters have been associated with profound fetal anemia leading to hydrops fetalis and fetal death. In any fetus that has ultrasonographic evidence of hydrops fetalis, the mother or fetus should be checked for parvovirus B19 infection. Because most women are unaware of their exposure to parvovirus B19, maternal IgG and IgM antibody determination should be used to establish an acute infection. Viral cultures of maternal blood are not useful in the diagnosis of parvovirus B19 infection.

Women in the second and third trimesters who have a documented parvovirus B19 infection should have ultrasonography to document fetal viability. Because fetal anemia can lead to hydrops fetalis and fetal death, ultrasonographic surveillance for evidence of fetal anemia is warranted. This is most often accomplished with weekly ultrasonography to detect signs of fetal anemia, accompanied by measurement of the peak systolic velocity of the middle cerebral artery. The optimal duration of the surveillance is controversial, but a maximum of 12 weeks appears to be the most reasonable duration.

Levy R, Weissman A, Blomberg G, Hagay ZJ. Infection by parvovirus B19 during pregnancy: a review. Obstet Gynecol Surv 1997;52:254–9.

Ramirez MM, Mastrobattista JM. Diagnosis and management of human parvovirus B19 infection. Clin Perinatol 2005;32:697–704.

Rodis JF, Quinn DL, Gary GW Jr, Anderson LJ, Rosengren S, Cartter ML, et al. Management and outcome of pregnancies complicated by human B19 parvovirus infection: a prospective study. Am J Obstet Gynecol 1990;163:1168–71.

6

Placenta accreta

A 38-year-old woman, gravida 5, para 3, with a history of three cesarean deliveries, comes to your office for a fetal anatomic survey. She has an anterior placenta. Which ultrasonographic image in Fig. 6-1 is most suspicious for a placenta accreta?

*   (A)
    (B)
    (C)
    (D)

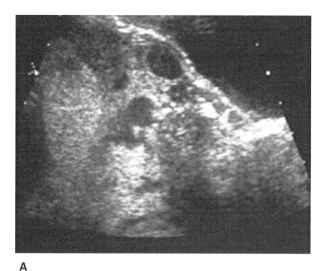

A

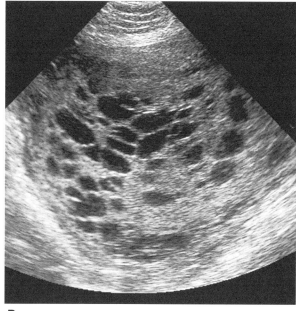

B

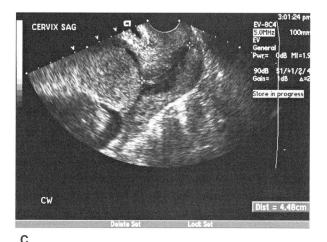

C

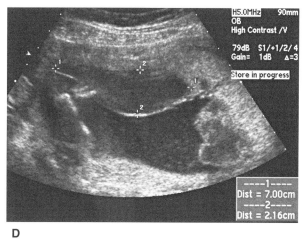

D

FIG. 6-1.

Placenta accreta develops when there is a defect in the decidua basalis leading to abnormal placental implantation. Placenta accreta is an abnormal adherence of the placenta to the myometrium, placenta increta involves placental invasion of the myometrium, and placenta percreta is placental invasion through the serosal surface of the uterus. Risk factors for placenta accreta include the following:

- Placenta previa
- Previous cesarean delivery
- Previous myomectomy
- Advanced maternal age
- Grand multiparity
- Asherman syndrome
- Submucous myoma

Placenta accreta is associated with significant maternal morbidity and even mortality. As a result, antenatal diagnosis can lead to improved intrapartum care. Such an antenatal diagnosis will allow an improved surgical approach with the involvement of appropriate consultations and the anticipation of possible significant blood loss requiring transfusion.

Both ultrasonographic and magnetic resonance imaging modalities have been used to evaluate abnormal placentation during pregnancy. The ultrasonographic findings suggestive of placenta accreta are placental lacunae, interruptions, or bulging of the border between the bladder and myometrium, lower uterine segment myometrial thickness of less than 1 mm, and turbulent blood flow by color Doppler ultrasonography that extends from the placenta into the surrounding tissue. Magnetic resonance imaging studies are most useful in the evaluation of a placenta percreta to determine the extent and location of placental invasion.

Image A demonstrates multiple placental lacunae, which give a "moth-eaten" appearance to the placenta. These lacunae usually have turbulent flow by color Doppler ultrasonography. When visualized on an ultrasonogram at 15–20 weeks of gestation, placental lacunae had a 79% sensitivity in the detection of placenta accreta. Thus, of the four ultrasonographic images in Fig. 6-1, Image A is most suspicious for a placenta accreta.

Image B shows a complete hydatidiform mole. The ultrasonographic image reveals a uterine cavity filled with multiple sonolucent areas. These sonolucent areas represent generalized trophoblastic hyperplasia and villous edema. Image C depicts a complete placenta previa. Even though placenta previa can be associated with placenta accreta, this ultrasonographic image has no suspicious findings for an accreta. Image D illustrates a placental lake. Placental lakes are common findings and are not associated with placenta accreta.

Comstock CH. Antenatal diagnosis of placenta accreta: a review. Ultrasound Obstet Gynecol 2005;26:89–96.

Comstock CH, Love JJ Jr, Bronsteen RA, Lee W, Vettraino IM, Huang RR, et al. Sonographic detection of placenta accreta in the second and third trimesters of pregnancy. Am J Obstet Gynecol 2004;190:1135–40.

Jauniaux E. Diagnosis and follow up of gestational trophoblastic disorders. In: Callen PW, editor. Ultrasonography in obstetrics and gynecology. 4th ed. Philadelphia (PA): WB Saunders; 2000. p. 847.

Palacios Jaraquemada JM, Bruno CH. Magnetic resonance imaging in 300 cases of placenta accreta: surgical correlation of new findings. Acta Obstet Gynecol Scand 2005;84:716–24.

7

Hemolysis, elevated liver enzymes, and low platelets (HELLP) syndrome

The antepartum use of high-dose dexamethasone in the management of hemolysis, elevated liver enzymes, and low platelets (HELLP) syndrome has been most consistently reported to

    (A) hasten the rate of recovery of transaminase values
*   (B) increase the rate of regional anesthesia use
    (C) reduce maternal mortality
    (D) reduce the need for blood product transfusion

The HELLP syndrome is a disorder within the clinical spectrum of preeclampsia. Multiple theories have been proposed to explain the etiology of HELLP syndrome, including oxidative stress, endothelial cell damage, an exaggerated maternal inflammatory response syndrome, and disordered angiogenesis. Although the HELLP syndrome affects liver function, red blood cell integrity, and platelet count, the most frequent cause of morbidity is lowered platelet count. Liver rupture can be catastrophic and a cause of maternal mortality but fortunately is rare. Thrombocytopenia, however, is not uncommon and frequently affects decisions relating to route of delivery and technique of anesthesia. Frank disseminated intravascular coagulation also may complicate HELLP syndrome and has been reported to occur in 20–40% of patients with HELLP.

In an effort to address the multisystemic nature of the clinical manifestations of HELLP syndrome, corticosteroids have been proposed as a means of ameliorating the course of the disease. Unfortunately, trials that suggest improved outcome with the administration of corticosteroids have been hampered by their nonrandomized methodology, multiple confounding variables, and lack of a standardized definition of the HELLP syndrome. A similar statement may be made with respect to the use of plasmapheresis in cases of HELLP. A recent randomized clinical trial failed to demonstrate the efficacy of maternally administered dexamethasone in improving the time to recovery of serum transaminase values, shortening length of hospitalization, or reducing the need for blood product administration. Additionally, dexamethasone treatment of HELLP syndrome has not been associated with a reduction in maternal mortality. A recent retrospective study has suggested that maternally administered corticosteroids may allow for increased use of regional anesthesia among patients with HELLP syndrome.

At this time, evidence does not support the routine use of either corticosteroids or plasmapheresis in the management of HELLP syndrome. A possible exception is in patients with borderline platelet counts, where modest corticosteroid-induced elevations of platelet count could favorably affect patient candidacy for regional anesthesia.

Fonseca JE, Mendez F, Catano C, Arias F. Dexamethasone treatment does not improve the outcome of women with HELLP syndrome: a double blind, placebo-controlled, randomized clinical trial. Am J Obstet Gynecol 2005;193:1591–8.

Martin JN Jr, Blake PG, Lowry SL, Perry KG Jr, Files JC, Morrison JC. Pregnancy complicated by preeclampsia–eclampsia with the syndrome of hemolysis, elevated liver enzymes, and low platelet count: how rapid is postpartum recovery? Obstet Gynecol 1990;76:737–41.

O'Brien JM, Shumate SA, Satchwell SL, Milligan DA, Barton JR. Maternal benefit of corticosteroid therapy in patients with HELLP (hemolysis, elevated liver enzymes, and low platelet count) syndrome: impact on the rate of regional anesthesia. Am J Obstet Gynecol 2002;186:475–9.

Sibai BM. Hypertension. In: Gabbe SG, Niebyl JR, Simpson JL, editors. Obstetrics: normal and problem pregnancies. 4th ed. New York (NY): Churchill Livingstone; 2002. p. 945–1004.

8

Causes of stillbirth

A 32-year-old woman, gravida 3, para 2, presents with decreased fetal movements at 36 weeks of gestation. Her prepregnancy weight was 99.8 kg (220 lb), height 1.5 m (60 in.), and body mass index (weight in kilograms divided by height in meters squared [kg/m^2]) 43. She has so far had uneventful antepartum care. Ultrasonography shows intrauterine fetal demise, and the estimated fetal weight was at the 20th percentile for 36 weeks of gestation. The most likely etiology is

* (A) unexplained stillbirth
  (B) abruptio placentae
  (C) aneuploidy
  (D) umbilical cord accident
  (E) fetal–maternal hemorrhage

In the United States in 2002, stillbirth occurred at a rate of 6.4 per 1,000 pregnancies and the neonatal death rate was 4.7 per 1,000 pregnancies. A database including 709 stillbirths among 88,651 births with a 97% autopsy rate has been used to track specific causes of stillbirth over three decades. The data showed a 95% reduction in stillbirths due to Rh isoimmunization as a result of Rh immune prophylaxis and also a 95% reduction in stillbirths caused by intrapartum asphyxia as a result of intrapartum fetal monitoring. Low rates of stillbirth due to preeclampsia and diabetes mellitus were felt to be the result of advances in medical care. After 28 weeks of gestation, the largest category of fetal demise was found to be deaths from unexplained causes, followed by intrauterine growth restriction and abruptio placentae.

Unexplained fetal demise is defined as fetal death that is unexplained by fetal, placental, maternal, or obstetric factors. The prevalence of unexplained fetal demise is affected by the thoroughness of the stillbirth evaluation and method of classification. A new classification system called ReCoDe (Relevant Condition at Death) has been shown to decrease the percentage of stillbirths classified as unexplained. Nevertheless, unexplained fetal demise is the most frequent type of fetal death, representing 15–60% of all such deaths in various studies. Risk factors for unexplained fetal demise include advanced maternal age, low educational attainment, obesity, and smoking. A large database from Norway showed that intrauterine growth restriction was the most important risk factor for sudden intrauterine fetal death. Approximately 40–50% of cases classified as unexplained stillbirth may be attributable to intrauterine growth restriction. Unexplained stillbirths increase as gestation advances, especially after 37–39 weeks of gestation.

A review of trends of late fetal deaths from 1982 to 2000 showed large reductions in stillbirths from intrapartum-related deaths, congenital anomalies, antepartum hemorrhage, and preeclampsia. However, unexplained fetal deaths, which occurred in approximately 50% of cases, remained largely unchanged over the years.

Umbilical cord accident, which includes prolapse, constricting loop, knot, or velamentous insertion, is not a common cause of stillbirth and has been reported in 0.9–3.4% of cases. Fetal anomalies and aneuploidy tend to occur more in early stillbirth. At 24–27 weeks of gestation, anomalies and abruptio placentae each occurred in 14% of pregnancies, with infections being the most common cause of stillbirth at 19% of pregnancies. Fetal–maternal hemorrhage is a rare cause and was reported to occur only in 0.6% of 3,886 late fetal deaths.

It is important to identify risk factors for stillbirth. Table 8-1 shows estimates of maternal risk factors and risk of stillbirth.

African-American women consistently have twice the risk of stillbirth that white women have. This may be related to socioeconomic disadvantages and to increased risks of diabetes mellitus, hypertension, abruptio placentae, and premature rupture of membranes.

Advanced maternal age is an independent risk factor for stillbirth even after adjusting for medical conditions and lethal anomalies. The risk for stillbirth reported for women younger than 35 years was 1.1 per 1,000; for women aged 35–39 years, risk was 3.6 per 1,000; and for women aged 40 years and over, risk was 4 per 1,000. The risk of fetal death in older women when compared with women younger than 35 years becomes significant in late pregnancy from 36 weeks of gestation onward.

Obesity is associated with increased frequency of smoking, diabetes mellitus, and preeclampsia. After controlling for these factors, obesity remains a consistently significant risk factor for stillbirth, and the association also increases with advancing gestational age. Investigators have suggested several hypotheses for the increased risk of stillbirths in obese women independent of associated medical

TABLE 8-1. Estimates of Maternal Risk Factors and Risk of Stillbirth*

Condition	Prevalence (%)	Estimated Rate of Stillbirth (per 1,000 Pregnancies)	Odds Ratio
All pregnancies		6.4	1.0
Low-risk pregnancies	80	4.0–5.5	0.86
Chronic hypertension	6–10	6–25	1.5–2.7
Mild PIH	5.8–7.7	9–51	1.2–4.0
Severe PIH	1.3–3.3	12–29	1.8–4.4
Diabetes mellitus treated with diet	2.5–5	6–10	1.2–2.2
Diabetes mellitus requiring insulin	2.4	6–35	1.7–7.0
SLE	Less than 1	40–150	6–20
Renal disease	Less than 1	15–200	2.2–30
Thyroid disorders	0.2–2	12–20	2.2–3.0
Thrombophilia	1–5	18–40	2.8–5.0
Cholestasis of pregnancy	Less than 0.1	12–30	1.8–4.4
Smoking more than 10 cigarettes per day	10–20	10–15	1.7–3.0
Twins	2.7	12	1.0–2.8
Triplets	0.14	34	2.8–3.7
Previous growth-restricted infant (less than 10%)	6.7	12–30	2–4.6
Previous stillbirth	0.5–1.0	9–20	1.4–3.2

PIH, pregnancy-induced hypertension; SLE, systemic lupus erythematosus.

*There were 709 stillbirths among 88,651 births with an autopsy rate of 97%.

Modified from Fretts RC. Etiology and prevention of stillbirth. Am J Obstet Gynecol 2005;193:1928. Copyright Elsevier 2005.

complications. Obese women may not feel decreased fetal movements. Women who are obese are more likely to have hyperlipidemia and increased endothelial dysfunction, platelet aggregation, and atherosclerosis, all of which may be a predisposition to uterine underperfusion. Obese pregnant women may snore longer and experience more apnea–hypoxic episodes and more oxygen desaturation events than nonobese women. These factors may predispose obese women to fetal hypoxia and fetal death. Delivery of a previous small-for-gestational-age infant, especially if the infant was preterm, also has been shown to be an important predictor for stillbirth, associated with a fivefold increased risk.

Bell R, Parker L, MacPhail S, Wright C. Trends in the cause of late fetal death, 1982–2000. BJOG 2004;111:1400–7.

Fretts RC. Etiology and prevention of stillbirth. Am J Obstet Gynecol 2005;193:1923–35.

Froen JF, Gardosi JO, Thurmann A, Francis A, Stray-Pedersen B. Restricted fetal growth in sudden intrauterine unexplained death. Acta Obstet Gynecol Scand 2004;83:801–7.

Gardosi J, Kady SM, McGeown P, Francis A, Tonks A. Classification of stillbirth by relevant condition at death (ReCoDe): population-based cohort study. BMJ 2005;331:1113–7.

Smith GC, Pell JP, Dobbie R. Caesarean section and risk of unexplained stillbirth in subsequent pregnancy. Lancet 2003;362:1779–84.

Surkan PJ, Stephansson O, Dickman PW, Cnattingius S. Previous preterm and small-for-gestational-age births and the subsequent risk of stillbirth. N Engl J Med 2004;350:777–85.

9

Use of vibroacoustic stimulation in pregnancy

A 26-year-old woman, gravida 3, para 2, is seen in the labor and delivery department at 38 weeks of gestation complaining of decreased fetal movements. She has no history of ruptured membranes or vaginal bleeding. The bimanual pelvic examination reveals an engaged fetal head and a long and closed cervix. External fetal heart rate monitoring shows a baseline of 135 beats per minute, with decreased variability, and with no accelerations or decelerations. The best next step to induce fetal movements should be

    (A) glucose administration (eg, orange juice)

    (B) turning the patient on her left side

    (C) induced labor

*   (D) vibroacoustic stimulation

    (E) fetal scalp stimulation

A reactive nonstress test (NST) result is defined as a fetal heart rate tracing that shows two or more fetal heart-rate accelerations of at least 15 beats per minute, lasting at least 15 seconds during a 20-minute period, as a result of fetal movements, which may or not be perceived by the patient. A reactive NST result indicates that the fetus is not acidotic or neurologically depressed. However, a nonreactive NST is not necessarily the result of fetal acid–base abnormalities. A nonreactive NST result may be normal with early gestational age, in the presence of structural heart or conduction defects, or as a result of medications. However, the most common association of the nonreactive NST is with fetal sleep–wake states. At term, four distinct fetal behavioral states have been described (Table 9-1). The healthy term fetus may spend up to 40% of the day in a quiet sleep state (1F or 3F). The fetus usually stays in state 1F for approximately 40 minutes; however, this state may persist for as long as 2 hours. A nonreactive nonstress test result during periods of fetal sleep or quiescence is not associated with fetal compromise.

Investigators have used a variety of external stimuli to induce fetal movements. Techniques have included changing maternal position, physical activity, glucose administration, sound stimulation, light stimulation, and manual fetal manipulation in an effort to arouse the fetus sufficiently and in turn reduce the incidence of falsely nonreactive NST results. A group of investigators looked at the efficacy of administering orange juice to decrease the time to a reactive NST; however, they were unable to confirm that orange juice influences the outcome of the NST. Similarly, changing position does not influence outcome. Fetal scalp stimulation similarly would not influence outcome. Inductin of labor is not indicated.

The most effective technique to arouse a fetus from a sleep cycle has proved to be vibroacoustic stimulation (VAS) using the artificial larynx. Fetal heart rate accelerations as a result of vibroacoustic stimulation appear to be valid in the prediction of fetal well-being without compromising the detection of the acidotic fetus (Fig. 9-1).

The vibroacoustic stimulation is performed with an artificial larynx with a vibrating disc, optimally one specifically designed for fetal stimulation. The artificial larynx is positioned on the maternal abdomen and a stimulus is applied. It transmits brief sounds through the

TABLE 9-1. Characteristics of Fetal Behavioral States

State	Eyes	Body Movements	Fetal Heart Rate Pattern	Breathing
1F	No eye movement	Isolated	No accelerations, except with a startle	Regular (if present)
2F	Frequent eye movements	Frequent	Frequent accelerations with movements	Irregular (if present)
3F	Frequent eye movements	Absent	No accelerations	Not defined
4F	Frequent eye movements	Vigorous	Large and long accelerations, often fused into a sustained tachycardia	Irregular (if present)

Modified from Nijhuis JG, Nijhuis IJM. Neurobehavioral development of the fetal brain. In: Timor-Tritsch IE, Monteagudo A, Cohen HL, editors. Ultrasonography of the prenatal and neonatal brain. 2nd ed. New York (NY): McGraw-Hill; 2001. p. 491.

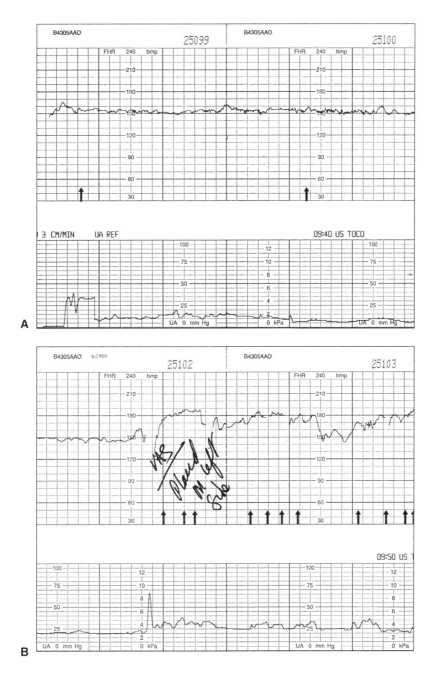

FIG. 9-1. A segment of a nonstress test before and after the application of vibroacoustic stimulation. **A.** This segment shows a nonreactive nonstress test result with a baseline of 150 beats per minute with no accelerations. **B.** This shows the point in time when the vibroacoustic stimulation was applied with the resulting accelerations.

maternal abdominal wall to the fetus. As standard protocol, this stimulus may be repeated up to three times for progressively longer durations of up to 3 seconds to elicit fetal heart rate accelerations.

Vibroacoustic stimulation improves the efficiency of antenatal nonstress testing by reducing the number of nonreactive nonstress tests due to sleep states. It also shortens the overall testing time and thus allows perinatal resources to be used more efficiently.

Eglinton GS, Paul RH, Broussard PM, Walla CA, Platt LD. Antepartum fetal heart rate testing. XI. Stimulation with orange juice. Am J Obstet Gynecol 1984;150:97–9.

Marden D, McDuffie RS Jr, Allen R, Abitz D. A randomized controlled trial of a new fetal acoustic stimulation test for fetal well-being. Am J Obstet Gynecol 1997;176:1386–8.

Nijhuis JG, Nijhuis IJM. Neurobehavioral development of the fetal brain. In: Timor-Tritsch IE, Monteagudo A, Cohen HL, editors. Ultrasonography of the prenatal and neonatal brain. 2nd ed. New York (NY): McGraw-Hill; 2001.

Tan KH, Smyth R. Fetal vibroacoustic stimulation for facilitation of tests of fetal wellbeing. Cochrane Database of Systematic Reviews 2001, Issue 1. Art. No.: CD002963. DOI: 10.1002/14651858.CD002963.

Zimmer EZ, Divon MY. Fetal vibroacoustic stimulation. Obstet Gynecol 1993;81:451–7.

10

Disseminated intravascular coagulopathy

A 30-year-old primigravid woman presents at 30 weeks of gestation with regular painful uterine contractions and vaginal bleeding. On examination, her pulse is 120 beats per minute, her blood pressure is 150/95 mm Hg, and she is afebrile. She is placed on a fetal monitor and is having regular uterine contractions approximately every 3 minutes. The fetal heart rate is nonreactive. On speculum examination, 250 mL of clots are immediately expelled. Her cervix appears to be dilated approximately 3 cm. Membranes and vertex are visible through the os. On review of her prenatal record, you note that she has had previous ultrasonography, which confirmed her dates and showed a fundal placenta. The most useful laboratory test for disseminated intravascular coagulopathy to support your clinical impression of abruptio placentae is

*   (A) fibrinogen level
     (B) whole blood clotting time
     (C) partial thromboplastin time (PTT)
     (D) hematocrit
     (E) platelet count

Patients who present with preterm labor may have abruptio placentae as an underlying cause. In patients in whom abruptio placentae is significant, there is an increased risk for disseminated intravascular coagulation (DIC). These patients are at increased risk for fetal distress in labor and, therefore, are at increased risk for cesarean delivery. In this setting, DIC is a common clinical diagnosis and reflects reaction to the entry of thromboplastins into the maternal circulation from the site of the abruptio placentae. This in turn causes intravascular fibrin formation, fibrinolysis, and the formation of fibrin degradation products with ensuing coagulopathy. Simultaneously, there is a consumption of platelets and plasma factors that leads to plasma factor deficiency and thrombocytopenia.

Disseminated intravascular coagulation is diagnosed when there is bleeding from puncture sites or uncontrollable hemorrhage at surgery in a typical clinical scenario such as the presumed abruptio placentae in this patient. However, the clinical picture may be confusing or there may not be signs of excessive hemorrhage in the patient known to have abruptio placentae and, therefore, is at risk for DIC. In such cases, laboratory testing may be useful. Laboratory values may be normal in early stages of disease, and serial testing to monitor for the changes in factor levels may be more useful than testing at any one static point.

A bedside whole blood clotting time may be useful if the DIC is severe, but is positive only after more than 50% of all the clotting factors have been consumed. For the same reason, prothrombin time and PTT are unlikely to be abnormal in these patients. An abnormal hematocrit reading reflects the amount of bleeding the patient has experienced but is not directly related to the degree of coagulopathy. Fibrinogen is a sensitive indicator of DIC, but because the serum fibrinogen level is elevated in normal pregnancy, an initial value may not be in the abnormal range. Serial testing may be very helpful, and an abnormal test result is diagnostic in a patient with a typical scenario such as the patient described. The most sensitive and specific test for DIC is for the presence of fibrin degradation products such as D-dimer. An abnormal result using this test confirms the presence of a coagulopathy; however, it is not a quantitative test that gives an idea of the degree of severity of the coagulopathy. The platelet count generally decreases in cases of DIC and often parallels the decrease in fibrinogen. Because normal platelet counts vary widely in pregnancy and a single value may not be in the abnormal range, the result may not reflect the degree of ongoing coagulopathy.

Most patients who have DIC in an obstetric setting are best treated by treating the underlying cause. In many cases, delivery alone will correct the problem; however, it is anticipated that this patient may need to have an operative delivery. In that case, she may need to have specific treatment to correct the abnormalities in blood counts and coagulation. This could include aggressive volume replacement, transfusion of red blood cells, cryoprecipitate to correct fibrinogen levels and clotting factors, fresh frozen plasma also for clotting factors and volume, and, in cases where the platelet count is severely decreased, platelet transfusions. In general, platelets are not given unless the platelet count has decreased below 20,000/mm^3, but they would be replaced more aggressively if a cesarean delivery is anticipated.

Bick RL. Disseminated intravascular coagulation current concepts of etiology, pathophysiology, diagnosis, and treatment. Hematol Oncol Clin North Am 2003;17:149–76.

Bick RL, Arun B, Frenkel EP. Disseminated intravascular coagulation: clinical and pathophysiological mechanisms and manifestations. Haemostasis 1999;29:111–34.

Clark SL. Placenta previa and abruptio placentae. In: Creasy RK, Resnik R, editors. Maternal-fetal medicine: principles and practice. 5th ed. Philadelphia (PA): WB Saunders; 2004. p. 707–22.

11

Hemoglobinopathy screening

A healthy, primigravid African-American woman comes to the office for prenatal care. In addition to doing a complete blood count, the best test to screen for hemoglobinopathies is

    (A) solubility test for hemoglobin S (Sickledex)
    (B) high-performance liquid chromatography to detect abnormal hemoglobin
*   (C) hemoglobin electrophoresis
    (D) DNA-based test for hemoglobin chain gene deletions

Hemoglobin is a complex molecule made up of four chains. Human hemoglobins consist of gene clusters with the α chains on chromosome 16 and the β chains on chromosome 11. The hemoglobinopathies are classified into five categories (Box 11-1).

Hemoglobinopathies predominate in areas where malaria is endemic and probably are of some evolutionary adaptive survival significance. For example, children with α-thalassemia may be more vulnerable to *Plasmodium vivax* infection but are less susceptible to the more lethal *P falciparum* form of malaria.

Worldwide, the thalassemias are the most predominant hemoglobinopathy. Approximately 15% of African Americans are silent carriers of α-thalassemia, and α-thalassemia is found among individuals of West Indian and Southeast Asian descent. Beta-thalassemia affects approximately 15% of individuals of Mediterranean or Southeast Asian descent.

Sickle cell anemia is a specific hemoglobinopathy that involves alteration of the β-globin gene with substitution of thymine for adenine, which leads to an amino acid change from valine for glutamate and gives rise to hemoglobin S. A heterozygote contains both hemoglobin A and hemoglobin S components. In sickle cell anemia, hemoglobin A has been replaced by hemoglobin S.

A number of tests have been used to screen for the presence of abnormal hemoglobins, including isoelectric focusing, high-performance liquid chromatography, the solubility test (Sickledex), and hemoglobin electrophoresis. In situations where rapid identification of hemoglobinopathies is critical for proper patient care, solubility testing may be of some value, but such testing is inadequate for screening for other potentially important gene abnormalities that might affect fetal outcome. The expense and lack of availability of high-performance liquid chromatography to detect abnormal hemoglobin do not make it a viable option.

Therefore, hemoglobin electrophoresis is the most appropriate initial test to include, along with a complete blood count, to screen for hemoglobinopathies. The complete blood count is of importance in that red blood cell indices may aid in making certain diagnoses, eg, β-thalassemia trait, when used in conjunction with hemoglobin electrophoresis results (Fig. 11-1). In situations where screening for α-thalassemia trait is warranted, hemoglobin electrophoresis is not sufficient, and DNA-based testing is useful and may be used as part of a prenatal fetal diagnostic strategy.

BOX 11-1

Classification of Hemoglobinopathies

1. Structural hemoglobinopathies
2. Thalassemias
3. Thalassemia hemoglobin variants
4. Hereditary persistence of fetal hemoglobin
5. Acquired hemoglobinopathies

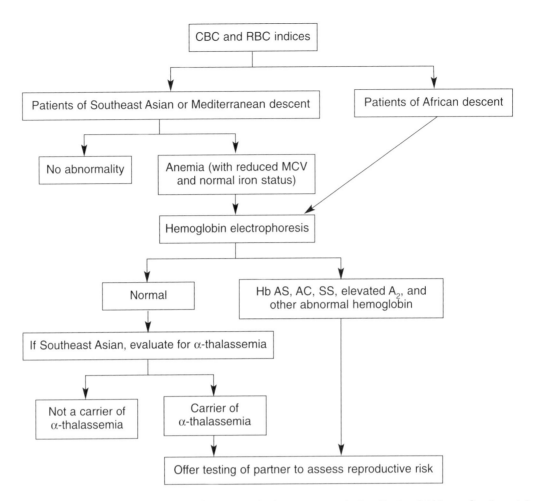

FIG. 11-1. Specialized antepartum evaluation for hematologic assessment of patients of African, Southeast Asian, or Mediterranean descent. Patients of Southeast Asian or Mediterranean descent should undergo electrophoresis if their blood test results reveal anemia. CBC, complete blood count; Hb, hemoglobin; MCV, mean corpuscular volume; RBC, red blood cell. (Hemoglobinopathies in pregnancy. ACOG Practice Bulletin No. 78. American College of Obstetricians and Gynecologists. Obstet Gynecol 2007;109:229–37.)

Benz EJ. Hemoglobinopathies. In: Kasper DL, Braunwald E, Fauci AS, Hauser SL, Longo DL, Jameson JH, editors. Harrison's principles of internal medicine. 16th ed. New York (NY): McGraw-Hill; 2005. p. 593–601.

Hemoglobinopathies in pregnancy. ACOG Practice Bulletin No. 78. American College of Obstetricians and Gynecologists. Obstet Gynecol 2007;109:229–37.

12

Recurrent spontaneous abortion

A 35-year-old woman, gravida 3, presents after her third consecutive spontaneous first trimester pregnancy loss. All pregnancy losses have occurred before 10 weeks of gestation. No karyotypes of the products of conception have been determined, but maternal and paternal karyotypes are 46,XX and 46,XY, respectively. A sonohysterogram has revealed a normal uterine cavity. Her evaluation also should include

        (A) inherited thrombophilia assessment
        (B) mycoplasma genital culture
        (C) Hegar dilator test
        (D) alloimmunization test
*   (E) antiphospholipid antibodies assessment

Pregnancy loss usually is defined as a spontaneous loss of pregnancy from conception to 19 6/7 weeks of gestation. The term spontaneous abortion is equivalent, but should be avoided because women associate negative feelings with this term. Miscarriage is a lay term for pregnancy loss. Anembryonic pregnancy loss occurs when no embryo is identified (eg, missed abortion, blighted ovum). Embryonic pregnancy loss occurs when an embryo is identified but is nonviable.

A first-trimester pregnancy loss is a loss that occurs from conception to 13 6/7 weeks of gestation. An early first-trimester pregnancy loss occurs between conception and 9 6/7 weeks, whereas a late first-trimester pregnancy loss occurs between 10 and 13 6/7 weeks. Recurrent pregnancy loss is defined as three or more consecutive losses, although some studies define it as two or more losses.

Initial workup for a recurrent spontaneous first-trimester pregnancy loss consists of a detailed history (smoking, alcohol and caffeine use, illicit drug use, environmental exposures, working conditions, as well as detailed obstetric and gynecologic history) and physical examination including a pelvic examination.

Approximately 3–15% of women with recurrent early pregnancy losses have antiphospholipid antibodies. Antiphospholipid antibodies to be tested in these women are anticardiolipin antibodies, lupus anticoagulant, and anti-β_2 glycoprotein-1 antibodies. Two positive test results more than 12 weeks apart should be obtained because isolated false-positive tests are common. The presence of antiphospholipid antibodies on these two occasions and recurrent first-trimester loss is diagnostic for the antiphospholipid syndrome. Screening for these antibodies is cost-effective and beneficial because an intervention is available that can improve the outcome. Low-dose aspirin and prophylactic heparin therapy for antiphospholipid syndrome with either three or more

unexplained consecutive pregnancy losses at less than 10 weeks of gestation or one or more unexplained fetal deaths at more than 10 weeks of gestation has been associated with a higher number of live births than placebo.

Inherited thrombophilic mutations have not been consistently associated with recurrent early first-trimester losses. A stronger association appears to exist between these thrombophilias with later (after 10 weeks of gestation) pregnancy losses. One trial studied women with both a previous fetal loss after 10 weeks of gestation and a thrombophilic defect such as heterozygous factor V Leiden, prothrombin 20210, or protein S deficiency. Women who received daily enoxaparin experienced a 10-fold increase in live births.

Ureaplasma urealyticum or *Mycoplasma hominis* colonization of the cervicovaginal tract is common in pregnancy, and has been associated with a possible increased risk of preterm birth, but not usually of early pregnancy losses. There are no trials to show that screening for and treating *Ureaplasma* or *Mycoplasma* in early pregnancy prevent early losses. Oral azithromycin and metronidazole every 4 months for the treatment of *Ureaplasma* or *Mycoplasma* infections after a preterm birth and before the next conception do not significantly reduce the incidences of subsequent miscarriage before 15 weeks of gestation or preterm birth.

All prepregnancy evaluations of the cervix (eg, hysterosalpingography, no. 8 Hegar dilator passage, catheter traction test) have usually been studied for women with possible cervical insufficiency or prior preterm birth, and not in women with recurrent first-trimester losses. The cervix does not appear to have a significant role in most women with recurrent first-trimester losses. Moreover, these cervical evaluations either have been inadequately studied or have been shown not to be sufficiently predictive to be useful in any prevention program. To date, these tests have not been studied in a randomized trial.

Testing for alloimmunization has not been consistently associated with a higher risk for first-trimester pregnancy losses. The various forms of immunotherapy studied so far include paternal cell immunization, third party donor cell immunization, trophoblast membranes infusion, and intravenous immune globulin (IVIG). None of these interventions has been associated with significant differences between the treatment and control groups in terms of subsequent live births. In fact, in addition to no benefit, these interventions are associated with increased risks. Immunization using viable mononuclear cells carries the risk of any blood transfusion such as transmission of hepatitis B virus or human immunodeficiency virus (HIV). Women who receive lymphocyte immune therapy may have a higher incidence of subsequent miscarriage than women who do not receive such cellular products. The U.S. Food and Drug Administration (FDA) issued a directive in January 2002 that injectable products used for lymphocyte immune therapy to prevent pregnancy loss do not have FDA approval and are considered investigational drugs that pose significant safety concerns.

Intravenous immune globulin therapy is expensive and in relatively short supply. Women should be spared the pain and grief associated with false expectations that an ineffective treatment might work. These therapies should no longer be offered as treatment for unexplained recurrent pregnancy loss.

Often obstetric history is complicated, with early pregnancy losses as well as second-trimester losses, preterm birth, or fetal deaths. Thus, the workup may necessitate a range of tests.

Andrews WW, Goldenberg RL, Hauth JC, Cliver SP, Copper R, Conner M. Interconceptional antibiotics to prevent spontaneous preterm birth: a randomized clinical trial. Am J Obstet Gynecol 2006;194:617–23.

Farquharson RG, Quenby S, Greaves M. Antiphospholipid syndrome in pregnancy: a randomized, controlled trial of treatment [published erratum appears in Obstet Gynecol 2002;100:1361]. Obstet Gynecol 2002;100:408–13.

Gris JC, Mercier E, Quere I, Lavigne-Lissalde G, Cochery-Nouvellon E, Hoffet M, et al. Low-molecular-weight heparin versus low-dose aspirin in women with one fetal loss and a constitutional thrombophilic disorder. Blood 2004;103:3695–9.

Kutteh WH. Antiphospholipid antibody-associated recurrent pregnancy loss: treatment with heparin and low-dose aspirin is superior to low-dose aspirin alone. Am J Obstet Gynecol 1996;174:1584–9.

Porter TF, LaCoursiere Y, Scott JR. Immunotherapy for recurrent miscarriage. Cochrane Database of Systematic Reviews 2006, Issue 2. Art. No.: CD000112. DOI: 10.1002/14651858.CD000112.pub2.

Rai R, Cohen H, Dave M, Regan L. Randomised controlled trial of aspirin and aspirin plus heparin in pregnant women with recurrent miscarriage associated with phospholipid antibodies (or antiphospholipid antibodies). BMJ 1997;314:253–7.

13
External version

A 33-year-old multigravid woman, with a body mass index (weight in kilograms divided by height in meters squared [kg/m^2]) of 24, is seen at 38 weeks of gestation for an external cephalic version of her current breech presenting fetus. She has a negative past medical and surgical history. A recent ultrasonogram revealed a singleton fetus in breech presentation and a posterior placenta. The nonstress test result is reactive. Informed consent has been obtained. The next step is to

* (A) confirm adequate volume of amniotic fluid
  (B) relax the uterus using a β-adrenergic receptor agonist
  (C) provide regional analgesia
  (D) disengage the breech from the pelvis
  (E) initiate pushing actions on the fetus's back

Cesarean delivery of a live singleton fetus in a breech presentation is becoming increasingly common. Therefore, the alternatives available to a woman at term with such a presentation are limited to watchful waiting for spontaneous version, cesarean delivery, or external cephalic version. Performed with ultrasonographic guidance and appropriate fetal monitoring, after the 36th gestational week, external cephalic version is a safe alternative to routine cesarean delivery and has been demonstrated to reduce the rate of breech presentation at the time of labor.

In studies of external cephalic version, multivariate analysis has confirmed that absence of oligohydramnios, relaxed uterine tone, and placental location were significant predictors of success. For successful and atraumatic version to occur, there must be an adequate volume of amniotic fluid within which the passage of the fetus from nonvertex to vertex presentation can be accomplished. Currently, therefore, the presence of an adequate amount of amniotic fluid is a primary prerequisite for version. As a corollary to confirming the presence of an adequate volume of amniotic fluid, rupture of membranes must be ruled out before initiating the procedure. Use of external cephalic version in the face of ruptured membranes has rarely been reported and is controversial.

Once an adequate amniotic fluid volume has been confirmed, uterine relaxation may be established with a tocolytic agent. Although there is sufficient evidence to recommend routine tocolysis for all patients, it may particularly benefit multiparous patients. The most commonly used tocolytic agents to reduce uterine tone to facilitate external cephalic version have been the β-mimetic drugs, specifically terbutaline. Several randomized controlled trials have demonstrated enhanced external cephalic version success rates with this category of tocolytic. Terbutaline is administered as a subcutaneous injection, and the external cephalic version is started approximately

5 minutes after drug administration. Common side effects of terbutaline include maternal and fetal tachycardia and maternal hyperglycemia. Uncommonly, maternal cardiac arrhythmia and myocardial ischemia have occurred. More recently, investigators have studied nitroglycerin for use in external cephalic version; however, results do not show improved rates of success and some studies reveal a trend toward higher rates of some side effects such as headache and hypotension.

Epidural analgesia has been suggested as an adjuvant to enhance the version success rate. Evidence is insufficient to show benefit during external cephalic version events. In one retrospective study of epidural analgesia to aid external cephalic version, versions done with an epidural were successful in 19 of 32 women (59%) versus 9 of 37 women (24%) without anesthesia (P <.05). In a prospective randomized trial of epidural during version, 69% of women with epidural analgesia had a successful external cephalic version compared with 32% in controls (P <.05). There were no apparent detrimental effects related to epidural use in either investigation. The previous results notwithstanding, many external cephalic versions are performed in units other than hospital labor and delivery areas; thus, regional analgesia would not be expected to be available. Therefore, although a valuable adjunct, regional analgesia is neither required nor is its absence a contraindication to the procedure. Moreover, one must be alert that the analgesic effect of the epidural may result in more forceful attempts at external cephalic version, compared with procedures done without it. Excessive force during version can cause direct fetal or maternal trauma. It is important to remember that the purpose of analgesia is to relax the maternal abdominal musculature, not to allow for force.

Once all preparatory actions have been taken, the procedure begins with the disengagement of the breech presenting fetus from the pelvis. Two alternatives are available to the clinician: manual uplifting of the breech presenting fetus by the vaginal route, similar to the uplifting applied to a deep pelvic arrest of the presenting part before a second stage cesarean delivery; or, if the breech fetus is not deep in the pelvis, as is more usual, manually uplifting the breech fetus by the extended fingers of both hands placed on the suprapubic area. Following success in disengagement, pushing actions are exerted upon the upper portion of the fetal back or lower portion of the fetal head to begin the rotational movement of a forward somersault.

If external cephalic version has been successfully performed, the patient should be told that she is still at greater risk for cesarean delivery than those with a spontaneous vertex presentation. Reasons for this remain unclear. Possible reasons that have been proposed include coexisting uterine anomalies, atypical maternal pelvis configuration, and a higher likelihood of an unengaged or asynclitic fetal head.

American College of Obstetricians and Gynecologists. External cephalic version. ACOG Practice Bulletin 13. Washington, DC: ACOG; 2000.

Aisenbrey GA, Catanzarite VA, Nelson C. External cephalic version: predictors of success. Obstet Gynecol 1999;94:783–6.

Brost BC, Adams JD, Hester M. External cephalic version after rupture of membranes. Obstet Gynecol 2000;95:1041.

El-Sayed YY, Pullen K, Riley ET, Lyell D, Druzin ML, Cohen SE, et al. Randomized comparison of intravenous nitroglycerin and subcutaneous terbutaline for external cephalic version under tocolysis. Am J Obstet Gynecol 2004;191:2051–5.

Mancuso KM, Yancey MK, Murphy JA, Markenson GR. Epidural analgesia for cephalic version: a randomized trial. Obstet Gynecol 2000;95: 648–51.

Vezina Y, Bujold E, Varin J, Marquette GP, Boucher M. Cesarean delivery after successful external cephalic version of breech presentation at term: a comparative study. Am J Obstet Gynecol 2004;190:763–8.

14

Fetal acid–base assessment

A 34-year-old healthy multigravid woman in the 37th week of gestation gives birth to an initially depressed newborn with a tight double nuchal cord and Apgar scores of 2, 4, and 7. Results of umbilical artery blood gas evaluation are as follows: pH, 7.05; P_{CO_2}, 90 mm Hg; P_{O_2}, 25 mm Hg; and base excess, –10 mEq/L. These results are most compatible with

       (A) normal blood gas values
*   (B) respiratory acidosis
       (C) metabolic acidosis
       (D) mixed acidosis
       (E) lactic acidosis

Umbilical cord arterial blood gas evaluation is a crucial element in the evaluation of a depressed newborn. However, confusion persists both in the need for or availability of a complete evaluation compared with an isolated pH determination and in the interpretation of results. Sampling umbilical arterial cord blood is necessary and often difficult. Umbilical arterial blood most accurately reflects fetal status because it has circulated throughout the fetus. In contrast, the umbilical vein carries blood from the placenta back to the fetus. As a consequence, umbilical venous blood gas measurements reflect maternal acid–base status and placental function acting upon blood that has circulated throughout the fetus. Therefore, if only one vessel is selected, it should be the umbilical artery rather than the vein. If there is confusion about the identity of a vessel, it is best to obtain samples from it and an immediate adjacent vessel. It is likely that one of those vessels will be an artery and in most instances the differences in individual elements will allow the correct vessel to be identified. Recently, the American College of Obstetricians and Gynecologists has suggested that both arterial and venous cord gases be obtained in the following circumstances:

- Cesarean delivery for fetal compromise
- Low 5-minute Apgar score
- Severe growth restriction
- Abnormal fetal heart rate tracing
- Maternal thyroid disease
- Intrapartum fever
- Multiple gestations

To appreciate the complexities of abnormal umbilical cord blood pH and blood gas values noted among newborns, it is first necessary to appreciate the variety of normal ranges. Table 14-1 summarizes these norms. Among all alert, term newborns in a large Swedish cohort study, the mean umbilical cord artery pH was 7.238 plus or minus

TABLE 14-1. Normal Umbilical Cord Blood pH and Blood Gas Values in Full-Term Newborns

Arterial Blood	Normal Ranges
pH	7.24–7.28 plus or minus 0.07
Po_2	14–32 mm Hg
Pco_2	49.2–56.3 plus or minus 8 mm Hg
Hco_3	22.0–24.1 plus or minus 2.2 mEq/L
Base excess	–2.7 to –3.6 plus or minus 2.7 mEq/L

pH, hydrogen ion concentration; Po_2, partial oxygen pressure; Pco_2, partial carbon dioxide pressure; Hco_3, bicarbonate ion.

0.081. Of note, this value decreased linearly with each successive gestational week between 37 and 42 weeks of gestation. The lower cutoff level (mean –2 SD) at 37 weeks was 7.10 and at 42 weeks it was 7.06. The physiologic mechanisms explaining the continuous decrease of cord artery pH are not known. In the above case, the arterial cord pH is not normal and is in the acidotic range.

Fetal acidemias are classified as metabolic, mixed, or respiratory. The former two impart a prognosis of more concern than pure respiratory acidosis. Metabolic acidemia is primarily caused by hypoxia, leading to anerobic metabolism to meet energy needs, which results in the production and accumulation of lactic acid. Lactic acid combines with and thereby decreases bicarbonate concentration resulting in an increase (higher negative value) in base excess. A growing body of evidence from laboratory and clinical studies shows that the threshold for a significant metabolic acidosis is a base deficit between –12 mmol/L and –16 mmol/L. In the patient described, oxygen levels are within normal limits, as is base excess. There is no evidence for metabolic or mixed acidosis nor is there evidence of accumulation of lactic acid.

Respiratory acidosis is caused by an accumulation of carbon dioxide, such as occurs when the cord compresses. This may be due to any labor complication such as uterine contraction compression of an umbilical cord around a fetus's body or a tight loop of umbilical cord around the fetal neck. This compression inhibits transfer of carbon dioxide across the placenta. In this patient, the markedly elevated carbon dioxide concentration identifies this acidosis as respiratory.

The World Federation of Neurology formed a task force for the prevention of cerebral palsy and related neurologic disorders. The task force defined asphyxia as a condition of impaired gas exchange leading, if it persists, to progressive hypoxemia, hypercapnia, and a significant metabolic acidosis. The American College of Obstetricians and Gynecologists supports the use of an umbilical arterial pH of less than 7 as a clinically useful cutoff for such acidosis.

American Academy of Pediatrics, American College of Obstetricians and Gynecologists. Neonatal encephalopathy and cerebral palsy: defining the pathogenesis and pathophysiology. Elk Grove Village (IL): AAP; Washington, DC: ACOG; 2003. p. 25–38.

Umbilical cord blood gas and acid-base analysis. ACOG Committee Opinion No. 348. American College of Obstetricians and Gynecologists. Obstet Gynecol 2006;108:1319–22.

Gilstrap LC. Fetal acid-base balance. In: Creasy RK, Resnik R, Iams JD, editors. Maternal–fetal medicine: principles and practice. 5th ed. Philadelphia (PA): WB Saunders Co.; 2004. p. 434.

Low JA. Intrapartum fetal asphyxia: definition, diagnosis, and classification. Am J Obstet Gynecol 1997;176;957–9.

Kitlinski ML, Kallen K, Marsal K, Olofsson P. Gestational age-dependent reference values for pH in umbilical cord arterial blood at term. Obstet Gynecol 2003;102:338–45.

Nodwell A, Carmichael L, Ross M, Richardson B. Placental compared with umbilical cord blood to assess fetal blood gas and acid-base status. Obstet Gynecol 2005;105:129–38.

Thorp JA, Dildy GA, Yeomans ER, Meyer EA, Parisi VM. Umbilical cord blood gas analysis at delivery. Am J Obstet Gynecol 1996; 175:517–22.

15

Use of peak flow meter in asthma

You are counseling a pregnant patient with moderate persistent asthma on the use of her peak flow meter. You explain to her that peak expiratory flow rate (PEFR) results between 60% and 80% of baseline indicate

* (A) a mild to moderate asthma exacerbation
  (B) a normal fluctuation in baseline
  (C) a severe asthma exacerbation
  (D) a malfunction of her peak flow meter

Asthma may be the most common potentially serious medical complication of pregnancy, affecting 4–8% of pregnancies. The National Asthma Education and Prevention Program Working Group on Asthma and Pregnancy categorizes asthma severity as mild intermittent, mild persistent, moderate persistent, and severe persistent, according to symptomatic exacerbations and objective tests of pulmonary function (Table 15-1). The care and treatment of patients with asthma are organized around several components, of which patient education and assessment and monitoring of asthma, including objective measures of pulmonary function, play a central role. Although severe asthma may increase the risk of perinatal complications, adequately controlled asthma is associated with outcomes that are not significantly different from those of the nonasthmatic population. It is recommended that asthmatic patients, even with mild or well-controlled disease, have pulmonary function monitoring during pregnancy. The most commonly used measures of pulmonary function are the peak expiratory flow rate (PEFR) and forced expiratory volume in 1 second (FEV_1).

The FEV_1 after a maximal inspiration is the single best measure of pulmonary function. When adjusted for confounders, a mean FEV_1 less than 80% predicted has been found to be significantly associated with increased preterm delivery and birth weight less than 2,500 g. However, measurement of FEV_1 requires a spirometer. The PEFR correlates well with the FEV_1 and can be measured reliably with inexpensive, disposable, portable peak flow meters.

Home peak flow monitoring can be used for both the short- and long-term monitoring of asthma control, as well as in the detection and management of acute asthma exacerbations. Peak flow monitoring during exacerbations of asthma can help determine the severity of the exacerbation and guide therapeutic decisions. Patients with persistent asthma should be evaluated at least monthly. Those with moderate to severe asthma should have daily PEFR monitoring to detect early changes in disease status that may require treatment or evaluation of responses to changes in therapy.

In women, normal PEFR values range from 380 L/min to 550 L/min. However, it is recommended that each

TABLE 15-1. Asthma Severity and Peak Expiratory Flow Rate Characteristics

Asthma Classification	PEFR Characteristics
Mild intermittent Symptoms twice per week or less Nocturnal symptoms twice per month or less	PEFR or FEV_1 80% predicted or more, variability less than 20%
Mild persistent Symptoms more than twice per week but not daily Nocturnal symptoms more than twice per month	PEFR or FEV_1 80% predicted or more, variability less than 20–30%
Moderate persistent Daily symptoms Nocturnal symptoms more than once per week	PEFR or FEV_1 more than 60% to less than 80% predicted, variability more than 30%
Severe Continuous symptoms and frequent exacerbations Frequent nocturnal symptoms	PEFR or FEV_1 60% predicted or less, variability more than 30%

FEV_1, forced expiratory volume in 1 second; PEFR, peak expiratory flow rate.

National Asthma Education and Prevention Program. Working group report on managing asthma during pregnancy: recommendations for pharmacologic treatment—update 2004. Bethesda (MD): U.S. Department of Health and Human Services; National Institutes of Health; National Heart, Lung, and Blood Institute; 2004.

woman determine her "personal best" PEFR when her asthma is well controlled. Patients should therefore be instructed on use of the peak flow meter and maintenance when they are at normal pulmonary function. A PEFR result of 80–100% of a woman's personal best signals good control, whereas a result in the range of 50–79% signals a worsening in her asthma, and PEFR values below 50% of personal best indicate a severe exacerbation. Many patients with asthma have structured writing action plans to guide them through management of an acute exacerbation, including criteria for hospital or emergency department visits (Fig. 15-1). A Cochrane analysis concluded that training in asthma self-care that involves self-monitoring by peak flow, coupled with regular medical review

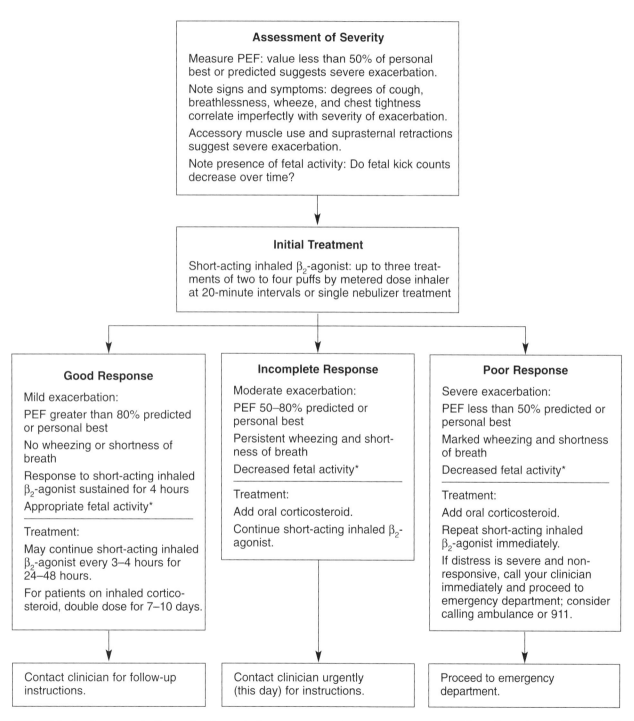

FIG. 15-1. Acute exacerbations of asthma during pregnancy: home management. PEF, peak expiratory flow. *Fetal activity is monitored by observing whether fetal kick counts decrease over time. (Modified from National Asthma Education and Prevention Program. Working group report on managing asthma during pregnancy: recommendations for pharmacologic treatment—update 2004. Bethesda (MD): U.S. Department of Health and Human Services; National Institutes of Health; National Heart, Lung, and Blood Institute; 2004. p. 8.)

and a written action plan, appears to improve health outcomes for adults with asthma. Patients who adopted PEFR measures with a written action plan demonstrated reduced asthma-related hospital admissions and emergency department visits.

Incorrect peak flow meter readings may be related to poor technique, misinterpretation, or device failure. Periodic inspection and calibration will ensure proper functioning of peak flow meters.

American College of Obstetricians and Gynecologists, American College of Allergy, Asthma and Immunology. The use of newer asthma and allergy medications during pregnancy [position statement]. Ann Allergy Asthma Immunol 2000;84:475–80.

Dombrowski MP. Asthma and pregnancy. Obstet Gynecol 2006;108: 667–81.

Gibson PG, Powell H, Coughlan J, Wilson AJ, Abramson M, Haywood P, et al. Self-management education and regular practitioner review for adults with asthma [Systemic Review] Cochrane Airways Group. Cochrane Database of Systematic Reviews 2002, Issue 3. Art. No.: CD001117. DOI: 10.1002/14651858.CD001117, 4, 2006.

National Asthma Education and Prevention Program. Expert panel report: guidelines for the diagnosis and management of asthma—update on selected topics 2002. Bethesda (MD): U.S. Department of Health and Human Services; National Institutes of Health; National Heart, Lung, and Blood Institute; 2003.

National Asthma Education and Prevention Program. Working group report on managing asthma during pregnancy: recommendations for pharmacologic treatment—update 2004. Bethesda (MD): U.S. Department of Health and Human Services; National Institutes of Health; National Heart, Lung, and Blood Institute; 2004.

16

Diagnostic accuracy in fetal distress

A 28-year-old primigravid woman at 38 weeks of gestation is in the first hour of the second stage of labor. Uterine contractions occur every 3 minutes, lasting 50 seconds. You note mild variable decelerations, minimal variability, a baseline fetal heart rate of 170 beats per minute, and accelerations. Usually, a fetal cord pH of 7.20 or more is assured due to the presence of

* (A) accelerations
  (B) variable decelerations
  (C) minimal variability
  (D) baseline fetal heart rate of 170 beats per minute

Continuous electronic fetal heart rate (FHR) monitoring is used today to assess fetal tolerance of labor in the majority of hospitals in the United States. This technology was first developed in the 1950s and became widespread in the 1960s. During the 1960s, theories were developed in regard to the cause of FHR patterns, and a limited amount of experimental and empirical evidence was produced to support these theories. This gave rise to great enthusiasm for the technique, and many hospitals purchased FHR monitors for their delivery rooms, initially in limited numbers but later in sufficient numbers so that all laboring mothers could be monitored electronically. Despite the lack of standard interpretation, once FHR monitoring was used extensively, evidence began to accumulate regarding its predictability and efficacy. The initial data noted positive results (virtual disappearance of intrapartum stillbirths). However, larger and better controlled prospective studies provided results that were less heartening. It had been hoped that intrapartum FHR surveillance would be effective and accurate in predicting and diagnosing fetal hypoxia and metabolic acidosis during

labor, which in turn would decrease the incidence of hypoxic brain injury. When compared with intermittent auscultation of FHR in low-risk women, continuous electronic FHR monitoring was associated with a reduction in the risk of neonatal seizures, but at the expense of an increased rate of cesarean delivery and operative vaginal births and without evidence of a reduction in the risk of cerebral palsy or hypoxic brain injury. Nonetheless, the use of this modality remains high, and there is agreement that consistency in interpretation and the use of common definitions and language would be beneficial. Appendix B shows the National Institute of Child Health and Human Development (NICHD) Research Planning definitions of FHR patterns.

An acceleration of the FHR is defined as an increase of baseline FHR of 15 beats per minute amplitude over at least a 15-second interval. To evaluate for the absence of acidemia, both digital scalp stimulation and vibroacoustic stimulation are used. Digital scalp stimulation is gentle digital stroking of the fetal scalp for at least 15 seconds during a vaginal examination. Vibroacoustic stimulation can be applied continuously for 3 seconds to the maternal abdominal skin over the fetal head. Data show that both techniques, when they provoke an acceleration in the FHR, are equivalent in predicting the absence of fetal acidemia. Caution is necessary because the fetal status may change over time; this modality predicts only the current acid–base status. In one study of 108 women with FHR pattern suggestive of acidosis, digital scalp stimulation was performed as described. It was followed within 1–2 minutes by scalp pH sampling. In all 51 instances of accelerations, the scalp pH was equal to or greater than 7.20.

In a study using computerized recordings of a fetal monitor, the umbilical artery pH failed to show significant correlation with FHR decelerations during the last hour of labor, confirming the relative insensitivity of decelerations for predicting pH.

A descriptive study to assess the relationship between the FHR monitoring pattern and fetal acid–base balance, interpreted according to NICHD guidelines, demonstrated that baseline variability did have clinical significance. Decreased variability (less than five beats per minute), characterized visually as either minimal or absent, was more frequently associated with lower pH values than was moderate variability. In the described case, minimal variability, although not diagnostic of abnormally low fetal pH, cannot be used for reassurance.

The normal range of baseline FHR is 110–160 beats per minute, regardless of the stage of labor. A baseline FHR of greater than 160 beats per minute is considered tachycardia, is abnormal, and requires a clinical evaluation to determine its cause. It is not diagnostic of an abnormal pH but it is also not reassuring of a normal pH.

Agrawal SK, Doucette F, Gratton R, Richardson B, Gagnon R. Intrapartum computerized fetal heart rate parameters and metabolic acidosis at birth. Obstet Gynecol 2003;102:731–8.

Elimian A, Figuero R, Tejani N. Intrapartum assessment of fetal well-being: a comparison of scalp stimulation with scalp blood pH sampling. Obstet Gynecol 1997;89:373–6.

Intrapartum fetal heart rate monitoring. ACOG Practice Bulletin No. 70. American College of Obstetricians and Gynecologists. Obstet Gynecol 2005;106:1453–61.

Parer JT, King T. Fetal heart rate monitoring: is it salvageable? Am J Obstet Gynecol 2000;182:982–7.

Sameshima H, Ikenoue T, Ikeda T, Kamitomo M, Ibara S. Unselected low-risk pregnancies and the effect of continuous intrapartum fetal heart rate monitoring on umbilical blood gases and cerebral palsy. Am J Obstet Gynecol 2004;190:118–23.

Skupski DW, Rosenberg CR, Eglinton GS. Intrapartum fetal stimulation tests: a meta-analysis. Obstet Gynecol 2002;99:129–34.

17

Smoking cessation

A 22-year-old primigravid woman comes in for her first prenatal visit at 12 weeks of gestation. She reports smoking two packs of cigarettes per day and expresses a willingness to quit. The best initial step in the care of this patient is to

   (A) prescribe bupropion hydrochloride (Zyban)

   (B) recommend use of a nicotine patch

   (C) recommend use of nicotine gum

*   (D) provide pregnancy-specific educational materials about smoking cessation

The need for patients to quit smoking is increasingly emphasized by health care practitioners. Pregnancy is an ideal time to address smoking cessation because pregnant women may be more motivated to make significant lifestyle changes than nonpregnant women. Nearly 50% of prepregnancy smokers quit during pregnancy. Unfortunately, 60–80% of those who quit during pregnancy resume smoking within 1 year postpartum.

Smoking during pregnancy increases the risk of both maternal and neonatal complications—including abruptio placentae, placenta previa, growth restriction, low birth weight, preterm premature rupture of membranes, and perinatal mortality. In addition, smoking during pregnancy is associated with increased risks of sudden infant death syndrome and offspring with asthma.

Smoking cessation programs have been tested in pregnancy in terms of their effect on infant outcomes. In a recent Cochrane review of randomized clinical trials of smoking cessation in pregnancy, compared with patients who received "usual care," women in smoking cessation programs had a reduced risk of low birth weight (pooled odds ratio [OR] = 0.81, 95% confidence interval (CI), 0.70–0.94) and preterm birth (pooled OR = 0.84, 95% CI, 0.72–0.98); a small improvement in mean birth weight was also observed.

A five-step intervention, known as the 5 A's, takes 5–15 minutes and should be performed as a routine part of prenatal care:

1. Ask about smoking status.
2. Advise patients about the benefits of quitting smoking.
3. Assess the patient's willingness to attempt to quit smoking within 30 days.
4. Assist patients who are interested in quitting by providing pregnancy-specific, self-help educational materials about smoking cessation.
5. Arrange follow-up visits to track the progress of the patient's attempt to quit smoking.

The initial step in the care of a woman who smokes cigarettes and who is willing to quit is to provide pregnancy-specific smoking cessation educational materials. The patient can be provided with the Internet addresses of helpful web sites to enable her to gain access to information provided by the American College of Obstetricians and Gynecologists, the National Cancer Institute, and other organizations (see Box 17-1). It is also important to explain the symptoms of nicotine withdrawal, such as irritability and cravings. This can be done either verbally or through printed or electronic materials.

BOX 17-1	
Web Site Resources for Smoking Cessation in Pregnant Patients	
Name of Organization	**Web Address**
American Cancer Society	http://www.cancer.org
The American Heart Association	http://www.american heart.org
The National Cancer Institute	http://www.cancer.gov
National Partnership to Help Pregnant Smokers Quit	http://www.helppregnantsmokersquit.org/quit
Smoke-Free Families	http://www.smokefreefamilies.org
Smokefree.gov	http://www.smokefree.gov

Bupropion hydrochloride (Zyban), nicotine patches, and nicotine gum are inappropriate for initial management of smoking cessation because there is insufficient evidence to support the efficacy and safety of their use during pregnancy. Bupropion is an antidepressant in the aminoketone class, and is currently categorized as a Class B drug in pregnancy. It should be recognized, however, that the safety data on this drug during pregnancy are sparse. Likewise, neither the efficacy nor safety of nicotine replacement has been adequately assessed in pregnant women. Some have suggested that if the nicotine replacement is used, products with intermittent dosages, such as gum or inhaler, be tried first. If the nicotine patch is used, it can be removed at night to reduce fetal exposure. Based on the relative paucity of information on pharmacologic methods of smoking cessation in pregnancy, the use of such treatments should be considered only after nonpharmacologic methods of smoking cessation have failed.

Castles A, Adams EK, Melvin CL, Kelsch C, Boulton ML. Effects of smoking during pregnancy. Five meta-analyses. Am J Prev Med 1999; 16:208–15.

Lumley J, Oliver SS, Chamberlain C, Oakley L. Interventions for promoting smoking cessation during pregnancy. Cochrane Database of Systematic Reviews 2004, Issue 4. Art. No.: CD001055. DOI: 10.1002/14651858.CD001055.pub2.

Melvin CL, Dolan-Mullen P, Windsor RA, Whiteside HP Jr, Goldenberg RL. Recommended cessation counselling for pregnant women who smoke: a review of the evidence. Tob Control 2000;9(suppl 3):III80–4.

Smoking cessation during pregnancy. ACOG Committee Opinion No. 316. American College of Obstetricians and Gynecologists. Obstet Gynecol 2005;106:883–8.

18

Expectant management in the latent phase of labor

A 24-year-old primigravid woman presents at 39 weeks of gestation with frequent uterine contractions for the past 6 hours. On repeated examinations, the cervix is 1 cm dilated and 70% effaced, with the fetal presentation at –3 station. The fetal heart rate tracing is reassuring. The best next step in management is

    (A) oxytocin administration
    (B) prostaglandin administration
    (C) artificial rupture of membranes
*   (D) expectant management

The patient described is in the latent phase of labor. This phase is defined as the time from the onset of regular uterine contractions until active labor (approximately 4 cm cervical dilation). The course and duration of labor have been traditionally described by the Friedman curve. This curve is based on 500 primigravid subjects at term who presented in spontaneous labor and graphs the duration of labor versus cervical dilation and station. The course and duration of labor varies by several factors, the most important of which is parity. Based on data from the Friedman curve, the duration of the latent phase of labor in nulliparous patients is less than 20 hours, and in multiparous patients it is less than 14 hours. Importantly, these cutoffs describe the fifth percentile for labor progression, meaning that 95% of parturients will progress more quickly than described in the Friedman curve.

Recently, some have questioned whether the Friedman curve, which was generated in the 1950s, is applicable in modern obstetric practice. A recent study of 1,329 nulliparous women in spontaneous labor at term reassessed labor curves. Although the latent phase was not strictly redefined, this study did suggest that the cutoffs for protraction disorders defined in the Friedman curve may be too stringent for modern obstetric practice.

The best choice in the care of this patient is expectant management to await active labor. If the patient is extremely uncomfortable, administration of a narcotic or sleeping medication may be useful (ie, so-called "therapeutic rest"). Labor induction with oxytocin, prostaglandin, or artificial rupture of membranes is not indicated in the management of a normal latent phase of labor because it may increase the risk of cesarean delivery.

A prolonged latent phase is more problematic because patients in the latent phase of labor often are markedly uncomfortable and frustrated. The care of a patient with a prolonged latent phase should be individualized. Important factors to consider in management of such cases include the gestational age, cervical examination, and parity. In general, it is reasonable to manage a prolonged latent phase expectantly as well because the prognosis for vaginal delivery is still good. Alternatively, in cases of prolonged latent phase, it may also be reasonable to consider labor induction.

Dystocia and augmentation of labor. ACOG Practice Bulletin No. 49. American College of Obstetricians and Gynecologists. Obstet Gynecol 2003;102:1445–54.

Zhang J, Troendle JF, Yancey MK. Reassessing the labor curve in nulliparous women. Am J Obstet Gynecol 2002;187:824–8.

19

Recurrence of gestational diabetes mellitus

A 24-year-old woman, gravida 1, para 1, is seen for an annual examination. She is planning her next pregnancy and is concerned because she had gestational diabetes mellitus (GDM) in her first pregnancy. She weighs 90.7 kg (200 lb) and is 1.6 m (5 ft 3 in.) tall; her body mass index (weight in kilograms divided by height in meters squared [kg/m^2]) is 35. She weighed 88.5 kg (195 lb) at the beginning of her last pregnancy. Because of a positive family history during her last pregnancy, she was screened for GDM at 12 weeks of gestation and had a normal test result. A follow-up glucose tolerance test at 30 weeks showed GDM. She was placed on a diet and home glucose monitoring and ultimately gave birth to a 3,628 g (8 lb) baby at term. Her greatest risk factor for recurrence of GDM is

* (A) obesity
  (B) gestational age at diagnosis
  (C) maternal age
  (D) parity

Gestational diabetes mellitus complicates 3–6% of all pregnancies and is a marker for the development of diabetes mellitus in later life. Risk factors for the development of GDM include the following:

- Maternal obesity
- Maternal age older than 25 years
- Family history of diabetes mellitus
- Previous child with macrosomia

Members of certain racial or ethnic groups have a high prevalence of diabetes mellitus and these patients also have a higher incidence of GDM. High-risk groups include patients of Native American, Hispanic, African, and South and Eastern Asian ancestry.

Patients who develop GDM are at risk in a subsequent pregnancy for recurrence of the condition. The magnitude of the recurrence risk is 35–70%. Most studies have found recurrence rates at the higher end of that range. Studies have found a variety of risk factors to be associated with recurrence of GDM including the following:

- Maternal age
- Maternal weight
- Weight gain between pregnancies
- Values on the glucose tolerance test
- Gestational age at diagnosis

In most studies, patients with recurrent GDM are older than patients in whom the disease did not recur. In some studies, however, there is no difference in the age of the patients with recurrence compared with patients with no recurrence. A younger maternal age is not a risk factor in any study and is protective in some. Therefore, the described patient's young age is not associated with an increased risk of GDM.

Parity has been examined in a few studies as a risk factor for recurrence; patients with recurrent GDM are of higher parity than patients without recurrence. This is therefore not a risk factor for the patient described.

Severity of GDM has been examined in several ways as a possible marker for increased recurrence risk. Early gestational age at diagnosis, need for insulin therapy, and higher values on the abnormal glucose tolerance test have all been associated with recurrence. Macrosomia has been associated with recurrence in some studies but not others. The weight of this patient's neonate was appropriate for gestational age and, therefore, is not a risk factor. Because she required only diet therapy, and the diagnosis was made in the third trimester, these are not factors associated with recurrence.

In almost all studies, heavier maternal weight is associated with an increased risk of recurrence. This has been measured by body mass index (BMI) and weight gain between pregnancies. Although this patient has not had an excessive weight gain between pregnancies, she is obese as measured by her BMI. This is a strong, consistently found risk factor for recurrent GDM. Weight gain between pregnancies greater than 6.8 kg (15 lb) has been found to be a risk factor in most studies.

The described patient, who has come to the office for preconception counseling, can be assessed for risk factors for recurrent GDM and counseled about weight loss. However, no prospective trials have been done of weight loss to demonstrate a decrease in recurrence of GDM through weight loss. There is compelling evidence in the nonpregnant population that weight loss decreases the development of type 2 diabetes mellitus. She should be counseled that weight loss may help to decrease her risk

of recurrent GDM but will certainly decrease her risk of developing type 2 diabetes mellitus in later life.

Foster-Powell KA, Cheung NW. Recurrence of gestational diabetes. Aust N Z J Obstet Gynaecol 1998;38:384–7.

MacNeill S, Dodds L, Hamilton DC, Armson BA, VandenHof M. Rates and risk factors for recurrence of gestational diabetes. Diabetes Care 2001;24:659–62.

Nohira T, Kim S, Nakai H, Okabe K, Nohira T, Yoneyama K. Recurrence of gestational diabetes mellitus: rates and risk factors from initial GDM and one abnormal GTT value. Diabetes Res Clin Pract 2006;71:75–81.

Tuomilehto J, Lindstrom J, Eriksson JG, Valle TT, Hämäläinen H, Ilanne-Parikka P, et al. Prevention of type 2 diabetes mellitus by changes in lifestyle among subjects with impaired glucose tolerance. Finnish Diabetes Prevention Study Group. N Engl J Med 2001;344: 1343–50.

20

Vaginal birth after cesarean delivery

The major contraindication to vaginal birth after a cesarean delivery is

*   (A) prior history of transfundal uterine surgery
       (B) two prior cesarean deliveries and one prior term vaginal delivery
       (C) one prior low-vertical cesarean delivery
       (D) estimated fetal weight of 4,000 g
       (E) prior one-layer uterine closure

Vaginal birth after cesarean delivery (VBAC) became an increasingly popular procedure in the 1980s and early 1990s as a response to the national increase in cesarean delivery rates. Numerous studies have been performed in an attempt to quantify better the maternal and fetal risks associated with VBAC. Among the variables that have been investigated are interpregnancy interval, estimated fetal weight of more than 4,000 g, type of uterine incision (low vertical versus low transverse), type of uterine closure, a history of postpartum endomyometritis, success rates after 41 weeks of gestation, role of labor induction, and appropriateness in multiple gestations. It has also been debated whether or not women with an unknown type of prior uterine incision should be permitted a trial of VBAC. From a risk management perspective, other than the obvious issue of providing and obtaining full informed consent regardless of which route of delivery is chosen, it is also essential that VBAC be attempted only in facilities that have the capability to perform an emergency cesarean delivery should the need arise.

Available data suggest that VBAC is acceptable in patients who have had a prior vaginal delivery and not

more than two prior cesarean deliveries. Although fetal weight estimates of greater than 4,000 g may be associated with a slightly lower success rate for VBAC, this is not a contraindication. Preliminary data suggest that single-layer closure and history of postpartum endometritis may be associated with increased risk of uterine rupture in a subsequent VBAC attempt. However, these data are insufficient to affect management decisions at this time. Patients who have had a prior classical cesarean delivery or who have undergone other transfundal uterine surgery are not considered candidates for VBAC because of an elevated risk of uterine rupture. Moreover, recent data suggest a possible role of VBAC in women who have undergone more than one prior cesarean delivery without having had a prior vaginal delivery.

Landon MB, Spong CY, Thom E, Hauth JC, Bloom SL, Varner MW, et al. Risk of uterine rupture with a trial of labor in women with multiple and single prior cesarean delivery. National Institute of Child Health and Human Development Network of Maternal–Fetal Medicine Units. Obstet Gynecol 2006;108:12–20.

Vaginal birth after previous cesarean delivery. ACOG Practice Bulletin No. 54. American College of Obstetricians and Gynecologists. Obstet Gynecol 2004;104:203–12.

21

Hydramnios

A 31-year-old woman, gravida 3, para 2, presents at 29 weeks of gestation with abdominal distention, difficulty catching her breath, and irregular uterine contractions. Her fundal height measures 37 cm, and hydramnios is suspected. An ultrasonogram at 19 weeks of gestation revealed a singleton fetus with no apparent anomalies. The patient's last child was anemic and received a blood transfusion in the nursery. Screening test results for gestational diabetes mellitus and viral infections are negative. The indirect Coombs test result is positive for anti-C with a titer of 1:256. The ultrasonographic image shown in Fig. 21-1 that you would most likely see in this patient is

   (A) double-bubble
   (B) congenital cystic adenomatoid malformation
 * (C) abdominal ascites and skin edema
   (D) anencephaly
   (E) normal stomach bubble

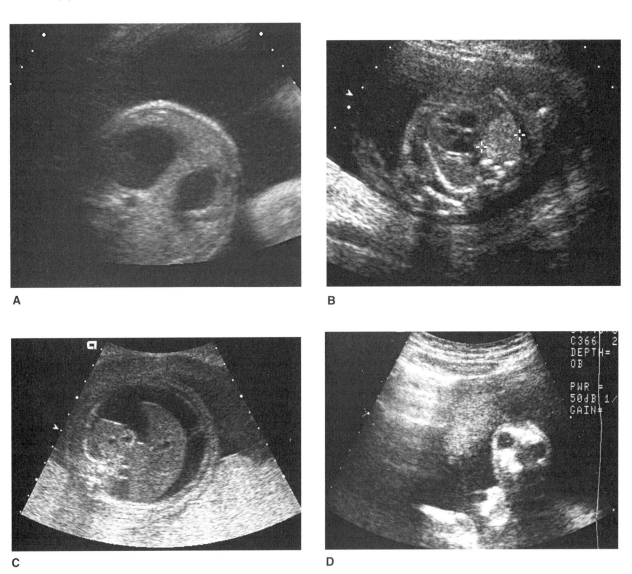

A   B

C   D

FIG. 21-1.

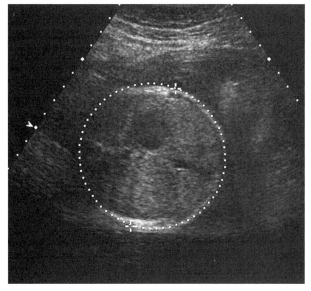

E

Hydramnios is defined as an excess of amniotic fluid. A number of ultrasonographic techniques are used to evaluate amniotic fluid volume. To determine the amniotic fluid index (AFI), the maternal abdomen is partitioned into four equal quadrants, and the deepest vertical pocket in each quadrant is measured in centimeters; the sum of the four deepest vertical pocket measurements yields the overall AFI. Significant hydramnios often is defined as an AFI greater than 25 cm, the deepest vertical pocket of 8 cm or more, or an AFI that exceeds the 95th percentile for gestational age. Hydramnios may be mild with a deep vertical pocket of 8–11 cm, moderate if 12–15 cm, and severe if greater than 15 cm. Both maternal and fetal conditions may cause hydramnios. The extent of hydramnios and the fetal prognosis are associated with its cause. Hydramnios has many etiologies, the most common being idiopathic (Box 21-1). In severe cases, workup is needed. Diabetes mellitus is a common cause of hydramnios; drug exposures constitute a less common cause. Fetal structural abnormalities that affect fetal swallowing by compression or obstruction often are implicated in hydramnios. Fetuses with anencephaly and esophageal atresia usually have some degree of hydramnios. Twin–twin transfusion, rhesus alloimmunization, and fetal viral infections also are associated with increased amniotic fluid.

Once hydramnios is confirmed, a detailed medical history is elicited focusing on current or past diabetes mellitus, drug exposures, recent travel, possible viral infections, personal or family history of skeletal dysplasias, and history of alloimmunization. A targeted fetal anatomic survey is performed to evaluate for fetal structural anomalies and possible genetic syndromes. In fetuses with hydramnios or growth restriction, a karyotypic abnormality may be identified. Additionally, ultrasonography can be used to detect signs of fetal infection and

fetal anemia. One diagnostic algorithm to evaluate hydramnios is listed in Box 21-2.

Patients with hydramnios should be counseled about possible pregnancy complications associated with this condition. Preterm labor and uterine irritability are often seen, both of which may result in preterm birth. Premature rupture of membranes occurs more frequently in the setting of hydramnios with the additional risks of umbilical cord prolapse and abruptio placentae from rapid decompression. There is an increased risk of cesarean delivery because of the unstable fetal presentation and postpartum hemorrhage from uterine atony.

Patients with mild hydramnios usually are managed expectantly. With severe hydramnios, maternal pulmonary compromise may ensue, requiring therapeutic reduction amniocentesis. Patients generally give birth at a facility equipped to manage their particular problem.

Alloimmunization is a common cause of fetal anemia with resultant fetal ascites, hydrops fetalis, and hydramnios. In women with an elevated antibody titer, serial ultrasonographic evaluations are performed to assess for fetal anemia. Hydrops fetalis and hydramnios may be reversed after the fetal anemia has been corrected. The

---

BOX 21-2

Diagnostic Evaluation of Hydramnios

History-taking with emphasis on maternal symptoms, diabetes mellitus, red blood cell alloimmunization, and maternal drug ingestion

High-resolution ultrasonography to assess

- The degree of hydramnios (amniotic fluid index)
- Presence of multiple gestation, growth deficiency, or macrosomia
- Fetal thorax
- Fetal central nervous system (midline structures, neural tube, tone)
- Fetal gastrointestinal system (mouth, stomach, small bowel, abdominal wall)
- Fetal bladder dynamics
- Middle cerebral artery peak systolic velocity (for suspected fetal anemia)
- Chorionicity in multiple gestation

Fetal specimens for karyotyping and diagnosis of viral infection

---

Modified from Taylor FO, Fisk NM. Hydramnios and oligohydramnios. In: James DK, Steer PJ, Weiner CP, Gonik B, editors. High risk pregnancy management options. 3rd ed. Philadelphia (PA): Elsevier Saunders; 2006. p. 274. Copyright 2006 by Elsevier.

---

most likely ultrasonographic finding in this scenario is abdominal ascites and skin edema (image C).

The other ultrasonographic images depicted show: double-bubble—an enlarged fluid-filled stomach and proximal duodenum as a result of duodenal atresia with a lack of normal duodenal canalization leading to a partial or complete obstruction (image A); congenital cystic adenomatoid malformation of the lung—benign lung hematoma with proliferation of terminal bronchioles and lack of normal alveoli (image B); anencephaly—an absence of cranial bone cephalad to the orbits (image D); and normal stomach bubble (image E).

Disorders of amniotic fluid volume. In: Cunningham FG, Leveno KJ, Bloom SL, Hauth JC, Gilstrap L 3rd, Wenstrom KD, editors. Williams obstetrics. 22nd ed. New York (NY): McGraw-Hill; 2005. p. 525–34.

Taylor FO, Fisk NM. Hydramnios and oligohydramnios. In: James DK, Steer PJ, Weiner CP, Gonik B, editors. High risk pregnancy management options. 3rd ed. Philadelphia (PA): Elsevier Saunders; 2006. p. 272–90.

Woodward PJ, Kennedy A, Sohaey R, Byrne JL, Oh KY, Puchalski MD, editors. Diagnostic imaging obstetrics. Salt Lake City (UT): Amirsys; 2005. p. 17:2–5.

22

Thyroid nodule in a pregnant woman

On initial physical examination of a 32-year-old woman, gravida 3, para 2, at 16 weeks of gestation, you palpate a small thyroid nodule. Ultrasonography shows a cystic mass measuring 1.5×1.9 cm, and thyroid function test results are within normal limits. The next step in management is

      (A) postpartum evaluation
*   (B) fine-needle aspiration
      (C) radionuclide scan
      (D) computerized tomography (CT) scan
      (E) wide local excision

Thyroid tumors are the most common endocrine neoplasm. The frequency of thyroid tumors increases throughout life, with half of these manifesting as single benign hyperplastic (or colloid) nodules. Three out of four thyroid tumors occur in women, and half of those occur during the reproductive years. Only 1 in 1,000 are found to be malignant.

Pregnancy does not appear to alter the course of thyroid cancer, and evaluation of a thyroid nodule found in pregnancy should follow similar principles as that found in a nonpregnant woman. Delaying evaluation until after delivery is not recommended. Any thyroid nodule discovered during pregnancy should be diagnostically evaluated at the time of identification. Serum thyroid-stimulating hormone (TSH) and free thyroxine (T_4) should first be obtained. Nodules that are 1 cm in diameter or larger usually can be palpated unless they lie deep within the neck. Although imaging studies often are the first diagnostic test, they cannot reliably distinguish malignant and benign nodules and are unnecessary in most patients. Ultrasonography categorizes nodules as solid, cystic, or mixed with more than 90% accuracy and is the best method to determine the volume of a nodule. Ultrasonography is particularly useful during follow-up because it can distinguish nodular growth from intranodular hemorrhage. However, benign and malignant nodules cannot be differentiated reliably by ultrasonography.

Fine-needle aspiration (FNA) biopsy should be the first test performed in a euthyroid patient with a solitary thyroid nodule. Aspirates are then sent for cytologic interpretation. It is possible that FNA may cure a cystic nodule. Almost half of such nodules disappear permanently after one or more aspirations. Nodules that recur are usually greater than 4 cm in size, and their aspiration tends to yield bloody fluid but insufficient material for diagnosis. These nodules should be considered for surgical removal. Timing of surgical removal of a thyroid nodule in pregnancy will depend on the findings of the cytologic evaluation. If cytology findings are suspicious for malignancy in a nodule discovered early in pregnancy, surgical exploration and possible thyroidectomy may be indicated in the second trimester. Delaying surgical treatment until the postpartum period may be reasonable, especially in cases found later in pregnancy or in cases of a recurrent nodule with intermediate cytology results (Fig. 22-1).

Radionuclide scans can be particularly useful in nonpregnant patients with indeterminate cytologic results, but they are not indicated as an initial diagnostic tool. Moreover, radionuclide scanning is contraindicated during pregnancy. There is little information on the use of CT scans for differentiating between a benign and a malignant nodule. Wide local excision has no role in evaluation of a nodule that has not been first biopsied to assess for malignancy. Surgery, whether a lobectomy and isthmectomy or a total thyroidectomy and local excision of involved lymph nodes, is reserved for treatment of biopsy-proven malignant lesions.

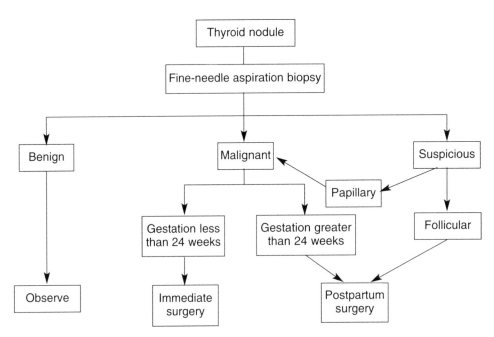

FIG. 22-1. Algorithm for approach to thyroid nodules in pregnant women. (Tan G, Gharib H, Goellner J, van Heerden J, Bahn R. Management of thyroid nodules in pregnancy. Arch Intern Med 1996;156:2317–20.)

Mazzaferri EL. Management of a solitary thyroid nodule. N Engl J Med 1993;328:553–9.

Nader S. Thyroid disease and pregnancy. In: Creasy RK, Resnik R, Iams JD, editors. Maternal–fetal medicine: principles and practice. 5th ed. Philadelphia (PA): WB Saunders; 2004. p. 1076.

Neale D, Burrow G. Thyroid disease in pregnancy. Obstet Gynecol Clin North Am 2004;31:893–905, xi.

Tan GH, Gharib H, Goellner JR, van Heerden JA, Bahn RS. Management of thyroid nodules in pregnancy. Arch Intern Med 1996; 156:2317–20.

Thyroid disease in pregnancy. ACOG Practice Bulletin No. 37. American College of Obstetricians and Gynecologists. Obstet Gynecol 2002;100:387–96.

23

Neural tube defects

A 27-year-old primigravid woman has a first-trimester screen at 11 weeks of gestation. Her risk for trisomy 21 is 1 in 3,000. The most appropriate screening for open neural tube defects is

    (A) no further testing needed
    (B) an amniocentesis for serum alpha-fetoprotein and acetylcholinesterase
    (C) a quadruple screen and a fetal anatomic survey
*   (D) a serum alpha-fetoprotein and a fetal anatomic survey
    (E) serum inhibin and a fetal anatomic survey

Neural tube defects (NTDs) occur in 1.4–2 in 1,000 pregnancies, making them the second most common congenital malformation. Screening for NTDs occurs in the second trimester. A serum screen and a fetal anatomic survey are the major components of the screening paradigm. However, with the advent of early aneuploidy screening in the first trimester, it is important to remember second-trimester NTD screening.

From 16 to 21 weeks of gestation, a maternal serum alpha-fetoprotein (MSAFP) greater than 2.5 multiples of the median (MoM) has a sensitivity of 85%. A fetal anatomic survey performed by experienced operators has a sensitivity of 97% and a specificity of 100% in detecting NTDs. When inexperienced operators perform ultrasonography, it has a high false-negative rate in the detection of NTDs. The ultrasonographic findings diagnostic for an NTD include abnormalities in the cranium and the spine. The classic cranial defect is an Arnold Chiari malformation II. The cerebellar vermis, fourth ventricle, and the medulla oblongata are herniated through the cisterna magna, and there is usually hydrocephalus. The "banana sign" (Fig. 23-1) is used to describe the posterior fossa ultrasonographic findings. The other cranial sign for NTDs is a concave contour of the fetal calvarium, known as the "lemon sign" (Fig. 23-2). A lemon sign is not as accurate as the banana sign, and around 1–2% of normal fetuses will display a concave contour of the fetal calvarium. The spinal ultrasonographic findings include disruption of the normal sagittal parallel lines representing the spine or splaying of the vertebra in transverse section. Figures 23-3 and 23-4 show spina bifida transverse and sagittal sections of the sacral spine, respectively.

If a patient has a normal result from a first-trimester aneuploidy screen, it is important to recommend an MSAFP test in the second trimester. Other components of a quadruple screen (inhibin, human chorionic gonadotropin [hCG], and estriol) are not screening tests for NTDs, either individually or collectively.

An amniocentesis for amniotic fluid AFP and acetylcholinesterase are the diagnostic tests for NTDs. Elevated amniotic fluid AFP in the presence of amniotic fluid acetylcholinesterase is used to diagnose almost 100% of open NTDs. The false-positive rate of an amniocentesis is

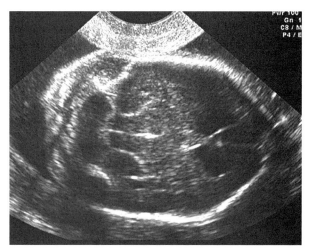

FIG. 23-1. *Banana sign*: posterior fossa with the cerebellar vermis, fourth ventricle, and the medulla oblongata herniated through the cisterna magna. (Courtesy of Ana Monteagudo, MD).

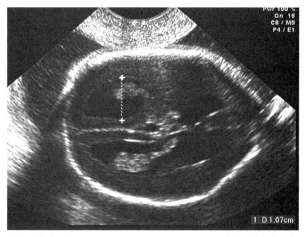

FIG. 23-2. *Lemon sign*: concave contour of the fetal calvarium. The image also shows mild ventriculomegaly. (Courtesy of Ana Monteagudo, MD).

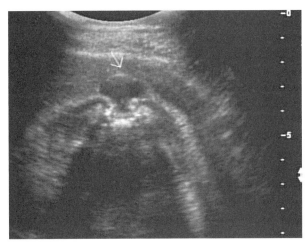

FIG. 23-3. Spina bifida, transverse section of sacral spine. (Courtesy of Ana Monteagudo, MD).

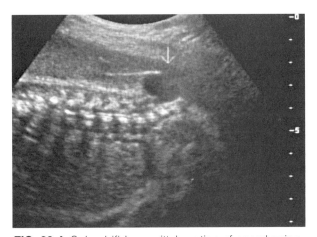

FIG. 23-4. Spina bifida, sagittal section of sacral spine. (Courtesy of Ana Monteagudo, MD).

2.2 per 1,000 procedures. A diagnostic test is indicated when one of the screening test results is positive. After a normal first-trimester screen result, an amniocentesis is not indicated unless there are abnormal ultrasonographic findings or an elevated MSAFP level.

Bradley LA, Palomaki GE, McDowell GA. Technical standards and guidelines: prenatal screening for open neural tube defects. ONTD Working Group; ACMG Laboratory Quality Assurance Committee. Genet Med 2005;7:355–69.

Driscoll DA. Second trimester maternal serum screening for fetal open neural tube defects and aneuploidy. Professional Practice and Guidelines Committee. Genet Med 2004;6:540–1.

Neural tube defects. ACOG Practice Bulletin No. 44. American College of Obstetricians and Gynecologists. Obstet Gynecol 2003;102:203–13.

Screening for fetal chromosomal abnormalities. ACOG Practice Bulletin No. 77. American College of Obstetricians and Gynecologists. Obstet Gynecol 2007;109:217–27.

24

Influenza vaccination

A 24-year-old primigravid woman at 9 weeks of gestation asks you whether she should receive the intramuscular influenza vaccination that is being offered at work. You advise her that she

    (A) should not take the vaccine

*   (B) may receive the vaccine now

    (C) should take the vaccine when she is in her second trimester

    (D) should take the nasal vaccine instead of the intramuscular vaccine

Influenza is characterized by sore throat, cough, fever, headache, myalgia, and weakness. The influenza viruses are members of the Orthomyxoviridae family. There are three types of influenza viruses: A, B, and C. Type A is more severe than B and is subdivided on the basis of surface hemagglutinin and neuraminidase antigens. Influenza C virus appears to be a minor cause of disease in humans. Complications of influenza include primary influenza pneumonia, secondary bacterial pneumonia, exacerbation of chronic obstructive pulmonary disease and asthma, rhabdomyolysis, myocarditis, and pericarditis. Reye's syndrome may be seen in children with influenza who are given aspirin therapy.

It is recognized that influenza is more severe in pregnancy. In both the 1918 and 1957 influenza epidemics, increased mortality occurred in pregnant women. Recent studies confirm increased hospitalization rates of pregnant women during influenza epidemics.

Vaccination of pregnant women aims to prevent influenza and its complications as well as to provide passive protection for the neonate. The American College of Obstetricians and Gynecologists (ACOG) supports the Centers for Disease Control and Prevention (CDC) recommendation that all women in the United States who will be pregnant during the influenza season (October to May) should be vaccinated. Ideally, the vaccine is given in October and November; however, it may be given throughout the influenza season as long as the supply of vaccine lasts. The intramuscular, inactivated vaccine is not teratogenic and may be used in all trimesters.

Before 2004, first-trimester vaccination had been limited to pregnant women with high-risk medical conditions (eg, diabetes mellitus, asthma) to avoid coincidental association with spontaneous abortion. In May 2004, the CDC Advisory Committee on Immunization Practice published simplified recommendations that advised vaccination in any trimester for healthy pregnant women and pregnant women with high-risk medical conditions. Breastfeeding is not a contraindication to vaccination.

The influenza vaccine is made up of inactivated viruses that are likely to circulate in the upcoming winter. The vaccine is 70–90% effective depending on the accuracy of predicting the viral antigens. A recent study found that only 44% of obstetrician–gynecologists provided influenza vaccinations during pregnancy. In contrast to the intramuscular vaccine, the intranasal vaccine is a live, attenuated influenza virus and is not recommended for use in pregnant women.

Couch RB. Prevention and treatment of influenza. N Engl J Med 2000; 343:1778–87.

Dolin R. Influenza. In: Kasper DL, Braunwald E, Fauci AS, Hauser SL, Longo DL, Jameson JH, eds. Harrison's principles of internal medicine. 16th ed. New York (NY): McGraw-Hill; 2005. p. 1066–71.

Influenza vaccination and treatment during pregnancy. ACOG Committee Opinion No. 305. American College of Obstetricians and Gynecologists. Obstet Gynecol 2004;104:1125–6.

Influenza vaccination in pregnancy: practices among obstetrician–gynecologists—United States, 2003–04 influenza season. Centers for Disease Control and Prevention (CDC). MMWR Morb Mortal Wkly Rep 2005;54:1050–2.

Schrag SJ, Fiore AE, Gonik B, Malik T, Reef S, Singleton JA, et al. Vaccination and perinatal infection prevention practices among obstetrician–gynecologists. Obstet Gynecol 2003;101:704–10.

25

Headaches

A 29-year-old woman, gravida 3, para 2, at 27 weeks of gestation presents to the emergency department with a 12-hour history of what she describes as "the worst headache of her life." Her blood pressure is 145/80 mm Hg; heart rate 100 beats per minute; and respirations are 16 breaths per minute. Other than mild photophobia, the physical examination is within normal limits and the uterine size is consistent with her dates. The fetal heart rate is 150 beats per minute. Urinalysis reveals 1+ proteinuria by dipstick. Urine drug screen result is negative. Complete blood count and tests of renal function and electrolytes are normal. Cranial computed tomography (CT) scan without contrast material is normal. Lumbar puncture reveals xanthochromic cerebrospinal fluid with elevated red blood cell count unchanged from tube 1 to tube 4. The most likely diagnosis is

   (A) severe preeclampsia
   (B) pseudotumor cerebri
   (C) transformed migraine
 * (D) cerebral aneurysm
   (E) sagittal sinus venous thrombosis

The obstetrician–gynecologist evaluates many patients with headaches. About one third of pregnant women have headaches, which are usually migraine, tension-type, sinus-related, or secondary to hypertension.

Subarachnoid hemorrhage complicates between 1 and 5 per 10,000 pregnancies and accounts for 5% of maternal deaths. In pregnancy, approximately 80% of subarachnoid hemorrhages are due to ruptured saccular aneurysms and the other 20% are primarily due to arteriovenous malformations. The initial hemorrhage may be fatal, may result in devastating sequelae, or may produce only transient, minor symptoms. The patient with the smallest bleed is the hardest to diagnose (normal physical examination and CT scan), yet is the one to benefit the most from early treatment (eg, endovascular coiling or surgical clipping of the aneurysm before rebleeding or symptomatic vasospasm occurs). In nonpregnant patients with subarachnoid hemorrhage, 25–50% receive the wrong initial diagnosis. Pitfalls in the diagnosis of subarachnoid hemorrhage fall into three patterns: failure to appreciate the spectrum of clinical presentation, failure to understand the limitations of computed tomography, and failure to perform or correctly interpret the results of lumbar puncture. Of patients with the "worst headache of their lives" and a normal neurologic examination, about 12% have subarachnoid hemorrhage.

A CT scan does not definitively rule out subarachnoid hemorrhage. If there is a high index of suspicion, a lumbar puncture should be performed. Up to 20% of lumbar punctures are "traumatic taps" and must be distinguished from true hemorrhage. Therefore, it is important to perform a red cell count on tubes 1 and 4 and to look for xanthochromia (yellow supernatant owing to red cell breakdown) both visually and by means of spectrophotometry.

Reasons for a false-negative CT scan with subarachnoid hemorrhage include lower sensitivity with increasing time between onset of headache and scanning, small volume bleeding, variations in expertise of physician reading the scan, thickness of slices taken, motion artifact, and subarachnoid blood hematocrit of less than 30%. Figure 25-1 shows a diagnostic algorithm for the condition.

Differentiating subarachnoid hemorrhage from preeclampsia may be difficult. Hypertension and proteinuria may be seen in one third of patients with subarachnoid hemorrhage; however, subarachnoid blood should not be found with preeclampsia. Pseudotumor cerebri is associated with elevated opening pressure on lumbar puncture, normal cerebrospinal fluid analysis, and normal CT scan. This patient has no history of previous migraine or use of headache medications to suggest transformed migraine. Sagittal sinus venous thrombosis usually is seen in the puerperium and may be associated with preeclampsia, sepsis, or thrombophilia. The CT scan may be normal with the diagnosis being made by magnetic resonance imaging (MRI), magnetic resonance venography, or cerebral angiography. Subarachnoid blood is not usually found with cerebral venous sinus thrombosis.

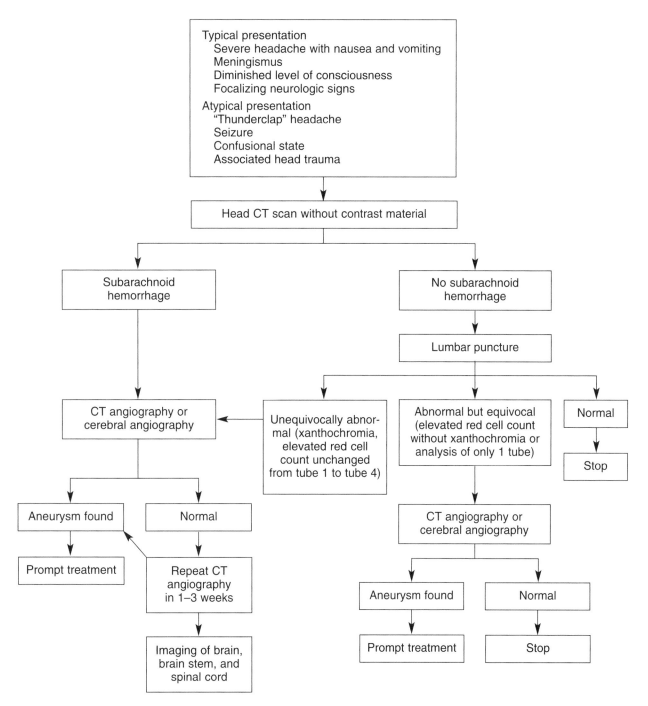

FIG. 25-1. Diagnostic algorithm for subarachnoid hemorrhage. CT, computed tomography. (Suarez JI, Tarr RW, Selman SR. Aneurysmal subarachnoid hemorrhage [review]. N Engl J Med 2006;354:389. Copyright © 2006 Massachusetts Medical Society. All rights reserved.)

Berg CJ, Chang J, Callaghan WM, Whitehead SJ. Pregnancy-related mortality in the United States, 1991–1997. Obstet Gynecol 2003;101: 289–96.

Dias MS, Sekhar LN. Intracranial hemorrhage from aneurysms and arteriovenous malformations during pregnancy and the puerperium. Neurosurgery 1990;27:855–65; discussion 865–6.

Edlow JA, Caplan LR. Avoiding pitfalls in the diagnosis of subarachnoid hemorrhage. N Engl J Med 2000;342:29–36.

Martin SR, Foley MR. Approach to the pregnant patient with headache. Clin Obstet Gynecol 2005;48:2–11.

Suarez JI, Tarr RW, Selman WR. Aneurysmal subarachnoid hemorrhage [review]. N Engl J Med 2006;354:387–96.

26

Postpartum depression

You have decided to institute postpartum depression screening in your clinic, which serves a population predominantly African American and Hispanic, and has a significant portion of patients who do not speak English. Your major concern with the accuracy of such testing in your patients is

* (A) lack of trials in non-Caucasian patients
  (B) low specificity
  (C) that it is less predictable than nonpregnant screening
  (D) that it is a better predictor of minor depression than major depression

Postpartum depression has received significant media attention in the past few years, in part in response to high-profile stories in the news. Suggested approaches to this disorder begin with screening; many cases are unidentified and thus not referred for treatment. A number of tools exist for the purpose of screening. All consist of patient self-administered questionnaires, which are then scored. A number of studies have looked at the usefulness of these screening tools in terms of diagnostic accuracy.

An ideal screening tool is both sensitive and specific when compared with diagnostic tests. Sensitivity is the proportion of patients with the condition who test positive using the screening tool. Specificity is the proportion of patients without the condition with negative test results using the screening tool. The screen, therefore, has to be compared with a criterion standard, which is the diagnostic test. Diagnostic testing for depression is performed either with clinical assessment to see if the patient meets *Diagnostic and Statistical Manual of Mental Disorders*, 4th edition (DSM-IV), or other diagnostic criteria, or with structured interviews, such as the Goldberg Standardized Psychiatric Interview (SPI). To adequately assess a screening tool for postpartum depression, a population should be screened and then all patients assessed with a diagnostic test. The results are then compared. In an ideal test that is 100% sensitive, all patients who have depression will screen positive. In addition, all patients who have a negative diagnostic test result for depression would screen negative, making the test 100% specific. In more realistic, less ideal circumstances, for most screening tests, it is preferable that some patients who have a negative diagnosis should screen positive than to have a substantial number of affected patients screen negative. Therefore, sensitivity is often more important than specificity.

Several screening tools exist such as the Edinburgh Postnatal Depression Scale, the Beck Depression Inventory, the Pitt scale, and the General Health Questionnaire (GHQ). Some screening tools have been modified from tools used in nonpregnant populations; others were developed for pregnancy but have also been used in nonpregnant populations. In general, it is not more difficult to screen in pregnancy and postpartum than in nonpregnant populations. The accuracy of screening, that is, the sensitivity and specificity, is similar to depression screening in nonpregnant populations.

Although there are many studies that use these screening tools to identify and characterize populations of depressed women, far fewer studies have carefully validated these scales in a variety of populations. In many studies, the ethnic and socioeconomic characteristics of the population have not been reported. Most studies of screening accuracy are in Caucasian populations or are unspecified in the study. The two largest U.S. studies involving perinatal patients were in predominantly or completely Caucasian groups. If depression screening tools are affected by cultural or socioeconomic differences, this is likely to be a factor in the accuracy in other unstudied populations. Therefore, your major concern with the accuracy of depression screening in the patient population described would be the lack of trials in non-Caucasian patients.

Although these tools were developed to screen for major depression, they have been tested for accuracy in both major and minor depression. As expected, they work better with more severe disease, that is, major depression, and less well with minor depression.

Most of these tests have high specificity, but are not as sensitive. Therefore, most patients who screen positive have depression, but all tests miss some patients with depression. The magnitude of this depends on the prevalence of depression in the population being studied.

Gavin NI, Gaynes BN, Lohr KN, Meltzer-Brody S, Gartlehner G, Swinson T. Perinatal depression: a systematic review of prevalence and incidence. Obstet Gynecol 2005;106:1071–83.

Gaynes BN, Gavin N, Meltzer-Brody S, Lohr KN, Swinson T, Gartlehner G, et al. Perinatal depression: prevalence, screening accuracy, and screening outcomes. Evidence Report/Technology Assessment No. 119. (Prepared by the RTI–University of North Carolina Evidence-based Practice Center, under Contract No. 290-02-0016.) AHRQ Publication No. 05-E006-2. Rockville (MD): Agency for Healthcare Research and Quality; 2005.

Leverton TJ, Elliott SA. Is the EPDS a magic wand? 1. A comparison of the Edinburgh Postnatal Depression Scale and health visitor report as predictors of diagnosis on the Present State Examination. J Reprod Infant Psychol 2000;18:279–96.

27

Complications of gastric bypass in the obese parturient

A 24-year-old primigravid woman had a successful Roux-en-Y gastric bypass surgery approximately 2 years ago. Her body mass index (weight in kilograms divided by height in meters squared [kg/m^2]) is now 24. She comes to your office for prenatal counseling about the potential pregnancy complications associated with gastric bypass surgery. You advise her that the most likely pregnancy complication associated with her gastric bypass surgery is

    (A) gestational diabetes mellitus
    (B) gestational hypertension
    (C) macrosomia
    (D) cesarean delivery
*   (E) vitamin deficiency

Obesity is a significant risk factor for increased maternal mortality and morbidity. In patients with morbid obesity, gastric bypass surgery may be indicated. Gastric bypass surgery uses either a malabsorption operation or a restrictive operation. An illustrated guide to weight-loss procedures using gastric bypass surgery is shown (Fig. 27-1 A–C; see color plates).

The malabsorption operation restricts both food intake and the amount of calories and nutrients the body absorbs. In this procedure, the stomach wall is stapled at the fundus and a 40-cm Roux-en-Y loop of jejunum is anastomosed to the remaining gastric pouch near the gastroesophageal junction. The stomach contents then drain directly into the distal jejunum, bypassing the distal stomach, duodenum, and proximal jejunum. This procedure is associated with electrolyte abnormalities and deficiencies in iron, vitamin B_{12}, and fat-soluble vitamins.

The restrictive operations include the vertical-banded gastroplasty and adjustable gastroplasty. The adjustable gastric banding produces early satiety and decreased food intake. Subsequent nonoperative adjustments of the gastric band alters the lumen size and quantity of food consumed. This procedure is preferred in reproductive-aged women because of concern about significant weight loss, nausea, and vomiting or intrauterine growth restriction. In the vertical-banded gastroplasty, stapling is used to create a small gastric pouch (15–20 mL) that empties into the residual stomach through a narrow channel in the lesser curvature of the stomach. A prosthetic band maintains the circumference, and preservation of gastroduodenal continuity limits micronutrient deficiencies.

Gastric bypass surgery to reduce the woman's weight appears to decrease the incidence of obesity related comorbidities. Review of current literature shows that, compared to their obese counterparts, women with gastric bypass surgery have less gestational hypertension, gestational diabetes mellitus, macrosomia, and the need for cesarean delivery. Vitamin deficiencies due to malabsorp-

tion, especially severe iron and cobalamin deficiencies, have been reported and thus the patient will require close monitoring and treatment. Box 27-1 shows clinical considerations for care following gastric bypass surgery. Box 27-2 lists recommendations for prenatal care of the obese pregnant woman.

BOX 27-1

Clinical Considerations for Care After Gastric Bypass Surgery

- Provide preoperative and preconception counseling regarding surgical complications, including vitamin and metabolic disturbances with possible effects on the growing fetus.
- Determine need for vitamin supplementation.
- Determine appropriate timing after surgery to conceive, preferably after the initial period of rapid weight loss, approximately 12–18 months.
- Screen for vitamin deficiencies and electrolyte abnormalities, specifically vitamin B_{12}, folate, and iron.
- Obtain a nutrition consultation with recommendations for vitamin supplements.
- Closely monitor weight gain or loss.
- Monitor for appropriate fetal growth.
- Do not perform first-degree Glucola (Ames Diagnostic) because of poor absorption and development of dumping syndrome.
- Consider the following regimen for screening for gestational diabetes mellitus: Fasting and 1-hour postprandial blood sugars at 22–24, 28, 32, and 35 weeks of gestation
- Continue vitamin supplements in puerperium, especially breastfeeding.

Hall LF, Neubert AG. Obesity and pregnancy. Obstet Gynecol Surv 2005;60:253–60.

BOX 27-2

Recommendations for Prenatal Care of the Obese Patient

Preconception

- Prescribe prenatal vitamins and folic acid 1 mg every day.
- Obtain a thorough medical history and screen for existing conditions such as diabetes mellitus and hypertension.
- Encourage weight loss.
- Consult on nutrition needs.

First trimester

- Perform 1-hour 50-g glucose screen, and repeat at 28 weeks if normal.
- Screen for medical conditions (ie, chronic hypertension, diabetes mellitus) and treat appropriately, if not done so preconceptionally.
- Perform early ultrasound examination to confirm estimated delivery dates.
- Discuss optimal weight gain.
- Administer folic acid 2 mg every day.

Second and third trimesters

- Screen serum to determine risk for neural tube defect and chromosomal abnormalities.
- Perform second-trimester anatomy evaluation (transumbilical ultrasonography may improve visualization).
- Schedule more frequent prenatal visits to detect conditions such as preeclampsia.
- Consider antenatal testing as a result of increased risk of stillbirth.

Delivery and postpartum

- Consult on anesthesia needs in early labor.
- Consider increased incidence of shoulder dystocia.
- Review incision options if operative delivery is planned.
- Consider the use of subcutaneous drain or closure.
- Anticipate increased blood loss.
- Take antithrombotic precautions.

Hall LF, Neubert AG. Obesity and pregnancy. Obstet Gynecol Surv 2005;60:253–60.

Gurewitsch ED, Smith-Levitin M, Mack J. Pregnancy following gastric bypass surgery for morbid obesity. Obstet Gynecol 1996;88:658–61.

Hall LF, Neubert AG. Obesity and pregnancy. Obstet Gynecol Surv 2005;60:253–60.

Saravanakumar K, Rao SG, Cooper GM. Obesity and obstetric anesthesia. Anesthesia 2006;61:36–48.

Wittgrove AC, Jester L, Wittgrove P, Clark GW. Pregnancy following gastric bypass for morbid obesity. Obes Surg 1998;8:461–4; discussion 465–6.

28

Anemia

A 22-year-old woman, gravida 3, para 1, at 33 weeks of gestation, has a hemoglobin level of 9.7 g/dL, with a mean corpuscular volume (MCV) of 77.2 fL and a ferritin level of 13 mcg/L. She states that she has been taking daily prenatal vitamins as prescribed. You advise her that in addition to her prenatal vitamins she should take

* (A) oral elemental iron
  (B) subcutaneous erythropoietin
  (C) intravenous iron dextran
  (D) oral folic acid
  (E) vitamin B$_{12}$

During the second and third trimesters of pregnancy, the expansion of blood volume by approximately 35% and the growth of the fetus, placenta, and other maternal tissues increase the demand for iron threefold, to approximately 5.0 mg per day. Although iron absorption increases during pregnancy and menstruation ceases, most pregnant women who do not take iron supplements to meet increased iron requirements during pregnancy cannot maintain adequate iron stores, particularly during the second and third trimesters. Iron-deficiency anemia during the first two trimesters of pregnancy is associated with an increased risk for preterm delivery and for delivery of a low birth weight infant. Evidence from randomized control trials indicates that iron supplementation decreases the incidence of iron-deficiency anemia during pregnancy. The Centers for Disease Control and Prevention emphasizes the need for sound iron nutrition screening for anemia among women of childbearing age, as well as the importance of low-dose iron supplementation for pregnant women.

Low-dose supplementation regimens that meet pregnancy requirements and reduce unwanted side effects are as effective as higher dose regimens in preventing iron-deficiency anemia. Most prenatal vitamins contain at least the required 30-mg suggested dose of elemental iron supplementation. Secondary prevention of iron deficiency in pregnancy involves screening for, diagnosing, and treating iron-deficiency anemia. Recommendations include treatment of anemia with 60–120 mg of oral elemental iron per day. When the hemoglobin concentration or hematocrit becomes normal for the stage of gestation, the dose of iron can be decreased. It is important to recognize that only a small fraction of oral elemental iron is absorbed and bioavailable.

Subcutaneous erythropoietin with or without oral iron therapy or intravenous iron sucrose has been used successfully to treat severe iron-deficiency anemia in pregnancy with no significant risks to the mother. This option is limited by cost and is rarely indicated. It should be reserved for patients with a malabsorption syndrome or those who are significantly anemic (hemoglobin less than 8.5 g/dL) and absolutely will not take oral iron.

Parenteral administration of iron dextran can also be used to treat iron-deficiency in pregnancy. However, the potential for systemic adverse effects limits its use, and it should be reserved for the small number of patients in whom oral treatment fails or for whom iron loss exceeds intake that can be met by oral therapy. Because unpredictable anaphylactic reactions can occur with intravenous administration of iron dextran, when indicated, a test dose is required before the first administration.

Folate and vitamin B$_{12}$ deficiencies also can produce anemia in pregnancy. However, these anemias are typically macrocytic in nature as opposed to the microcytic anemia seen with iron deficiency. Folic acid is a water-soluble vitamin, available through diet, but folate supplementation is necessary in the first trimester. Such supplementation is recommended to reduce the occurrence of neural tube defects in all women considering pregnancy. The most common causes of vitamin B$_{12}$ deficiency are pernicious anemia and malabsorption after gastric bypass surgeries. Neither folic acid nor vitamin B$_{12}$ supplementation is recommended in the treatment of iron-deficiency anemia.

Al RA, Unlubilgin E, Kandemir O, Yalvac S, Cakir L, Haberal A. Intravenous versus oral iron for treatment of anemia in pregnancy: a randomized trial. Obstet Gynecol 2005;106:1335–40.

Kilpatrick SJ, Laros RK. Maternal hematologic disorders. In: Creasy RK, Resnik R, Iams JD, editors. Maternal–fetal medicine: principles and practice. 5th ed. Philadelphia (PA): WB Saunders Co.; 2004. p. 977–84.

Recommendations to prevent and control iron deficiency in the United States. Centers for Disease Control and Prevention. MMWR Recomm Rep 1998;47(RR-3):1–29.

Tefferi A. Anemia in adults: a contemporary approach to diagnosis. Mayo Clin Proc 2003;78:1274–80.

29

Steroid use in pregnancy

A 29-year-old woman with systemic lupus erythematosus (SLE) received low-dose prednisone for 1 week at 18 weeks of gestation for a lupus flare. She had no other steroid therapy during pregnancy except this single episode. She presents at 37 weeks of gestation with ruptured membranes and occasional contractions. She has normal vital signs. The best approach to management regarding her previous steroid intake is to prescribe

      (A) oral steroids
      (B) single-dose intravenous steroids
*   (C) no steroids
      (D) multiple-dose intravenous steroids for 24 hours

Steroid use is not uncommon during pregnancy. It occurs more often in women with either SLE or asthma. The potential dangers of chronic steroid use for perioperative patients were first described in 1952. A single case report described a steroid-dependent patient who died of intractable hypotension after undergoing major orthopedic surgery. Based on this association, "stress-dose" steroids have been advocated by some at the time of labor and delivery for women on chronic steroids. The aim is to avoid this "addisonian crisis," ie, a perioperative adrenal insufficiency characterized by hypotension.

The true incidence of perioperative adrenal insufficiency in patients treated with steroids is unknown, but probably averages around 1–2% even in patients on high doses of steroids for long periods. Reviews of the literature have shown that only three cases of perioperative hypotension attributed to adrenal insufficiency secondary to chronic steroid use have sufficient clinical and biochemical data to support this diagnosis. Only two randomized trials in nonpregnant patients address the use of perioperative stress steroids; no randomized trials in pregnant women have addressed the use of such steroids. The two studies on nonpregnant patients included only 38 patients and failed to show any difference in outcomes between patients who received perioperative stress-dose steroids versus those who did not. The investigators concluded that there is no evidence that supraphysiologic doses of corticosteroids are necessary to prevent hypotension secondary to adrenal insufficiency in the perioperative period.

Additional evidence from nonpregnant patients comes from a randomized trial of patients with congenital adrenal hyperplasia (CAH). The authors found that patients with classic CAH do not benefit from additional hydrocortisone during short-term, high-intensity exercise.

Patients considered not to have suppression of their hypothalamic–pituitary–adrenal (HPA) axis are those who had:

- Any dose of corticosteroid for less than 3 weeks
- Dosages of less than 5 mg per day of prednisone or its equivalent
- Alternate-day corticosteroid therapy

In contrast, patients who should be assumed to have suppression of HPA function are those who have:

- Received more than 20 mg per day of prednisone or its equivalent for more than 3 weeks. Equivalent doses are 16 mg per day of methylprednisolone, 2 mg per day of dexamethasone, or 80 mg per day of hydrocortisone.

Several recent reviews in the surgical literature have concluded that in patients who are receiving long-term corticosteroids, the combination of the patient's baseline exogenous steroid plus endogenous steroid production is able to meet the demands of the stress of surgery. Biochemical testing of the hypothalamic–adrenal axis is not recommended. If a patient is on chronic steroids at the time of labor or delivery, continuing the usual daily dose is suggested, without need for "stress" steroids.

The patient described was on steroids for only 1 week remote (more than 1 month) before presenting for delivery. Biochemical recovery from adrenal suppression from steroid intake has been reported to occur within 5 days in patients who use low-dose prednisone (less than 30 mg) for 1 week or less. The risk of adrenal suppression usually occurs only with long-term steroid use (ie, 3 weeks or more).

Therefore, the use of stress steroids in this patient at 37 weeks with only 1 week of use in the second trimester is unnecessary. Intravenous or oral corticosteroids are associated with complications (Box 29-1), and should not be

---

BOX 29-1

Major Side Effects Associated With Corticosteroid Therapy

Dermatologic and soft tissue
Skin thinning and purpura
Cushingoid appearance
Alopecia
Acne
Hirsutism
Striae
Hypertrichosis

Eye
Posterior subcapsular cataract
Elevated intraocular pressure or glaucoma
Exophthalmos

Cardiovascular
Hypertension
Perturbations of serum lipoproteins
Premature atherosclerotic disease
Arrhythmias with pulse infusions

Gastrointestinal
Gastritis
Peptic ulcer disease
Pancreatitis
Steatohepatitis
Visceral perforation

Renal
Hypokalemia
Fluid volume shifts

Genitourinary and reproductive
Amenorrhea and infertility
Intrauterine growth restriction

Bone
Osteoporosis
Avascular necrosis

Muscle
Myopathy

Neuropsychiatric
Euphoria
Dysphoria or depression
    Insomnia or akathisia
    Psychosis
    Pseudo tumor cerebri

Endocrine
Diabetes mellitus
Hypothalamic–pituitary–adrenal insufficiency

Infectious disease
Heightened risk of typical infections
Herpes zoster
Opportunistic infections

Modified from Saag KG, Furst DE. Major side effects of systemic glucocorticoids. In: Rose BD, editor. UpToDate. Wellesley (MA): UpToDate; 2007.

---

recommended in this scenario. Steroid tapering is unnecessary because the steroid use was more than 1 month before delivery.

The obstetrician, anesthesiologist, and nurse who care for a woman who was on chronic steroids in pregnancy must be aware of the necessity to closely monitor vital signs, in particular blood pressure, during labor and delivery. The use of stress-dose steroids may be necessary in cases with volume refractory hypotension. In these rare cases, or in cases in which blood pressure monitoring peripartum is less than ideal, intravenous hydrocortisone can be given every 8 hours for one to three doses peripartum.

Brown CJ, Buie WD. Perioperative stress dose steroids: do they make a difference? J Am Coll Surg 2001;193:678–86.

Glowniak JV, Loriaux DL. A double-blind study of perioperative steroid requirements in secondary adrenal insufficiency. Surgery 1997;121:123–9.

Saag KG, Furst DE. Major side effects of systemic glucocorticoids. In: Rose BD, editor. UpToDate. Wellesley (MA): UpToDate; 2007.

Thomason JM, Girdler NM, Kendall-Taylor P, Wastell H, Weddel A, Seymour RA. An investigation into the need for supplementary steroids in organ transplant patients undergoing gingival surgery. A double-blind, split-month, cross-over study. J Clin Periodontal 1999;26:577–82.

Weise M, Drinkard B, Mehlinger SL, Holzer SM, Eisenhofer G, Charmandari E, et al. Stress dose of hydrocortisone is not beneficial in patients with classic congenital adrenal hyperplasia undergoing short-term, high-intensity exercise. J Clin Endocrinol Metab 2004;89:3679–84.

30

Bacterial vaginosis

A 25-year-old woman, gravida 1, para 0, is seen at 14 weeks of gestation for her second prenatal visit. Cytologic screening reveals normal cytology, with an incidental finding of bacterial vaginosis. She is asymptomatic. The most appropriate next step in care related to bacterial vaginosis is to

    (A) initiate metronidazole therapy
    (B) perform confirmatory wet mount
    (C) initiate clindamycin therapy
*   (D) counsel about the increased risk of preterm birth
    (E) perform transvaginal ultrasonography at 16 weeks of gestation

Bacterial vaginosis is a massive overgrowth of organisms such as anaerobes, *Gardnerella*, and *Mycoplasma* in the vagina. Most of these organisms are normally present in the vagina, but their concentrations are increased in bacterial vaginosis, and levels of predominant normal flora such as lactobacilli are decreased.

The diagnosis of bacterial vaginosis usually is made clinically based on the presence of at least three out of four Amsel's criteria (ie, particularly pH greater than 4.5, wet mount showing clue cells, thin homogenous discharge, and a positive amine test), or on the basis of Nugent criteria (7 or greater on Gram stain). No special expertise is required for this clinical diagnosis, so the test does not usually need to be repeated. Cytologic screening by means of a Pap test can detect bacterial vaginosis by Gram stain. Diagnosis by Amsel's criteria is well correlated with the Gram stain results and, therefore, a wet mount to confirm Gram stain results is not clinically indicated.

With the use of either set of criteria, the diagnosis of asymptomatic bacterial vaginosis has been associated with a 1.3- to 2-fold increase in the risk of spontaneous preterm birth. Therefore, counseling about the increased risk for preterm birth is justified. Counseling should include the fact that screening for asymptomatic bacterial vaginosis is not very accurate in predicting preterm birth, with positive predictive values that range from 6% to 49% depending on the prevalence of preterm birth in the specific patient population. In nonselected women, as the one described, the positive predictive value for preterm birth is usually less than 30%, and more than 70–80% of women who have asymptomatic bacterial vaginosis give birth at term without therapy.

Antibiotic treatment for bacterial vaginosis in asymptomatic pregnant women is not effective in reducing the incidence of preterm birth, or of preterm premature rupture of membranes (preterm PROM). In women with a previous preterm birth, treatment does not seem to affect the risk of recurrent preterm birth. In two recent meta-analyses, a 17–25% nonsignificant trend toward benefit was observed. Antibiotic treatment may decrease the risk of preterm PROM and low birth weight in these high-risk women, but limited long-term follow-up data are available. In the meta-analyses, subgroup analysis has shown that treatment with metronidazole or clindamycin does not alter the incidence of preterm birth before 37 weeks of gestation, even though individual studies demonstrate conflicting results.

Measurement of cervical length by transvaginal ultrasonography is a screening test used to predict preterm birth. Although asymptomatic bacterial vaginosis is associated with a modest risk of spontaneous preterm birth, transvaginal ultrasonography of the cervix has not been sufficiently studied in a population of women with bacterial vaginosis. The presence of both a short cervical length and bacterial vaginosis increases the risk of preterm birth beyond the risk attributable to each factor, but there is no evidence that an intervention may modify this risk of preterm birth. No intervention has been studied in this particular clinical situation.

Leitich H, Bodner-Adler B, Brunbauer M, Kaider A, Egarter C, Husslein P. Bacterial vaginosis as a risk factor for preterm delivery: a meta-analysis. Am J Obstet Gynecol 2003;189:139–47.

McDonald HM, Brocklehurst P, Gordon A. Antibiotics for treating bacterial vaginosis in pregnancy. Art. No.: CD000262. DOI: 10.1002/14651858.CD000262.pub3.

Nugent RP, Krohn MA, Hillier SL. Reliability of diagnosing bacterial vaginosis is improved by a standardized method of gram stain interpretation. J Clin Microbiol 1991;29:297–301.

Okun N, Gronau KA, Hannah ME. Antibiotics for bacterial vaginosis or Trichomonas vaginalis in pregnancy: a systematic review. Obstet Gynecol 2005;105:857–68.

Surbek DV, Hoesli IM, Holzgreve W. Morphology assessed by transvaginal ultrasonography differs in patients in preterm labor with vs. without bacterial vaginosis. Ultrasound Obstet Gynecol 2000;15:242–5.

31

Epidemiology of cytomegalovirus

A 25-year-old primigravid woman at 19 weeks of gestation has a fetal anatomic survey significant for echogenic bowel without other malformations. A cystic fibrosis carrier screening test result was negative. On her quadruple screen, her risk for Down syndrome was 1 in 6,350 and her risk for trisomy 18 was less than 1 in 10,000. Her cytomegalovirus (CMV) titers are positive for both immunoglobulin G (IgG) and immunoglobulin M (IgM). The next laboratory evaluation should be

      (A) amniocentesis for CMV polymerase chain reaction (PCR)
      (B) repeat testing of CMV titers in 1 month
  * (C) CMV IgG avidity testing
      (D) cordocentesis for CMV IgM
      (E) maternal CMV urine culture

Cytomegalovirus infection is the most common intrauterine viral infection, affecting 1% of all live births in the United States. It is a DNA virus and a member of the herpesvirus family. Congenital CMV infection causes sensorineural hearing loss, mental retardation, motor deficits, seizures, and chorioretinitis. A pregnant woman who develops a primary CMV infection has an overall 40% risk of vertical transmission to the fetus. Of these neonates, 10–15% will be symptomatic at birth, 20% will die, and 90% of the survivors will develop severe sequelae. Approximately 85–90% of infected neonates are asymptomatic at birth and of these, 5–15% will develop sequelae.

A pregnant woman with a recurrent infection has a reduced risk for an affected infant. Although some case reports exist of pregnant women who have recurrent CMV infection and who have severely affected symptomatic neonates at birth, most women with recurrent infection have a small risk for having an infected neonate. Most of these infants will be asymptomatic; however, if they develop long-term sequelae, they are more likely to develop sensorineural hearing loss (Fig. 31-1).

Mean rates of vertical transmission increase with gestational age at infection. Mean vertical transmission rates by gestational age at infection are 36% in the first trimester, 44% in the second trimester, and 77.6% in the third trimester. Earlier fetal infection can lead to a more severe congenital CMV infection.

Because of the differential in vertical transmission and the severity of affected neonates, a primary CMV infection must be differentiated from a recurrent CMV infection. Maternal serologies can be confusing and not diagnostic. A pregnant woman with a primary or recurrent infection may produce IgM antibodies. The peak production of CMV IgM is in the first 1–3 months of a primary infection. Convalescent titers are present for the next 6–9 months. Some individuals will have persis-

tent IgM titers for more than a year. A small percentage of women with a recurrent infection will produce IgM antibodies. Testing for IgG avidity provides additional data to distinguish between primary and recurrent CMV infections. Avidity is the strength with which an IgG antibody attaches to its antigen; IgG avidity matures with the length of time the antibody has been exposed to the antigen. The IgG produced within the first 3–5 months following a primary infection exhibits low avidity whereas IgG produced several months or years later exhibit high avidity. As a result, CMV avidity testing helps differentiate primary from recurrent infection and will allow improved patient counseling. Repeat CMV titers in 1 month do not help differentiate primary CMV infection from recurrent CMV infection in the patient described, because she has both IgG and IgM antibodies.

Amniocentesis for CMV PCR is a very useful diagnostic test to determine fetal infection. The accuracy of the test varies with the gestational age at which it is performed. When amniocentesis is performed before 21 weeks of gestation, the sensitivity is approximately 65%; when it is performed after 21 weeks of gestation, the sensitivity is greater than 95%. In the clinical scenario, the patient is at 19 weeks of gestation with IgG and IgM antibodies. At this stage of pregnancy, an amniocentesis is not as sensitive a test as it would be later in gestation. It would be preferable to obtain an IgG avidity index, determine if she has a primary or recurrent infection, counsel the patient regarding the neonatal outcomes depending on the type of maternal infection, and then offer the patient an amniocentesis to determine fetal infection. After waiting for the avidity index, the patient will be at greater than 21 weeks of gestation and, at that time, the sensitivity of an amniocentesis will improve.

Cordocentesis for CMV IgM antibodies in fetal blood is another diagnostic test to identify fetal infection. Cordocentesis after 20 weeks of gestation has sensitivity

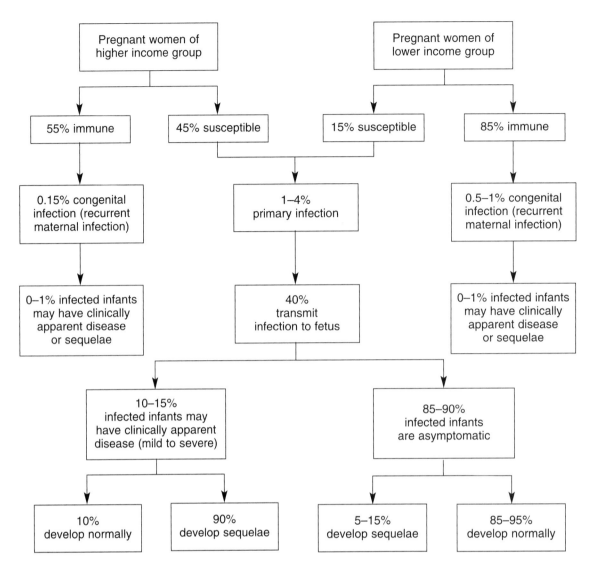

FIG. 31-1. Progression of human cytomegalovirus infection in pregnancy. (Stagno S, Whitley RJ. Herpesvirus infection of pregnancy. Part I: Cytomegalovirus and Epstein-Barr virus infections. N Engl J Med 1985;313:1270–4. Copyright © 1985 Massachusetts Medical Society. All rights reserved.)

of 50–60%. When compared with amniocentesis with the new nested PCR technique, cordocentesis is not as accurate a test. In addition, cordocentesis has a higher procedure-related pregnancy loss rate. As a result, an amniocentesis is a superior test to diagnose fetal infection.

A maternal CMV urine culture does not differentiate between a primary infection and a recurrent infection. Women with recurrent infections can shed virus in their blood, saliva, and urine. Thus, a maternal CMV urine culture would not be useful. Although research is ongoing, there is no currently accepted treatment for intrauterine CMV infection.

Bodeus M, Hubinont C, Goubau P. Increased risk of cytomegalovirus transmission in utero during late gestation. Obstet Gynecol 1999;93:658–60.

Fowler KB, Stagno S, Pass RF. Maternal immunity and prevention of congenital cytomegalovirus infection. JAMA 2003;289:1008–11.

Lazzarotto T, Gabrielli L, Lanari M, Guerra B, Bellucci T, Sassi M, et al. Congenital cytomegalovirus infection: recent advances in the diagnosis of maternal infection. Hum Immunol 2004;65:410–5.

Liesnard C, Donner C, Brancart F, Gosselin F, Delforge ML, Rodesch F. Prenatal diagnosis of congenital cytomegalovirus infection: prospective study of 237 pregnancies at risk. Obstet Gynecol 2000;95:881–8.

Revello MG, Gerna G. Diagnosis and management of human cytomegalovirus infection in the mother, fetus, and newborn infant. Clin Microbiol Rev 2002;15:680–715.

32

Peripartum cardiomyopathy

A 33-year-old woman, gravida 3, para 2, at 38 weeks of gestation, comes to the labor and delivery department because of shortness of breath. Her respiratory rate is 30 breaths per minute. Her blood pressure is 130/80 mm Hg, heart rate is 110 beats per minute, and oxygen saturation is 85%. Her arterial blood gas (ABG) on room air is pH 7.35, P_{CO_2} 25 mm Hg, P_{O_2} 55 mm Hg, and H_{CO_3} –20 mmol/L. She is immediately started on oxygen therapy. In other findings, a chest X-ray shows bilateral pulmonary edema with cardiomegaly confirmed by spiral computed tomography (CT); an electrocardiogram (ECG) shows sinus tachycardia; and an echocardiogram shows an ejection fraction of 25%. In addition to a diuretic and a positive inotropic agent, the best therapy is

       (A) verapamil hydrochloride
       (B) captopril (Capoten, Capozide)
  *   (C) hydralazine hydrochloride
       (D) enoxaparin sodium (Lovenox)

Peripartum cardiomyopathy is a pregnancy-associated cardiomyopathy. In the United States, the incidence is approximately 1 in 3,000 to 1 in 15,000 pregnancies. This condition is diagnosed by the following four criteria:

1. Development of cardiac failure in the last month of pregnancy or within 5 months after delivery
2. Absence of a demonstrable cause for the cardiac failure
3. Absence of a demonstrable heart disease before the last month of pregnancy
4. Documented echocardiographic left ventricular systolic dysfunction

This definition excludes preexisting cardiac conditions that may worsen as pregnancy evolves (Box 32-1).

The evaluation of a pregnancy in a patient who is tachycardic, tachypneic, and hypoxic includes chest X-ray, ECG, ABG, spiral CT, and echocardiography. These studies help differentiate between peripartum cardiomyopathy, a pulmonary embolus, pulmonary edema from diastolic dysfunction, and noncardiogenic pulmonary edema. The patient's history and presentation will dictate the order in which the studies should be carried out. For example, a patient who becomes acutely short of breath after a cross-country trip is more likely to have a pulmonary embolus, and a spiral CT should be done first. However, a patient who develops more insidious symptoms of worsening dyspnea over a few weeks is more likely to have cardiac dysfunction, and, in these circumstances, echocardiography should be obtained first.

The treatment for peripartum cardiomyopathy includes diuretics and vasodilators. Digoxin is an inotropic agent used to improve cardiac output. Its use has become controversial. Carvedilol, a β-adrenergic blocker with an α–blocking activity, decreases mortality and improves left ventricular function in patients with heart failure. There has been no direct comparison of carvedilol and digoxin in patients with peripartum cardiomyopathy. As a result, some cardiologists would still recommend digoxin as part of the primary therapy for peripartum cardiomyopathy, although other cardiologists may recommend carvedilol as part of the primary regimen. In a pregnant patient, vasodilation is achieved with hydralazine hydrochloride and nitrates. Angiotensin-converting enzyme (ACE) inhibitors such as captopril are contraindicated in pregnancy because of their adverse effects on the fetal kidneys. A recent study also linked first-trimester ACE inhibitor use to cardiovascular and central nervous

---

BOX 32-1

Definition of Peripartum Cardiomyopathy

Classic
- Development of cardiac failure in the last month of pregnancy or within 5 months of delivery
- Absence of an identifiable cause for the cardiac failure
- Absence of recognizable heart disease before the last month of pregnancy

Additional
- Left ventricular systolic dysfunction demonstrated by classic echocardiographic criteria:
  —Ejection fraction, less than 45%
  —Fractional shortening less than 30%
  —End-diastolic dimension greater than 2.7 cm/m² body surface area

Ro A, Frishman WH. Peripartum cardiomyopathy. Cardiol Rev 2006;14:36.

system malformations. However, these medications can be added to a postpartum medication regimen. In addition, breastfeeding women can safely take captopril and enalapril. Thus, in combination with furosemide, the most appropriate treatment for this patient is hydralazine.

Verapamil hydrochloride is a calcium channel blocker that can regulate blood pressure; however, it has negative inotropic effects and, as a result, should not be used in patients with systolic dysfunction. The one exception is amlodipine, a dihydropyridine calcium channel blocker that does not have negative inotropic effects and has been demonstrated to improve survival in patients with nonischemic cardiomyopathy. Enoxaparin sodium (Lovenox) is a low molecular weight heparin used for anticoagulation in patients considered to be at high risk for embolic events. Patients with peripartum cardiomyopathy are at risk for embolic events from the combination of the hypercoagulable state of pregnancy and the stasis and turbulent blood flow in a dilated heart. Anticoagulation should be considered in these patients, but it is not a first-line therapy.

Cooper WO, Hernandez-Diaz S, Arbogast PG, Dudley JA, Dyer S, Gideion PS, et al. Major congenital malformations after first-trimester exposure to ACE inhibitors. N Engl J Med 2006;354:2443–51.

Elkayam U, Akhter MW, Singh H, Khan S, Bitar F, Hameed A, et al. Pregnancy-associated cardiomyopathy: clinical characteristics and a comparison between early and late presentation. Circulation 2005; 111:2050–5.

Metra M, Cas LD, di Lenarda A, Poole-Wilson P. Beta-blockers in heart failure: are pharmacological differences clinically important? Heart Fail Rev 2004;9:123–30.

Murali S, Baldisseri MR. Peripartum cardiomyopathy. Crit Care Med 2005;33(suppl):S340–6.

Ro A, Frishman WH. Peripartum cardiomyopathy. Cardiol Rev 2006; 14:35–42.

33

Amniotic fluid embolism

A 17-year-old primigravid adolescent presents in labor at 39 weeks of gestation. Her prenatal course and labor course have been uncomplicated. She has no medical problems except for a history of atopy. The cervix is 3 cm dilated, 50% effaced, and fetal presentation is at −1 station. During the cervical examination, the patient has shortness of breath followed quickly by whole body petechia and bleeding from her gums and intravenous site. As blood is being drawn for the presence of a coagulopathy, the patient has a cardiopulmonary arrest. The cervical examination is unchanged and the fetus is bradycardic. She has no other medical problems. Along with basic supportive therapy, the next most appropriate action is

*   (A) immediate cesarean delivery
     (B) administration of coagulation factor replacement
     (C) internal fetal monitoring
     (D) perform cardiac pacing

The symptoms described match the scenario for amniotic fluid embolus. The first case of amniotic fluid embolus was described in 1926. Although the diagnosis was originally based on the finding of fetal squamous cells or fetal debris in the maternal pulmonary vasculature, animal study results have varied. Although most animal models show some untoward effect of the injection of heterologous amniotic fluid, this has not been universal. The pathophysiology in humans has not been fully explained, but there are stark similarities to anaphylaxis. A more accurate term that has been suggested is anaphylactoid syndrome of pregnancy.

The clinical presentation of amniotic fluid embolus is varied but the most common scenario is that the patient experiences an acute episode of hypoxia and hypotension followed by cardiopulmonary arrest shortly before or after delivery or after pregnancy termination. Coagulopathy complicates most cases of amniotic fluid embolus, but it must be emphasized that any part of the common trilogy of hypoxia, hypotension, and coagulopathy may be missing. The diagnosis of amniotic fluid embolus is a clinical one. The presence of fetal cellular elements in the maternal vasculature need not be present to make the diagnosis of amniotic fluid embolus. In fact, 25–50% of women who met criteria for the diagnosis of amniotic fluid embolus did not have evidence of fetal debris in their pulmonary vasculature.

The maternal outcome for a patient with diagnosed amniotic fluid embolus is grim: approximately 80% of women die. Treatment of women with amniotic fluid embolus before delivery is difficult. If the patient has not had cardiopulmonary arrest, supportive therapy should begin, with close attention to monitoring the fetal condition. However, in the face of an unstable mother and a nonreassuring fetal condition, the decision to perform a cesarean delivery is difficult because of the potential for worsening the mother's condition. Perimortem cesarean delivery is usually performed if cardiopulmonary resuscitation is not successful within 4 minutes. However, because of the dismal prognosis in women with the diagnosis of amniotic fluid embolus who have a cardiopulmonary arrest, if the fetus is still alive, cardiopulmonary resuscitation should be performed and immediate cesarean delivery should be done.

In the patient who has already given birth and amniotic fluid embolus is diagnosed, initial supportive treatment should include oxygen therapy and volume expansion. In the face of hypotension, adding an inotrope may be beneficial. The use of invasive monitoring such as pulmonary artery catheterization may be of benefit especially to guide treatment. Some investigators have suggested addition of corticosteroids in patients with amniotic fluid embolus; however, their use remains controversial.

Clark SL, Hankins GD, Dudley DA, Dildy GA, Porter TF. Amniotic fluid embolism: analysis of the national registry. Am J Obstet Gynecol 1995;172:1158–67; discussion 1167–9.

Plauche WC. Amniotic fluid embolism. Am J Obstet Gynecol 1983;147:982–3.

34

Vaginal breech delivery of a second twin

A 32-year-old woman, gravida 5, para 4, is in active labor at 34 weeks of gestation with twins. On examination, the cervix is 6 cm dilated with twin A at +1 station. Ultrasonography shows that twin A is in the vertex presentation and twin B is in the transverse lie. The patient is counseled and accepts vaginal breech extraction of twin B. The most important factor to consider in this case for the breech extraction of twin B is

      (A) gestational age
      (B) parity
  * (C) perform ultrasonography to estimate fetal weights
      (D) need for oxytocin

The increased rate of multiple gestations in the United States as a result of new reproductive technologies has resulted in a dramatic increase in the number of twin gestations during the past decade. Although twin gestations were once uncommon events, the obstetrician is now frequently faced with the intrapartum management of preterm twin gestations.

Twin gestations can present as vertex–vertex, vertex–nonvertex, nonvertex–nonvertex, or nonvertex–vertex. Approximately 80% will present as vertex–vertex or vertex–nonvertex with most being both vertex. In addition to twin positions in utero, intrapartum management is dictated by several factors:

- Estimated fetal weights
- Resources to perform concomitant fetal heart rate monitoring
- Availability of real time ultrasonography
- Appropriate anesthesia support
- Availability of a pediatrician at delivery
- A ready operating room
- Staff familiar with twin deliveries and complications

When presented with a vertex–vertex twin gestation in labor, it appears safe to allow them both to be delivered vaginally. Conversely, it is more common to perform a cesarean delivery on any twin gestation in which the presenting twin is nonvertex. Although there is no good evidence to support this approach, there is no evidence to support the safety of a vaginal delivery in this instance.

When the second twin is nonvertex, evidence indicates that in most cases the delivery of the second fetus either by external cephalic version or breech extraction appears safe. One large study noted that although there were no neonatal deaths in the group of second nonvertex twins greater than 1,500 g, 38% (6/16) of neonates weighing less than 1,500 g died. Other retrospective studies that have looked at second twins weighing less than 1,500 g

have noted improved outcomes, but this finding remains controversial.

Because most of the information on second-twin gestations and mode of delivery comes from descriptive studies or retrospective studies, it is difficult to recommend one particular management schema. However, the most common initial intrapartum approach to the vertex–nonvertex twin gestation is to confirm presentation, viability, and estimated fetal weights with ultrasonographic examination on admission. Guidelines to ensure proper management of the vertex–nonvertex twin pregnancy are listed in Box 34-1.

It has been recommended that the estimated fetal weights be between 2,000 g and 3,500 g, which allows for the error in ultrasonographic measurement of estimated fetal weights, before attempted vaginal delivery of a nonvertex second twin. Early in preparation for delivery, the patient is moved to the operating room and the staff is

---

BOX 34-1

Guidelines for Management of the Vertex–Nonvertex Twin Pregnancy

- Informed consent of patient
- Ultrasonographic examination at admission to confirm presentation, viability, and estimated fetal weights
- Intravenous access
- Concomitant electronic fetal heart rate monitoring and uterine contraction monitoring
- Hematocrit and platelet count
- Confirmation of the quick availability of blood products
- An experienced obstetrician (preferably two)
- Experienced nursing staff
- Availability of an operating suite
- Consultation with anesthesiology
- Availability of regional anesthesia

organized. Fetal heart rate and contraction monitoring continues in the operating suite. Once twin A has been delivered, confirmation of fetal presentation and heart rate of twin B by ultrasonography should occur. If the heart rate is reassuring and the fetus is in a nonvertex presentation, external version may be attempted. Alternatively, it has been recommended to not delay delivery and to perform a breech extraction.

Chervenak FA, Johnson RE, Berkowitz RI, Grannum P, Hobbins JC. Is routine cesarean section necessary for vertex–breech and vertex–transverse twin gestations? Am J Obstet Gynecol 1984;148:1–5.

Chervenak FA, Johnson RE, Youcha S, Hobbins JC, Berkowitz RL. Intrapartum management of twin gestation. Obstet Gynecol 1985; 65:119–24.

Healy AJ, Gaddipati S. Intrapartum management of twins: truths and controversies. Clin Perinatol 2005;32:455–73, vii.

35

Motor vehicle accident

A 19-year-old primigravid woman at 35 weeks of gestation was a restrained passenger in an automobile accident. During her evaluation in the emergency department, the study that is most likely to detect a clinically significant concealed abruptio placentae is

    (A) an ultrasonographic examination
*   (B) electronic fetal cardiac and uterine activity monitoring
    (C) serum fibrinogen
    (D) a Kleihauer–Betke test
    (E) a platelet count

Approximately 3% of pregnant women are involved in motor vehicle accidents during their pregnancy. Of these women, approximately 80% are wearing seat belts at the time of the accident. Seat belts have been shown to decrease adverse maternal and fetal outcomes. One major factor that determines fetal outcome in a motor vehicle accident is maternal condition. Fetal loss rates are high with life-threatening maternal injuries, such as severe head injury, pelvic fractures, and ruptured intraabdominal viscera. Therefore, aggressive diagnosis and treatment of the mother is the best way to ensure fetal survival. Nevertheless, fetal loss has been seen in non–life-threatening injuries, many of which were considered trivial.

Tests performed in the emergency department that are specific for evaluating fetal condition include the following:

- Cardiotocographic monitoring
- Abdominal ultrasonography
- Kleihauer–Betke test
- Blood type and Rh

Abruptio placentae is the main cause of fetal death in abdominal trauma with maternal survival. The incidence in pregnant women with non–life-threatening abdominal trauma is approximately 2%. Abruptio placentae may be difficult to diagnose because bleeding is often concealed. An ultrasonographic examination may show evidence of abruptio placentae, but it is not sensitive. Coagulation studies are insensitive for abruptio placentae.

The role of a routine Kleihauer–Betke test after trauma in predicting adverse outcomes is not clear. It is not sensitive for the diagnosis of abruptio placentae. A negative test result does not rule out abruptio placentae and a positive test result does not confirm it. In a retrospective case–control study, the incidence of a positive Kleihauer–Betke test result (5.1%) in low-risk pregnancies did not differ from results in maternal trauma patients (2.6%). Therefore, a positive Kleihauer–Betke test result alone does not necessarily indicate pathologic fetal–maternal hemorrhage in patients with trauma. However, one team of investigators found that a Kleihauer–Betke test result showing fetal cells of 0.1% or greater was predictive of preterm labor in maternal trauma patients. The Kleihauer–Betke test is most useful for evaluating trauma in Rh-negative women to determine the dose of Rho (D) immune globulin to be administered. All Rh-negative women should receive at least one dose because only 0.01 mL of fetal blood may cause sensitization. This amount would not be detected by Kleihauer–Betke staining.

The best test to diagnose abruptio placentae is electronic fetal heart rate and uterine contraction monitoring. The fetal heart rate monitor may show baseline tachycardia, decreased variability, and late decelerations. Uterine contractions may be a sign of abruptio placentae. The recommended duration of monitoring ranges from 4 to 24 hours. If up to six contractions per hour are seen during the first 4 hours of continuous monitoring, abruptio placentae is unlikely. If in the first 4 hours the patient experiences uterine contractions, a nonreassuring fetal heart rate pattern, vaginal bleeding, or significant uterine tenderness, prolonged monitoring may be necessary.

Dahmus M, Sibai BM. Blunt abdominal trauma: are there any predictive factors for abruptio placentae or maternal-fetal distress? Am J Obstet Gynecol 1993;169:1054–9.

Hyde LK, Cook LJ, Olson LM, Weiss HB, Dean JM. Effect of motor vehicle crashes on adverse fetal outcomes. Obstet Gynecol 2003;102: 279–86.

Kissinger DP, Rozycki GS, Morris JA Jr, Knudson M, Copes WS, Bass SM, et al. Trauma in pregnancy. Predicting pregnancy outcome [published erratum appears in Arch Surg 1991;126:1524]. Arch Surg 1991; 126:1079–86.

Pearlman MD, Tintinalli JE. Evaluation and treatment of the gravida and fetus following trauma during pregnancy. Obstet Gynecol Clin North Am 1991;18:371–81.

Williams JK, McClain L, Rosemurgy AS, Colorado NM. Evaluation of blunt abdominal trauma in the third trimester of pregnancy: maternal and fetal considerations. Obstet Gynecol 1990;75:33–7.

36

Gestational diabetes mellitus

Gestational diabetes mellitus (GDM) was diagnosed in a 24-year-old woman at 24 weeks of gestation. She initiated a daily 1,800-calorie American Diabetes Association diet and a 30-minute walk after each meal. Four weeks later, her home fasting blood glucose level is 100–105 mg/dL, and her 2-hour postprandial glucose level is 160–180 mg/dL. The best management for this patient is

        (A) increased exercise activity
        (B) metformin hydrochloride (Glucophage) therapy
*   (C) split-dose insulin therapy
        (D) insulin pump
        (E) decreased caloric intake to 1,200 calories per day

In patients with GDM, it is reasonable to allow a 1- to 2-week trial of dietary adjustments in the attempt to attain the preferred glycemic control. Approximately 50% of patients will achieve glycemic control by 2 weeks of dietary therapy, and only an additional 10% will have achieved acceptable control by the fourth week of therapy. In studies of fetuses with abdominal circumferences above the 75th percentile at 28 weeks of gestation, insulin therapy has been shown to reduce macrosomia and neonatal obesity. Given that the period of maximum fetal growth velocity and fat deposition is between 28 and 33 weeks of gestation, there is no reason to delay appropriate pharmacologic therapy. Increasing exercise activity is unlikely to be beneficial in this patient.

A 1,200-kcal diet in pregnancy is ketogenic. Maternal ketonemia resulting in maternal acidemia is probably unfavorable to mother and fetus. Although a diet based on body mass index is used, the empirical result is usually between 1,800 kcal and 2,200 kcal daily.

Patients with GDM who fail diet therapy should be started on subcutaneous short-acting and intermediate-acting insulin. Table 36-1 shows insulin preparations and pharmacokinetics for GDM.

Continuous subcutaneous insulin infusion often is reserved for women with pregestational diabetes mellitus who are poorly controlled on intermittent insulin administration. A properly designed insulin pump infusion allows convenient tailoring of the insulin administration profile to the patients' individual metabolic profile and lifestyle. Because of the risks of pump malfunctions, precipitation of insulin inside pump mechanism, abscess formation, and poor intake, therapy with the insulin pump requires a compliant patient and a knowledgeable provider with emergency counseling and maintenance available on a 24-hour basis.

When pharmacotherapy is required, a possible alternative is oral therapy with glyburide. In a large randomized study that compared insulin to glyburide therapy in women with GDM, only 4% of the glyburide group required conversion to insulin. However, published clinical experience suggests that 10–20% of women who take glyburide may require conversion to insulin. In some centers, glyburide has become part of the therapy for women with GDM. Other centers have not supported this practice because of the limited availability of controlled data.

Metformin hydrochloride increases insulin sensitivity, which would be beneficial in the treatment of GDM. However, because metformin crosses the placenta, there is concern about its safety in the fetus. Metformin has been shown to be useful in the treatment of polycystic ovary

TABLE 36-1. Insulin Preparations and Pharmacokinetics for Gestational Diabetes Mellitus

Insulin Preparation	Time to Peak Action (hours)	Total Duration of Action (hours)	Comments
Lispro (Humalog) Aspart (NovoLog)	1	2	Onset within 10 minutes of injection. No need to delay meal after injection
Regular insulin	2	4	Good coverage of individual meals if injected 20 minutes before eating. Increase risk of postprandial hypoglycemia with unopposed action 2–3 hours after eating
Neutral protamine Hagedorn insulin Lente insulin	4	8	Provides intermediate-acting control Give on rising and at bedtime. Risk of 3:00 AM hypoglycemia.
Ultralente	8	20	High risk of nocturnal hypoglycemia. Does not cover a full 24 hours in pregnancy.
Insulin glargine (Lantus)	5	Less than 24	Prolonged flat action profile. Limited pregnancy experience. Increased risk of nocturnal hypoglycemia or under treatment during the day.

Modified from Moore TR. In: Creasy RK, Resnik R, Iams JD, editors. Maternal–fetal medicine: principles and practice. 5th ed. Philadelphia (PA): WB Saunders Co.; 2004. p. 1023–61. Copyright 2004 by Elsevier.

syndrome but is not yet accepted as treatment for GDM. Observational studies have not shown any adverse effects of metformin when used in pregnancy. Currently, trials are underway to investigate the role of metformin in GDM.

Hawthorne G. Metformin use and diabetic pregnancy—has its time come? Diabet Med 2006;23:223–7.

Langer O, Conway DL, Berkus MD, Xanakis MJ, Gonzales O. A comparison of glyburide and insulin in women with gestational diabetes mellitus. N Engl J Med 2000;343:1134–8.

Moore TR. Diabetes in pregnancy. In: Creasy RK, Resnik R, Iams JD, editors. Maternal–fetal medicine: principles and practice. 5th ed. Philadelphia (PA): WB Saunders Co.; 2004. p. 1023–61.

Saade G. Gestational diabetes mellitus: a pill or a shot? Obstet Gynecol 2005;105:456–7.

Schaefer-Graf UM, Kjos SL, Fauzan OH, Buhling KJ, Siebert G, Buhrer C, et al. A randomized trial evaluating a predominantly fetal growth-based strategy to guide management of gestational diabetes in Caucasian women. Diabetes Care 2004;27:297–302.

37

Management of episiotomy breakdown

A 25-year-old patient is 4 days postpartum from an uncomplicated vaginal delivery and repair of a spontaneous second-degree perineal laceration. She reports increased perineal pain and purulent discharge. On examination, it is apparent that the repair of the perineum has broken down and has become infected. The patient has normal sensation and minimal induration. The best next step in management is

      (A) immediate return to operating room for repair and subsequent antibiotic therapy
      (B) débridement and discharge to home until perineum has healed via granulation
*   (C) antibiotic therapy and return to operating room in 72–96 hours for perineal repair
      (D) wide excision of infected tissue to prevent necrotizing fasciitis

The management of postpartum perineal breakdown challenges the obstetrician to choose a course of action most likely to result in a speedy and complete recovery. Traditionally, perineal breakdowns were allowed to heal by granulation, and any necessary surgical revisions were done at least 3–4 months after the initial event. Although this approach ultimately does result in a good outcome, the prolonged recovery time involved is not always beneficial to the patient who now has increased demands on her time with a newborn child.

In general, after an episiotomy or perineal wound breakdown, it is best to wait at least until the patient is afebrile with no further evidence of cellulitis and with any purulent exudates replaced by healthy appearing granulation tissue. Immediate return to the operating room in the setting of acute infection and wound breakdown is not likely to lead to a favorable result.

Inordinate perineal pain can signal the potentially fatal entity of necrotizing fasciitis, which requires wide excision of infected tissue. However, in the absence of clinical findings suggestive of this diagnosis such as marked induration, often described as "woody" in texture, with loss of sensation, such radical excision should not be performed as a prophylactic measure.

Either débridement and discharge to home for healing by secondary intention or antibiotic treatment with repair in 3–4 days after infection has resolved would be acceptable modes of management. The preferred mode would be early closure rather than healing by secondary intention because the long-term outcomes are equivalent but the speed of recovery is much greater with early closure.

Hankins GD, Hauth JC, Gilstrap LC 3rd, Hammond TL, Yeomans ER, Snyder RR. Early repair of episiotomy dehiscence. Obstet Gynecol 1990;75:48–51.

Ramin SM, Ramus RM, Little BB, Gilstrap LC 3rd. Early repair of episiotomy dehiscence associated with infection. Am J Obstet Gynecol 1992;167:1104–7.

Uygur D, Yesildaglar N, Kis S, Sipahi T. Early repair of episiotomy dehiscence. Aust N Z J Obstet Gynaecol 2004;44:244–6.

38

Breast mass in pregnancy

A 36-year-old primigravid woman at 30 weeks of gestation reports a painless mass in her right breast, first noted 3 weeks earlier. Physical examination confirms a nontender, mobile, 3-cm mass in the upper outer quadrant of the right breast without axillary or supraclavicular adenopathy. Ultrasonographic examination shows that the mass is solid, 3 cm in diameter, and has irregular margins. The patient reports a history of fibrocystic change diagnosed after a previous biopsy performed when she was 25 years old. She denies any family history of breast cancer. The best next step in her care is

* (A) core needle biopsy of the mass
  (B) needle aspiration of the mass
  (C) genetic studies for *BRCA1* and *BRCA2* mutations
  (D) mammography
  (E) reexamination of the breast mass 6 weeks postpartum

The workup of a breast mass in pregnancy should include a history and physical, selective imaging, and biopsy. When a breast mass is detected by the physician or by patient self-examination, a careful medical history should be taken and a physical examination should be performed. In addition to the chronology and description of the mass, the history should address some of the epidemiologic risk factors for breast cancer: current age, age at menarche, age at first pregnancy, family history of breast cancer, carriage of *BRCA1* or *BRCA2* gene mutations, history of benign breast disease, alcohol intake, and exposure to radiation. The physical examination should include size of the mass, consistency, mobility, skin changes, regional adenopathy, and findings in the examination of the other breast. The differential diagnosis of a breast mass in pregnancy includes lactating adenoma, fibroadenoma, cystic disease, lobular hyperplasia, galactocele, abscess, lipoma, hamartoma, phyllodes tumor, and cancer.

The first imaging study of a breast mass found during pregnancy should be ultrasonography to determine if the mass is cystic or solid. Ultrasonography also can detect other signs suspicious for malignancy such as noncompressability, irregular margins, both cystic and solid components, and thick walls. If the mass is cystic and has no other ultrasonographic characteristics of malignancy, a fine-needle aspiration may be done. If the cyst fluid is clear or yellow and the cyst resolves, no other treatment is required. The patient may be followed to see if the cyst recurs. If the fluid is bloody or a residual solid mass is present, a core needle biopsy or excisional biopsy should be done. The role of diagnostic mammography in pregnancy is controversial. The fetus can be shielded from most of the radiation; however, breast tissue is denser in

pregnancy and mammography is associated with a false-negative rate of 35–40%. If a solid mass is found on ultrasound examination, it will require histologic evaluation to rule out cancer irrespective of mammographic findings.

Stage-for-stage, the prognosis is the same for breast cancer diagnosed in age-matched pregnant and nonpregnant women. However, many case series report more advanced disease at diagnosis in pregnant women. Proposed explanations for the late stage at presentation include difficulty in palpating a breast mass, reluctance to biopsy, enhancement of breast cancer growth by pregnancy-related hormones, and potential enhancement of tumor metastases by the rich blood supply and lymphatics in pregnancy. The workup of a breast mass should not be delayed because of pregnancy.

In the patient described, a core needle biopsy should be done. This will provide enough tissue for a histologic diagnosis. A fine-needle aspiration may not provide enough tissue for diagnosis and requires a skilled and experienced pathologist to read it. Genetic studies for *BRCA1* and *BRCA2* mutations would be important to consider if the patient had a family history of breast cancer with onset before age 40 years or breast cancer in three or more relatives on the same side of the family. Wide local excision used to be the criterion for evaluating a breast mass. It has the advantage of combining diagnosis and treatment in the same procedure. It usually requires an operating room and anesthesia and is not as cost-effective as a core-needle biopsy. Complications are uncommon but include bleeding, infection, scarring, and a milk fistula. Reexamination of the breast mass 6 weeks postpartum would introduce too much delay in the diagnosis.

Cunningham FG, Leveno KJ, Bloom SL, Hauth JC, Gilstrap LC, Wenstrom KD, editors. Williams obstetrics. 22nd ed. New York (NY): McGraw-Hill; 2005. p. 1259–61.

Hogge JP, de Paredes ES, Magnant CM, Lage J. Imaging and management of breast masses during pregnancy and lactation. Breast J 1999; 5:272–83.

Lippman ME. Breast cancer. In: Kasper DL, Braunwald E, Fauci AS, Hauser SL, Longo DL, Jameson JH, editors. Harrison's principles of internal medicine. 16th ed. New York: McGraw-Hill; 2005. p. 516–23.

Sorosky JI, Scott-Conner CE. Breast disease complicating pregnancy. Obstet Gynecol Clin North Am 1998;25:353–63.

Woo JC, Yu T, Hurd TC. Breast cancer in pregnancy: a literature review. Arch Surg 2003;138:91–8; discussion 99.

39

Fetal premature atrial contractions

A 31-year-old healthy, multiparous woman at 30 weeks of gestation is referred for targeted ultrasonography after an irregular fetal heart rhythm was auscultated in the office. She does not smoke cigarettes nor drink alcohol. Ultrasonography revealed a normal fetal anatomic survey. Frequent fetal premature atrial contractions (PACs) are identified by motion mode (M-mode) echocardiography, and the fetal cardiac anatomy appears normal. There is no evidence of a fetal tachyarrhythmia, abdominal ascites, or hydrops fetalis. The next step in evaluation is to

    (A) refer for fetal echocardiography
    (B) refer for genetic counseling
*   (C) inquire about caffeine intake and medications
    (D) order a urine drug screen
    (E) order screen for anti-SSA (anti-Ro) and anti-SSB (anti-La) antibodies

Arrhythmias are identified in approximately 1–3% of all fetuses and often are discovered at routine obstetric visits. Most cardiac rhythm abnormalities are composed primarily of transient, isolated ectopic beats or extrasystoles, which may be of atrial, junctional, or ventricular origin. Most extrasystoles are of atrial origin (PACs) with premature ventricular contractions representing less than 4% of extrasystoles. Premature atrial contractions may be conducted to the ventricle, partially conducted, or may be blocked resulting in varying ventricular responses. Most PACs are of little clinical significance, and the majority resolve spontaneously either prenatally or early in the postnatal period. Fetal cardiac abnormalities associated with atrial extrasystoles are rare and are found in only 0.3–2% of fetuses.

Premature atrial contractions are typically idiopathic, but some investigators speculate that redundancy of the foramen ovale flap may contribute to atrial extrasystolic beats. Extrasystoles also are attributed to immature conducting pathways in the fetal heart. Maternal exposures and conditions that may trigger PACs are caffeine, alcohol, smoking, and hyperthyroidism. Despite being relatively benign, PACs have the potential to induce a supraventricular tachyarrhythmia in susceptible fetuses, which may lead to fetal hydrops fetalis, cardiac failure, and intrauterine demise.

When an arrhythmia is identified, the physician should determine the etiology and evaluate for fetal cardiac abnormalities and associated fetal anomalies. Targeted ultrasonography is an excellent tool to evaluate fetal anatomy. Fetal echocardiography is the primary diagnostic tool to characterize and monitor fetal arrhythmias. M-mode echocardiography can be used to evaluate the relationship between atrial and ventricular contractions by positioning the cursor through the atrial wall, atrioventricular valve, and ventricular wall to obtain simultaneous recordings (Fig. 39-1). Premature atrial contractions can be conducted to the ventricle or may be blocked.

In this case, an irregular fetal heartbeat was auscultated in the office. Frequent PACs were demonstrated with M-mode during targeted ultrasonography. The fetal cardiac anatomy appeared normal, and there was no evidence of a tachyarrhythmia or hydrops fetalis. At this initial screening, the patient should be questioned about caffeine intake, tobacco use, alcohol intake, and use of prescription and nonprescription medications because many of these exposures are associated with PACs in adults. When fetal PACs are identified, pregnant women are cautioned to avoid such exposures. With suspected PACs, definitive evaluation is performed with either real-time ultrasonography or fetal echocardiography. If there is the capability of performing an M-mode evaluation of the arrhythmia in

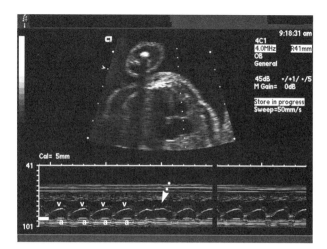

FIG. 39-1. Premature atrial contractions. Motion-mode, two-dimensional image of the four-chamber heart is obtained. The M-mode cursor intersects the right ventricle anteriorly and the right atrium posteriorly. The straight arrow represents a premature atrial contraction that was conducted to the ventricle (dotted arrow). a = atrial contraction; v = ventricular contraction.

a fetus with normal cardiac examination, as in this case, a fetal echocardiogram is not necessary. Genetic counseling typically is not warranted unless associated fetal anomalies are present. Without a history of illicit drug use, a urine drug screen is not indicated as an initial evaluation. Anti-SSA (anti-Ro) and anti-SSB (anti-La) antibodies are obtained when fetal bradyarrhythmias or complete heart block are identified. Elevated antibody titers may be present in women with collagen vascular disease, and these antibodies can cross the placenta and cause a fetal myocarditis, immune-complex mediated inflammatory damage to the conduction system, and fibrous replacement of conducting tissue.

Patients in which fetal PACs are identified may undergo weekly auscultation or electronic fetal monitoring to evaluate for fetal tachycardia. Alternatively, in the presence of an intermittent arrhythmia, weekly ultrasonographic evaluation to assess for the development of an intermittent or sustained tachyarrhythmia, hydramnios, and fetal hydrops fetalis may be preferred. In the presence of a sustained tachyarrhythmia, a fetal echocardiogram is warranted. Additional management options include assessing the frequency of fetal movement and avoidance of caffeine and medications that may precipitate ectopy.

Copel JA, Liang RI, Demasio K, Ozeren S, Kleinman CS. The clinical significance of the irregular fetal heart rhythm. Am J Obstet Gynecol 2000;182:813–7; discussion 817–9.

Larmay HJ, Strasburger JF. Differential diagnosis and management of the fetus and newborn with an irregular or abnormal heart rate. Pediatr Clin North Am 2004;51:1033–50, x.

Simpson LL. Fetal supraventricular tachycardias: diagnosis and management. Semin Perinatol 2000;24:360–72.

Snyder CS, Copel JA. Fetal cardiac arrhythmias: diagnosis and therapy. In: James DK, Steer PJ, Weiner CP, Gonik B, editors. High risk pregnancy management options. 3rd ed. Philadelphia (PA): Elsevier Saunders; 2006. p. 325–40.

40

Lupus and pregnancy

A 25-year-old woman with systemic lupus erythematosus (SLE), for which she takes hydroxy-chloroquine (Plaquenil), is contemplating pregnancy. She seeks advice regarding pregnancy risks associated with SLE. You explain that SLE has been associated with an increased risk of

    (A) infertility
* (B) prematurity
    (C) cervical incompetence
    (D) macrosomia
    (E) gestational diabetes mellitus

Systemic lupus erythematosus is a multisystem autoimmune disease that disproportionately affects women in their childbearing years. The peak incidence of SLE occurs between the ages of 15 and 40 years, with an estimated female-to-male SLE incidence of 9:1. Women with SLE usually have normal fertility rates, and pregnancy is common.

In patients who do not have hypertension, renal impairment, or antiphospholipid syndrome in conjunction with SLE, pregnancy outcomes are often good, with few adverse sequelae for mother or infant. In addition, those who have been in remission for 6 months or more before conception have reported better outcomes. However, pregnancies in patients with SLE are at risk for several specific poor outcomes. Numerous studies have shown an increase in lupus flares, preeclampsia, neonatal lupus syndrome, and stillbirth in these patients. The reported stillbirth rate in pregnancies complicated by SLE ranges from 4% to 22%.

Systemic lupus erythematosus is associated with an increased risk for pregnancy loss, most commonly in association with antiphospholipid antibody syndrome, a condition often found in conjunction with SLE. Studies have also reported an increased rate of prematurity among live births in women with SLE, with a high proportion of these due to preterm premature rupture of membranes (preterm PROM) (70%). This increased risk of preterm PROM is found to be more prominent in patients receiv-

ing corticosteroid therapy. Pregnancy loss and premature delivery in subjects with SLE are not caused by an increased rate of cervical incompetence. There are no reports of SLE being associated with increased risk of cervical incompetence.

Most investigators have reported higher rates of intrauterine growth restriction in patients with SLE. Macrosomic or large-for-gestational-age infants have not been associated with SLE-complicated pregnancies. Pregnant women with SLE on chronic oral steroid therapy may develop insulin resistance. However, patients with SLE not on oral steroid therapy are at no increased risk for developing gestational diabetes mellitus.

Chakravarty EF, Colon I, Langen ES, Nix DA, El-Sayed YY, Genovese MC, et al. Factors that predict prematurity and preeclampsia in pregnancies that are complicated by systemic lupus erythematosus. Am J Obstet Gynecol 2005;192:1897–904.

Clowse ME, Magder LS, Witter F, Petri M. The impact of increased lupus activity on obstetric outcomes. Arthritis Rheum 2005;52:514–21.

Dhar JP, Essenmacher LM, Ager JW, Sokol RJ. Pregnancy outcomes before and after a diagnosis of systemic lupus erythematosus. Am J Obstet Gynecol 2005;193:1444–55.

Hankins GDV, Suarez VR. Rheumatologic and connective tissue disorders. In: Creasy RK, Resnik R, Iams JD, editors. Maternal–fetal medicine: principles and practice. 5th ed. Philadelphia (PA): WB Saunders; 2004. p. 1150–9.

Yasmeen S, Wilkins EE, Field NT, Sheikh RA, Gilbert WM. Pregnancy outcomes in women with systemic lupus erythematosus. J Matern Fetal Med 2001;10:91–6.

41

Thrombophilia

Left femoral deep vein thrombosis is diagnosed in a 25-year-old primigravid woman at 22 weeks of gestation. She was started on heparin 2 days ago. The thrombophilia assessment that can be reliably performed at this time is

      (A) lupus anticoagulant
*   (B) factor V Leiden mutation
      (C) antithrombin III
      (D) protein S
      (E) protein C

The Virchow triad of venous stasis, hypercoagulability, and vascular trauma increases the risk of thrombosis and is present in pregnancy, thus making pregnancy and the postpartum period a hypercoagulable state. Venous stasis of the lower extremities occurs as a result of direct compression by the enlarging uterus and venodilation secondary to hormonal effect. A 20–200% increase occurs in concentration of the procoagulants of fibrinogen, prothrombin, and factors VII, VIII, X, and XII. A decrease takes place in the endogenous anticoagulant protein S with a progressive rise in resistance to activated protein C, but antithrombin III and protein C are largely unchanged. The fibrinolytic system also is affected with an increase in the levels of antifibrinolytic plasminogen activator inhibitor types 1 and 2 (PAI-1, PAI-2). Delivery is associated with vascular damage. This increase in coagulability reduces the risk of bleeding during pregnancy but is responsible for an increased risk of venous thromboembolism in pregnancy. This risk for venous thromboembolism is increased further in patients with acquired or inherited thrombophilia.

The pregnancy-associated changes of coagulation assays may influence appropriate ordering and accurate interpretation of tests. The basic laboratory evaluation of coagulation in pregnancy is unchanged and includes prothrombin time (PT), activated partial thromboplastin time (APTT), platelet count, and fibrinogen level. The PT and APTT evaluate components of the extrinsic, intrinsic, and common pathways of the clotting cascade. Platelet count tends to be lower during pregnancy, but in normal pregnancies without gestational thrombocytopenia, platelet counts should still be at least $150 \times 10^3/mm^3$. Fibrinogen levels usually increase by approximately 50% in pregnancy.

Women with venous thromboembolism in pregnancy should be considered to be at high risk for having a thrombophilia. However, there are specific caveats for the interpretation of thrombophilia tests especially in pregnancy. Acute thromboembolic events may influence laboratory investigations or make the interpretation difficult for plasma tests (ie, for protein S, protein C, antithrombin III, and activated protein C resistance). Furthermore, heparin given to treat venous thromboembolism may affect results of tests such as lupus anticoagulant. As a consequence, it is recommended that tests on plasma not be performed during an acute thrombosis, and investigation should wait until after discontinuation of anticoagulant treatment for at least 2–3 weeks. Repeat confirmation of a low plasma protein result at a separate time is advisable. Furthermore, not all tests can be interpreted accurately during pregnancy. For example, protein S activity is decreased in pregnancy, thus testing is not reliable. However, some use a value less than 35% of protein S activity in pregnancy to make a diagnosis of protein S deficiency (Table 41-1).

A factor V Leiden polymerase chain reaction test is the most reliable test that can be performed on this patient because results are not altered by pregnancy, anticoagulant therapy, or acute thrombosis.

TABLE 41-1. Influence of Pregnancy, Acute Thrombosis, Heparin, and Warfarin on Thrombophilia Test Results

Abnormality	Prevalence in Patients With Thrombosis	Testing Methods	Is the Test Reliable During Pregnancy?	Is the Test Reliable During Acute Thrombosis?	Is the Test Reliable While Patient Is Taking Heparin?	Is the Test Reliable While Patient Is Taking Vitamin K Antagonist?
Factor V Leiden	40–70%*	APC resistance assay	No	Yes	Yes	Yes
		DNA analysis	No	Yes	Yes	Yes
Prothrombin gene mutation G20210A	8–30%†	DNA analysis	Yes	Yes	Yes	Yes
Antiphospholipid antibody	10–15%‡	Lupus anticoagulant (eg, dilute Russell viper venom time)	Yes	Yes	No	No
		Anticardiolipin antibodies	Yes	Yes		
		β₂-Glycoprotein-1 antibodies	Yes	Yes	Yes	Yes
Protein C deficiency	–	Protein C activity	Yes	No	Yes	No
Protein S deficiency	10–15%§	Protein S total and free antigen	No	No	Yes	No
Antithrombin-III deficiency	–	Antithrombin-III activity	Yes	No	No	No
Hyperhomocystinemia	8–25%	Fasting plasma homocystine	Yes	Yes	Yes	Yes

*Bokarewa MI, Bremme K, Blombäck M. Arg⁵⁰⁶-Gln mutation in factor V and risk of thrombosis during pregnancy. Br J Haematol 1996;92:473–8; Hellgren M, Svensson PJ, Dahlbäck B. Resistance to activated protein C as a basis for venous thromboembolism associated with pregnancy and oral contraceptives. Am J Obstet Gynecol 1995;173:210–13; *and* Faioni EM, Razzari C, Martinelli I, Panzeri D, Franchi F, Mannucci PM. Resistance to activated protein C in unselected patients with arterial and venous thrombosis. Am J Hematol 1997;55:59–64.

†Grandone E, Margaglione M, Colaizzo D, D'Andrea G, Cappucci G, Brancaccio V, et al. Genetic susceptibility to pregnancy-related venous thromboembolism: roles of factor V Leiden, prothrombin G20210A, and methylenetetrahydrofolate reductase C677T mutations. Am J Obstet Gynecol 1998;179:1324–8; Martinelli I, Taioli E, Bucciarelli P, Akhavan S, Mannucci PM. Interaction between the G20210A mutation of the prothrombin gene and oral contraceptive use in deep vein thrombosis. Arterioscler Thromb Vasc Biol 1999;19:700–3; *and* Salomon O, Steinberg DM, Zivelin A, Gitel S, Dardik R, Rosenberg N, et al. Single and combined prothrombotic factors in patients with idiopathic venous thromboembolism: prevalence and risk assessment. Arterioscler Thromb Vasc Biol 1999;19:511–18.

‡Ginsberg JS, Wells PS, Brill-Edwards P, Donovan D, Moffat K, Johnston M, et al. Antiphospholipid antibodies and venous thromboembolism. Blood 1995;86:3685–91.

§Aiach M, Borgel D, Gaussem P, Emmerich J, Alhenc-Gelas M, Gandrille S. Protein C and protein S deficiencies. Semin Hematol 1997;34:205–16; De Stefano V, Leone G, Mastrangelo S, Tripodi A, Rodeghiero F, Castaman G, et al. Clinical manifestations and management of inherited thrombophilia: retrospective analysis and follow-up after diagnosis of 238 patients with congenital deficiency of antithrombin III, protein C, or protein S. Thromb Haemost 1994;72:352–8; *and* Pabinger I, Schneider B. Thrombotic risk in hereditary antithrombin III, protein C, or protein S deficiency. A cooperative, retrospective study. Gesellschaft fur Thrombose- und Hamostaseforschung (GTH) Study Group on Natural Inhibitors. Arterioscler Thromb Vasc Biol 1996;16:742–8.

Modified from Moll S. Thrombophilias—practical implications. J Thromb Thrombolysis 2006;21:7–15.

Prevention of deep vein thrombosis and pulmonary embolism. ACOG Practice Bulletin 84. American College of Obstetricians and Gynecologists. Obstet Gynecol 2007;110:429–40.

Lockwood CJ. Inherited thrombophilias in pregnant patients: detection and treatment paradigm. Obstet Gynecol 2002;99:333–41.

Moll S. Thrombophilias—practical implications. J Thromb Thrombolysis 2006;21:7–15.

Tripodi A, Mannucci PM. Laboratory investigation of thrombophilia. Clin Chem 2001;47:1597–606.

42

Acute appendicitis in pregnancy

A 26-year-old woman, gravida 3, para 1, at 28 weeks and 6 days of gestation comes to the labor and delivery department reporting abdominal pain for the past 12 hours. On further questioning, she states that she has nausea and has vomited twice. Her past obstetric history is significant for a cesarean delivery at term for a transverse presentation. On admission, the patient's vital signs are blood pressure 98/56 mm Hg, pulse 92 beats per minute, and oral temperature of 37.2°C (98.9°F). The physical examination is significant for diffuse abdominal pain with rebound and guarding especially in the right mid to lower quadrant. The external fetal monitor shows a baseline of 165 beats per minute, but is otherwise reassuring. Bedside transabdominal ultrasonography revealed the fetus to be in a cephalic presentation, with an amniotic fluid index of 9 cm. A urine dipstick was negative for glucose, protein, and blood. A complete blood count revealed a hematocrit of 38% and a white blood cell count of 16.4×10^9/L with 84% neutrophils. The most likely diagnosis for this patient is

> (A) uterine rupture
> (B) renal stones
> (C) abruptio placentae
> * (D) appendicitis
> (E) diverticulitis

Acute appendicitis is the leading cause of nonobstetric surgery during pregnancy. It has been a long-held belief that the incidence of appendicitis was the same in pregnant and in nonpregnant women. However, a recent study from the Swedish Inpatient Register found that there is an inverse relationship between gestational age and appendicitis. Ruptured appendix occurs two to three times more often during pregnancy and is associated with increased fetal mortality. This increase in ruptured appendix may be a result of delayed diagnosis in the pregnant patient.

The false-positive rate (surgery for suspected appendicitis when the appendix is actually normal) has been reported to be 34–36%, with the lowest rate during the first trimester of the pregnancy. This is in contrast to the nonpregnant patient, in which the rate of false-positive diagnosis is approximately 15%. This increased rate in pregnancy may be related to the gradual upward displacement of the appendix by the growing uterus, causing it to move above the iliac angle by the fourth month of the pregnancy, therefore making the diagnosis more difficult.

Diagnosis of appendicitis in pregnancy is a challenge because many of the classical signs and symptoms of appendicitis occur in the "normal" pregnant patient. Typical signs and symptoms of appendicitis include abdominal pain, anorexia, nausea and vomiting, mild to moderate leukocytosis, and low-grade fever. Classically, in the nonpregnant patient, the pain of appendicitis starts periumbilically and subsequently migrates to the right lower quadrant. Similarly, pain in the right lower quadrant is the most common symptom during pregnancy regardless of the gestational age. Other locations of pain include the left lower quadrant, midabdomen, epigastric region, and a combination of locations.

The diagnosis of appendicitis remains clinical. Leukocytosis is common; however, up to 30% of patients with acute appendicitis may have a normal white blood cell count. A urinalysis result can be confusing because the inflamed appendix is often in close proximity to the bladder and ureter; as a consequence, microscopic hematuria and pyuria can be present in up to one third of patients with acute appendicitis.

In this patient, the most likely diagnosis is acute appendicitis. In cases of uterine rupture, one of the most common signs is a nonreassuring fetal heart rate, which is not present in this case. In patients with renal stones, the pain is sharp and in the back, and the urinalysis will demonstrate blood. Diverticulitis usually occurs in older patients, especially those older than 60 years; therefore, it is unlikely in this young patient. Abruptio placentae typically presents with vaginal bleeding as well as irregular contractions. In addition, there are risk factors associated with an increased risk of abruptio placentae, such as preterm premature rupture of membranes, preeclampsia or eclampsia, hydramnios, and chronic hypertension, which the patient does not have.

In the nonpregnant patient with suspected appendicitis, the imaging modality of choice is computed tomography with contrast. Computed tomography is estimated to deliver approximately 30 milligray (mGy) of ionizing radiation to the uterus. In contrast, in the pregnant patient with suspected appendicitis, ultrasonography with graded compression is the modality of choice because of its wide availability and lack of ionizing radiation. In institutions in which magnetic resonance imaging (MRI) is accessible, MRI is the alternative test of choice for those cases in which the ultrasound findings are not clear. In contrast to computed tomography, MRI does not use ionizing radiation or contrast and has excellent soft-tissue contrast resolution as well as multiplanar imaging capabilities. All of these imaging techniques are hampered by poor sensitivity and therefore would not be the best choice for diagnosis.

Andersson RE, Lambe M. Incidence of appendicitis during pregnancy. Int J Epidemiol 2001;30:1281–5.

Flum DR, McClure TD, Morris A, Koepsell T. Misdiagnosis of appendicitis and the use of diagnostic imaging. J Am Coll Surg 2005;201: 933–9.

Mazze RI, Kallen B. Appendectomy during pregnancy: a Swedish registry study of 778 cases. Obstet Gynecol 1991;77:835–40.

Mourad J, Elliott JP, Erickson L, Lisboa L. Appendicitis in pregnancy: new information that contradicts long-held clinical beliefs. Am J Obstet Gynecol 2000;182:1027–9.

Oto A, Ernst RD, Shah R, Koroglu M, Chaljub G, Gei AF, et al. Right-lower-quadrant pain and suspected appendicitis in pregnant women: evaluation with MR imaging—initial experience. Radiology 2005;234: 445–51.

Pedrosa I, Levine D, Eyvazzadeh AD, Siewert B, Ngo L, Rofsky NM. MR imaging evaluation of acute appendicitis in pregnancy. Radiology 2006;238:891–9.

43

Expectant management in a patient with vaginal bleeding

A 31-year-old primigravid woman, with the date of her last menstrual period unknown, comes to the office for her first prenatal visit. A week ago, she presented to her local emergency department with vaginal spotting. An ultrasound examination performed during the emergency department visit revealed a single live intrauterine pregnancy with a crown–rump length of 24 mm consistent with 9 weeks of gestation and a fetal heart rate of 153 beats per minute. A subchorionic hematoma was seen measuring 2.2 × 2.1 × 2.5 cm at the right side of the chorionic sac not involving and extending to the area of the placenta. You inform her that the most common outcome in patients who present with subchorionic hematoma or vaginal bleeding during the first trimester is

*   (A)   term delivery
       (B)   spontaneous abortion
       (C)   intrauterine growth restriction (IUGR)
       (D)   preterm delivery
       (E)   abruptio placentae

During the first trimester of pregnancy, bleeding is the most common indication for an ultrasonographic evaluation of the pregnancy. Vaginal bleeding during the first trimester of pregnancy is a relatively common occurrence seen in approximately 14–25% of all pregnant women. If bleeding occurs before ultrasonographic evaluation of viability, approximately 50% of these pregnancies will result in a spontaneous abortion. However, if a viable fetus is seen on an ultrasonogram after bleeding, approximately 95–98% of those pregnancies will continue beyond 20 weeks of gestation.

A subchorionic hematoma is defined as a fluid-filled collection in the uterine cavity between the chorion and the decidua. When viewed using ultrasonography, the hematoma typically appears as an anechoic crescent-shaped fluid collection that separates the chorion from the inner aspect of the uterus. The reported incidence of intrauterine hematomas ranges from 0.5% to 22%, depending on the population that was studied, and most of these hematomas are associated with vaginal bleeding. Subchorionic hematomas have been associated with pre-existing medical conditions, such as autoimmune diseases and immunologic factors.

Vaginal bleeding and the presence of a subchorionic hematoma have been reported to convey some risk to the pregnancy. However, in a study of women referred for vaginal bleeding or spotting who had viable pregnancies and intrauterine hematoma, most patients had a favorable outcome (Table 43-1).

In a recent study of 16,506 patients, who were enrolled in the First and Second Trimester Evaluation of Risk (FASTER) trial, 14,160 patients had no vaginal bleeding (control group), 2,094 patients had light bleeding (spotting), and 252 patients had heavy bleeding. All patients were scanned at the time of enrolling into the trial and all had a viable pregnancy. The overall spontaneous abortion rate before 24 weeks was 0.4% for the control group, 1% for patients who experienced light bleeding, and 2% for the women with heavy bleeding. In other words, if a viable fetus was seen after 10 weeks of gestation, and the patient had symptoms of threatened abortion, 98% of the pregnancies reached 24 weeks of gestation. However, when compared with the control group, the patients with light or heavy bleeding were more likely to experience a fetal loss before 24 weeks of gestation. In women with bleeding, the heavier the vaginal bleeding during the first trimester, the greater the risk of fetal loss when compared with light bleeding for an odds ratio of 4.2 versus 2.5, respectively. The obstetric outcomes were not significantly different between the controls and the groups with bleeding in the incidence of IUGR, gestational hyperten-

TABLE 43-1. Intrauterine Hematoma and Associated Clinical Conditions

Outcome of Pregnancy	% of Cases
Term delivery*	61.5
Spontaneous abortion	14.3
Intrauterine growth restriction	7.7
Threatened preterm delivery	7.1
Preterm delivery	6.6
Abruptio placentae	1.1
Fetal distress	1.6
Total	100

*Excludes other items listed in the table.

Modified from Maso G, D'Ottavio G, De Seta F, Sartore A, Piccoli M, Mandruzzato G. First-trimester intrauterine hematoma and outcome of pregnancy. Obstet Gynecol 2005;105:339–44.

sion, prolonged premature rupture of membranes, or placenta previa. However, the patients with vaginal spotting were more likely to have preeclampsia, preterm delivery, abruptio placentae, or cesarean deliveries (Table 43-2).

TABLE 43-2. Obstetric Complications by Amount of Vaginal Bleeding

Outcome	Light Bleeding vs Control Adjusted OR (95% CI)	P Value	Heavy Bleeding vs Control Adjusted OR (95% CI)	P Value
IUGR	1.4 (0.9–2.1)	.09	2.6 (1.2–5.6)	.02
Gestational hypertension	1.0 (0.9–1.3)	.67	1.5 (0.9–2.4)	.09
Preterm delivery	1.3 (1.1–1.7)	.01	3.0 (1.9–4.5)	<.01
Prolonged PROM	1.3 (0.9–1.9)	.06	3.2 (1.8–5.7)	.01
Abruptio placentae	1.6 (1.1–2.6)	.03	3.6 (1.6–7.9)	<.01
Placenta previa	0.9 (0.5–1.8)	.89	2.5 (0.9–6.9)	.08
Cesarean delivery	1.1 (1.01–1.3)	.03	1.4 (1.04–1.8)	.02

OR, odds ratio; CI, confidence interval; IUGR, intrauterine growth restriction; PROM, premature rupture of membranes.

Weiss JL, Malone FD, Vidaver J, Ball RH, Nyberg DA, Comstock CH, et al. Threatened abortion: a risk factor for poor pregnancy outcome, a population-based screening study. FASTER Consortium. Am J Obstet Gynecol 2004;190:745–50. Copyright 2004 by Elsevier.

Maso G, D'Ottavio G, De Seta F, Sartore A, Piccoli M, Mandruzzato G. First-trimester intrauterine hematoma and outcome of pregnancy. Obstet Gynecol 2005;105:339–44.

Weiss JL, Malone FD, Vidaver J, Ball RH, Nyberg DA, Comstock CH, et al. Threatened abortion: a risk factor for poor pregnancy outcome, a population-based screening study. FASTER Consortium. Am J Obstet Gynecol 2004;190:745–50.

44

Elective cesarean delivery

A 41-year-old woman, gravida 1, comes to the office at 36 weeks of gestation for a routine prenatal visit. She conceived through in vitro fertilization (IVF). Ultrasonograms have shown a normally growing fetus in vertex presentation without gross anomalies. She desires a cesarean delivery, although she has no medical indications for cesarean delivery. She also would like a tubal ligation at the time of the cesarean delivery because she is not interested in further childbearing. You inform her that, compared with planned vaginal delivery, planned cesarean delivery is associated with a higher risk of

      (A) postpartum hemorrhage
*   (B) longer hospital stay
      (C) urinary incontinence
      (D) sexual dysfunction
      (E) neonatal mortality

Cesarean delivery on maternal request is defined as a cesarean delivery for a singleton pregnancy based solely on maternal request at term, in the absence of medical or obstetric indications. The true incidence of cesarean delivery on maternal request is unknown and probably varies widely in different countries. In the United States, the true incidence of cesarean delivery on maternal request has been estimated to be approximately 4–18% of all cesarean deliveries.

No randomized studies have compared planned vaginal delivery to cesarean delivery on maternal request for the woman carrying a singleton gestation at term. The only randomized trial data comes from term breech gestations. Compared with planned vaginal delivery, planned cesarean delivery for the full-term breech fetus is associated with a decrease in perinatal death or serious neonatal morbidity, but no difference in death or neurodevelopmental delay at 2 years after delivery. Maternal outcomes at 2 years are similar, with constipation significantly more common in the cesarean delivery group (27% versus 20%), but self-reported urinary incontinence is not significantly different (18% versus 22%).

The evidence to compare planned vaginal delivery with cesarean delivery in term vertex gestations is of either poor or moderate quality. Compared with planned vaginal delivery, planned cesarean delivery is associated with less postpartum hemorrhage but longer hospitalization and slightly worse neonatal respiratory morbidity, with all other outcomes based on weak evidence. Insufficient evidence is available to assess any effect of mode of delivery on urinary incontinence, sexual dysfunction, or neonatal mortality. Large randomized trials are needed to answer these questions. The necessary data are unavailable to recommend planned cesarean delivery compared with planned vaginal delivery for the singleton gestation at term. Therefore, it does not have to be discussed with all patients.

If a woman inquires regarding a cesarean delivery on maternal request, the risks and benefits of both approaches need to be discussed, with counseling tailored to each woman based on her personal and clinical situation. Factors such as the number of children planned, obesity, other medical and surgical history, and psychology can influence the risks of planned vaginal or cesarean delivery for the woman. Planned cesarean delivery may not be beneficial in a woman younger than 25 years who desires a large family (more than three children). The higher the number of cesarean deliveries, the higher the risk of significant complications, in particular from placenta previa or placenta accreta (Table 44-1). If the woman is fearful of labor, pain management strategies and reassurance should be addressed.

After proper individualized review and counseling, the woman may still request cesarean delivery based on her wishes alone. In this situation, most authorities and a recent National Institutes of Health statement agree that cesarean delivery on maternal request is a reasonable alternative to planned vaginal delivery. When a health care provider cannot support this request, it is appropriate to refer the woman to another health care provider.

Most women prefer a vaginal birth; others prefer the convenience and control of being able to plan the time of birth. Although some obstetrician–gynecologists have argued that there is no autonomy-based obligation to offer elective cesarean delivery, most likely the overall health and welfare of the woman will be promoted by proper counseling and discussion and by support of her final request.

TABLE 44-1. Risk of Complications (%) With Multiple Cesarean Deliveries

Complication	Cesarean Delivery (%)					
	First	**Second**	**Third**	**Fourth**	**Fifth**	**Sixth or More**
Hysterectomy (overall)	0.7	0.4	0.9	2.4	3.5	9.0
Placenta accreta (overall)	0.2	0.3	0.6	2.1	2.3	6.7
Placenta accreta (with known previa)	3	11	40	61	67*	

*Five or more cesarean deliveries.

Data from Silver RM, Landon MB, Rouse DJ, Leveno KJ, Spong CY, Thom EA, et al. Maternal morbidity associated with multiple repeat cesarean deliveries. Obstet Gynecol 2006;107:1226–32.

Hannah ME, Hannah WJ, Hewson SA, Hodnett ED, Saigal S, Willan AR. Planned caesarean section versus planned vaginal birth for breech presentation at term: a randomised multicentre trial. Term Breech Trial Collaborative Group. Lancet 2000;356:1375–83.

Hannah ME. Planned elective cesarean section: a reasonable choice for some women? CMAJ 2004;170:813–4.

Hofmeyr GJ, Hannah ME. Planned caesarean section for term breech delivery. Cochrane Database of Systematic Reviews 2003, Issue 2. Art. No.: CD000166. DOI: 10.1002/14651858.CD000166.

Minkoff H, Powderly KR, Chervenak F, McCullough LB. Ethical dimensions of elective primary cesarean delivery. Obstet Gynecol 2004; 103:387–92.

National Institutes of Health state-of-the-science conference statement: cesarean delivery on maternal request March 27-29, 2006. Obstet Gynecol 2006;107:1386–97.

Silver RM, Landon MB, Rouse DJ, Leveno KJ, Spong CY, Thom EA, et al. Maternal morbidity associated with multiple repeat cesarean deliveries. National Institute of Child Health and Human Development Maternal-Fetal Medicine Units Network. Obstet Gynecol 2006;107: 1226–32.

45

Cervical length

A 25-year-old primigravid woman, at 19 weeks of gestation, has a short cervical length of 20 mm documented on an anatomic ultrasonographic examination, confirmed by transvaginal ultrasonography. She is asymptomatic and has no risk factor for preterm birth. The most appropriate care is

    (A) cervical cerclage
    (B) monitoring for uterine contractions
    (C) tocolysis
    (D) hospitalization
*   (E) counseling regarding risks

Approximately 10% of all pregnant women screened in the second trimester by transvaginal ultrasonography have a cervical length less than 25 mm. This finding is associated with an increased risk of preterm birth. The shorter the cervical length, the higher is the risk of preterm birth. The earlier in gestation the short cervical length is detected, the higher the risk of preterm birth. The risk of preterm birth also depends on other patient characteristics, in particular other major risk factors (Appendix C). A woman with a cervical length less than 25 mm and no other risk factor for preterm birth should be counseled that she has approximately an 18–30% risk of preterm birth, which represents an increase over the risk in the general U.S. population (12%).

No intervention has been shown to decrease the risk of preterm birth in otherwise low-risk women with a short cervical length. Cerclage has been the only intervention tested by randomized trials. A meta-analysis of four trials on cerclage for short cervical length showed a nonsignificant 24% decrease in preterm birth in low-risk women who carry singleton gestations with a short cervical length. The largest randomized trial on this population failed to show a benefit from cerclage in prevention of preterm birth.

Women with a short cervical length in the second trimester have been shown to have asymptomatic uterine contractions. This association does not prove by itself clinical effectiveness of uterine monitoring in this population. In fact, there is no evidence that monitoring of uterine contractions is beneficial. No intervention has been studied aimed at women with a short cervical length and asymptomatic contractions.

No clinical trial has assessed the efficacy of tocolytic therapy in women with short cervical length. A meta-analysis based on cerclage trials showed no benefit of tocolysis for women with short cervical length in decreasing preterm birth before 35 weeks of gestation. Randomized clinical trials are needed before tocolysis can be recommended as a beneficial clinical intervention in asymptomatic women with short cervical length.

Hospitalization has not been studied specifically in women with a short cervical length by transvaginal ultrasonography. Hospitalization has not been shown to be associated with preterm birth prevention in any population in which it was assessed. In some populations at risk for preterm birth, such as women with multiple gestations, prophylactic hospitalization to prevent preterm birth actually is associated with an increase in preterm birth. There is insufficient evidence that bed rest, at home or in the hospital, is beneficial in women at risk of preterm birth in preventing preterm delivery. Bed rest can be associated with significant complications in pregnancy, including venous thromboembolism and decreased physical fitness. Bed rest is also associated with significant personal, institutional, and societal costs. In the absence of benefits and in the presence of potential risks, bed rest should not be suggested lightly in pregnancy, and should be recommended very rarely, if at all.

A recent placebo-controlled randomized clinical trial assessed the role of vaginal progesterone for the prevention of preterm birth at less than 34 weeks of gestation in women with a transvaginal cervical length of 1.5 cm or less. This finding suggested a benefit from treatment with vaginal progesterone. The study included a heterogeneous group of patients (twins, those with a prior preterm birth), so it is unclear whether this treatment should be offered in routine clinical care to women with a short cervix. The National Institute of Child Health and Human Development Maternal-Fetal Medicine Units (MFMU) Network currently is undertaking a study to assess the role of 17α-hydroxyprogesterone caproate in reducing the risk of preterm birth in women with a short cervix.

Berghella V, Obido AO, To MS, Rust OA, Althiusius SM. Cerclage for short cervix on ultrasonography: meta-analysis of trials using individual patient-level data. Obstet Gynecol 2005;106:181–9.

Berghella V, Rust OA, Althuisius SM. Short cervix on ultrasound: does indomethacin prevent preterm birth? Am J Obstet Gynecol 2006;195: 809–13.

Fonseca EB, Celik E, Parra M, Singh M, Nicolaides KH. Progesterone and the risk of preterm birth among women with a short cervix. Fetal Medicine Foundation Second Trimester Screening Group. N Engl J Med 2007;357:462–9.

Lewis D, Pelham JJ, Done E, Sawhney H, Talucci M, Berghella V. Uterine contractions in asymptomatic pregnant women with a short cervix on ultrasound. J Matern Fetal Neonatal Med 2005;18:325–8.

To MS, Alfirevic Z, Heath VC, Cicero S, Cacho AM, Williamson PR, et al. Cervical cerclage for prevention of preterm delivery in women with short cervix: randomised controlled trial. Fetal Medicine Foundation Second Trimester Screening Group. Lancet 2004;363:1849–53.

Vermeulen GM, Bruinse HW. Prophylactic administration of clindamycin 2% vaginal cream to reduce the incidence of spontaneous preterm birth in women with an increased recurrence risk: a randomised placebo-controlled double-blind trial. Br J Obstet Gynaecol 1999; 106:652–7.

46

Neonatal outcomes

A 25-year-old primigravid woman who has had an uncomplicated pregnancy presents to the labor and delivery department at 28 weeks of gestation with leaking fluid. On examination, you confirm ruptured membranes. Ultrasonography shows an amniotic fluid index (AFI) of 3.4 cm, a vertex-presenting fetus with a normal anatomic survey, and an estimated fetal weight of 1,100 g. You counsel her that if the baby is delivered in the next few days, there is a greater than 50% chance of

      (A) necrotizing enterocolitis
*   (B) postnatal growth delay
      (C) chronic lung disease
      (D) intracranial hemorrhage
      (E) periventricular leukomalacia

Patients with premature rupture of membranes can be expected to give birth within a short time. With expectant management, some will have a long latent period, but approximately 75% will give birth within a week. Therefore, an important component of the care of these patients is to prepare for the delivery of a preterm infant, including counseling the parents about outcome. Although pediatrics or neonatology consults are helpful, obstetrician input is also important to the family.

Neonatal morbidity and mortality can be either weight-based or gestational age-based. Mortality is uncommon at this gestational age and fetal weight. If the pregnancy continues, risk of morbidity and mortality will decrease further. The mortality in most centers at 28 weeks of gestation or 1,100 g is approximately 5%. The main medical and counseling issues therefore involve morbidities.

The most common immediate morbidity in this age and weight category is respiratory distress syndrome, with an incidence of approximately 44%. In a recent collaborative report, the incidence in participating centers ranged from 23% to 63%. Antenatal therapy with corticosteroids is indicated in this patient in order to minimize this risk.

Other common complications of very low birth weight (VLBW) neonates include necrotizing enterocolitis, with an incidence of 5% at this gestational age and weight, and patent ductus arteriosus, with an incidence of 25%. Periventricular leukomalacia has an incidence of 4%. The true incidence of intraventricular hemorrhage is harder to ascertain. By grade of intraventricular hemorrhage, the data from a large National Institutes of Health collaborative report show an incidence of 8% for grades 3 and 4, 4% for grade 2, and 15% for grade 1. However, the ranges between centers were wide, and protocols for ultrasonographic diagnosis were not uniform. Therefore, intraventricular hemorrhage may be underreported. This morbidity in the neonate is also reduced with use of antenatal corticosteroids, which was given to 74% of fetuses in this cohort at this weight category.

Unlike respiratory distress syndrome, chronic lung disease is not reduced with corticosteroid use in the mother before birth. The incidence of chronic lung disease is 15% in this weight group. Chronic lung disease has been measured in a number of ways, including the neonate's need for oxygen at discharge and at 28 days of life, and the fetus at 36 postmenstrual weeks. Depending on which calculated method is used, the incidence is approximately 10–25%.

Postnatal growth delay is defined as weight below the 10th percentile at 36 weeks postmenstrual age. This is a much more common problem than those described above with an incidence of 97%. This is true in all weight categories and is not decreased in incidence with increasing gestational age or weight at delivery in VLBW babies. Some studies have attempted to look at the reasons for this morbidity. In the National Institute of Child Health and Human Development Neonatal Research Network data, postnatal growth during hospitalization was not affected by race or sex, but was related to in-hospital morbidities. Newborns who had the highest weight gain were those who did not develop severe complications, such as chronic lung disease, severe intraventricular hemorrhage, necrotizing enterocolitis, or sepsis. Rapid weight gain was associated with less need for parenteral nutrition and earlier initiation of enteral feedings. As a result, investigators identify two issues: 1) the overall severity of the neonate's condition; and 2) nutritional. As one might expect, babies who are able to feed normally at an earlier age gain weight more rapidly.

Ehrenkranz RA, Younes N, Lemons JA, Fanaroff AA, Donovan EF, Wright LL, et al. Longitudinal growth of hospitalized very low birth weight infants. Pediatrics 1999;104:280–9.

Lemons JA, Bauer CR, Oh W, Korones SB, Papile L, Stoll BJ, et al. Very low birth weight outcomes of the National Institute of Child Health and Human Development Neonatal Research Network, January 1995 through December 1996. NICHD Neonatal Research Network. Pediatrics 2001;107:E1.

Premature rupture of membranes. ACOG Practice Bulletin No. 80. American College of Obstetricians and Gynecologists. Obstet Gynecol 2007;109:1007–19.

47

Cerebral palsy

A 34-year-old primigravid woman presents in spontaneous preterm labor at 34 weeks of gestation. Her pregnancy to date has been uncomplicated. She remains afebrile during the course of labor. During the second stage of labor, the fetal monitor shows an 11-minute end-stage bradycardia. She pushes effectively and spontaneously gives birth to a newborn weighing 1,899 g (4 1b 3 oz) and having Apgar scores of 6 and 9. The infant requires minimal resuscitation. Umbilical arterial cord blood gases include a pH of 7.15, a P_{CO_2} of 70 mm Hg, and a base excess of –8 mmol/L. The neonatal course was uncomplicated. During early childhood, cerebral palsy is diagnosed. The most likely cause of this diagnosis is

* (A) developmental defect
* (B) prematurity
* (C) chorioamnionitis
* (D) intrauterine fetal stroke
* (E) acidemia

The erroneous view that neonatal brain injury is uniform and results primarily from acquired insults such as birth asphyxia is slowly being modified by advances in neuroimaging and diagnostic laboratory techniques. Cerebral palsy is a chronic central nervous system disorder of movement or posture, which manifests early in life, and is not the result of progressive disease. The condition is frequently accompanied by seizure disorders, sensory impairment, and cognitive limitations. For singleton pregnancies, most commonly, cerebral palsy is a developmental event that is not preventable given the current state of knowledge and technology.

Extreme prematurity, birth weight less than 1,000 g, and multiple gestation are significant risk factors for the later development of cerebral palsy. In this very low birth weight category, the rate of subsequent cerebral palsy is in the range of 8–10%. The criteria to define an acute intrapartum event sufficient to cause cerebral palsy are shown in Box 47-1.

Neonatal brain injury in the very premature infant often eludes diagnosis because obvious signs are lacking or because signs that are present are attributed to developmental immaturity. In the case described, the newborn is only 3 weeks premature and of satisfactory birth weight. Cerebral palsy due to prematurity would not be expected to occur.

Recent data confirm the observation that a diagnosis of chorioamnionitis during pregnancy is associated with an increased risk of cerebral palsy in infants who weigh 2,500 g or more at birth. In very premature infants, the association of infection with cerebral palsy has been less consistent and, when present, less strong. Intrauterine exposure to infections other than toxoplasmosis, rubella, cytomegalovirus, and herpes simplex virus (TORCH) infections has been estimated to result in approximately 12% of otherwise unexplained spastic cerebral palsy in nonmalformed singleton infants of normal birth weight.

BOX 47-1

Essential Criteria Sufficient to Cause Cerebral Palsy (Must Meet All Four Criteria)

1. Evidence of a metabolic acidosis in fetal umbilical cord arterial blood obtained at delivery (pH less than 7 and base deficit 12 mmol/L or more)
2. Early onset of severe or moderate neonatal encephalopathy in infants born at 34 or more weeks of gestation
3. Cerebral palsy of the spastic quadriplegic or dyskinetic type*
4. Exclusion of other identifiable etiologies such as trauma, coagulation disorders, infectious conditions, or genetic disorders

---

*Spastic quadriplegia and, less commonly, dyskinetic cerebral palsy are the only types of cerebral palsy associated with acute hypoxic intrapartum events. Spastic quadriplegia is not specific to intrapartum hypoxia. Hemiparetic cerebral palsy, hemiplegic cerebral palsy, spastic diplegia, and ataxia are unlikely to result from acute intrapartum hypoxia. (Nelson KB, Grether JK. Potentially asphyxiating conditions and spastic cerebral palsy in infants of normal birth weight. Am J Obstet Gynecol 1998;179:507–13.)

Modified from MacLennan A. A template for defining a casual relation between acute intrapartum events and cerebral palsy: international consensus statement. BMJ 1999;319:1054–9.

Randomized trials of the use of antibiotics during pregnancy have been designed to investigate the outcomes of pregnancy or birth. Such trials have not been large enough nor have they monitored children long enough to examine whether such therapy can reduce the risk of cerebral palsy. In this patient, however, there was no antenatal or intrapartum history or signs of infection.

Perinatal stroke, with an incidence of one in 4,000 term infants, is not synonymous with cerebral palsy; however, in some neonates who have strokes, hemiparetic cerebral palsy does develop. The presenting sign of such a complication is unilateral weakness or paralysis, which was not described in the above case, making arterial ischemic stroke unlikely. Factors that contribute to the vulnerability of the fetus or infant to stroke are inherited or acquired thrombophilia in the mother or infant, placental thrombosis, infection, and the use of intravascular catheters.

Umbilical artery base excess measurements are the most direct method to rule out fetal metabolic acidosis. To establish a threshold of metabolic acidosis that is associated with newborn central nervous system complications, the course of 174 full term newborns with a range of umbilical artery base excess was examined. Ten percent of infants with a base excess of −12 mmol/L to −16 mmol/L developed moderate and severe newborn encephalopathy and respiratory complications. This increased to 80% among infants with the most severe metabolic acidosis (buffer base less than −22 mmol/L). A 14% incidence of major deficits and a 27% incidence of minor deficits at 1 year of age was found among infants with a newborn buffer base of less than −34 mmol/L. Therefore, most cases of newborn encephalopathy resolve and do not lead to permanent injury. The elevated PCO_2 allows the conclusion that the acidemia in the above case is respiratory in origin and the base excess values in the above case rule out metabolic acidosis. Respiratory acidosis alone is generally not associated with newborn complications and is not the cause of the subsequent cerebral palsy.

American College of Obstetricians and Gynecologists. Neonatal encephalopathy and cerebral palsy: defining the pathogenesis and pathophysiology. Washington, DC: ACOG; 2003.

Clark SL, Hankins GD. Temporal and demographic trends in cerebral palsy—fact and fiction. Am J Obstet Gynecol 2003;188:628–33.

Ferriero DM. Neonatal brain injury. N Engl J Med 2004;351:1985–95.

Nelson KB. Can we prevent cerebral palsy? N Engl J Med 2003;349: 1765–9.

Ross MG, Gala R. Use of umbilical artery base excess: algorithm for the timing of hypoxic injury. Am J Obstet Gynecol 2002;187:1–9.

48

Cocaine use

A 32-year-old woman who is a known cocaine user is seen in the obstetric triage area at 30 weeks of gestation with palpitations, chest pain, abdominal pain, and vaginal bleeding. The common link between her cocaine use and these specific symptoms is drug-induced

*   (A) vasoconstriction of myocardial and uterine blood vessels
    (B) direct myocardial and uterine cellular toxic effect
    (C) displacement of carrier-bound thyroxine (T_4) and triiodothyronine (T_3)
    (D) corticotropin secretion
    (E) acute thrombocytopenia

Cocaine (benzoylecgonine) is an alkaloid extracted from the leaf of the coca bush (*Erythroxylon coca*). It is available as pure cocaine or "coke" powder, which is inhaled and passes through the nasal mucosa and as "crack" cocaine, which is made by adding cocaine powder to water and baking soda, and boiling the water off. The resulting mixture is smoked with special glass pipes or silver foil, although it can be injected after rediluting with water. It is rapidly absorbed into the bloodstream producing a "high" in approximately 6–8 minutes.

Cocaine use is found in all socioeconomic groups. Incidence varies widely, from 0.8% to 16%, depending on the population studied. With the greater availability of less expensive forms of cocaine, use has increased. Thus, many clinicians will treat patients who have complications from use of this illegal recreational drug.

The major clinical effects of cocaine are mediated by alterations in synaptic transmission. Cocaine blocks the presynaptic reuptake of norepinephrine and dopamine, producing an excess of these neurotransmitters at the site of the postsynaptic receptor. In short, cocaine acts as a powerful sympathomimetic vasoconstrictor agent, with resulting hypertension. Such acute increases in hypertension are directly related to abruptio placentae and to myocardial ischemia and infarction. The signs and symptoms in this patient reflect the frequently observed association of acute hypertension and abruptio placentae and the pathologic cardiac consequences of acute increases in after-load pressure.

In long-term users, other cardiac complications of cocaine use result from thrombus formation within the coronary arteries, left ventricular hypertrophy, and systolic dysfunction. Therefore, cardiac and uterine complications are not due to direct toxic effects of cocaine on myocardial or uterine tissue.

Many of the signs and symptoms described are found in association with hyperthyroidism. Pregnancy-associated hormone changes, specifically increasing estrogen levels, are associated with changes in thyroid function but not a release of or an increase in clinically significant amounts of free thyroid hormones. Thyroid storm may result from untreated or uncontrolled hyperthyroidism; however, there is no evidence of a relationship between cocaine use and hyperthyroidism or thyroid storm.

Cocaine does induce a rapid increase in corticotropin secretion that modulates responsivity to stress and sexual behavior. This process speeds the enhancement of perceived pleasure and diminution of concern about environmental stressors. The action and its acknowledged consequences are not associated with the described signs and symptoms.

Thrombocytopenia was studied within a cohort of 1,900 women screened for substance use in pregnancy at the Yale–New Haven prenatal clinic. Of these women, 709 subjects had platelet counts performed and 19 of the 709 (2.6%) exhibited a low platelet count (range, $35–148 \times 10^9$/L). The results indicate that cocaine use is an independent risk factor for thrombocytopenia in an inner-city parturient population. The mechanism resulting in cocaine-associated thrombocytopenia is unknown. In isolation, this finding would not be expected to be clinically associated with the described signs and symptoms.

Ecker JL, Musci TJ. Thyroid function and disease in pregnancy. Curr Probl Obstet Gynecol Fertil 2000;23:110–22.

Kain ZN, Mayes LC, Pakes J, Rosenbaum SH, Schottenfeld R. Thrombocytopenia in pregnant women who use cocaine. Am J Obstet Gynecol 1995;173:885–90.

Lange RA, Hillis LD. Cardiovascular complications of cocaine use [published erratum appears in N Engl J Med 2001;345:1432]. N Engl J Med 2001;345:351–8.

Mendelson JH, Mello NK. Management of cocaine abuse and dependence. N Engl J Med 1996;334:965–72.

49

Labor induction

A 34-year-old woman, gravida 3, para 1, comes to the office at 39 weeks of gestation for a prenatal visit. Her previous delivery was by low transverse cesarean breech delivery. Her cervix is long, closed, posterior, midposition, and soft. The patient is interested in a trial of labor. The best approach is

* (A) await spontaneous labor
  (B) begin cervical ripening with the Foley catheter
  (C) perform a cesarean delivery
  (D) begin cervical ripening with misoprostol

As the rate of cesarean deliveries in the United States continues to climb, the number of women who are candidates for vaginal birth after cesarean delivery (VBAC) can be expected to increase. With subsequent pregnancies after a cesarean delivery, the patient must choose between a repeat cesarean delivery and VBAC. The rate of VBAC rose from 3.1% in 1981 to 31% in 1998, but reports of worse outcomes associated with VBAC may have contributed to the drop in use of VBAC to 10.6% in 2003.

It has been standard management to consider induction of labor safe in women who have a history of a low transverse cesarean delivery. However, a recent publication suggested a marked increased risk of uterine rupture in women with a prior cesarean delivery who receive prostaglandins for labor induction. This publication was based on birth certificate data and, therefore, has serious methodological limitations. Two large observational studies have shed light on the relationship between labor induction, augmentation, and uterine rupture. Taken together, the results of these studies suggest a small increase in the risk of uterine rupture with labor induction. One study suggested a substantial increase in risk when sequential prostaglandins and oxytocin are used. The Foley catheter has become a popular preinduction cervical ripening agent and, in some studies, has not been associated with an increased risk of uterine rupture in women who had a previous cesarean delivery and induction of labor versus women who were in spontaneous labor.

A recent study showed that the risk for uterine rupture was higher when the Foley catheter was used for preinduction cervical ripening than when women entered spontaneous labor. All of the uterine ruptures occurred after extrusion of the catheter and after the beginning of oxytocin. The Society of Obstetricians and Gynaecologists of Canada has stated that "a Foley catheter may be safely used to ripen the cervix in a woman planning a trial of labor after cesarean section."

A much more compelling case can be made for the avoidance of misoprostol as an induction agent in women who have a previous cesarean delivery. After several reports of uterine scar disruption in women who had a previous cesarean delivery and were given misoprostol, the American College of Obstetricians and Gynecologists stated that "until reassuring studies are available, misoprostol is not recommended for cervical ripening in patients who have had prior cesarean delivery."

Women who have a previous low transverse cesarean delivery who desire VBAC and require induction of labor should be counseled that their risk of uterine scar disruption is higher than if they entered spontaneous labor. If they require preinduction cervical ripening, this increases the risk. The Foley catheter may represent a safer method for preinduction cervical ripening than prostaglandin preparations. Furthermore, it should be noted that among women who require induction of labor who have had a previous cesarean delivery, the rate of cesarean delivery remains high at approximately 60%.

Hoffman MK, Sciscione A, Srinivasana M, Shackelford DP, Ekbladh L. Uterine rupture in patients with a prior cesarean delivery: the impact of cervical ripening. Am J Perinat 2004;21:217–22.

Induction of labor for vaginal birth after cesarean delivery. ACOG Committee Opinion No. 342. American College of Obstetricians and Gynecologists. Obstet Gynecol 2006;108:465–7.

Landon MB, Hauth JC, Leveno KJ, Spong CY, Leindecker S, Varner MW, et al. Maternal and perinatal outcomes associated with a trial of labor after prior cesarean delivery. N Engl J Med 2004;351:2581–9.

Lydon-Rochelle M, Holt V, Easterling TR, Martin D. Risk of uterine rupture during labor among women with a prior Cesarean delivery. N Engl J Med 2001;345:3–8.

Macones GA, Peipert J, Nelson DB, Odibo A, Stevens EJ, Stamilio DM, et al. Maternal complications with vaginal birth after cesarean delivery: a multicenter study. Am J Obstet Gynecol 2005;193:1656–62.

Ravasia DJ, Wood SL, Pollard JK. Uterine rupture during induced trial of labor among women with previous cesarean delivery. Am J Obstet Gynecol 2000;183:1176–9.

Vaginal birth after previous cesarean delivery. ACOG Practice Bulletin No. 54. American College of Obstetricians and Gynecologists. Obstet Gynecol 2004;104:203–12.

50

Migraine

A 28-year-old woman, gravida 2, para 1, at 8 weeks of gestation comes to the emergency department because of a severe, right-sided, throbbing headache accompanied by photophobia, nausea, and repeated vomiting. The headache began 20 hours ago, and she has taken 3 g of oral acetaminophen and 50 mg of oral promethazine hydrochloride (Phenergan). She has a 10-year history of similar headaches, which occur about once per month. Physical and neurologic examinations are normal. The best next step in her management is to prescribe

* (A) intravenous morphine
  (B) subcutaneous sumatriptan succinate (Imitrex)
  (C) oral propranolol (Inderal)
  (D) intravenous dihydroergotamine
  (E) oral codeine

The patient has severe migraine without aura. The diagnosis is based on a 10-year history of recurrent headaches that are unilateral, throbbing, last for hours, and are accompanied by photophobia, nausea, vomiting, and a normal examination.

Approximately 20% of pregnant women have migraine headaches. Migraine improves during pregnancy approximately 70% of the time, usually after the first trimester. Migraine itself seems to have no effect on the course and outcome of pregnancy. It is a complex, recurrent syndrome, the pathogenesis of which is poorly understood. The most common types of migraine are migraine with and without aura. Examples of rare types are hemiplegic migraine, aura without headache, and basilar migraine.

Drug treatment of migraine may be classified under two headings, nonspecific and migraine-specific (Box 50-1). Ergot alkaloids are nonselective serotonin receptor agonists and should not be used in pregnancy because of their oxytocic, vasoconstrictor, and teratogenic effects. Isometheptene is a sympathomimetic drug whose efficacy and safety in pregnancy are unclear. The selective serotonin receptor agonists or triptans have revolutionized the short-term treatment of migraine. The triptans have been available for more than 10 years, but their use in pregnancy is still controversial. Among the triptans, data are most available for sumatriptan because it is the triptan that has been on the market the longest, is the most widely used, and is available for oral, nasal, rectal, and subcutaneous administration. The data so far consist of case–control studies, prescription-linkage studies, open-label pharmacovigilance studies, and pregnancy registries. The studies have been reviewed and criticized as being retrospective, observational, containing small sample sizes, having unknown dose and duration of sumatriptan exposure, and for the absence of data regarding concomitant medication use or exposure to other terato-

---

BOX 50-1

Selected Medications for the Treatment of Acute Migraine

Nonspecific
Acetaminophen
Nonsteroidal antiinflammatory drugs
    Aspirin
    Ibuprofen
    Naproxen
Caffeine
Butalbital
Antiemetics
    Promethazine
    Prochlorperazine
    Metoclopramide
Narcotics
    Morphine
    Meperidine
    Codeine
    Hydrocodone
    Butorphanol

Migraine-specific
Ergot alkaloids (contraindicated in pregnancy)
    Ergotamine
    Dihydroergotamine
Sympathomimetics
    Isometheptene
5-HT agonists

Shorter half-life
    Sumatriptan
    Rizatriptan
    Zolmitriptan
    Almotriptan
    Eletriptan

Longer half-life
    Naratriptan
    Frovatriptan

gens. Caution should be exercised in recommending use of sumatriptan during pregnancy.

For this patient, the best choice of treatment would be intravenous morphine. She needs parenteral therapy for prolonged, severe migraine headache that is accompanied by repeated vomiting. There are problems with narcotic use for migraine headache, such as drug-seeking behavior and differentiating narcotic withdrawal headache from migraine. Narcotic use in migraine should be limited to patients with severe, intractable headaches.

Insufficient evidence is available to recommend sumatriptan in this patient. Propranolol, a nonselective β-blocker, has been used for migraine prophylaxis in pregnancy. Because the patient is in the first trimester and the probability of spontaneous remission after the first trimester approaches 70%, one would not commence prophylactic medication. In addition, a history of two or more severe migraine attacks per month is a generally accepted indication for migraine prophylaxis, and this patient has only one attack per month. Intravenous dihy-

droergotamine is contraindicated in pregnancy. Oral codeine is a poor choice because the patient is vomiting.

Briggs GG, Freeman RK, Yaffe SJ. Drugs in pregnancy and lactation. 7th ed. Philadelphia (PA): Lippincott Williams & Wilkins; 2005. p. 1515–8.

Fox AW, Diamond ML, Spierings EL. Migraine during pregnancy: options for therapy. CNS Drugs 2005;19:465–81.

Hilaire ML, Cross LB, Eichner SF. Treatment of migraine headaches with sumatriptan in pregnancy. Ann Pharmacother 2004;38:1726–30.

Loder E. Safety of sumatriptan in pregnancy: a review of data so far. CNS Drugs 2003;17:1–7.

Maggioni F, Allessi C, Maggino T, Zanchin G. Headache during pregnancy. Cephalalgia 1997;17:765–9.

Snow V, Weiss K, Wall EM, Mottur-Pilson C. Pharmacologic management of acute attacks of migraine and prevention of migraine headache. American Academy of Family Physicians, American College of Physicians—American Society of Internal Medicine. Ann Intern Med 2002;137:840–9.

Von Wald T, Walling AD. Headache during pregnancy. Obstet Gynecol Surv 2002;57:179–85.

51

Diagnosis of placenta previa

A 30-year-old woman, para 3, gravida 2, at 34 weeks of gestation, with a history of one previous cesarean delivery for a breech presentation, reports vaginal bleeding. At 20 weeks of gestation, she had an ultrasound examination that revealed a complete placenta previa. On transvaginal ultrasound examination today (Fig. 51-1), the placental location is most consistent with a

    (A) complete placenta previa
    (B) partial placenta previa
*   (C) marginal placenta previa
    (D) low-lying placenta
    (E) placenta accreta

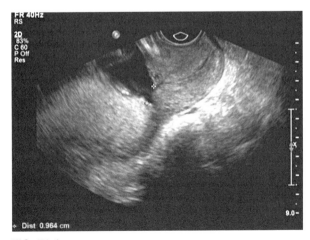

FIG. 51-1.

Transvaginal ultrasonography is a powerful tool in the diagnosis of placenta previa. It uses higher ultrasound frequencies than transabdominal ultrasonography does, and such higher frequencies provide better resolution or a clearer ultrasonographic image. In addition, the transvaginal probes can be placed closer to the region of interest, namely the cervix and placenta, therefore yielding high-quality images of the relationship between the placenta and the internal cervical os.

The incidence of placenta previa has been estimated to be approximately 0.5% at delivery and 1.1% at 15–20 weeks of gestation using transvaginal ultrasonography. Therefore, most of the cases of placenta previa diagnosed during the second trimester of pregnancy will resolve by the time term approaches. However, in patients with a previous cesarean delivery, the incidence of placenta previa is directly related to the number of previous cesarean deliveries (Table 51-1).

In placenta previa, the placenta is implanted low in the uterine cavity and covers the internal cervical os. Four different subtypes of placenta previa are recognized (Box 51-1).

Placenta accreta occurs when there is an absence of the normal intervening decidua basalis and the fibrinoid Nitabuch layer resulting in an abnormally adherent placenta. This is the most common type of the abnormally adherent placenta.

In placenta increta, the abnormally adherent placenta has invaded into the myometrium. This constitutes the second most common type of abnormally adherent placenta.

The less commonly encountered form of abnormally adherent placenta is the placenta percreta. In this situation, the placenta invades through the entire myometrial wall and serosa and may involve other organs such as the bladder.

The incidence of abnormally adherent placentas is increasing as numbers of cesarean deliveries and placenta previa increase. In the 1930s to 1950s, the rate of placenta accreta was estimated to be 1 in 30,000; in the 1980s, the rate was 1 in 2,500; and, more recently, it has been estimated at 1 in 533. In a study done in the 1980s, the investigators found the risk of a placenta previa in the unscarred uterus was 0.26% and that it increased almost linearly with the number of prior cesarean deliveries to 10% in patients with four or more prior cesarean deliveries. But with a placenta previa and one previous cesarean delivery, the risk of placenta accreta was 24%; this risk continued to increase to 67% with a placenta previa and four or more cesarean deliveries. More recently, another group of investigators found that the most important risk factors for placenta accreta besides a previous cesarean delivery were placenta previa, followed by two or more cesarean deliveries, and advancing maternal age (Table 51-2).

TABLE 51-1. Relationship of Placenta Previa to Number of Previous Cesarean Deliveries

No. of Previous Cesarean Deliveries	Incidence of Placenta Previa* (%)
0	0.3
1	0.8
2	2
3 or more	4.2

*All differences are statistically significant ($P < .01$).

Miller DA, Chollet JA, Goodwin TM. Clinical risk factors for placenta previa–placenta accreta. Am J Obstet Gynecol 1997; 177:211.

BOX 51-1

Classification of Placenta Previa*

1. *Complete.* The internal cervical os is completely covered by placenta; the term is commonly applied to placentas centrally implanted over the internal os.
2. *Partial.* As the name implies, the placenta only partially covers the internal cervical os.
3. *Marginal.* The inferior-most edge of the placenta reaches but does not cover the internal cervical os. When imaged by transvaginal ultrasonography, the distance between the lowest-most edge and the placenta and the internal cervical os can be measured; if this measurement is 2 cm or less, the placenta is considered to be a marginal previa.
4. *Low-lying.* The placenta is in the lower uterine segment and is located a minimum of 2 cm from the internal cervical os.

Adapted from Oyelese Y, Smulian JC. Placenta previa, placenta accreta, and vasa previa. Obstet Gynecol 2006; 107:927–41.

TABLE 51-2. Risk Factors for Placenta Accreta, Identified Using Conditional Logistic Regression, in University of Chicago Hospitals, 1982–2002

Risk Factor	Odds Ratio	95% Confidence Interval	P Value
Age (years)	1.14	1.08–1.19	<.0001
Previous cesarean deliveries			
One	2.2	0.96–4.86	0.064
Two or more	8.6	3.53–21.07	<.0001
Placenta previa	51.4	10.65–248.39	<.0001

Wu S, Kocherginsky M, Hibbard JU. Abnormal placentation: twenty-year analysis. Am J Obstet Gynecol 2005;192:1460.

Clark SL, Koonings PP, Phelan JP. Placenta previa/accreta and prior cesarean section. Obstet Gynecol 1985;66:89–92.

Miller DA, Chollet JA, Goodwin TM. Clinical risk factors for placenta previa-placenta accreta. Am J Obstet Gynecol 1997;177:210–4.

Oyelese Y, Smulian JC. Placenta previa, placenta accreta, and vasa previa. Obstet Gynecol 2006;107:927–41.

Silver RM, Landon MB, Rouse DJ, Leveno KJ, Spong CY, Thom EA, et al. Maternal morbidity associated with multiple repeat cesarean deliveries. National Institute of Child Health and Human Development Maternal-Fetal Medicine Units Network. Obstet Gynecol 2006;107: 1226–32.

Wu S, Kocherginsky M, Hibbard JU. Abnormal placentation: twenty-year analysis. Am J Obstet Gynecol 2005;192:1458–61.

52

Herpesvirus and preterm premature rupture of membranes

A woman with a known history of recurrent genital herpes is admitted to the hospital at 28 weeks of gestation with preterm premature rupture of membranes (preterm PROM). On hospital day 1, she develops a herpes lesion on her left labium. The most appropriate next step is

    (A) immediate induction of labor
    (B) immediate cesarean delivery
*   (C) immediate antiviral treatment
    (D) antiviral treatment at 34 weeks of gestation
    (E) delivery at 34 weeks of gestation

Most genital herpes infections are due to the herpes simplex virus type 2 (HSV-2) and are characterized by recurrent, painful vesicular and ulcerative lesions in the genital and anal areas. Although herpes simplex virus type 1 (HSV-1) also can result in genital infection, it is more typical that infection with HSV-1 will manifest as recurrent orolabial and facial lesions. A recent study that assessed data from the National Health and Nutrition Examination Survey (NHANES) indicated that the seroprevalence of HSV-2 in the United States decreased by 19% in persons aged 14–49 years between 1994 and 2004, in contrast to prior study findings that HSV-2 seroprevalence was increasing. Nonetheless, approximately 17% of pregnant women are seropositive for HSV-2, and an additional 2% will become seropositive during pregnancy. Although recurrent infections rarely result in serious maternal sequelae, both HSV-1 and HSV-2 genital infection can result in neonatal infection.

Neonatal HSV infection occurs in up to 1 in 3,200 live births, with an estimated incidence of 1,500 cases in the United States annually. Neonatal HSV infection causes disseminated or central nervous system (CNS) disease in approximately 50% of cases. Up to 30% of these infants will die, and up to 40% of survivors will have neurologic damage, despite antiviral therapy. Most cases of neonatal HSV infection are the consequence of vaginal delivery of a neonate through an infected birth canal. In patients with recurrent HSV infection, vertical transmission can occur in up to 3% of neonates who are delivered vaginally. Therefore, induction of labor at any gestational age in a patient with active genital herpes is generally contraindicated.

In patients with active HSV infection and ruptured membranes at or near term, cesarean delivery is indicated. However, the decision to perform a cesarean delivery depends on whether active lesions are present at the time of delivery. In pregnancies with preterm PROM remote from term and active HSV, especially in women with recurrent disease, the risk of prematurity must be weighed against the potential risk of neonatal disease. In such patients, an expectant management approach is increasingly favored, to allow time for maturation of the fetus, as opposed to immediate delivery. If the pregnancy is continued, treatment with an antiviral agent is indicated. Although delivery at 34 weeks might be a feasible management option with preterm PROM remote from term, in this case where there is an active herpes lesion, delivery at 34 weeks would not be the most appropriate next step in management of this patient. Treatment of an active lesion in the context of ruptured membranes should occur at the time of the outbreak to decrease risk to the fetus.

Several antiviral agents are commercially available for treatment of herpes (Appendix D). Acyclovir, a pregnancy category B medication, has been shown to reduce viral shedding, reduce pain, and heal lesions faster than placebo. Numerous studies have demonstrated its safety when used during pregnancy. The newer antiherpetic drugs, valacyclovir and famciclovir, are also pregnancy risk category B medications and are both approved for the treatment of primary genital herpes, the treatment of episodes of recurrent disease, and the daily treatment for suppression of outbreaks of recurrent genital herpes. Although these new agents are not well studied in pregnancy, small studies have been done with similar beneficial effects in decreasing viral shedding and decreasing cesarean birth rates in patients with genital herpes, also with similar safety profiles. The decision of which agent is used will depend on cost, availability, and physician preference.

Brown ZA, Gardella C, Wald A, Morrow RA, Corey L. Genital herpes complicating pregnancy [published errata appear in Obstet Gynecol 2006;107:428; Obstet Gynecol 2007;109:207]. Obstet Gynecol 2005;106:845–56.

Brown ZA, Selke S, Zeh J, Kopelman J, Maslow A, Ashley R, et al. The acquisition of herpes simplex virus during pregnancy. N Engl J Med 1997;337:509–15.

Major CA, Towers CV, Lewis DF, Garite TJ. Expectant management of preterm premature rupture of membranes complicated by active recurrent genital herpes. Am J Obstet Gynecol 2003;188:1551–4; discussion 1554–5.

Management of herpes in pregnancy. ACOG Practice Bulletin Number 82. American College of Obstetricians and Gynecologists. Obstet Gynecol 2007;109:1489–98.

Sheffield JS, Hollier LM, Hill JB, Stuart GS, Wendel GD. Acyclovir prophylaxis to prevent herpes simplex virus recurrence at delivery: a systematic review. Obstet Gynecol 2003;102:1396–403.

Xu F, Sternberg MR, Kottiri BJ, McQuillan GM, Lee FK, Nahmias AJ, et al. Trends in herpes simplex virus type 1 and type 2 seroprevalence in the United States. JAMA 2006;296:964–73.

53

Preterm birth

A 36-year-old woman, gravida 4, comes to the office for a prenatal visit at 12 weeks of gestation. She has a history of two first-trimester spontaneous pregnancy losses, without dilation and curettage (D&C), followed by a spontaneous preterm birth at 30 weeks of gestation. She works 40 hours per week and remarried before this conception. Her most significant risk factor for recurrent preterm birth is

      (A) maternal age 35 years or older
*   (B) prior preterm birth
      (C) prior first-trimester losses
      (D) workload of 40 hours per week
      (E) new father of the baby

Preterm birth remains the number one cause of perinatal mortality in the United States, with more than 500,000 births between 20 and 36 6/7 weeks of gestation in 2005 (incidence, 12.7%). Although its pathophysiology remains unclear, a number of factors have been associated with spontaneous preterm birth (Appendix E). It is important to make a complete assessment of each patient's risk for this occurrence because preventive strategies may vary depending on the risk factor(s) present. For example, weekly injections of 17α-hydroxyprogesterone caproate have been shown to decrease the risk of recurrent spontaneous preterm birth in women with a prior preterm birth. However, this approach has not been tested extensively among women with other risk factors.

An accurate medical history should be taken in all pregnant women regarding risk factors for spontaneous preterm birth, including obstetric and gynecologic history, maternal lifestyle, and prepregnancy weight. Even combinations of clinical risk factors do not have a high predictive accuracy for delivery within a week, especially in asymptomatic women. Interventions based on combinations of risk factors or a "risk score" have not been efficacious in prevention of preterm birth.

Of all risk factors for preterm birth (Appendix E), the one usually most significantly associated with an increased risk of preterm birth is a prior preterm birth, with odds ratios of around 3–5. Maternal age of 35 years or more, usually referred to as advanced maternal age, is associated with an increased risk of preterm birth, with odds ratios of around 1.5–2. This risk is less than that associated with prior preterm birth.

A prior first spontaneous trimester loss usually has not been associated with an increased risk for preterm birth by itself. Multiple pregnancy losses, with D&Cs, are associated with an increased risk of preterm birth, with odds ratios of around 1.3–1.5. The risk of preterm birth increases with the number of D&Cs, especially when performed for voluntary terminations.

Number of hours at work has been shown to be associated with preterm birth in some but not the majority of studies. Physically demanding work, prolonged standing, and night and shift work have been associated with an increased risk of preterm birth, usually with odd ratios around 1.2–1.4. New father of the baby is not associated with an effect on the risk of preterm birth.

Goldenberg RL, Iams JD, Mercer BM, Meis PJ, Moawad AH, Copper RL, et al. The preterm prediction study: the value of new vs standard risk factors in predicting early and all spontaneous preterm births. NICHD MFMU Network. Am J Public Health 1998;88:233–8.

Martin JA, Hamilton BE, Sutton PD, Ventura SJ, Menacker F, Kirmeyer S. Births: final data for 2004. Natl Vital Stat Rep 2006;55(1):1–101.

Macones GA, Segel SY, Stamilio DM, Morgan MA. Prediction of delivery among women with early preterm labor by means of clinical characteristics alone. Am J Obstet Gynecol 1999;181:1414–8.

Meis PJ, Klebanoff M, Thom E, Dombrowski MP, Sibai B, Moawad AH, et al. Prevention of recurrent preterm delivery by 17 alpha-hydroxyprogesterone caproate. National Institute of Child Health and Human Development Maternal-Fetal Medicine Units Network [published erratum appears in N Engl J Med 2003;349:1299]. N Engl J Med 2003;348:2379–85.

Mozurkewich EL, Luke B, Avni M, Wolf FM. Working conditions and adverse pregnancy outcome: a meta-analysis. Obstet Gynecol 2000;95:623–35.

54

Hypertension in pregnancy

A 29-year-old nulliparous woman had a blood pressure reading of 143/90 mm Hg in the first trimester but required no antihypertensive medications during the pregnancy. She has struggled with weight gain over the past 5 years and has a prepregnancy body mass index (weight in kilograms divided by height in meters squared [kg/m²]) of 30. She was referred to the labor and delivery suite at 32 weeks of gestation because of a frontal headache and visual blurriness. She has an initial blood pressure reading of 162/91 mm Hg and 2+ urinary protein. She reports excellent fetal movement. Her cervix is 2 cm dilated and 50% effaced. Ultrasonography for biometrics yields an estimated fetal weight of less than the 3rd percentile with an amniotic fluid index of 4.2 cm. A nonstress test is reactive, uterine contractions are noted every 4 minutes, and corticosteroids are initiated. The best next step in management is

    (A) tocolysis
    (B) methyldopa
    (C) observation
*   (D) magnesium sulfate therapy and delivery

There are five types of hypertensive disorders that may complicate pregnancy, each with different diagnostic criteria: gestational hypertension, preeclampsia, eclampsia, superimposed preeclampsia (on chronic hypertension), and chronic hypertension. Chronic hypertension, according to the National High Blood Pressure Working Group on High Blood Pressure in Pregnancy, is defined as hypertension present before 20 weeks of gestation or hypertension that antedates pregnancy; chronic hypertension is also present in women with hypertension first diagnosed after 20 weeks of gestation and persistent after 12 weeks postpartum. Chronic hypertension occurs in up to 5% of pregnant women and may result in maternal, fetal, or neonatal morbidity and mortality. Specific criteria for diagnosis of chronic hypertension in pregnancy are listed in Box 54-1.

Chronic hypertension may have significant adverse effects on the pregnancy. Women with longstanding chronic hypertension often have end-organ damage that may worsen with pregnancy. Essential hypertension is the cause of underlying vascular disease in the majority of pregnant women. Box 54-2 lists additional underlying causes of chronic hypertension.

Much of the increased perinatal morbidity and mortality related to chronic hypertension centers around superimposed preeclampsia and intrauterine growth restriction. Depending on the duration of hypertension, ventricular hypertrophy and cardiac decompensation, renal damage, and cerebrovascular accidents may occur. Superimposed preeclampsia may develop in up to 25% of pregnant women with chronic hypertension, and complications occur more frequently in this group. Abruptio placentae is substantially more common in women with chronic

---

BOX 54-1

Criteria for Diagnosis of Chronic Hypertension in Pregnancy

Mild: Systolic blood pressure 140 mm Hg or higher
           Diastolic blood pressure 90 mm Hg or higher
Severe: Systolic blood pressure 180 mm Hg or higher
           Diastolic blood pressure 110 mm Hg or higher

Use of antihypertensive medications before pregnancy
Onset of hypertension before 20 weeks of gestation
Persistence of hypertension beyond the usual postpartum period

Chronic hypertension in pregnancy. ACOG Practice Bulletin No. 29. American College of Obstetricians and Gynecologists. Obstet Gynecol 2001;98:177–92.

---

hypertension and superimposed preeclampsia. Iatrogenic preterm birth, stillbirth, oligohydramnios, and intrauterine growth restriction represent additional pregnancy complications that may occur with chronic hypertension.

Associated risk factors portending a poorer outcome include:

- Long-standing hypertension
- Advanced maternal age (especially older than 40 years)
- Severe hypertension in early pregnancy

- Pregestational diabetes mellitus
- Preexisting renal disease
- Cardiomyopathy
- Connective tissue diseases such as lupus, antiphospholipid syndrome, and scleroderma

The patient in this scenario has mild chronic hypertension that did not require treatment during pregnancy. Her hypertension may be associated with her obesity. Her presentation is consistent with a diagnosis of superimposed severe preeclampsia. Elevated blood pressure, proteinuria, and central nervous system irritability are present. Fetal effects of the disease process are marked growth restriction and oligohydramnios. Criteria for diagnosis of severe preeclampsia and superimposed preeclampsia on chronic hypertension are listed in Box 54-3. The most appropriate next step is initiation of magnesium sulfate therapy for seizure prophylaxis and delivery. Tocolytic therapy to abate the contractions and prolong pregnancy would be inappropriate in this situation with evidence of severe preeclampsia and fetal compromise. Maintenance antihypertensive therapy would not be started at this time. Intravenous hydralazine or labetalol, however, may be needed during the intrapartum and early postpartum period for

---

BOX 54-2

Underlying Causes of Chronic Hypertensive Disorders

Essential familial hypertension (hypertensive
  vascular disorder)
Obesity
Arterial abnormalities
  Renovascular hypertension
  Coarctation of the aorta
Endocrine disorders
  Diabetes mellitus
  Cushing syndrome
  Primary aldosteronism
  Pheochromocytoma
  Thyrotoxicosis
Glomerulonephritis (acute and chronic)
Renoprival hypertension
  Chronic glomerulonephritis
  Chronic renal insufficiency
  Diabetic nephropathy
Connective tissue diseases
  Lupus erythematosus
  Systemic sclerosis
  Periarteritis nodosa
Polycystic kidney disease
Acute renal failure

Cunningham FG, Leveno KJ, Bloom SL, Hauth JC, Gilstrap LC 3rd, Wenstrom KD, editors. Williams obstetrics. 22nd ed. New York (NY): McGraw-Hill; 2005. p. 764. (Copyright 2005 by McGraw-Hill)

BOX 54-3

Diagnosis of Severe Preeclampsia

Preeclampsia is considered severe if one or more of the following criteria are present:
- Blood pressure of 160 mm Hg systolic or higher or 110 mm Hg or higher on two occasions at least 6 hours apart while the patient is on bed rest
- Proteinuria of 5 g or higher in a 24-hour urine specimen or 3 g or more on two random urine samples collected at least 4 hours apart
- Oliguria of less than 500 mL in 24 hours
- Cerebral or visual disturbances
- Pulmonary edema or cyanosis
- Epigastric or right upper quadrant pain
- Impaired liver function
- Thrombocytopenia
- Intrauterine growth restriction

Diagnosis of superimposed preeclampsia (on chronic hypertension):

In women with hypertension and no proteinuria at 20 weeks of gestation or less
- New-onset proteinuria of 300 mg or more in 24 hours

In women with hypertension and proteinuria at 20 weeks of gestation or less
- Sudden increase in blood pressure
- Sudden increase in proteinuria
- Platelet count less than $100,000/mm^3$
- An increase in alanine transaminase or aspartate transaminase to abnormal levels

Modified from Diagnosis and management of preeclampsia and eclampsia. ACOG Practice Bulletin No. 33. American College of Obstetricians and Gynecologists. Obstet Gynecol 2002;99:159–67 and Report of the National High Blood Pressure Education Program Working Group on High Blood Pressure in Pregnancy. Am J Obstet Gynecol 2000;183(suppl 1):S1–22.

---

systolic blood pressure of 180 mm Hg or more or diastolic blood pressure of 110 mm Hg or more. Expectant management or observation of women with severe preeclampsia is reserved for women remote from term.

Chronic hypertension in pregnancy. ACOG Practice Bulletin No. 29. American College of Obstetricians and Gynecologists. Obstet Gynecol 2001;98:177–92.

Diagnosis and management of preeclampsia and eclampsia. ACOG Practice Bulletin No. 33. American College of Obstetricians and Gynecologists. Obstet Gynecol 2002;99:159–67.

Hypertensive disorders in pregnancy. In: Cunningham FG, Leveno KJ, Bloom SL, Hauth JC, Gilstrap LC 3rd, Wenstrom KD, editors. Williams obstetrics. 22nd ed. New York (NY): McGraw-Hill; 2005. p. 761–808.

Report of the National High Blood Pressure Education Program Working Group on High Blood Pressure in Pregnancy. Am J Obstet Gynecol 2000;183:S1–22.

Walfisch A, Hallak M. Hypertension. In: James DK, Steer PJ, Weiner CP, Gonik B, editors. High risk pregnancy management options. 3rd ed. Philadelphia (PA): Elsevier Saunders; 2006. p. 772–97.

55

Complications of neonatal circumcision

A 26-year-old woman who gave birth to a healthy, term male infant 24 hours ago requests a neonatal circumcision. After the procedure, persistent oozing is observed. The first step in management is

    (A) application of silver nitrate
    (B) application of Gelfoam
    (C) suture ligation
*   (D) application of direct pressure
    (E) electrocautery

The American Academy of Pediatrics 1999 Policy Statement on neonatal circumcision reports that existing scientific evidence demonstrates potential medical benefits to neonatal circumcision, but the current evidence is insufficient to recommend routine male neonatal circumcision. This position is supported by the American College of Obstetricians and Gynecologists. Nevertheless, it is estimated that more than 1 million newborn males undergo circumcision each year in the United States. This elective surgical procedure, which involves excising the foreskin to the level of the coronal sulcus, usually is safe when performed by a trained operator using sterile technique. Contraindications to newborn circumcision include prematurity, an unstable infant, family history of bleeding disorders, abnormal body temperature or abnormal feeding, and penile abnormalities such as hypospadias, epispadias, webbed penis, ambiguous genitalia, micropenis, and megalourethra, in which the foreskin may be needed to reconstruct the penis at a later time.

The exact incidence of complications from neonatal circumcision is unknown, but estimates range from approximately 0.2% to 0.6%. Most complications are minor, with the most frequent being postoperative bleeding (0.1% of circumcisions) followed by local infection. Additional complications of newborn circumcision may include phimosis, wound separation, adhesion formation, unsatisfactory cosmesis with either excess or insufficient skin removal, skin bridges, urinary retention, urethral fistula, meatitis, meatal stenosis, chordee, injury to the glans, and inclusion cysts.

In this neonate, persistent oozing is encountered following circumcision. In most cases, postoperative bleeding can be controlled with direct pressure. If the bleeding continues, hemostatic agents such as Gelfoam or silver nitrate may be used to achieve hemostasis. Occasionally vessel ligation or suturing of superficial tissues may be required to control minor postoperative bleeding. Electrocautery may cause significant damage to the glans and surrounding tissues. If postoperative bleeding does not respond to initial management, the pediatrician or pediatric urologist should be notified for appropriate workup and management.

Local infection, the next most common complication, is usually evident by redness and purulence of the surgical site and can be treated by local wound care or antibiotics.

Alanis MC, Lucidi RS. Neonatal circumcision: a review of the world's oldest and most controversial operation. Obstet Gynecol Surv 2004;59:379–95.

Circumcision. ACOG Committee Opinion No. 260. American College of Obstetricians and Gynecologists. Obstet Gynecol 2001;98:707–8.

Circumcision policy statement. American Academy of Pediatrics. Task Force on Circumcision. Pediatrics 1999;103:686–93.

Mastrobattista JM, Swaim LS. Circumcision. In: Gilstrap LC 3rd, Cunningham FG, VanDorsten JP, editors. Operative obstetrics. 2nd ed. New York (NY): McGraw-Hill; 2002. p. 655–69.

56

Ultrasonography for intrauterine growth restriction

A 32-year-old primigravid woman at 34 6/7 weeks of gestation with an ultrasound-confirmed estimated date of delivery (EDD) is seen for a routine prenatal visit. However, because she is obese, with body mass index (weight in kilograms divided by height in meters squared [kg/m^2]) of 41, it is difficult to obtain an adequate assessment of the fundal height using the physical examination. Her ultrasound examination today reveals the following measurements: biparietal diameter, 85 mm = 34 1/7 weeks (37%); head circumference, 309 mm = 34 3/7 weeks (38%); abdominal circumference, 270 mm = 31 weeks (4%); femur length, 62 mm = 32 weeks (10%); estimated fetal weight, 1,878 g (less than 10%); amniotic fluid index of 8.1 cm with a biophysical profile of 8/8. The next step in the care of this patient should be

      (A) fetal heart rate monitoring
      (B) oxytocin challenge test
      (C) amniocentesis
*   (D) Doppler velocimetry

Assessment of fetal growth plays a vital role in the evaluation of fetal well-being. A small-for-gestational-age fetus is defined as a fetus that is less than the cutoff weight for a given population, as a result of constitutional factors. In contrast, a growth-restricted fetus is one that has not been able to attain its full growth potential. A number of factors influence normal fetal growth, such as genetic disposition, parental influence, ethnic differences, environment (altitude), fetal sex, maternal weight gain, and maternal medical conditions (Box 56-1).

BOX 56-1

Risk Factors for Intrauterine Growth Restriction

Maternal medical conditions
- Hypertension
- Restrictive lung disease
- Diabetes mellitus (with microvascular disease)
- Cyanotic heart disease
- Antiphospholipid syndrome
- Collagen vascular disease
- Hemoglobinopathies

Smoking and substance abuse
Severe malnutrition
Primary placental disease
Multiple gestation
Infections (viral, protozoal)
Genetic disorders
Exposure to teratogens

American College of Obstetricians and Gynecologists. Intrauterine growth restriction. ACOG Practice Bulletin 12. Washington, DC: ACOG; 2000.

Fetal weight is estimated by numerous published formulas based on measurements of different fetal parts. The most commonly used fetal biometric parameters are the biparietal diameter, head circumference, femur length, and abdominal circumference. All formulas that estimate fetal weights using these parameters have an inherent absolute error of approximately 10%, ie, the fetal weight is plus or minus 10% of the estimated weight. Of the ultrasonographic biometric measurements, the abdominal circumference is the most sensitive measure of fetal growth. Hence, an abdominal circumference within the normal range essentially excludes intrauterine growth restriction (IUGR) with a false-negative rate of less than 10%.

Amniotic fluid volume needs to be measured any time IUGR is suspected because chronic hypoxemia often produces oligohydramnios as well as IUGR. The amniotic fluid volume may be normal in some cases of IUGR; however, when the fluid volume is normal, it is indicative of a noncompromised fetus. Amniotic fluid volume can be estimated in two ways: 1) using the deepest (largest) vertical pocket or 2) using the amniotic fluid index (AFI). When using the single largest pocket, oligohydramnios is considered when the pocket is 2 cm or less. The AFI is obtained by measuring the largest vertical pocket (free of umbilical cord and fetal parts) in the four abdominal quadrants and then adding them together. When using the AFI, the amniotic fluid volume is considered to be abnormal if it is 5 cm or less.

Flow indices that have been used to assess blood flow in arterial vessels include the systolic-to-diastolic ratio, the pulsatility index, and the resistance index. Of these, the pulsatility index can be calculated even in the absence of diastolic flow. In the normal scenario, the umbilical flow velocity waveform is characterized by high-velocity diastolic flow. This is a result of decreased resistance to blood flow in the umbilical artery due to the reservoir effect of the placenta. However, in cases of IUGR, diastolic flow in the umbilical artery is decreased as a result of increased resistance to blood flow within the placenta; therefore, the systolic-to-diastolic ratio increases. In severely compromised fetuses, absent or reverse diastolic flow may be seen (Fig. 56-1; see color plate).

How can a normal but small-for-gestational-age (SGA) fetus be differentiated from a small-but-growth-restricted fetus? Umbilical artery flow studies can help differentiate between those fetuses that are "constitutionally small" from those in which there is placental dysfunction leading to "pathologic" growth restriction. In addition, Doppler ultrasonographic studies of fetuses with IUGR or suspected IUGR are helpful in the management of the pregnancy. For example, a fetus with IUGR with absent or reverse end-diastolic flow would most likely need maternal hospitalization with daily fetal monitoring or delivery depending on the gestational age and the result of the biophysical profile.

In pregnancies complicated by IUGR, Doppler ultrasonography reduces the odds of perinatal death by 38%. Fetal heart rate and biophysical profile abnormalities are late findings and are usually present in preterminal states. However, abnormalities seen by Doppler ultrasonography, such as absent end-diastolic flow, usually are observed before the occurrence of fetal decompensation. Thus, early delivery of these fetuses before the fetal decompensation improves the perinatal morbidity and mortality.

In the case presented, fetal heart rate monitoring would not add any further information in view of the biophysical profile of 8/8, which essentially demonstrates a nonasphyxiated fetus with a low risk of fetal death within the week. The addition of Doppler velocimetry in assessment of IUGR is useful because it has been associated with a reduction in perinatal death. If the Doppler studies are normal, this information can be used to delay delivery or admission to the hospital with some reassurance. Once the diagnosis of IUGR has been made, periodic assessment of the fetus can be achieved by Doppler velocimetry, biophysical profile (BPP), or a modified BPP (nonstress test and amniotic fluid volume), or an oxytocin challenge. Amniocentesis for a fetal karyotype is not routinely recommended for IUGR fetuses unless a structural anomaly is seen by ultrasound examination or the IUGR occurs early in pregnancy or is severe. Approximately 10% of fetuses with IUGR and structural anomaly will have an abnormal karyotype. In cases remote from term, if all fetal surveillance testing is normal, a repeat scan in 2–4 weeks is suggested to reassess fetal growth.

Alfirevic Z, Neilson JP. Doppler ultrasonography in high-risk pregnancies: systematic review with meta-analysis. Am J Obstet Gynecol 1995; 172:1379–87.

American College of Obstetricians and Gynecologists. Antepartum fetal surveillance. ACOG Practice Bulletin 9. Washington, DC: ACOG; 1999.

American College of Obstetricians and Gynecologists. Intrauterine growth restriction. ACOG Practice Bulletin 12. Washington, DC: ACOG; 2000.

Growth, Doppler and fetal assessment. In: Nyberg DA, McGahan JP, Pretorius DH, Pilu G, editors. Diagnostic imaging of fetal anomalies. Lippincott Williams & Wilkins; 2003. p. 31–58.

Soothill PW, Ajayi RA, Campbell S, Nicolaides KH. Prediction of morbidity in small and normally grown fetuses by fetal heart rate variability, biophysical profile score and umbilical artery Doppler studies. Br J Obstet Gynaecol 1993;100:742–5.

Soothill PW, Bobrow CS, Holmes R. Small for gestational age is not a diagnosis [editorial]. Ultrasound Obstet Gynecol 1999;13:225–8.

57

Hepatitis C screening in pregnancy

The population group that should be routinely screened for hepatitis C virus (HCV) in pregnancy is

    (A) health care workers
    (B) all pregnant women
    (C) household (nonsexual) contacts of an HCV-positive person
*   (D) current intravenous drug users
    (E) recent immigrants from Southeast Asia

Hepatitis C, previously referred to as non-A, non-B hepatitis, was so renamed after being reported in 1989 as a new viral agent with its own uniquely sequenced viral genome. It is a 9600-nucleotide RNA virus configured in a linear, single strand, positive sense. Because it is an RNA virus, it does not replicate through a DNA intermediate and therefore does not incorporate itself into the host genome. Hepatitis C exists in at least six genotypes with multiple subtypes. It is also capable of rapid mutation so that neutralizing antibodies to hepatitis C are not long-lasting and host susceptibility to reinfection with even the same strain of virus is possible.

Hepatitis C does not seem to be as efficiently transmitted as hepatitis B. Its less efficient transmission has led to fewer predictable infection patterns and less consensus on screening guidelines. Sexual or perinatal transmission is estimated to occur at a rate of approximately 5% or less. Breastfeeding does not appear to increase the risk of infection from mother to infant, and HCV infection among health care workers is equivalent to that seen in the general population.

The Centers for Disease Control and Prevention (CDC) has issued guidelines regarding the screening, diagnosis, and treatment of hepatitis C. Prior reports from case–control studies had listed a number of risk factors for hepatitis C infection, including blood transfusion, intravenous drug use, working in the health care industry, living with a person with positive hepatitis C serology, body piercing, and foreign travel. As data continued to be collected, it became apparent that a better focus for screening would be needed. Based on these data, the population best served by routine screening is individuals who inject illegal intravenous drugs. Routine screening of all pregnant women is not warranted, nor is screening of health care workers unless they have sustained a needlestick injury or other mucosal exposure from a known HCV-seropositive individual. Currently, nonsexual household contacts of HCV-positive individuals do not warrant routine screening because it has yet to be determined whether or not long-term sex partners of known HCV-positive individuals benefit from HCV testing. In some parts of Southeast Asia, especially before the introduction of hepatitis B vaccine, hepatitis B infection was endemic, but screening individuals from this region for hepatitis C is not indicated unless they have some other accepted risk factor.

Dienstag JL, Isselbacher KJ. Acute viral hepatitis. In: Kasper DL, Braunwald E, Fauci AS, Hauser SL, Longo DL, Jameson JH, editors. Harrison's principles of internal medicine. 16th ed. New York (NY): McGraw-Hill; 2005. p. 1822–38.

Recommendations for prevention and control of hepatitis C virus (HCV) infection and HCV-related chronic disease. Centers for Disease Control and Prevention. MMWR Recomm Rep 1998;47(RR-19):1–39.

58
Cholestasis

The greatest perinatal risk from cholestasis in pregnancy is

      (A) preeclampsia
      (B) postterm delivery
*   (C) fetal loss
      (D) gestational diabetes mellitus

Cholestasis is a condition in which, for various reasons, clearance of bile acids and bilirubin is impaired. The etiologies of cholestasis are numerous and may be subdivided into intrahepatic and extrahepatic cholestasis (Box 58-1).

Intrahepatic cholestasis of pregnancy complicates approximately 0.5–1.8% of otherwise normal uncomplicated pregnancies. The etiology is not entirely clear. Some evidence of familial and geographic clustering of cases points to at least a partial genetic basis for this disorder. Some data suggest that in approximately 10–16% of cases, the mode of transmission may be autosomal dominant. Cholestasis is associated with cholelithiasis in nearly one quarter of cases, but most cases of cholestasis reveal no underlying etiology. Patients frequently present with itching in the third trimester without apparent rash or other dermatologic manifestations. Bile acids will be elevated and treatment is generally targeted initially at

alleviation of symptoms, but may then progress to therapies to reduce bile acid formation or enhance bile acid clearance. Agents such as cholestyramine and ursodiol have been used successfully for this purpose. It has been proposed that bile salt deposition in the placenta may result in deterioration of placental function.

Although liver disease can be associated with other disorders of glucose metabolism, there is no evidence that gestational diabetes mellitus leads to or is altered by the development of cholestasis. Likewise, although liver function abnormalities may be seen in preeclampsia, no studies link intrahepatic cholestasis to the development of preeclampsia. Most often intrahepatic cholestasis of pregnancy has been linked to an increased risk of prematurity and to fetal death, the latter possibly resulting in deterioration of placental function secondary to bile salt deposition, although this association remains unclear. One recent study suggested that pruritus gravidarum was not associated with adverse perinatal outcome, although the study was not methodologically rigorous in its distinction between pruritus that was secondary to cholestasis and pruritus that was secondary to some other cause. For these reasons, these pregnancies may be considered high risk. As term approaches, heightened fetal surveillance is warranted and has led some to recommend delivery at term.

BOX 58-1

Common Etiologies of Cholestasis

Intrahepatic cholestasis
- Viral hepatitis
- Alcoholic hepatitis
- Toxicity of drugs, including oral contraceptives
- Biliary cirrhosis
- Inherited disorders of bilirubin metabolism
- Cholestasis of pregnancy

Extrahepatic cholestasis
- Malignancy
- Choledocholithiasis
- Chronic pancreatitis
- AIDS cholangiopathy

AIDS, acquired immunodeficiency syndrome.

Kaaja RJ, Greer IA. Manifestations of chronic disease during pregnancy. JAMA 2005;294:2751–7.

Pratt DS, Kaplan MM. Jaundice. In: Kasper DL, Braunwald E, Fauci AS, Hauser SL, Longo DL, Jameson JH, editors. Harrison's principles of internal medicine. 16th ed. New York (NY): McGraw-Hill; 2005. p. 238–43.

Samuels P. Hepatic disease. In: Gabbe SG, Niebyl JR, Simpson JL, editors. Obstetrics: normal and problem pregnancies. 4th ed. New York (NY): Churchill Livingstone; 2002. p. 1218–21.

Sheiner E, Ohel I, Levy A, Katz M. Pregnancy outcome in women with pruritus gravidarum. J Reprod Med 2006;51:394–8.

59

Triplets

A 33-year-old woman, gravida 1, comes to the office for her first prenatal care visit in the first trimester at 10 weeks of gestation. Office ultrasonography to confirm her expected date of delivery demonstrated that she has triplets. At this gestational age, the clinical finding that is most important in helping to counsel the patient regarding her triplet gestation is

      (A) baseline cervical length
*   (B) chorionicity
      (C) nuchal translucency of each fetus
      (D) fasting blood sugar

A 500% increase has been seen in the frequency of triplet gestation in the United States since 1980, from 37 per 100,000 live births to 184 per 100,000 live births. Most of this increase results from assisted reproductive technology (ART). Spontaneous triplet gestation occurs in 1 in 6,000 to 1 in 8,000 gestations. Only 19% of the triplet gestations are a result of spontaneous conceptions.

Triplet gestations have a higher rate of both neonatal and maternal morbidity. The average age at birth for triplet gestation is 32 weeks. Approximately 20% of all triplet gestations will produce at least one child with cerebral palsy and around 50–60% of triplet gestations will be complicated by intrauterine growth restriction. The incidence of cerebral palsy in premature growth restricted infants is significantly greater. Three quarters of all triplet gestations will require neonatal intensive care unit admissions, and the average length of stay is 30 days. Women with triplet gestations have a higher rate of preeclampsia, preterm labor, preterm premature rupture of membranes (preterm PROM), abruptio placentae, gestational diabetes mellitus, and postpartum hemorrhage.

Monochorionic gestations are at increased risk for perinatal morbidity and mortality. The background rate of monochorionicity is 0.4%. The rate increases to 1–5% after ART. Dichorionic triamniotic triplets (1 monochorionic diamnionic pair and one fetus with a separate chorion and amnion) have a higher rate of perinatal death, preterm birth at less than 30 weeks of gestation, preterm PROM, low birth weight, and twin–twin transfusion syndrome compared with trichorionic triplets.

Mothers with triplet gestations should have a discussion to review multifetal pregnancy reduction (MFPR), and the risks of preterm birth, preterm PROM, abruptio placentae, gestational diabetes mellitus, preeclampsia, and postpartum hemorrhage. Once a decision has been made regarding MFPR, an antenatal management plan can be developed.

The MFPR technique reduces the number of fetuses in a high-order multiple gestation to decrease the risk of loss prior to viability and preterm birth, especially preterm birth between 24 and 28 weeks of gestation. A transabdominal approach is used at 10–13 weeks of gestation. Before the procedure, chorionicity, crown–rump length, and nuchal translucency measurements are made for each fetus. If the crown–rump length or the nuchal translucency is abnormal for a fetus, that fetus is chosen for reduction; otherwise the easiest fetal target is chosen for reduction. This technique reduces the rate of loss prior to viability and the rate of extreme preterm birth by 50% (Table 59-1).

This procedure is contingent on each fetus having its own chorion and amnion; MFPR cannot be performed on a fetus in a monochorionic twin gestation secondary to immediate risk of death to the second fetus.

The first step in managing a triplet pregnancy is to determine the chorionicity. Based on the chorionicity, the patient can be adequately counseled regarding MFPR. In dichorionic triplet gestation, MFPR of the monochorionic diamnionic pair should be strongly considered because of the increased risk of loss before viability, twin–twin transfusion syndrome, and preterm birth before 30 weeks of gestation.

The nuchal translucencies are used to determine each fetus's individual risk for aneuploidy. At 11–14 weeks of gestation, determination of nuchal translucencies is an important early step in the evaluation of multiple gestation but it follows the identification of chorionicity. In addition, discordant nuchal translucencies in monochorionic gestations increase the risk for developing twin–twin transfusion syndrome. Triplet gestations are at risk for preterm birth, and the average age of delivery is 32 weeks of gestation. A baseline transvaginal cervical length may be obtained in the second trimester. Although cervical length is an indicator for preterm labor and the risk of preterm birth, no intervention has been found to be effective. A recent study has demonstrated that a prophylactic cervical cerclage does not improve perinatal outcome in triplet gestations. Women with triplet gestations are at

TABLE 59-1. Summary of Eight Studies* Comparing Outcome of Expectantly Managed Triplet Gestations, With Triplet Gestations Reduced to Twins, and Nonreduced Gestations

Outcome	Triplets, Expectantly Managed	Twins, Reduced From Triplets	Twins, Nonreduced
No. of pregnancies	381	412	778
Pregnancy loss rate at less than 24 weeks (%)	13	7	5
Preterm delivery rate at 24–28 weeks (%)	8	3	7
Gestational age at delivery (weeks)	33.1	35.4	34.6
Birth weight (g)	1,879	2,553	2,187
Perinatal mortality rate (per 1,000)	80	46	35

Studies by year of publication: Porreco RP, Burke MS, Hendrix ML. Multifetal reduction of triplets and pregnancy outcome. Obstet Gynecol 1991;78(3 Pt 1):335–9; Melgar CA, Rosenfeld DL, Rawlinson K, Greenberg M. Perinatal outcome after multifetal reduction to twins compared with nonreduced multiple gestations. Obstet Gynecol 1991;78(5 Pt 1):763–7; Macones GA, Schemmer G, Pritts E, Weinblatt V, Wapner RJ. Multifetal reduction of triplets to twins improves perinatal outcome. Am J Obstet Gynecol 1993;169:982–6; Lipitz S, Reichman B, Uval J, Shalev J, Achiron R, Barkai G, et al. A prospective comparison of the outcome of triplet pregnancies managed expectantly or by multifetal reduction to twins. Am J Obstet Gynecol 1994;170:874–9; Smith-Levitin M, Kowalik A, Birnholz J, Skupski DW, Hutson JM, Chervenak FA, et al. Selective reduction of multifetal pregnancies to twins improves outcome over nonreduced triplet gestations. Am J Obstet Gynecol 1996;175(4 Pt 1):878–82; Yaron Y, Bryant-Greenwood PK, Dave N, Moldenhauer JS, Kramer RL, Johnson MP, et al. Multifetal pregnancy reductions of triplets to twins: comparison with nonreduced triplets and twins. Am J Obstet Gynecol 1999;180:1268–71; Boulot P, Vignal J, Vergnes C, Dechaud H, Faure JM, Hedon B. Multifetal reduction of triplets to twins: a prospective comparison of pregnancy outcome. Hum Reprod 2000 Jul;15:1619–23; Leondires MP, Ernst SD, Miller BT, Scott RT. Triplets: outcomes of expectant management versus multifetal reduction for 127 pregnancies. Am J Obstet Gynecol 2000;183:454–9.

Malone FD, D'Alton ME. Multiple gestation: clinical characteristics and management. In: Creasy RK, Resnik R, Iams JD, editors. Maternal–fetal medicine: principles and practice. 5th ed. Philadelphia (PA): WB Saunders Co.; 2004. p. 532. Copyright 2004 by Elsevier.

increased risk for gestational diabetes mellitus. These women are monitored closely for this condition especially in the early third trimester. However, no additional evaluation is required in the first trimester unless extenuating circumstances exist.

Bajoria R, Ward SB, Adegbite AL. Comparative study of perinatal outcome of dichorionic and trichorionic iatrogenic triplets. Am J Obstet Gynecol 2006;194:415–24.

Chasen ST, Al-Kouatly HB, Ballabh P, Skupski DW, Chervenak FA. Outcomes of dichorionic triplet pregnancies. Am J Obstet Gynecol 2002;186:765–7.

Geipel A, Berg C, Katalinic A, Plath H, Hansmann M, Germer U, et al. Prenatal diagnosis and obstetric outcomes in triplet pregnancies in relation to chorionicity. BJOG 2005;112:554–8.

Malone FD, D'Alton ME. Multiple gestation: clinical characteristics and management. In: Creasy RK, Resnik R, Iams JD, editors. Maternal–fetal medicine: principles and practice. 5th ed. Philadelphia (PA): WB Saunders Co.; 2004. p. 515–36.

Multiple gestation: complicated twin, triplet, and high-order multifetal pregnancy. ACOG Practice Bulletin No. 56. American College of Obstetricians and Gynecologists. Obstet Gynecol 2004;104:869–83.

Rebarber A, Roman AS, Istwan N, Rhea D, Stanziano G. Prophylactic cerclage in the management of triplet pregnancies. Am J Obstet Gynecol 2005;193:1193–6.

60

Cervical ripening

A 21-year-old woman, gravida 2, para 1, presents at 41 weeks of gestation for induction of labor. Her cervix is unfavorable. You discuss induction of labor with her. Intravaginal misoprostol is chosen as the preinduction cervical ripening agent. The most common complication of this ripening agent is

      (A) chorioamnionitis
*   (B) uterine tachysystole
      (C) maternal nausea
      (D) vaginal bleeding

Misoprostol is a prostaglandin E_1 analog that is marketed for the prevention of gastric ulcers in patients taking nonsteroidal antiinflammatory drugs (NSAIDs). Soon after its introduction, it was found to be a powerful uterotonic agent and studies confirmed its use as a method to induce labor. The mechanism of action of misoprostol is complex but appears to be related to an increase in calcium transport across cellular membranes, which increases cyclic adenosine monophosphate (cAMP) within uterine muscle triggering muscle cells to contract. Additionally, it appears to lead to the activation of collagenases, which results in breakdown in the collagen network of the cervix leading to softening and effacement of the cervix.

Misoprostol has been used for induction of labor by multiple routes including oral, vaginal, and sublingual. Multiple studies have documented the effectiveness of vaginal misoprostol to induce labor. Misoprostol, when compared to placebo, increased vaginal delivery within 24 hours and uterine tachysystole. When compared with intracervical prostaglandin (PG) E_2 gel and oxytocin, misoprostol was associated with a lower rate of epidural use, increase in the rate of vaginal delivery within 24 hours, increase in meconium stained fluid, and uterine tachysystole. However, when compared with the use of a Foley catheter and oxytocin, no difference was observed in the rate of vaginal delivery. There was, however, an increased risk of uterine tachysystole and passage of meconium with misoprostol use. The use of higher doses of vaginal misoprostol is associated with higher rates of vaginal delivery within 24 hours, decreased need for oxy-

tocin, and decreased induction to delivery intervals, but is also associated with higher rates of uterine tachysystole and uterine hyperstimulation.

Oral misoprostol has been shown to decrease delivery times in women with rupture of membranes. However, compared with oxytocin, no difference was found. Oral misoprostol does not appear to be a greater benefit than vaginal misoprostol for induction of labor with intact membranes.

Although variability exists in the definition of uterine tachysystole and uterine hyperstimulation between studies, it is the primary complication of misoprostol, but may be less common in women who receive the lower dosage. Also, increased passage of meconium in pregnancies exposed to misoprostol has been reported in multiple studies.

American College of Obstetricians and Gynecologists. Induction of labor with misoprostol. ACOG Committee Opinion 228. Washington, DC: ACOG; 1999.

American College of Obstetricians and Gynecologists. Induction of labor. ACOG Practice Bulletin 10. Washington, DC: ACOG; 1999.

Sanchez-Ramos L, Chen AH, Kaunitz AM, Gaudier FL, Delke I. Labor induction with intravaginal misoprostol in term premature rupture of membranes: a randomized study. Obstet Gynecol 1997;89:909–12.

Sciscione AC, Nguyen L, Manley J, Pollock M, Maas B, Colmorgen G. A randomized comparison of transcervical Foley catheter to intravaginal misoprostol for preinduction cervical ripening. Obstet Gynecol 2001;97:603–7.

Wing DA, Rahall A, Jones MM, Goodwin TM, Paul RH. Misoprostol: an effective agent for cervical ripening and labor induction. Am J Obstet Gynecol 1995;172:1811–6.

61

Peripartum cardiomyopathy

A 35-year-old African-American multiparous woman experienced peripartum cardiomyopathy 4 months following delivery in her previous pregnancy. Acute treatment was lifesaving. The most important test to perform for future reproductive counseling is

  (A) chest X-ray
 * (B) echocardiography
  (C) endomyocardial biopsy
  (D) molecular investigation for cardiotoxic viral genomes

Peripartum cardiomyopathy is a disorder of unknown cause in which initial left ventricular systolic dysfunction and symptoms of heart failure occur during the last month of pregnancy and the first 5 months postpartum. Some clinicians have described an identical clinical condition that appeared earlier in pregnancy, at 17–36 weeks of gestation, as "pregnancy-associated" cardiomyopathy. The signs and symptoms did not differ clinically from those in women with the usual presentation of peripartum cardiomyopathy. Some reports also include women who presented with first heart failure within 6 months postpartum. All these conditions may be part of the same clinical entity, with an expanded time interval for onset of heart failure. Most patients recover partially or completely; however, the mortality rate is approximately 15–20%. Because many patients with peripartum cardiomyopathy may consider future pregnancy, it is important to be able to provide them with information about relapse. Postpartum and posttreatment predictors of patient well-being or potential mortality will allow clinicians to counsel patients for future pregnancies.

The criteria for the diagnosis of peripartum cardiomyopathy were established in 1971. At that time, conventional chest X-ray was used to analyze the natural history of the disease. Resolution of cardiomegaly, by X-ray evaluation, was associated with the absence of mortality from congestive heart failure, whereas patients with persistent cardiomegaly had a probability of dying of heart failure within 4.7 years, on average. This modality is no longer used to predict mortality.

Echocardiography is the modern diagnostic test of choice for current clinical management and counseling. One study evaluated a cohort of 92 women with a history of peripartum cardiomyopathy. Clinical and echocardiographic information was available for 44 women. Normalization of left ventricular ejection fraction to at least 50% was documented in 28 women, whereas 16 did not achieve normalization. In the first subsequent pregnancy following the index "cardiomyopathy pregnancy," symptoms of heart failure occurred in 26% of those with

a normalized ejection fraction and in 50% of those without normalization. No deaths occurred in those with normalization of their ejection fraction, whereas death did occur in 25% of those without normalization.

Increasing evidence suggests that peripartum cardiomyopathy is a type of myocarditis that arises from infectious, autoimmune, or idiopathic processes. Numerous studies have reported histologic evidence of myocarditis in endomyocardial biopsy samples obtained from patients with peripartum cardiomyopathy. Unfortunately, in spite of the implication of these reports, endomyocardial biopsy cannot be relied on for prognosis or even to make the clinical diagnosis of myocarditis. The difficulty lies in the high rate of false-negative results because of the focal nature of the inflammatory infiltrates. In patients with autopsy-proven myocarditis, the diagnosis would be made by endomyocardial biopsy in only 63% of subjects. This test has limited predictive value for future pregnancies.

Some authorities recommend that myocardial biopsy be performed if there is no improvement after 2 weeks of adequate medical treatment. Information that may be gleaned from such biopsies includes the evaluation of cardiotoxic viral genomes (parvovirus B19, human herpesvirus 6, Epstein-Barr virus, and human cytomegalic virus) by polymerase chain reaction. Although potentially useful for acute care, this information will not be useful for counseling related to future pregnancies.

Brown CS, Bertolet BD. Peripartum cardiomyopathy: a comprehensive review. Am J Obstet Gynecol 1998;178:409–14.

Bultmann BD, Klingel K, Nabauer M, Wallwiener D, Kandolf R. High prevalence of viral genomes and inflammation in peripartum cardiomyopathy. Am J Obstet Gynecol 2005;193:363–5.

Elkayam U, Tummala PP, Rao K, Akhter M, Karaalp IS, Wani OR, et al. Maternal and fetal outcomes of subsequent pregnancies in women with peripartum cardiomyopathy [published erratum appears in N Engl J Med 2001;345:552]. N Engl J Med 2001;344:1567–71.

Sliwa K, Fett J, Elkayam U. Peripartum cardiomyopathy. Lancet 2006; 368:687–93.

Veille JC, Zaccaro D. Peripartum cardiomyopathy: summary of an international survey on peripartum cardiomyopathy. Am J Obstet Gynecol 1999;181:315–9.

62

Anemia

A 23-year-old African-American woman comes to the office for her first prenatal visit at 13 weeks of gestation. Initial prenatal laboratory test results indicate a hemoglobin level of 9.7 g/dL. Hemoglobin electrophoresis results show 98% hemoglobin A and red blood cell indices as follows: mean corpuscular volume (MCV), 78.5 fL; and serum ferritin concentration, 11.4 mcg/L. The most likely diagnosis is

 (A) dilutional (physiologic) anemia
* (B) iron-deficiency anemia
 (C) β-thalassemia trait
 (D) α-thalassemia trait
 (E) vitamin B$_{12}$ deficiency

Assessment of anemia during pregnancy requires an understanding of the physiologic changes that occur in pregnancy. Maternal hemoglobin concentration and hematocrit decline during the first and second trimesters because of expanding blood volume. As a result, a dilutional or physiologic anemia occurs due to an imbalance between the 50% increase in maternal plasma volume and the 25% increase in erythrocyte mass. This physiologic anemia of pregnancy usually is not associated with microcytosis.

The microcytic anemias are characterized by abnormal hemoglobin synthesis with normal red blood cell production. A low MCV test result (less than 80 fL) indicates some type of microcytic anemia, such as iron-deficiency anemia. Iron deficiency is among the most common causes of anemia in pregnant women and may be as prevalent as 47%. Iron status can be assessed through several laboratory tests; however, no single test can diagnose iron deficiency. Serum ferritin concentration is an early indicator of the status of iron stores and is the most specific indicator available of depleted iron stores, especially when used in conjunction with other tests to assess iron status. Among women who test positive for anemia on the basis of hemoglobin concentration or hematocrit, a serum ferritin concentration of 20 mcg/L or less confirms iron deficiency. The Institute of Medicine recommends that iron supplementation be offered only to women whose serum ferritin level is less than 20 mcg/L.

The thalassemias are named and classified by the type of chain that is inadequately produced. Alpha- and beta-thalassemia are the two most common thalassemias and range in severity dependent on the rate of production of α and β globulin chains. Alpha- and beta-thalassemia traits are characterized by mild anemia and microcytosis. In individuals with β-thalassemia trait, hemoglobin electrophoresis usually will reveal an increase in the level of hemoglobin A$_2$ from the normal value of 2% to a value of 3–6%. In contrast, hemoglobin electrophoresis results are normal in persons with α-thalassemia trait, and diagnosis is accomplished through polymerase chain reaction-based DNA tests. In both of these diseases, a normal or even elevated ferritin level would be expected.

Megaloblastic anemia is the second most common nutritional anemia seen during pregnancy, with folate deficiency being the most common cause. Vitamin B$_{12}$ deficiency also can occur, but this produces a macrocytic, normochromic anemia. The most common causes of vitamin B$_{12}$ deficiency are inadequate production of intrinsic factor (pernicious anemia), and malabsorption, as often seen after gastric bypass surgery. In the absence of iron deficiency, vitamin B$_{12}$ deficiency would be associated with a normal ferritin level.

Figure 62-1 shows steps to be considered in the evaluation of microcytic anemia in pregnancy. Pregnancy demands on iron often require supplementation in addition to diet changes. Supplementation with 30–60 mg of elemental iron per day during the second and third trimesters will meet the daily iron requirement of pregnancy.

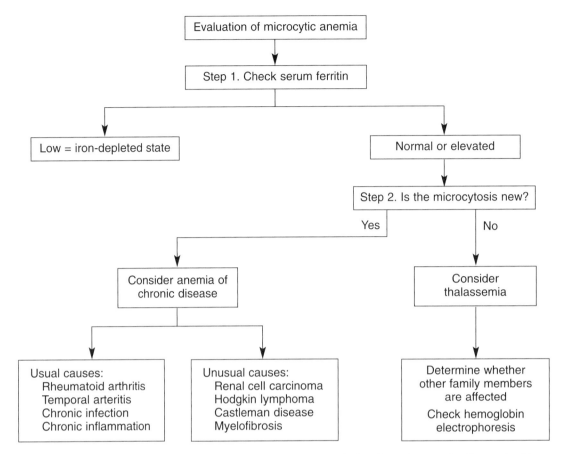

FIG. 62-1. Evaluation of microcytic anemia. (Tefferi A. Practical algorithms in anemia diagnosis. Mayo Clin Proc 2004;79:955–6.)

Hemoglobinopathies in pregnancy. ACOG Practice Bulletin No. 78. American College of Obstetricians and Gynecologists. Obstet Gynecol 2007;109:229–37.

Kilpatrick SJ, Laros RK. Maternal hematologic disorders. In: Creasy RK, Resnik R, Iams JD, editors. Maternal–fetal medicine: principles and practice. 5th ed. Philadelphia (PA): WB Saunders Co.; 2004. p. 977–84.

Tefferi A. Anemia in adults: a contemporary approach to diagnosis. Mayo Clin Proc 2003;78:1274–80.

Tefferi A. Practical algorithms in anemia diagnosis. Mayo Clin Proc 2004;79:955–6.

Recommendations to prevent and control iron deficiency in the United States. Centers for Disease Control and Prevention. MMWR Recomm Rep 1998;47(RR-3):1–29.

63

Preterm birth

A 29-year-old woman, gravida 2, with a history of a spontaneous preterm birth at 29 weeks of gestation, comes to the office for prenatal care at 12 weeks of gestation. The most effective intervention to decrease her risk of recurrent preterm birth is

* (A) weekly 17α-hydroxyprogesterone caproate injections starting at
       16 weeks of gestation
  (B) cervical cerclage at 12–14 weeks
  (C) measurement of cervical length by serial transvaginal ultrasonography
       at 16–24 weeks
  (D) reduction in maternal physical activity starting at 20–24 weeks of gestation
  (E) daily home uterine monitoring starting at 24 weeks of gestation

Prior spontaneous preterm birth is one of the strongest predictors of a future preterm birth, with an odds ratio of 3–5, and the earlier the preterm birth, the higher the risk of recurrence. Assuming a baseline preterm birth risk of 12% in the general U.S. population, the patient described has approximately a 36–60% risk of recurrent spontaneous preterm birth without intervention.

Weekly administration of intramuscular 17α-hydroxyprogesterone caproate "17P" from 16 to 20 weeks of gestation until 36 weeks of gestation reduces the risk of preterm birth by approximately 35% in women with singleton gestations who have a prior spontaneous preterm birth due to either preterm labor or preterm premature rupture of membranes between 20 and 36 6/7 weeks of gestation. The mechanism of action by which progesterone injections protect against preterm birth is unknown. The safety of progesterone therapy for the fetus and neonate has not been demonstrated with 100% certainty, but progesterone is known not to be a teratogen, and no long-term detrimental effects of prenatal progesterone therapy have been observed. Because of the paucity of data on the effectiveness of progesterone in other high-risk populations (eg, women with multiple gestations or other risk factors for preterm birth), the use of progesterone starting in the second trimester to reduce the risk of preterm birth cannot be recommended for conditions other than prior spontaneous preterm birth at 20–36 weeks of gestation.

Insufficient evidence exists to show that a cerclage would benefit a woman with one prior preterm birth. A history-indicated (ie, prophylactic or elective) cerclage, where placement is based solely on prior obstetric or gynecologic history, can prevent preterm birth in women with three or more second-trimester losses. However, clinical trials involving women at lower risk for preterm birth, such as those with one prior preterm birth, have not shown any benefit from history-indicated cerclage. The other possible clinical indication for history-indicated cerclage is cervical insufficiency, defined as prior painless cervical dilation leading to recurrent second-trimester loss. No trial has been conducted to confirm the efficacy of history-indicated cerclage in reducing preterm birth in women with a diagnosis of cervical insufficiency.

Cervical length, measured by transvaginal ultrasonography, has been shown to be predictive of preterm birth; however, cerclage indicated by a short cervical length (ie, ultrasonography-indicated cerclage) has not been definitively shown to be beneficial. Although a meta-analysis of four randomized trials of ultrasonography-indicated cerclage showed a decrease in preterm birth in women with a prior preterm birth and a short cervical length, these results need to be confirmed by a large randomized trial. Such a multicenter trial, sponsored by the National Institutes of Health, should report results in the next few years. Moreover, at 12 weeks of gestation, cervical length is normal in more than 95% of all patients, even in high-risk patients, and transvaginal ultrasonography to measure cervical length should not be initiated until 14–16 weeks of gestation, with the mean time of detection of cervical shortening in women destined to give birth preterm occurring at approximately 19 weeks of gestation.

No data suggest that decreased physical activity or bed rest can prevent preterm birth. In fact, data from the limited trials have shown an increase in the risk of preterm birth among women who are hospitalized prophylactically for bed rest.

Uterine contractions have been associated with preterm birth, but their predictive value is poor. An analysis of 14 trials showed that home uterine activity monitoring for 1 hour twice daily between 24 and 36 weeks of gestation is not associated with prevention of preterm birth. Therefore, such monitoring should not be routinely provided for prevention of preterm birth.

Crowther CA, Neilson JP, Verkuyl DA, Bannerman C, Ashurst HM. Preterm labour in twin pregnancies: can it be prevented by hospital admission? Br J Obstet Gynaecol 1989;96:850–3.

Dyson DC, Danbe KH, Bamber JA, Crites YM, Field DB, Maier JA, et al. Monitoring women at risk for preterm labor. N Engl J Med 1998; 338:15–9.

Final report of the Medical Research Council/Royal College of Obstetricians and Gynaecologists multicentre randomised trial of cervical cerclage. MRC/RCOG Working Party on Cervical Cerclage. Br J Obstet Gynaecol 1993;100:516–23.

Meis PJ, Klebanoff M, Thom E, Dombrowski MP, Sibai B, Moawad AH, et al. Prevention of recurrent preterm delivery by 17 alpha-hydroxyprogesterone caproate. National Institute of Child Health and Human Development Maternal-Fetal Medicine Units Network [published erratum appears in N Engl J Med 2003;349:1299]. N Engl J Med 2003;348:2379–85.

Rush RW, Issacs S, McPherson K, Jones L, Chalmers I, Grant A. A randomized controlled trial of cervical cerclage in women at high risk of spontaneous preterm delivery. Br J Obstet Gynaecol 1984;91: 724–30.

64

Use of heparin in the peripartum

A 31-year-old woman, gravida 2, para 1, presents in labor at 34 weeks of gestation. The fetus is in a frank breech presentation. The fetal heart rate tracing is reassuring. The cervix is 5 cm dilated with the presenting part at +1 station. The patient's medical history reveals that she is a compound heterozygote for factor V Leiden and prothrombin gene mutation and has had two previous episodes of thromboembolism, one 5 years ago and the other 3 years ago. Neither embolism was associated with pregnancy. She also has a strong family history of thromboses. She has been maintained throughout the pregnancy on therapeutic enoxaparin sodium (Lovenox), given subcutaneously twice daily. Her last injection was 4 hours ago. The decision is made to perform a cesarean delivery. The best choice of anesthesia for this patient is

    (A) spinal anesthesia

    (B) epidural anesthesia

    (C) protamine sulfate administration followed by epidural anesthesia

*   (D) general endotracheal anesthesia

The indication for therapeutic anticoagulation in this patient is her compound heterozygosity for two thrombophilias and two previous episodes of venous thromboembolism. The patient also has a family history of venous thromboembolism. When therapeutic anticoagulation is needed during pregnancy either adjusted-dose unfractionated heparin or adjusted-dose low molecular weight heparin may be used. The molecular weight of unfractionated heparin is 3,000–30,000 Daltons whereas the molecular weight of the second is 2,000–9,000 Daltons. Neither drug will cross the placenta because of its large molecular weight. Typically, unfractionated heparin is administered subcutaneously every 8–12 hours with the dose adjusted to target the midinterval partial thromboplastin time into the therapeutic range. Therapeutic low molecular weight heparin typically is administered twice daily in doses based on total body weight in the nonpregnant patient. However, in pregnancy, the dose usually is adjusted to produce an antifactor-Xa level between 0.5 and 1.2 units/mL measured 4 hours after the dose. There is no proven method for neutralizing low molecular weight heparin. Protamine appears to neutralize only about 60% of the antifactor-Xa activity of low molecular weight heparin. Low molecular weight heparin has less protein-binding, a longer half-life, and a more predictable response than unfractionated heparin. It also has the advantages of lower incidences of bleeding, osteoporosis, and heparin-induced thrombocytopenia. Another point to consider is that low molecular weight heparin is more expensive than unfractionated heparin.

The U.S. Food and Drug Administration has reported cases of epidural or spinal hematomas in nonpregnant patients with concurrent use of enoxaparin and spinal or epidural anesthesia. The hematomas have caused long-term or permanent paralysis. It is recommended that low molecular weight heparin be stopped 24 hours before regional anesthesia. The approach to peripartum low molecular weight heparin anticoagulation includes the following: 1) switch to unfractionated heparin at 36 weeks of gestation or 2) discontinue low molecular weight heparin 12–24 hours before planned induction of labor. Because the described patient is in preterm labor, this approach is not feasible. The best choice of anesthesia for this patient, who will undergo a cesarean delivery, is general endotracheal anesthesia.

American College of Obstetricians and Gynecologists. Thromboembolism in pregnancy. ACOG Practice Bulletin 19. Washington, DC: ACOG; 2000.

Bates SM, Greer IA, Hirsh J, Ginsberg J. Use of antithrombotic agents during pregnancy: the Seventh ACCP Conference on Antithrombotic and Thrombolytic Therapy. Chest 2004;126(suppl):627S–44S.

Hirsh J, Raschke R. Heparin and low-molecular-weight heparin: the Seventh ACCP Conference on Antithrombotic and Thrombolytic Therapy. Chest 2004;126(suppl):188S–203S.

65

Hyperemesis gravidarum

A 26-year-old woman, gravida 3, para 1, presents with a confirmed 9-week single intrauterine gestation with intense morning nausea and frequent vomiting throughout the day. Urine dipstick analysis is negative for ketones, and she is not tachycardic. The most appropriate initial treatment is

    (A) a tapered course of corticosteroids
    (B) intravenous fluids
    (C) ondansetron hydrochloride (Zofran)
*   (D) vitamin B_6

Nausea and vomiting of pregnancy, symptoms of the condition often referred to as "morning sickness," are some of the most common symptoms encountered in pregnancy. Nausea affects 70–80% of pregnant women; vomiting affects approximately 50%. Nausea and vomiting of pregnancy is a continuum classified into degrees of severity: mild disease (nausea only); moderate disease (nausea and vomiting); and severe disease (persistent vomiting leading to dehydration). Approximately 1–3% of women with nausea and vomiting of pregnancy experience a severe form known as hyperemesis gravidarum, which is characterized by intractable vomiting, weight loss of more than 5% of prepregnancy weight, dehydration, and electrolyte imbalances. Severe nausea and vomiting of pregnancy or hyperemesis gravidarum is the third most common indication for hospitalization during pregnancy.

Nausea and vomiting of pregnancy usually begins before 9 weeks of gestation. If a patient presents later than 9 weeks of gestation with new-onset nausea and vomiting, other conditions should be considered (Box 65-1). The exact etiology of nausea and vomiting of pregnancy remains unknown, although several theories have been proposed. Some have suggested that it is a result of increasing levels of human chorionic gonadotropin (hCG). Patients with increased placental mass, such as those with multiple gestations or a molar pregnancy, are at more risk for nausea and vomiting of pregnancy. Other risk factors include a family history of hyperemesis gravidarum, a prior pregnancy complicated by nausea and vomiting of pregnancy, history of motion sickness, and migraines.

If early symptoms are not treated, the likelihood of hospitalization for severe nausea and vomiting of pregnancy is increased. Early treatment helps to prevent the escalation of the disease. No uniform management scheme or evidence-based guidelines exist for management of nausea and vomiting of pregnancy. Nonpharmacologic thera-

---

BOX 65-1

Differential Diagnosis of Nausea and Vomiting of Pregnancy

Gastrointestinal conditions
- Gastroenteritis
- Gastroparesis
- Achalasia
- Biliary tract disease
- Hepatitis
- Intestinal obstruction
- Peptic ulcer disease
- Pancreatitis
- Appendicitis

Genitourinary tract conditions
- Pyelonephritis
- Uremia
- Ovarian torsion
- Kidney stones
- Degenerating uterine leiomyoma

Metabolic disease
- Diabetic ketoacidosis
- Porphyria
- Addison disease
- Hyperthyroidism

Neurologic disorders
- Pseudotumor cerebri
- Vestibular lesions
- Migraines
- Tumors of the central nervous system

Miscellaneous
- Drug toxicity or intolerance
- Psychologic

Pregnancy-related conditions
- Acute fatty liver of pregnancy
- Preeclampsia

Modified from Goodwin TM. Hyperemesis gravidarum. Clin Obstet Gynecol 1998;41:597–605.

pies center on prevention. Use of a multivitamin from the time of conception may be beneficial in preventing nausea and vomiting of pregnancy. Additional measures useful in managing symptoms of mild nausea and vomiting of pregnancy are listed in Box 65-2. Avoidance of offensive foods and smells and eating small, frequent meals are often recommended.

If conservative measures are ineffective, pharmacologic intervention for nausea and vomiting of pregnancy is recommended. A review of randomized trials concluded that antiemetic medications appear to decrease the frequency of nausea in early pregnancy. A pharmacologic treatment algorithm for nausea and vomiting of pregnancy is shown in Figure 65-1. The choice of medication is based on fetal safety and efficacy. Treatment begins with vitamin B_6 (pyridoxine) or a combination of vitamin B_6 and the antihistamine H_1-receptor blocker, doxylamine. These regimens are safe and effective and should be considered first-line therapies. Most studies also attest to the safety of phenothiazines. The use of 5-hydroxytryptamine 3 inhibitors (eg, ondansetron) is increasing in pregnancy partly because of the drug's efficacy in reducing chemotherapy-induced emesis. Droperidol in doses exceeding 25 mg has been associated with prolonged Q–T intervals leading to

fatal arrhythmias and should be used with caution. Corticosteroid use for nausea and vomiting of pregnancy should be avoided in gestations of less than 10 weeks because of the risk of oral clefts, but they may be used in extreme cases likely to require enteral or parenteral therapy. Recently, other treatments for nausea and vomiting of pregnancy, such as ginger and acupressure, have been suggested. In a recent trial, fresh ginger root was shown to be beneficial in reducing nausea and vomiting in pregnancy without adverse effects. Treatment with acupressure may work in decreasing nausea, but results from a recent review revealed equivocal results.

The first-line therapy for the woman with mild nausea and vomiting of pregnancy in this scenario is monotherapy with vitamin B_6 or vitamin B_6 plus doxylamine. A review of randomized trials concluded that pyridoxine on its own appears effective in reducing the severity of nausea and is least likely to cause side effects. Corticosteroids would not represent first-line therapy for nausea and vomiting of pregnancy and are not suggested in pregnancies less than 10 weeks of gestation. Intravenous hydration is reserved for women who have clinical signs and symptoms of dehydration and are unable to tolerate oral liquids or solids for an extended period. If ketosis is present, rehydration with a balanced salt solution with added dextrose and vitamins is recommended. Evidence is limited on the safety of ondansetron, but no developmental toxicity was found in animal studies at doses 70 times that given to humans. Ondansetron is not recommended as first-line therapy for nausea and vomiting of pregnancy because of its high cost.

BOX 65-2

Measures Useful in Managing Mild Symptoms of Nausea and Vomiting in Pregnancy

- Eating frequently in small amounts
- Eating high-carbohydrate, low-fat foods
- Eating protein-predominant meals
- Eating a bland, dry diet; try potato chips, crackers
- Drinking small amounts of cold, clear, carbonated, or sour liquids; drinking between meals rather than with meals
- Lying down as needed; getting plenty of rest
- Changing position slowly, especially when rising
- Going outside for fresh air as needed
- Avoiding offensive foods and smells
- Avoiding iron preparations
- Not brushing teeth after eating

Association of Professors of Gynecology and Obstetrics. Nausea and vomiting of pregnancy. APGO Educational Series on Women's Health Issues. Washington (DC): APGO; 2001. p. 17.

Association of Professors of Gynecology and Obstetrics. Nausea and vomiting of pregnancy. APGO Educational Series on Women's Health Issues. Washington, DC: APGO; 2001.

Jewell D, Young G. Interventions for nausea and vomiting in early pregnancy. Cochrane Database of Systematic Reviews 2003, Issue 4. Art. No.: CD000145. DOI: 10.1002/14651858.CD000145.

Koren G, Levichek Z. The teratogenicity of drugs for nausea and vomiting of pregnancy: perceived versus true risk. Am J Obstet Gynecol 2002;186(5 suppl understanding):S248–52.

Magee LA, Mazzotta P, Koren G. Evidence-based view of safety and effectiveness of pharmacologic therapy for nausea and vomiting of pregnancy (NVP). Am J Obstet Gynecol 2002;186(5 suppl understanding):S256–61.

Miller F. Nausea and vomiting in pregnancy: the problem of perception—is it really a disease? Am J Obstet Gynecol 2002;186(5 suppl understanding):S182–3.

Nausea and vomiting of pregnancy. ACOG Practice Bulletin No. 52. American College of Obstetricians and Gynecologists. Obstet Gynecol 2004;103:803–15.

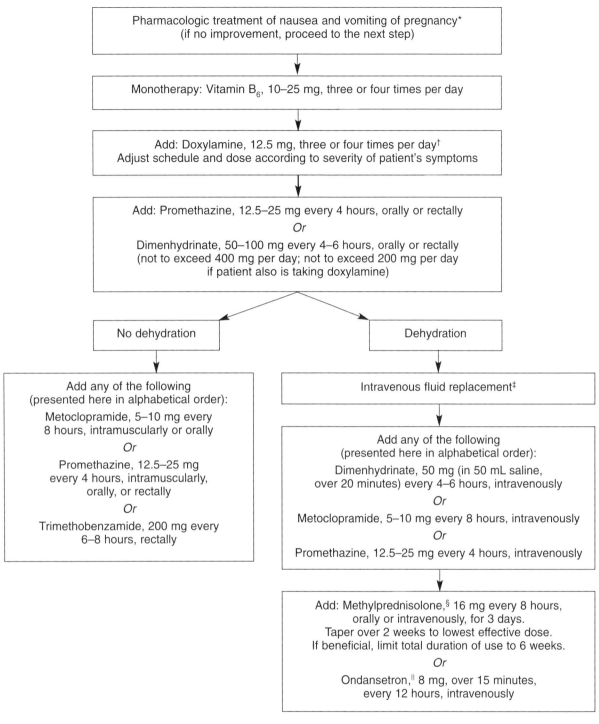

FIG. 65-1. Pharmacologic treatment of nausea and vomiting of pregnancy. (Nausea and vomiting of pregnancy. ACOG Practice Bulletin No. 52. American College of Obstetricians and Gynecologists. Obstet Gynecol 2004;103:803–15.)

66

Group B streptococci and penicillin allergy

A healthy 32-year-old woman, gravida 3, para 1, comes to the office for a prenatal visit at 36 weeks of gestation. She has received a positive test result from the vaginal and rectal culture for group B streptococci (GBS) that was obtained 1 week earlier. When you inquire about penicillin sensitivity, the patient reports that she had a mild allergic reaction to penicillin as a child. The next step in management is

       (A) intravenous clindamycin in labor
*   (B) intravenous cefazolin in labor
       (C) penicillin desensitization, then penicillin in labor
       (D) intravenous vancomycin in labor

Group B streptococci or *Streptococcus agalactiae* is an organism commonly found in the gastrointestinal tract of adults and is the likely source of vaginal colonization. Approximately 10–30% of pregnant women have GBS colonization of the vagina or rectum and most are asymptomatic. Nonpregnant carriers usually do not manifest disease. Pregnant carriers are at risk for urinary tract infection, chorioamnionitis, endometritis, sepsis, and in some instances, meningitis. Colonization of the lower genital tract with GBS may be transient, chronic, or intermittent; therefore, culture status may differ between pregnancies. If GBS is transmitted from the genital tract of a colonized woman to the fetus during labor or delivery, it can cause early-onset GBS disease, a severe invasive GBS infection that occurs during the neonate's first week of life. Early-onset disease may be reduced by using intrapartum chemoprophylaxis. In newborns, GBS can cause sepsis, pneumonia, and meningitis. Osteomyelitis, septic arthritis, and cellulitis are seen less frequently with neonatal GBS infection. However, proper peripartum identification and treatment of this organism can greatly reduce the risk of vertical transmission.

In 2002, the Centers for Disease Control and Prevention, the American Academy of Pediatrics, and the American College of Obstetricians and Gynecologists released revised national prevention guidelines recommending that obstetric providers adopt a universal antenatal culture-based screening approach to prevent early-onset GBS disease in the newborn (Fig. 66-1). All pregnant women should be screened for GBS colonization at 35–37 weeks of gestation unless GBS bacteriuria in any concentration is identified during the current pregnancy or if a previous infant had invasive GBS disease.

All women with a positive GBS screening culture result during the current pregnancy should receive intrapartum antibiotic prophylaxis. The only exception to this rule is women who undergo a planned a cesarean delivery

before the onset of labor or rupture of membranes. Other candidates for intrapartum antibiotic prophylaxis are listed in Figure 66-1. The criteria for prophylaxis for women with threatened preterm labor are summarized in Figure 66-2.

Recommended treatment regimens for intrapartum antibiotic prophylaxis for GBS prevention are listed in Table 66-1. The first-line medication for intrapartum GBS prophylaxis is penicillin. In a woman with a sensitivity or allergy to penicillin, the physician should carefully assess her history during the prenatal visit to determine whether she is at high risk for anaphylaxis. Women considered at high risk for anaphylaxis include those with a history of immediate hypersensitivity reactions to penicillin (eg, anaphylaxis, angioedema, or urticaria), as well as those with a history of asthma or other conditions that would make anaphylaxis more dangerous or more difficult to treat.

In women with a penicillin allergy who are at low risk for anaphylaxis, cefazolin is the recommended alternate therapy. In penicillin-sensitive women who are at high risk for anaphylaxis or whose anaphylaxis risk is uncertain, clindamycin and erythromycin susceptibility testing should be performed on GBS isolates. Women with isolates that are susceptible to clindamycin and erythromycin should be given intrapartum treatment with the appropriate drug. If the isolates are resistant to erythromycin or clindamycin, women can be given vancomycin.

The additional step of clindamycin and erythromycin sensitivity testing is recommended for penicillin-allergic women and those at high risk of anaphylaxis due to a recent increase in the proportion of GBS isolates that are resistant to second-line therapies. Administration of either clindamycin or erythromycin without sensitivity testing carries the risk of encountering a resistant GBS isolate and subsequent risk of GBS transmission to the neonate.

Vaginal and rectal GBS screening cultures at 35–37 weeks of gestation for *all* pregnant women (unless patient had GBS bacteriuria during the current pregnancy or a previous infant with invasive GBS disease)

Intrapartum prophylaxis indicated:

- Previous infant with invasive GBS disease
- GBS bacteriuria during current pregnancy
- Positive GBS screening culture during current pregnancy (unless a planned cesarean delivery, in the absence of labor or amniotic membrane rupture, is performed)
- Unknown GBS status (culture not done, incomplete, or results unknown) and any of the following:
  — Delivery at less than 37 weeks of gestation*
  — Amniotic membrane rupture at 18 hours or later
  — Intrapartum temperature 38.0°C (100.4°F) or higher[†]

Intrapartum prophylaxis not indicated:

- Previous pregnancy with a positive GBS screening culture (unless a culture was also positive during the current pregnancy)
- Planned cesarean delivery performed in the absence of labor or membrane rupture (regardless of maternal GBS culture status)
- Negative vaginal and rectal GBS screening culture in late gestation during the current pregnancy, regardless of intrapartum risk factors

FIG. 66-1. Indications for intrapartum antibiotic prophylaxis to prevent perinatal group B streptococci (GBS) disease under a universal prenatal screening strategy based on combined vaginal and rectal cultures collected from all pregnant women. *If onset of labor or rupture of amniotic membranes occurs before 37 weeks of gestation and there is a significant risk of preterm delivery (as assessed by the clinician), a suggested algorithm for GBS prophylaxis management is provided (see Fig. 66-2). [†]If amnionitis is suspected, broad-spectrum antibiotic therapy that includes an agent known to be active against GBS should replace GBS prophylaxis. (Prevention of perinatal group B streptococcal disease. Revised guidelines from CDC. MMWR Recomm Rep 2002;51(RR-11):1–22.)

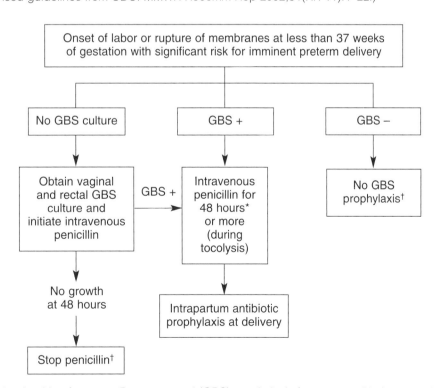

FIG. 66-2. Sample algorithm for group B streptococci (GBS) prophylaxis for women with threatened preterm delivery. This algorithm is not an exclusive course of management. Variations that incorporate individual circumstances or institutional preferences may be appropriate. (Schrag S, Gorwitz R, Fultz-Butts K, Schuchat A. Prevention of perinatal group B streptococcal disease. Revised guidelines from CDC. MMWR Recomm Rep 2002;51(RR-11):1–22.)

TABLE 66-1. Recommended Regimens for Intrapartum Antimicrobial Prophylaxis for Perinatal Group B Streptococcal Disease Prevention*

Prophylaxis	Regimen
Recommended	Penicillin G, 5 million units IV initial dose, then 2.5 million units IV every 4 hours until delivery
Alternative	Ampicillin, 2 g IV initial dose, then 1 g IV every 4 hours until delivery
If penicillin allergic[†]	
Patient not at high risk for anaphylaxis	Cefazolin, 2 g initial dose, then 1 g IV every 8 hours until delivery
Patient at high risk for anaphylaxis[‡]	
GBS susceptible to clindamycin and erythromycin[§]	Clindamycin, 900 mg IV every 8 hours until delivery *or* Erythromycin, 500 mg IV every 6 hours until delivery
GBS resistant to clindamycin or erythromycin or susceptibility unknown	Vancomycin,[‖] 1 g IV every 12 hours until delivery

GBS, group B streptococci; IV, intravenous.

*Broader-spectrum agents, including an agent active against GBS, may be necessary for treatment of chorioamnionitis.

[†]History of penicillin allergy should be assessed to determine whether a high risk for anaphylaxis is present. Penicillin-allergic patients at high risk for anaphylaxis are those who have experienced immediate hypersensitivity to penicillin including a history of penicillin-related anaphylaxis; other high-risk patients are those with asthma or other diseases that would make anaphylaxis more dangerous or difficult to treat, such as persons being threatened with β-adrenergic-blocking agents.

[‡]If laboratory facilities are adequate, clindamycin and erythromycin susceptibility testing should be performed on prenatal GBS isolates from penicillin-allergic women at high risk for anaphylaxis.

[§]Resistance to erythromycin is often but not always associated with clindamycin resistance. If a strain is resistant to erythromycin but appears susceptible to clindamycin, it may still have inducible resistance to clindamycin.

[‖]Cefazolin is preferred over vancomycin for women with a history of penicillin allergy other than immediate hypersensitivity reactions, and pharmacologic data suggest it achieves effective intraamniotic concentrations. Vancomycin should be reserved for penicillin-allergic women at high risk of anaphylaxis.

Schrag S, Gorwitz R, Fultz-Butts K, Schuchat A. Prevention of perinatal group B streptococcal disease. Revised guidelines from CDC. MMWR Recomm Rep 2002;51(RR-11):1–22.

In this scenario, the patient has a history of a mild penicillin reaction in childhood with no mention of anaphylaxis or asthma; therefore, in lieu of penicillin, intrapartum antibiotic prophylaxis with cefazolin should be initiated in labor. Because there are several alternatives to penicillin that can be used safely and effectively for intrapartum GBS prophylaxis, penicillin desensitization is not indicated. She should not be given vancomycin, because this medication should be reserved for those individuals who are penicillin-allergic, who have a high risk for anaphylaxis, and who have GBS isolates that are resistant to clindamycin and erythromycin.

Gibbs RS, Schrag S, Schuchat A. Perinatal infections due to group B streptococci. Obstet Gynecol 2004;104:1062–76.

Prevention of early-onset group B streptococcal disease in newborns. ACOG Committee Opinion No. 279. American College of Obstetricians and Gynecologists. Obstet Gynecol 2002;100:1405–12.

Schrag S, Gorwitz R, Fultz-Butts K, Schuchat A. Prevention of perinatal group B streptococcal disease. Revised guidelines from CDC. MMWR Recomm Rep 2002;51(RR-11):1–22.

67

Premature rupture of membranes at term

A 29-year-old woman, gravida 2, para 1, presents at 39 weeks of gestation with spontaneous rupture of membranes 6 hours before presentation. Her dates were confirmed by first-trimester ultrasonography. Her group B streptococci (GBS) culture was negative at 35 weeks of gestation. Rupture of membranes is confirmed by pooling, nitrazine, and ferning on speculum examination. Her cervix appears to be 1 cm dilated. Her vital signs are within normal limits. The ultrasonogram shows the fetus in vertex presentation. Monitoring reveals reassuring fetal status and no uterine contractions. The next best step in management is

* (A) induction of labor with oxytocin
  (B) discharge home to return when uncomfortable with uterine contractions
  (C) antibiotic prophylaxis
  (D) amniocentesis

The diagnosis of premature rupture of membranes (PROM) at term is based on pooling, ferning, and nitrazine tests. Direct visualization of pooling, which can be detected spontaneously or after asking the patient to perform a Valsalva maneuver, is considered diagnostic for PROM. The sensitivity, specificity, and positive and negative predictive values of nitrazine and ferning tests are all very high. There is no need to perform amniocentesis to confirm the diagnosis of PROM, especially when all three tests results are positive. Fetal maturity does not need to be assessed by amniocentesis in this patient because gestational age of 39 weeks has been confirmed by first-trimester ultrasonography.

The patient described shows no signs of intrauterine infection (chorioamnionitis). Chorioamnionitis usually is diagnosed at term by the presence of two or more of the following criteria: maternal tachycardia; fetal tachycardia; maternal fever; and fundal tenderness. Chorioamnionitis would be treated with antibiotics in a woman with PROM at term, without the need for an amniocentesis.

The most common complication of PROM at term is intrauterine infection; this incidence increases with duration of PROM, and, with longer latency, the risk of neonatal infection also increases. Maternal colonization with GBS is another risk factor for neonatal infection in women with term PROM; therefore, it is recommended that women with GBS colonization be induced immediately. Women whose test results were negative for GBS seen at 35–37 weeks of gestation and have a PROM of more than 18 hours do not need prophylaxis.

Approximately 50% of women with PROM at term give birth spontaneously within 6–12 hours, and approximately 70–90% give birth within 24 hours. Frequent digital cervical examinations should be avoided because they increase the risk of infection. Fetal presentation confirmed by ultrasonography, gestational age by records, and fetal status by external monitoring should be accurately checked and documented. Fetuses with nonreassuring heart testing should be delivered promptly.

Women with PROM at term should be hospitalized because management of PROM at term at home is associated with a 52% increase in need for maternal antibiotics for nulliparous women and with 97% more neonatal infections. Women with PROM at term should be induced with oxytocin within 6–12 hours of PROM. Compared with expectant management, induction of labor by oxytocin is associated with significant decreases in risks of maternal infection, endometritis, and neonatal infection. Compared with prostaglandins, oxytocin used to induce labor is associated with a decrease in maternal nausea or vomiting, numerous vaginal examinations, chorioamnionitis and neonatal infections, neonatal antibiotic therapy, and admission of the newborn to the neonatal intensive care unit, but increases in epidural analgesia and internal fetal heart rate monitoring. Cesarean delivery, endometritis, and perinatal mortality are not significantly different between the expectant management group and the induction with oxytocin group. Cost is less with oxytocin induction. Therefore, oxytocin induction for the woman with PROM at term is safe, effective, and cost-effective. Misoprostol induction is an alternative that is as effective, but data on its safety are insufficient. Foley catheter cervical ripening has not been sufficiently studied in randomized trials to assess its safety and efficacy for women with PROM at term. Most women with PROM at term, if given a choice, prefer induction.

The rate of maternal infection in this population is approximately 7% and even lower with immediate induction. It does not seem justifiable to expose all women with term PROM to antibiotics when treatment can be restricted to those who develop clinical indications for antibiotic treatment. All women with GBS colonization or a diagnosis of chorioamnionitis should receive appropriate antibiotics.

Dare MR, Middleton P, Crowther CA, Flenady VJ, Varatharaju B. Planned early birth versus expectant management (waiting) for prelabour rupture of membranes at term (37 weeks or more). Cochrane Database of Systematic Reviews 2006, Issue 1. Art. No.: CD005302. DOI: 10.1002/14651858.CD005302.pub2.

Davidson KM. Detection of premature rupture of membranes. Clin Obstet Gynecol 1991;34:715–22.

Hannah ME, Ohlsson A, Farine D, Hewson SA, Hodnett ED, Myhr TL, et al. Induction of labor compared with expectant management for

prelabor rupture of the membranes at term. TERMPROM Study Group. N Engl J Med 1996;334:1005–10.

Pereira L, Gould R, Pelham J, Goldberg J. Correlation between visual examination of the cervix and digital examination. J Matern Fetal Neonatal Med 2005;17:223–7.

Schrag S, Gorwitz R, Fultz-Butts K, Schuchat A. Prevention of perinatal group B streptococcal disease. Revised guidelines from CDC. MMWR Recomm Rep 2002;51(RR-11):1–22.

68

Fetal hyperthyroidism

A 34-year-old woman at 34 weeks of gestation has Graves disease. She takes propylthiouracil daily. Her thyroid-stimulating hormone (TSH) and free thyroxine (T_4) levels are within normal limits. Her thyroid-stimulating immunoglobulin level is elevated. Ultrasonography shows a homogenous anterior fetal neck mass. The estimated fetal weight is at approximately the 7th percentile for 34 weeks of gestation. The fetal heart rate is 180–190 beats per minute. The amniotic fluid index is 24 cm. You note evidence of fetal scalp edema and ascites. The most likely diagnosis is

    (A) anterior cystic hygroma
    (B) fetal hypothyroidism
*   (C) fetal hyperthyroidism
    (D) fetal supraventricular arrhythmia
    (E) immune hydrops

Fetal thyroid dysfunction can be caused by TSH receptor antibodies of maternal origin. These autoantibodies are immunoglobulin G (IgG) antibodies and can cross the placenta. Women with Graves disease have thyroid-stimulating immunoglobulin. If IgG crosses the placenta, it can stimulate the fetal thyroid and potentially cause fetal thyrotoxicosis. Maternal-to-fetal IgG transport tends to occur after 24–26 weeks of gestation and maternal–fetal IgG levels equilibrate; thus, maternal levels are indicative of fetal risks. The synthesis of thyroid hormones in the fetus remains limited up to 20 weeks of gestation; therefore, the effects of autoantibodies on the fetal thyroid do not become important until after 24 weeks of gestation.

The incidence of fetal–neonatal hyperthyroidism is not related to maternal thyroid function but to circulating levels of autoantibodies. In fact, neonates of women who have surgical or radioactive treatment and require no thioamide treatment are at higher risk because they lack suppressive thioamide protection. In a mother with Graves disease, fetal hyperthyroidism can be suspected based on the findings of a fetal neck mass, intrauterine growth restriction, or tachycardia. Hyperdynamic circulation associated with thyrotoxicosis can cause congestive

heart failure and hydrops in the fetus. It has been estimated that 1–5% of these neonates develop hyperthyroidism as a result of transplacental passage of maternal thyroid-stimulating immunoglobulin. If the maternal thyroid-stimulating immunoglobulin is normal, the likelihood of fetal hypothyroidism is low.

Fetal hypothyroidism also can develop as a result of placental transfer of IgG antibodies. Patients with Graves disease or other autoimmune thyroid disease can produce TSH-receptor blocking antibodies or TSH-binding inhibiting immunoglobulin, which can cause transient fetal–neonatal hypothyroidism. Thioamides (eg, propylthiouracil or methimazole) used to treat Graves disease also cross the placenta and can cause clinically evident fetal thyroid suppression. In addition, inadvertent maternal radioiodine treatment for Graves disease in pregnancy causes fetal hypothyroidism. Hypothyroidism is suspected when fetal goiter is noted; delayed bone maturation also may be observed. Hydrops fetalis as a result of fetal hypothyroidism has been reported.

The incidence of fetal thyroid dysfunction is low because there is usually a balance between stimulatory and inhibitory antibodies with thioamide treatment. Nevertheless, fetuses and neonates of women with Graves disease, autoimmune thyroiditis, or circulating thyroid antibodies and those on antithyroid therapy are at risk for thyroid dysfunction. Serial ultrasonographic assessment for a fetal goiter may be considered in these high-risk groups. Nomograms are available for fetal thyroid measurements. Recently, three-dimensional ultrasonography combined with power Doppler angiography has been shown to be useful in the evaluation and management of a fetus with a goiter.

Hyperthyroidism in the fetus is treated by administering propylthiouracil to the mother. The dose is adjusted to maintain the fetal heart rate at 140 beats per minute.

Fetal hypothyroidism in the presence of maternal propylthiouracil administration initially can be treated by decreasing the dose. If there is no resolution of the fetal goiter, fetal thyroxine therapy is required, by means of intraamniotic injections at 7- to 10-day intervals, because thyroxine crosses the placenta in limited amounts. The literature shows resolution of the fetal goiter and achievement of euthyroid fetal status before delivery in most cases treated with intraamniotic thyroxine. Table 68-1 shows placental permeability for substances that affect thyroid function.

Anterior cystic hygroma is a rare condition that presents with a multicystic mass and thus is unlikely in this patient. Fetal hypothyroidism is less likely because of the fetal tachycardia in this case. Fetal supraventricular arrhythmia is associated with fetal heart rates of 220 beats per minute or more. Immune hydrops fetalis is doubtful because of the fetal neck mass and no history for isoimmunization is provided.

TABLE 68-1. Placental Permeability for Substances Affecting Thyroid Function

Substance	Placental Permeability
Iodide	++++
Thyrotropin-releasing hormone	++++
Thyroid-stimulating hormone	0
Triiodothyronine (T_3)	0
Thyroxine (T_4)	+
Thioureylenes	+++
Thyroid IgG autoantibodies	+++

IgG, immunoglobulin G.

Adapted from Fisher DA. Fetal thyroid function: diagnosis and management of fetal thyroid disorders. Clin Obstet Gynecol 1997;24:16–31 and Mitsuda N, Tamaki, Amino N, Hosono T, Miyai K, Tanizawa O. Risk factors for developmental disorders in infants born to women with Graves disease. Obstet Gynecol 1992;80:359–64.

Brand F, Liegeois P, Langer B. One case of fetal and neonatal variable thyroid dysfunction in the context of Graves' disease. Fetal Diagn Ther 2005;20:12–5.

Fisher DA. Fetal thyroid function: diagnosis and management of fetal thyroid disorders. Clin Obstet Gynecol 1997;24:16–31.

Lembet A, Eroglu D, Kinik ST, Gurakan B, Kuscu E. Non-invasive management of fetal goiter during maternal treatment of hyperthyroidism in Graves disease. Fetal Diagn Ther 2005;20:254–7.

Nath CA, Oyelese Y, Yeo L, Chavez M, Kontopoulos EV, Giannina G, et al. Three-dimensional sonography in the evaluation and management of fetal goiter. Ultrasound Obstet Gynecol 2005;25:312–4.

Thyroid disease in pregnancy. ACOG Practice Bulletin No. 37. American College of Obstetricians and Gynecologists. Obstet Gynecol 2002;100:387–96.

Yanai N, Shveiky D. Fetal hydrops, associated with maternal propylthiouracil exposure, reversed by intrauterine therapy. Ultrasound Obstet Gynecol 2004;23;198–201.

69

Perinatal survival

A 22-year-old woman, gravida 4, presents at 23 1/7 weeks of gestation with uterine contractions. Gestational age has been confirmed by a first-trimester ultrasound examination. On examination, the cervix is 7 cm dilated, with delivery estimated to be imminent. The external fetal heart tracing is reassuring for gestational age. In counseling her, you should tell her that for the neonate, the most probable outcome regarding mortality and morbidity (for survivors) will be

    (A) low mortality with low morbidity
    (B) low mortality with high morbidity
    (C) high mortality with low morbidity
*   (D) high mortality with high morbidity

Up to about 10 years ago, there were no reports of survival before 24 weeks of gestation. This remains true in many countries. Advances in neonatal care have resulted in improved rates of morbidity and mortality in the very preterm neonate. Nonetheless, birth at gestational ages less than 32 weeks continues to be associated with significant morbidity and mortality, especially at the limits of viability, which in the United States is currently about 22–24 weeks of gestation.

At 23 weeks of gestation, U.S. academic tertiary care nurseries have recently reported survival rates as high as 11–40%. Therefore, a woman who presents at 23 weeks of gestation at high risk for imminent preterm birth should be counseled that survival is possible. Nonetheless, the most probable outcome is death (high mortality), not survival, for the fetus about to be born at 23 weeks of gestation.

The described patient also should be counseled regarding the fact that, if the neonate survives, the chance of intact survival is low, approximately 1–30%. Survival without disability at 6 years of age after being born at 23 weeks has been reported to be as low as 1%, despite the fact that most of these infants received steroids as fetuses and surfactant as neonates. The morbidities associated with preterm birth at less than 32 weeks of gestation, and at 23 weeks of gestation in particular, include respiratory distress syndrome (RDS), intraventricular hemorrhage, necrotizing enterocolitis, sepsis, and retinopathy. Therefore, even if this 23-week fetus survives the neonatal period, the chance of significant morbidity is high.

A neonatology consultation may be very useful in helping the patient and her family better understand the prognosis and management options. The most current rates of mortality and of morbidity for the survivors should be reviewed with the patient and her family.

Corticosteroids given before preterm birth (either spontaneous or indicated) at 24–33 6/7 weeks of gestation are effective in preventing RDS, intraventricular hemorrhage, and neonatal mortality. Antenatal administration of betamethasone or dexamethasone to women who are expected to give birth preterm is associated with significant (40%) reduction in mortality, 47% reduction in RDS, and 52% reduction in intraventricular hemorrhage in preterm infants. A trend for a 41% reduction in necrotizing enterocolitis has been observed, as has decreased need for surfactant, oxygen, and mechanical ventilation in the neonatal period. These benefits apply to gestational ages of at least 24–33 6/7 weeks, and are not limited by sex or race. The effects are significant mostly at 48 hours to 7 days from the first dose, but treatment should not be withheld even if delivery appears imminent. Such steroids should therefore be administered to any woman at these gestational ages at significant preterm birth risk on identification of the risk.

Insufficient data are available to assess steroid effect before or after these gestational ages. Although there has been no randomized trial on the use of steroids before 24 weeks, recent limited data have shown that the benefits described previously, observed at 24–34 weeks of gestation, may apply to patients at 22 and 23 weeks of gestation as well. At this point, however, insufficient information exists to recommend corticosteroids for fetal lung maturity before 24 weeks. Even with administration of betamethasone or dexamethasone, the prognosis of a neonate born at 23 1/7 weeks of gestation is one of high mortality, and high morbidity for the survivors.

Roberts D, Dalziel S. Antenatal corticosteroids for accelerating fetal lung maturation for women at risk of preterm birth. Cochrane Database of Systematic Reviews 2006, Issue 3. Art. No.: CD004454. DOI: 10.1002/14651858.CD004454.pub2.

Herber-Jonat S, Schulze A, Kribs A, Roth B, Lindner W, Pohlandt F. Survival and major neonatal complications in infants born between 22 0/7 and 24 6/7 weeks of gestation (1999–2003). Am J Obstet Gynecol 2006;195:16–22.

Marlow N, Wolke D, Bracewell MA, Samara M. Neurologic and developmental disability at six years of age after extremely preterm birth. EPICure Study Group. N Engl J Med 2005;352:9–19.

Vohr BR, Allen M. Extreme prematurity—the continuing dilemma [editorial]. N Engl J Med 2005;352:71–2.

70

Positive antibody screen

A 24-year-old woman, gravida 3, para 1, at 14 weeks of gestation, returns for her second prenatal care visit. Her antibody screen is positive with anti-D titers of 1:16. The next step in care is

    (A) repeat antibody screen in 1 month to reassess the anti-D titer
    (B) amniocentesis for fetal genotype
    (C) antenatal testing at 32 weeks of gestation
    (D) middle cerebral artery Doppler velocimetry
*   (E) determine paternal RhD status and zygosity

With the advent of Rh-immune globulin (RhIgG), rhesus alloimmunization has significantly decreased as a cause of perinatal morbidity and mortality. Currently the prevalence of this condition is 1–6 cases per 1,000 live births. Once sensitization occurs, RhIgG is no longer effective in preventing hemolytic disease. Currently, atypical antibodies cause 50% of alloimmunization. Management of a sensitized pregnancy involves making the following determinations:

- Whether the fetus is at risk for hemolytic disease
- Whether the affected fetus has a significant risk for hydrops fetalis
- When intervention is required

An antibody screen is an indirect Coombs test to determine the degree of alloimmunization. The first step in managing a patient with a positive antibody screen is to determine whether the antibody causes fetal hemolytic disease. Appendix F shows antigens that cause fetal hemolytic disease. Appendix G shows the atypical antibodies and their relationship to fetal hemolytic disease.

If the antibody can cause fetal hemolytic disease, the next step is to determine whether the fetus is at risk. Confirmation of paternity is a crucial part of this evaluation and requires a private conversation with the patient. Once the father of the baby is identified, his blood should be drawn for genotype. If he is homozygous for antibody-directed antigen, the fetus will carry the antigen. If he is heterozygous for the antibody-directed antigen, the fetus has a 50% chance of carrying the antigen.

If the fetus is at risk for hemolytic disease, maternal antibody titers should be checked every month until 24 weeks of gestation and then every 2 weeks for the remainder of the pregnancy. If a critical titer is reached (ie, 1:16 or greater), the fetus is at significant risk for hydrops fetalis. This titer will vary among institutions and is based on unique institutional clinical correlation. If the potential for fetal hydrops exists and the father is heterozygous, an amniocentesis can be performed to determine fetal genotype. Fetal genotype is determined by the polymerase chain reaction (PCR) test. Maternal and paternal blood needs to be compared with the PCR primers to prevent an incorrect fetal genotype evaluation.

If the fetus has the antibody-directed genotype, serial evaluations are required to determine if fetal anemia is present. Fetal anemia can be detected by middle cerebral artery Doppler velocimetry or amniotic fluid ΔOD_{450}. A middle cerebral artery Doppler greater than 1.5 MoM or an amniotic fluid ΔOD_{450} in the 80th percentile of zone II of the Liley curve or in the intrauterine transfusion zone of the Queenan curve indicates severe fetal anemia, and a fetal blood sampling is required. Doppler velocimetry is equivalent to amniotic fluid ΔOD_{450} and may offer advantages due to its noninvasive nature. If the fetal hematocrit is less than 30%, either a transfusion or delivery is required, depending on gestational age.

For the clinical scenario above, RhD is a major cause of fetal hemolytic disease. There are three rhesus antigen groups, D, C/c, and E/e. There are two rhesus genes, an *RhD* gene and an *RhCE* gene. These genes are found on the short arm of chromosome one. The genes are closely linked, and as a result with the appropriate antisera and gene frequency tables based on ethnicity, blood banks can predict paternal zygosity.

Antenatal testing usually is indicated for alloimmunized pregnancies at 32 weeks of gestation or at an earlier gestational age if an intrauterine transfusion has been performed. Appendix H shows an algorithm for overall clinical management of a sensitized pregnancy.

In the future, this management paradigm will change. Free fetal DNA has been isolated from maternal blood. The use of Rh genotyping on this free fetal DNA will eliminate the need for an invasive test.

Lipitz S, Many A, Mitrani-Rosenbaum S, Carp H, Frenkel Y, Achiron R. Obstetric outcome after RhD and Kell testing. Hum Reprod 1998; 13:1472–5.

Management of alloimmunization during pregnancy. ACOG Practice Bulletin No. 75. American College of Obstetricians and Gynecologists. Obstet Gynecol 2006;108:457–64.

Moise KJ Jr. Management of rhesus alloimmunization in pregnancy [published erratum appears in Obstet Gynecol 2002;100:833]. Obstet Gynecol 2002;100:600–11.

Zhou L, Thorson JA, Nugent C, Davenport RD, Butch SH, Judd WJ. Noninvasive prenatal RHD genotyping by real-time polymerase chain reaction using plasma from D-negative pregnant women. Am J Obstet Gynecol 2005;193:1966–71.

71

Tubal sterilization

A 27-year-old woman, gravida 4, para 3, is interested in sterilization after the birth of her current child. You advise her that the method with the lowest long-term failure rate is

    (A) interval sterilization using clips
* (B) immediate postpartum bilateral partial salpingectomy
    (C) interval sterilization using bipolar cautery
    (D) immediate postpartum sterilization using bipolar cautery

Sterilization is the most commonly used method of contraception in the United States, with nearly 750,000 tubal sterilization procedures performed annually. Such widespread use has led investigators to explore the most efficacious means to accomplish this procedure in a manner that maximizes patient safety and minimizes method failure. Approximately half of tubal sterilization procedures are performed as so-called interval procedures (unrelated in time to a pregnancy), with the remainder being performed either after delivery or after pregnancy termination.

Tubal sterilization should be undertaken only after the patient understands that the intent is for the procedure to be permanent. Selection of procedure, however, is frequently determined based on postpartum status, patient body habitus, estimated method-failure rate, and ease of reversibility. Techniques of female sterilization vary, and generally rely on occlusion of the fallopian tubes using cautery, clips, silastic bands, or suture. Intervening segments of tube are not always removed, depending on the technique employed. Recently, hysteroscopic tubal occlusion has been introduced, but long-term data on the efficacy of this method in the United States are not yet available.

The most commonly used laparoscopic method of tubal sterilization is bipolar electrocoagulation. At least 3 cm of isthmic tube should be destroyed, and use of a current meter is recommended to determine when the procedure is complete. Less thermal injury occurs using this method than occurs with unipolar cautery. Ectopic pregnancy risk is greatest after bipolar versus unipolar cautery, spring clip, or silicone band sterilization procedures. The timing of the procedure also has been investigated. In the U.S. Collaborative Review of Sterilization (CREST) study, the overall lowest cumulative failure rate of tubal sterilization at 5 and 10 years occurred with partial salpingectomy performed immediately postpartum (Table 71-1).

Benefits and risks of sterilization. ACOG Practice Bulletin No. 46. American College of Obstetricians and Gynecologists. Obstet Gynecol 2003;102:647–58.

Peterson HB, Xia Z, Hughes JM, Wilcox LS, Tylor LR, Trussell J. The risk of ectopic pregnancy after tubal sterilization. U.S. Collaborative Review of Sterilization Working Group. N Engl J Med 1997;336:762–7.

Peterson HB, Xia Z, Hughes JM, Wilcox LS, Tylor LR, Trussell J. The risk of pregnancy after tubal sterilization: findings from the U.S. Collaborative Review of Sterilization. Am J Obstet Gynecol 1996;174:1161–8; discussion 1168–70.

TABLE 71-1. Cumulative Probability of Ectopic Pregnancy Among Women Who Had Undergone Tubal Sterilization, According to Time Since Sterilization*

Method	No. of Women	No. of Ectopic Pregnancies†	No. per 1,000 Procedures (95% CI) by Years Since Sterilization		
			1	5	10
Bipolar coagulation	2,267	24	0.5 (0.0–1.3)	10.1 (5.4–14.7)	17.1 (9.8–24.4)
Unipolar coagulation	1,432	1	0.0	0.0	1.8 (0.0–5.2)
Silicone rubber-band application	3,329	10	0.6 (0.0–1.5)	2.5 (0.6–4.4)	7.3 (1.6–12.9)
Spring-clip application	1,595	7	1.3 (0.0–3.1)	3.6 (0.4–6.7)	8.5 (1.0–16.0)
Interval partial salpingectomy	425	3	4.9 (0.0–11.6)	7.5 (0.0–15.9)	7.5 (0.0–15.9)
Postpartum partial salpingectomy‡	1,637	2	0.0	1.5 (0.0–3.6)	1.5 (0.0–3.6)
All methods	10,685	47	0.7 (0.2–1.2)	4.0 (2.6–5.3)	7.3 (5.0–9.6)

*The probabilities were derived from life-table methods. CI, confidence interval.

†The number of ectopic pregnancies is that identified during 10 years of follow-up.

‡This category includes women undergoing sterilization after vaginal delivery (n = 1,166) or at the same time as a cesarean delivery (n = 471).

Peterson HB, Xia Z, Hughes JM, Wilcox LS, Tylor LR, Trussell J. The risk of ectopic pregnancy after tubal sterilization. U.S. Collaborative Review of Sterilization Working Group. N Engl J Med 1997;336:764. Copyright 1997 by the Massachusetts Medical Society.

72
Amnionitis

A 24-year-old woman, gravida 2, para 1, comes to the labor and delivery department at 28 weeks of gestation with leakage of vaginal fluid. Physical examination confirms rupture of membranes and, after further evaluation, she is considered a good candidate for expectant management. Over the next week, she remains hospitalized with reassuring fetal monitoring, no uterine contractions, and no signs or symptoms of chorioamnionitis.

One week later, you discover that she has symptoms of an upper respiratory infection, including rhinitis, nonproductive cough, and a headache. Later that morning, her temperature is 38°C (100.4°F). A complete blood count reveals an unchanged hematocrit and white blood cell count of 12,400 cells/mm^3. On examination, her uterus is nontender, her pulse rate is 120 beats per minute, and the fetal heart rate is 170 beats per minute. The differential diagnoses include chorioamnionitis and an upper respiratory infection. You perform an amniocentesis and obtain 10 mL of clear fluid. The amniotic fluid finding most sensitive and specific for chorioamnionitis is

* (A) positive Gram stain
   (B) white blood cell count of 25 cells/mm^3
   (C) glucose of 30 mg/dL
   (D) leukocyte esterase positive

The diagnosis of intraamniotic infection or chorioamnionitis is generally clinical and based on a number of parameters. The diagnosis is most commonly made and easiest to make in an at-risk patient such as one with premature rupture of membranes. The clinical criteria remain the same in patients with presenting symptoms that include uterine contractions and uterine tenderness. Patients frequently have tenderness on examination, foul-smelling vaginal discharge, fetal tachycardia, fever, and maternal tachycardia. In the setting of ruptured membranes or another high-risk factor such as advanced cervical dilatation, these findings usually are sufficient to institute therapy, including delivery.

In situations in which the clinical picture is confusing or ambiguous, the next step usually is an amniocentesis. In many cases, an amniocentesis is technically not possible because most of these patients have premature rupture of membranes and resulting oligohydramnios. If amniocentesis can be done, the criterion standard for diagnosis is culture. The results of an amniotic fluid culture are not available for several days. However, a variety of rapid tests are used for clinical management, including a glucose level, Gram stain, an interleukin-6 level, amniotic fluid white blood cell count, and leukocyte esterase activity. Use of the interleukin-6 level has been studied extensively; however, the interleukin-6 level is not clinically available in most centers. An elevated interleukin-6 level results in a very high sensitivity and good specificity with

an extremely high negative predictive level; positive predictive value is more modest and comparable to other tests. A Gram stain has good sensitivity and very good specificity resulting in high negative and positive predictive values, although a Gram stain is not diagnostic in all cases. A low glucose level has a high negative predictive value and modest positive predictive value. The cutoff used for glucose level in most studies is less than 14 mg/dL. A white blood cell count of greater than 50 cells/mm^3 is an excellent test if negative, but this test is not always reliable.

Leukocyte esterase activity has been tested on term patients with transvaginal collection and found to be highly sensitive and specific for the presence of chorioamnionitis defined clinically in laboring patients. Leukocyte esterase activity has not been confirmed in large studies, and it has not been tested in patients with preterm ruptured membranes who are undergoing amniocentesis.

Blackwell SC, Berry SM. Role of amniocentesis for the diagnosis of subclinical intra-amniotic infection in preterm premature rupture of the membranes. Curr Opin Obstet Gynecol 1999;11:541–7.

Odibo AO, Rodis JF, Sanders MM, Borgida AF, Wilson M, Egan JF, et al. Relationship of amniotic fluid markers of intra-amniotic infection with histopathology in cases of preterm labor with intact membranes. J Perinatol 1999;19:407–12.

Yoon BH, Romero R, Moon JB, Shim S, Kim M, Kim G, Jun JK. Clinical significance of intra-amniotic inflammation in patients with preterm labor and intact membranes. Am J Obstet Gynecol 2001;185:1130–6.

73

Pulmonary embolism

A 28-year-old woman, gravida 2, para 1, at 32 weeks of gestation has been admitted to the hospital and is on bed rest for preterm labor for 2 weeks. She develops a sudden onset of shortness of breath and chest pain. Her respiratory rate is 36 breaths per minute. An arterial blood gas shows a partial oxygen pressure (Po_2) of 52 mm Hg. The best diagnostic test for her condition is

    (A) D-dimer
    (B) electrocardiogram
 * (C) spiral computed tomography
    (D) pulmonary angiography
    (E) chest radiography

Pulmonary embolism is a leading cause of maternal death in the United States. During pregnancy, women have a fivefold increased risk of venous thromboembolism than do nonpregnant women. Survival from pulmonary embolism depends on early diagnosis and prompt treatment. The diagnosis in pregnancy is challenging because respiratory symptoms may be present in normal pregnancy or be due to respiratory or cardiovascular disease. Clinical pretest probability for pulmonary embolism is increased with risk factors such as immobilization or surgery in the preceding 4 weeks, family or personal history of venous thromboembolism, and coexisting medical or environmental conditions.

Dyspnea and tachypnea are the most common manifestations of pulmonary embolism. Tachycardia, sharp localized chest pain (usually pleuritic), cough, unexplained loss of consciousness, or hemoptysis may be present. Hypoxemia, hypotension, and syncope with or without cyanosis are seen in massive pulmonary embolism. Physical signs are nonspecific and include signs of right ventricular dysfunction, such as bulging neck veins, left parasternal shift, accentuation of the pulmonic component of the second heart sound, and a systolic murmur. Electrocardiography (ECG) and chest X-ray results may be suggestive but are usually normal and thus cannot confirm or refute the diagnosis. Respiratory alkalosis and hypoxemia may be present on arterial blood gas analysis.

Pulmonary embolism is mainly a radiologic diagnosis, and the use of compression ultrasonography, ventilation–perfusion scintigraphy, spiral (helical) computed tomography (CT), and angiography have been extensively studied in the nonpregnant population but have not been appropriately validated in pregnancy. Figure 73-1 shows an algorithm based on available data.

The ventilation–perfusion scan is designed to detect areas of the lung that are ventilated but not perfused. The presence of a mismatch suggests the possibility of pulmonary embolism. The ventilation–perfusion scan is diagnostic if it is normal (no perfusion defects) or if it demonstrates high probability (one or more segmental perfusion defects with normal ventilation or two or more large subsegmental perfusion defects). Approximately 35–40% in the nonpregnant population is nondiagnostic and further testing is required. Because pregnancy is associated with a younger healthier population, almost 75% of ventilation–perfusion scans are normal and, thus, can be used as a first-line modality. However, ventilation–perfusion scan is nondiagnostic in patients with abnormal chest radiogram or history of asthma or chronic obstructive pulmonary disease.

Spiral or helical CT is used to obtain images of pulmonary arteries after injection of radiopaque contrast material. This technique has several potential advantages over ventilation–perfusion scan. It is able to directly and noninvasively depict a thrombus as compared with the implication of the presence of a thrombus on ventilation–perfusion scan, and can determine other alternative explanations for patients' symptoms in the absence of pulmonary embolism. The ability to acquire multiple thin slices has improved visualization such that multislice spiral CT has comparable sensitivity to conventional pulmonary angiography and has been reported to be a cost-effective first-line diagnostic technique in pregnancy. Approximately 5–10% of tests are nondiagnostic in nonpregnant patients because of suboptimal contrast opacification, motion artifacts, and other technical issues. However, because of the hyperdynamic circulation and increased plasma volume, it is possible that an even higher percentage of patients may have a nondiagnostic scan in pregnancy.

Compression ultrasonography also may be used as first-line investigation for pulmonary embolism. A diagnosis of deep vein thrombosis (DVT) indirectly suggests a diagnosis of pulmonary embolism, and the treatment for both conditions is similar. It has been shown that approximately 10% of patients with a high clinical suspicion of

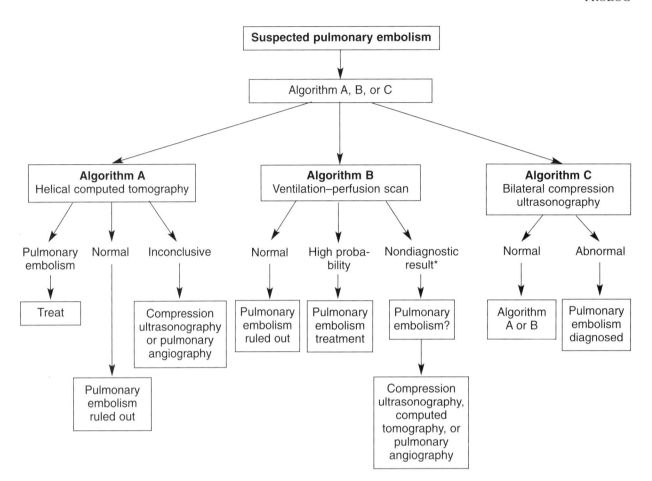

FIG. 73-1. Algorithm for clinically suspected pulmonary embolism in pregnancy. *ND, nondiagnostic result. Nondiagnostic results are those that indicate an intermediate or low-probability of pulmonary embolism, or that do not indicate a high probability. In patients with abnormal chest radiography, asthma, or chronic obstructive pulmonary disease (COPD), algorithm B cannot be used. (Nijkeuter M, Ginsberg JS, Huisman MV. Diagnosis of deep vein thrombosis and pulmonary embolism in pregnancy: a systematic review. J Thromb Haemost 2006;4:496–500.)

pulmonary embolism with negative results from lower limb ultrasonography have pulmonary embolism on angiography. Moreover, isolated iliac vein DVT is thought to be more common in pregnancy and is difficult to detect with compression ultrasonography.

Conventional pulmonary angiography has been long considered the criterion standard against which other imaging techniques were compared. However, it is now thought to be no more accurate than spiral CT. The technique is invasive, expensive, and has significant mortality with a significantly higher radiation dose. Because it is performed less frequently, the number of radiologists with sufficient experience in performing and interpreting pulmonary angiography is rapidly dwindling. Thus, pulmonary angiography has a limited role in evaluation of pulmonary embolism.

D-dimer, when negative, has been shown to have a high negative predictive value for suspected venous thromboembolism in nonpregnant patients. In pregnancy, D-dimer levels gradually increase until term, limiting

its use as a diagnostic test for pulmonary embolism in pregnancy.

The risk of radiation to fetus and mother is always a concern. The amount of fetal radiation exposure is low and is much lower than the threshold for induction of malignancies (100 mSv) and justifies the use of diagnostic tests involving radiation in pregnancy to exclude potentially fatal venous thromboembolism (Table 73-1). Fetal radiation from spiral CT appears to be slightly lower than with ventilation–perfusion scan. However, there is some theoretical uncertain risk of radiation dose to the breast during pregnancy from spiral or helical CT. It has been suggested that the average radiation received by the female breast during spiral CT is 20 mGy (2 rads). An exposure of 10 mGy to the breasts of a woman aged 35 years has been calculated to increase the risk of breast cancer by approximately 14% over the background rate for the general population. In addition, there is a small risk of an anaphylactic reaction to the intravenous contrast, which can endanger both mother and child.

TABLE 73-1. Radiation Dose to the Fetus by Radiologic Examination

Diagnostic Test	Fetal Radiation (mSv)	Maternal Radiation (mSv)
Unilateral venography without shielding	3.14	
Unilateral venography with shielding	Less than 0.5	
Pulmonary angiography via femoral route	2.21–3.74	
Pulmonary angiography via brachial route	Less than 0.5	5–30
Perfusion scintigraphy (99 mTc MAA, 200 MBq)	0.2–0.6	1.0
Perfusion scintigraphy (99 mTc MAA, 40 MBq)	0.11–0.20	
Ventilation scintigraphy (99 mTc aerosol)	0.1–0.3	0.5
Ventilation scintigraphy (81 mKr, 600 MBq)	0.0001	0.2
Single-detector row helical CT	0.026	1.6–4.0
Multi-detector row helical CT	0.013	4.0–6.0
CT venography	5.3	2.3–2.7

CT, computed tomography.

To convert mSv to rads: 1 mSv = 0.1 rad.

Estimates of radiation exposure are derived from Nijkeuter M, Ginsberg JS, Huisman MV. Diagnosis of deep vein thrombosis and pulmonary embolism in pregnancy: a systematic review. J Thromb Haemost 2006;4:496–500, and Scarsbrook AF, Evans AL, Owen AR, Gleeson FV. Diagnosis of suspected venous thromboembolic disease in pregnancy. Clin Radiol 2006;61:1–12.

Iodinated contrast media also may cross the placenta and has the potential to depress neonatal thyroid function, although any exposure is likely to be short in duration.

When confronted with a clinical suspicion of pulmonary embolism, a ventilation–perfusion scan, a spiral CT, or bilateral compression ultrasonography can be used depending on local availability and expertise (Fig. 73-1).

American College of Obstetricians and Gynecologists. Thromboembolism in pregnancy. Practice Bulletin No. 19. Washington, DC: ACOG; 2000.

Garcia D, Ageno W, Libby E. Update on the diagnosis and management of pulmonary embolism. Br J Haematol 2005;131:301–12.

Nijkeuter M, Ginsberg JS, Huisman MV. Diagnosis of deep vein thrombosis and pulmonary embolism in pregnancy: a systematic review. J Thromb Haemost 2006;4:496–500.

Scarsbrook AF, Evans AL, Owen AR, Gleeson FV. Diagnosis of suspected venous thromboembolic disease in pregnancy. Clin Radiol 2006; 61:1–12.

Stone SE, Morris TA. Pulmonary embolism during and after pregnancy. Crit Care Med. 2005;33(10 suppl):S294–300.

74

Cystic fibrosis screening

A 23-year-old African-American primigravid woman comes to the office at 9 weeks of gestation for her first prenatal visit. With regard to screening her for cystic fibrosis, the most appropriate recommendation is that carrier testing should

     (A) not be offered
*   (B) be offered
     (C) be offered only if there is a positive family history
     (D) be offered only in the presence of an abnormal fetal ultrasonogram

Cystic fibrosis is an autosomal recessive disorder with a frequency of 1 in 3,300 Caucasians. The frequency is lower in other populations such as African Americans (1 in 15,300) and Hispanics (1 in 8,000). Individuals with cystic fibrosis have multiple medical problems, including pulmonary complications, pancreatic insufficiency, and hepatobiliary disorders. Life expectancy is significantly shortened in people with cystic fibrosis, with a median survival of 30 years.

Cystic fibrosis is caused by a mutation in the cystic fibrosis transregulator (*CFTR*) gene. This gene is located on chromosome number seven, and was identified in 1989. The gene product protein *CFTR* functions as a cyclic adenosine monophosphate (cAMP)-regulated chloride channel in the apical membrane of epithelial cells. Mutations in the gene cause defective chloride transport, which results in high sweat chloride levels and tenacious mucus in the lungs and pancreas, leading to the major clinical features of cystic fibrosis. More than 1,300 mutations have been identified in the *CFTR* gene, although the frequency of specific mutations varies by population. For example, the ΔF508 mutation accounts for 70% of the cystic fibrosis mutations in Northern European Caucasians but only 30% of such mutations in persons of Ashkenazi Jewish descent. The carrier rate of cystic fibrosis varies by population, from

as high as 1 in 24 individuals of Ashkenazi Jewish descent to as low as 1 in 94 in Asian Americans (Table 74-1).

Because of the severity and prevalence of cystic fibrosis, the American College of Obstetricians and Gynecologists and the American College of Medical Genetics convened a task force to develop practice guidelines for preconception and prenatal screening of women. The goal of screening for carriers of cystic fibrosis is to identify couples at risk of having a child with cystic fibrosis.

The carrier screening test for cystic fibrosis is performed on DNA. The DNA can be extracted from various cells, although most laboratories use leukocytes from peripheral blood. Depending on the laboratory, it can take several weeks to obtain the carrier screening test results. The sensitivity of cystic fibrosis screening varies by population. Detection rates are highest in populations with the highest disease prevalence and lowest in those populations with the lowest disease prevalence. For example, the detection rate in Ashkenazi Jews is 94%, whereas in African Americans the detection rate is 65%. Given the imperfect sensitivity, even those with negative carrier testing results still have a small residual carrier risk (Table 74-1). It should be noted that current testing screens for approximately 34 known mutations, although there are more than 700 mutations.

TABLE 74-1. Cystic Fibrosis Detection and Carrier Rates Before and After Testing

Ethnic Group	Frequency	Detection Rate (%)	Carrier Rate Before Testing	Approximate Carrier Risk After Negative Test Result
Ashkenazi Jewish	1/3,300	94	1/24	1/400
Caucasian (non-Hispanic)	1/3,300	88	1/25	1/208
Hispanic	1/8,464	72	1/46	1/164
African American	1/16,900	65	1/65	1/186
Asian American	1/32,400	49	1/94	1/184

Modified from Update on carrier screening for cystic fibrosis. ACOG Committee Opinion No. 325. American College of Obstetricians and Gynecologists. Obstet Gynecol 2005;106:1465–8.

Despite these limitations, current guidelines recommend offering preconception cystic fibrosis carrier testing to all pregnant patients, regardless of ethnicity or other risk factors. An important factor underlying this recommendation is that it is increasingly difficult to assign ethnicity to an individual, due to population admixture. It would be inappropriate to offer screening only on the basis of a positive family history or an ultrasonographic finding associated with cystic fibrosis (eg, echogenic bowel) because these strategies would detect only a small proportion of affected fetuses.

Screening for carrier status for cystic fibrosis is best accomplished preconceptionally when possible, but it is recommended during pregnancy as well. Screening early in pregnancy will ensure that the couple receives the test results at a time when they can consider 1) having prenatal diagnosis if they are both carriers and 2) the option of terminating the pregnancy if the fetus is affected.

The most practical and cost-effective approach to cystic fibrosis screening is to perform initial carrier screening on the woman, and to screen the partner only if the woman is identified as a carrier (sequential screening). The other alternative is concurrent screening, where both partners are tested simultaneously. Depending on the gestational age, delay inherent in sequential screening may result in a more limited choice of reproductive options.

American College of Obstetricians and Gynecologists, American College of Medical Genetics. Preconception and prenatal carrier screening for cystic fibrosis: clinical and laboratory guidelines. Washington, DC: ACOG; Bethesda (MD): ACMG; 2001.

Correlation between genotype and phenotype in patients with cystic fibrosis. The Cystic Fibrosis Genotype–Phenotype Consortium. N Engl J Med 1993;329:1308–13.

Update on carrier screening for cystic fibrosis. ACOG Committee Opinion No. 325. American College of Obstetricians and Gynecologists. Obstet Gynecol 2005;106:1465–8.

75

Epidural complications

The greatest risk factor for hypotension with epidural anesthesia is

    (A) preeclampsia
*   (B) planned cesarean delivery
    (C) obesity
    (D) slow dosing of the epidural
    (E) Trendelenburg position

Epidural analgesia is widely used in the United States for labor-related pain relief. It is safe, effective, and can easily be converted to anesthetic levels to allow a cesarean delivery if necessary. Serious side effects from epidural analgesia are unusual. Less serious common side effects include pruritus, postdural puncture headache, fever, and maternal hypotension.

Maternal hypotension occurs in up to 31% of women who receive epidural analgesia. The percent of women who experience hypotension varies among studies as techniques to reduce it have evolved. In addition, the definition of hypotension varies among studies. In a smaller number of women, hypotension is associated with changes in the fetal heart rate, including bradycardia requiring emergent cesarean delivery.

A number of strategies have been used to avoid or minimize the risk of hypotension. Prehydration is the most common method used to prevent hypotension. Typically, 500–1,000 mL of crystalloid is infused intravenously before epidural placement. Although this may reduce the incidence of epidural-related hypotension, it does not prevent it.

Ephedrine administered to the mother is a common treatment of epidural-related hypotension. Ephedrine also is used as a prophylactic measure. The use of ephedrine reduces but does not eliminate maternal hypotension,

Supine hypotension is worsened by epidural analgesia, and positioning the patient is an important adjunct to prevention. The best position is not just a lateral tilt but the Trendelenburg position, which will reduce, not worsen, the blood pressure changes.

Patients with preeclampsia present a challenge to care. Epidurals are associated with a decrease in mean arterial pressure in all patients, including those with preeclampsia. However, the rate of hypotension is not increased from that seen in women without preeclampsia.

Some authors have advocated slow dosing of the epidural in order to help prevent hypotension. Therefore, it is not a risk factor for hypotension.

All studies have found that women undergoing cesarean delivery have the highest incidence of hypotension. This is likely to result from the higher dose of medication that must be given to patients who undergo cesarean delivery. In only a few cases is planned cesarean delivery associated with an adverse effect on fetal heart rate and subsequent condition of the neonate at delivery.

Bofill JA, Vincent RD, Ross EL, Martin RW, Norman PF, Werhan CF, et al. Nulliparous active labor, epidural analgesia, and cesarean delivery for dystocia. Am J Obstet Gynecol 1997;177:1465–70.

Obstetric analgesia and anesthesia. ACOG Practice Bulletin No. 36. American College of Obstetricians and Gynecologists. Obstet Gynecol 2002;100:177–91.

Olofsson C, Ekblom A, Ekman-Ordeberg G, Hjelm A, Irestedt L. Lack of analgesic effect of systemically administered morphine or pethidine on labour pain. Br J Obstet Gynaecol 1996;103:968–72.

Sharma SK, Sidawi JE, Ramin SM, Lucas MJ, Leveno KJ, Cunningham FG. Cesarean delivery: a randomized trial of epidural versus patient-controlled meperidine analgesia during labor. Anesthesiology 1997; 87:487–94.

76

Gastroesophageal reflux disease

A 38-year-old primigravid woman at 16 weeks of gestation has an 8-month history of heartburn and regurgitation, especially after she eats large or fatty meals. The symptoms have worsened with pregnancy and have been refractory to treatment with lifestyle modification, antacids, and H_2-receptor antagonists. The most appropriate next step in the care of this patient is

* (A) a trial of omeprazole (Prilosec)
  (B) 24-hour esophageal pH monitoring
  (C) an upper tract gastrointestinal (GI) endoscopy
  (D) esophageal manometry
  (E) a barium swallow

The patient has gastroesophageal reflux disease (GERD). Typical symptoms include heartburn and acid regurgitation. Atypical symptoms include anginalike chest pain, asthma, chronic cough, and chronic laryngitis. Complications of GERD include Barrett's esophagus (metaplasia of esophageal squamous epithelium to columnar epithelium, a precursor to esophageal cancer), esophageal erosion, stricture, hematemesis, anemia, and adenocarcinoma. It is rare to find any of these complications of GERD during pregnancy. Diagnosis of GERD is based on the history and response to acid suppressive therapy. Current guidelines recommend a trial of empiric medical therapy without diagnostic testing in patients with typical symptoms. A 2-week trial of a proton pump inhibitor has high sensitivity and specificity for diagnosing GERD. The effectiveness of the various treatments for GERD are as follows: antacids, 20%; lifestyle modification, 20–30%; H_2-receptor blocker, 50–60%; proton pump inhibitor, 80–85%; and surgical fundoplication, 80–90%. Lifestyle modification may include elevation of the head of the bed, decreased fat intake, cessation of smoking, avoiding recumbency for 2 hours postprandially, and weight loss if applicable.

The best next step in care of this patient should be a trial of omeprazole (Prilosec), a proton pump inhibitor. Any of the other four available proton pump inhibitors (lansoprazole, rabeprazole, pantoprazole, and esomeprazole) could be used instead of omeprazole, which is now an over-the-counter medication. The most common diagnostic tests for GERD are upper tract gastrointestinal endoscopy and ambulatory esophageal pH monitoring. Upper tract gastrointestinal endoscopy may show distal esophagitis and confirm the diagnosis. It also may rule out complications such as ulcer or stricture. Esophageal pH monitoring is the criterion standard for identifying abnormal acid exposure, but up to 20% of patients with GERD have a normal pH study. Esophageal manometry is used to diagnose such motility disorders as achalasia and to document effective esophageal peristalsis before antireflux surgery. Barium swallow is used to evaluate esophageal function and to assess for structural abnormalities of the esophagus. Barium radiographic studies are neither sensitive nor specific for diagnosing GERD or its complications.

DeVault KR, Castell DO. Updated guidelines for the diagnosis and treatment of gastroesophageal reflux disease. American College of Gastroenterology. Am J Gastroenterol 2005;100:190–200.

Pandak WM, Arezo S, Everett S, Jesse R, DeCosta G, Crofts T, et al. Short course of omeprazole: a better first diagnostic approach to noncardiac chest pain than endoscopy, manometry, or 24-hour esophageal pH monitoring. J Clin Gastroenterol 2002;35:307–14.

77

Postpartum fever

A 32-year-old woman, gravida 2, para 1, at 40 weeks of gestation underwent a repeat cesarean delivery for secondary arrest of the active phase of labor and failed vaginal birth after cesarean delivery. Labor had lasted 22 hours, and eight cervical examinations had been performed. At 35 weeks of gestation, results of culture for group B streptococci was negative. Prophylactic cefazolin was given after umbilical cord clamping. At 18 hours postpartum, the patient had a fever of 38.3°C (101°F) and was placed on intravenous clindamycin and gentamicin. Although the patient appeared well, multiple spiking fevers to 39.5°C (103°F) continued daily. Ninety-six hours postoperatively, physical examination was without localizing signs. Pelvic examination revealed a closed cervix, an 18 weeks of gestation-size uterus with appropriate tenderness, and no adnexal masses. Urinalysis was negative. Preoperative hematocrit and white blood cell count were 35% and 18,000 cells/mm³, respectively. Values drawn 96 hours postpartum were 31% and 23,600/mm³, respectively. Serum electrolytes, glucose, and creatinine were normal. Intravenous ampicillin was added to the antibiotic regimen but fever persisted. On postoperative day 5, a computed tomography (CT) scan of abdomen and pelvis with oral and intravenous contrast material was performed. The pathologic condition that the CT scan is most likely to reveal is

      (A) a retro-psoas abscess
      (B) a ruptured appendix
*   (C) an ovarian vein thrombosis
      (D) a retained laparotomy sponge
      (E) a ureteral ligation

The pathogenesis of ovarian vein thrombosis is thought to involve endometritis, which extends through the myometrium to the parametrium. The Virchow triad of factors that predispose to venous thrombosis includes stasis, hypercoagulability, and vessel wall injury. Infection presumably damages the vascular endothelium, and in the setting of stasis and the hypercoagulability of pregnancy, a clot forms. Risk factors for postpartum endometritis are shown in Box 77-1. Prophylactic antibiotics decrease the risk of postcesarean endometritis.

BOX 77-1

Risk Factors for Postpartum Endometritis

- Labor
- Multiple cervical examinations
- Rupture of membranes
- Internal fetal heart rate monitoring
- Chorioamnionitis
- Cesarean delivery
- Failed vaginal birth after cesarean delivery
- Low socioeconomic status
- Colonization of lower genital tract with
  —Gonorrhea
  —Group B streptococci
  —Bacterial vaginosis

Septic pelvic thrombophlebitis may present in two distinct forms. In the first, it may cause persistent fever, lower abdominal pain, uterine tenderness perhaps localized to one side, ileus, nausea, and vomiting. Tachypnea and dyspnea may be evident if pulmonary embolization has occurred. The second presentation is that of an enigmatic fever. The patient does not appear seriously ill but has persistent spiking fever. The diagnostic tests mostly used in evaluating patients for septic pelvic thrombophlebitis are CT scan, magnetic resonance imaging (MRI), and pelvic ultrasonography. The CT scan is the test most frequently used in postpartum women whose fever persists for 5 days despite broad-spectrum antibiotic therapy. Approximately 25% of such patients will be found to have unilateral or bilateral ovarian vein thrombosis. The thrombi may extend into the renal, iliac, or femoral veinsor into the inferior vena cava. The other 75% of patients have either septic pelvic thrombophlebitis, presumably with thrombi in small vessels that are not visualized by current imaging technology, or they have another cause of fever such as a wound infection, pelvic abscess, necrotizing fasciitis, pneumonia, or drug fever. In such cases, the ultimate diagnosis depends on a careful physical examination, search for other sources of fever, and the patient's response to a therapeutic trial of heparin. If the patient becomes afebrile after starting heparin, the presumptive diagnosis is septic pelvic thrombophlebitis. The response to heparin is variable. The patient may require more than 72 hours to become afebrile. A variety of empiric regimens are available for heparin dosage and duration of administration. The use of heparin in the treatment of septic pelvic thrombophlebitis is controversial. Some investigators argue that prolonged antibiotic therapy is all that is needed and that the use of heparin does not hasten recovery. If there is no decrease in the fever in a clinically ill patient and a remote source of infection is not identified, exploratory laparotomy may be considered.

Retro-psoas abscess is a severe infection that usually is associated with inoculation of bacteria via pudendal or paracervical block. Surgical drainage is often required. Ovarian vein thrombosis may be confused with appendicitis because the thrombosis is frequently right-sided. Sometimes the diagnosis is made at laparotomy for suspected appendicitis. Retained laparotomy sponge has a variable clinical presentation from an incidental finding on abdominal X-ray to acute bowel obstruction. Other presentations include a painless mass, abscess, peritonitis, or draining sinus. Recognition frequently is delayed weeks or months after the first surgery. Ureteral ligation

is a rare complication of cesarean delivery, but bladder and ureter injuries are more common with failed vaginal birth after cesarean delivery. Ureteral ligation has a variable presentation but usually is accompanied by flank pain, fever, and hydronephrosis on the affected side.

Brown CE, Stettler RW, Twickler D, Cunningham FG. Puerperal septic pelvic thrombophlebitis: incidence and response to heparin therapy. Am J Obstet Gynecol 1999;181:143–8.

Brumfield CG, Hauth JC, Andrews WW. Puerperal infection after cesarean delivery: evaluation of a standardized protocol. Am J Obstet Gynecol 2000;182:1147–51.

Duff P. Maternal and perinatal infection. In: Gabbe SG, Niebyl JR, Simpson JL, editors. Obstetrics: normal and problem pregnancies. 4th ed. New York (NY): Churchill Livingstone; 2002. p. 1293–1345.

Kominiarek MA, Hibbard JU. Postpartum ovarian vein thrombosis: an update. Obstet Gynecol Surv 2006;61:337–42.

Rodger MA, Avruch LI, Howley HE, Olivier A, Walker MC. Pelvic magnetic resonance venography reveals high rate of pelvic vein thrombosis after cesarean section. Am J Obstet Gynecol 2006;194:436–7.

Witlin AG, Sibai BM. Postpartum ovarian vein thrombosis after vaginal delivery: a report of 11 cases. Obstet Gynecol 1995;85:775–80.

Witlin AG, Mercer BM, Sibai BM. Septic pelvic thrombophlebitis or refractory postpartum fever of undetermined etiology. J Matern Fetal Med 1996;5:355–8.

78

Tuberculosis

A 37-year-old health care worker at 26 weeks of gestation reports a positive purified protein derivative (PPD) tuberculin skin test result. She was tested a year ago and had a negative PPD test result at that time. She has no respiratory symptoms, and a chest X-ray is within normal limits. In regard to prophylaxis with isoniazid and pyridoxine (vitamin B$_6$), you advise

* (A) antepartum prophylaxis
  (B) postpartum prophylaxis
  (C) no prophylaxis
  (D) prophylaxis only if acid-fast bacilli are present in sputum
  (E) prophylaxis only if respiratory symptoms develop

The Advisory Council for the Elimination of Tuberculosis recently recommended to the Centers for Disease Control and Prevention and the National Institutes of Health an aggressive approach to tuberculosis elimination in the United States. Because prenatal care is often the only contact that many women have with the health care system, screening during pregnancy for tuberculosis is recommended for women deemed to be at high risk (Box 78-1).

Tuberculin skin testing is the standard method for identifying infected persons. The Mantoux test, an intracuta-

neous administration of five units of PPD tuberculin, best detects infection. Skin testing with the PPD tuberculin test is considered valid and safe throughout pregnancy. Testing with the new whole blood test, QuantiFERON-TB Gold (QFT-G), has not been evaluated for use during pregnancy.

A guide to the interpretation of tuberculin skin test results is shown in Box 78-2. All pregnant women who have a positive tuberculin skin test result should undergo chest radiography with abdominal shielding to assess for evidence of disease. Most women with a positive

PPD test result in pregnancy are asymptomatic and without evidence of active disease. Once active disease is excluded, prophylaxis is recommended for pregnant women who have had conversion of their PPD test results within 2 years of pregnancy (when the risk of progression to active disease is highest), and for women who live with or are in close contact with a person with active disease. These women have a 2–4% risk of developing active tuberculosis in the first year after conversion. For women with a known recent conversion (less than 2 years) to a positive PPD test result and no evidence of active disease, the recommended prophylaxis is isoniazid, beginning after the first trimester and continuing for 6–9 months. Women with an unknown or prolonged (greater than 2 years) duration of PPD positivity and no evidence of active disease should receive postpartum prophylaxis. However, in the absence of active disease, postpartum isoniazid prophylaxis is not recommended for women older than 35 years who have an unknown or prolonged PPD positivity because there is an increased risk of hepatotoxicity (Fig. 78-1). Prophylaxis is indicated in patients who are recent converters regardless of age.

In patients who have suspected active pulmonary tuberculosis, three consecutive early-morning sputum specimens should be collected and submitted for acid-fast bacillus testing and mycobacteriology culture. Definitive diagnosis depends on the isolation and identification of *Mycobacterium tuberculosis* from a diagnostic specimen, such as sputum or tissue. For pregnant women with active tuberculosis, therapy with isoniazid and rifampin is recommended over isoniazid prophylaxis alone.

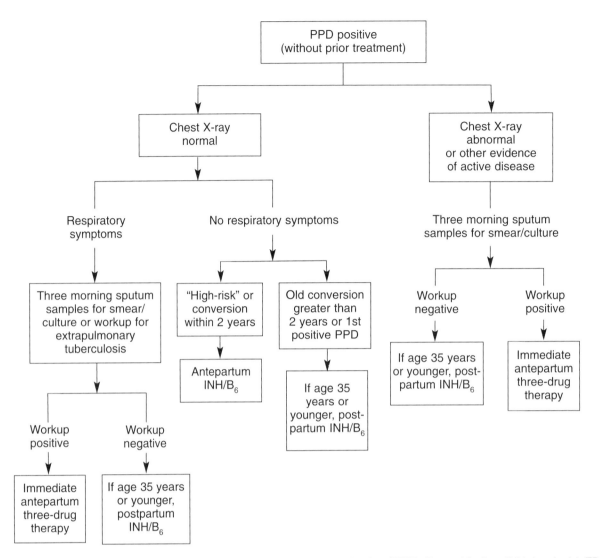

FIG. 78-1. Algorithm for management of positive purified protein derivative (PPD). B$_6$, pyridoxine; INH, isoniazid; TB, tuberculosis. (Whitty JE, Dombrowski MP. Respiratory diseases in pregnancy. In: Creasy RK, Resnik R, Iams JD, editors. Maternal–fetal medicine: principles and practice. 5th ed. Philadelphia [PA]: WB Saunders; 2004. p. 961. Copyright 2004 by Elsevier.)

Boggess KA, Myers ER, Hamilton CD. Antepartum or postpartum isoniazid treatment of latent tuberculosis infection. Obstet Gynecol 2000;96:757–62.

Essential components of a tuberculosis prevention and control program. Recommendations of the Advisory Council for the Elimination of Tuberculosis. Centers for Disease Control and Prevention. MMWR Recomm Rep 1995;44(RR-11):1–16.

Riley L. Pneumonia and tuberculosis in pregnancy. Infect Dis Clin North Am 1997;11:119–33.

Screening for tuberculosis and tuberculosis infection in high-risk populations. Recommendations of the Advisory Council for the Elimination of Tuberculosis. Centers for Disease Control and Prevention. MMWR Recomm Rep 1995;44(RR-11):19–34.

Whitty JE, Dombrowski MP. Respiratory diseases in pregnancy. In: Creasy RK, Resnik R, Iams JD, editors. Maternal–fetal medicine: principles and practice. 5th ed. Philadelphia (PA): WB Saunders; 2004. p. 959–62.

79

Seizure disorders in pregnancy

A 24-year-old nulligravid woman seeks preconception counseling. She has a seizure disorder that was diagnosed in childhood, and she reports good seizure control on her current antiepileptic medication, lamotrigine (Lamictal). Her last seizure was 8 months ago. She is planning to attempt conception in the next few months and wants to know if she should discontinue lamotrigine because she has read that it may harm a developing fetus. The best way to minimize the risks to both mother and fetus is to

     (A) increase the lamotrigine dose
     (B) discontinue lamotrigine until after delivery
*   (C) add folic acid to current regimen
     (D) add valproate sodium to current regimen
     (E) add vitamin K to current regimen

Administration of antiepileptic drugs during pregnancy is a complex issue. Certain antiepileptic drugs used in pregnancy have been associated with specific congenital malformations, such as neural tube defects (NTDs) or cleft lip and palate. However, untreated or poorly treated seizure disorder in pregnancy can result in significant maternal and fetal morbidity secondary to maternal and fetal hypoxia and acidosis associated with generalized tonic–clonic seizures.

Antiepileptic drug management is obviously a critical part of optimizing outcome for both mother and fetus in women with seizure disorders in pregnancy. However, because of the lack of randomized controlled trials in pregnancy, no level I evidence is available to guide the management of epilepsy during pregnancy.

Clearance of virtually all antiepileptic medications increases during pregnancy, resulting in a decrease in serum concentration. However, it is not recommended to increase doses without monitoring drug levels. With some antiepileptic drugs, baseline levels should be obtained before conception and repeated at the beginning of each trimester, with appropriate dose adjustments made to keep levels in therapeutic range. Monitoring drug levels may not be necessary in stable patients.

In a nonpregnant patient who has had no seizures during the past 2–5 years, the obstetrician may ask the neurologist to consider withdrawing anticonvulsant medications altogether. However, for most women with a seizure disorder, withdrawal of antiepileptic drugs before pregnancy is not a realistic option.

Many antiepileptic drugs are known to interfere with folic acid metabolism. Thus, patients taking these medications may develop folic acid deficiency, putting their fetuses at increased risk for NTDs. The American College of Obstetricians and Gynecologists recommends folic acid supplementation (0.4 mg per day) for all patients before conception and in the first trimester. However, dosing recommendations for women taking antiepileptic medications vary widely, from 0.4 mg to 5 mg per day, and the optimal dosing regimen for folic acid supplementation in these patients remains controversial. Because women taking these medications are considered at high risk for neural tube defects, the higher dose of 4 mg per day may be warranted, at least during organogenesis.

Changing antiepileptic drug regimens after conception is not routinely recommended because the patient often is in or past the critical period of organogenesis by the time pregnancy is confirmed. The risk of significant fetal malformation is approximately 3% when one drug is taken (slightly above the background risk) and up to 17% if two or more drugs are taken. If an antiepileptic drug is definitively needed for seizure control, monotherapy at the lowest effective dosage is preferred. Valproate sodium is reported to be significantly more teratogenic than other monotherapies, with NTDs being the single most common defect identified in those affected. The combination of valproate sodium and lamotrigine is reported to be even more teratogenic, thus avoiding valproate sodium, either as monotherapy or as a component of polytherapy, is recommended when possible.

Neonatal hemorrhage caused by decreased vitamin K-dependent clotting factors has occurred in infants born to mothers taking phenobarbital, phenytoin sodium (Dilantin), or primidone (Mysoline). These infants have been shown to respond to treatment with 1 mg vitamin K given intramuscularly at birth. Some investigators recommend maternal prophylactic oral vitamin K during the last month of pregnancy, although the utility of this approach in preventing neonatal hemorrhage has not been proved definitively.

Crawford P. Best practice guidelines for the management of women with epilepsy. Epilepsia 2005;46(suppl 9):117–24.

Guidelines for the care of women of childbearing age with epilepsy. Commission on Genetics, Pregnancy, and the Child, International League Against Epilepsy. Epilepsia 1993;34:588–9.

Pennell PB. Pregnancy in women who have epilepsy. Neurol Clin 2004; 22:799–820.

80

Abruptio placentae

A 21-year-old primigravid woman at 34 weeks of gestation was involved in a motor vehicle accident and is in the labor and delivery ward for continuous monitoring. She has persistent vaginal bleeding and has an average of four contractions per hour. Her pulse is 80 beats per minute and her blood pressure is 130/80 mm Hg. Her fundal height is 34 cm and her uterus is soft. The fetal heart rate is at 144 beats per minute with accelerations. There is a normal appearing anterior placenta on ultrasonography. She is Rh positive. A Kleihauer–Betke test result is negative and her D-dimer levels are normal. Serial cervical examinations demonstrate that the cervix is closed, long, and unchanged. The most likely diagnosis is

    (A) vasa previa
    (B) marginal placenta previa
*   (C) abruptio placentae
    (D) uterine rupture
    (E) preterm labor

It is estimated that abruptio placentae is a complication of 40–50% of pregnant women who sustain life-threatening maternal trauma and 1–5% of pregnant women who experience a non–life-threatening trauma. Uterine rupture is an infrequent but life-threatening complication of trauma that occurs in only 0.6% of all injuries complicating pregnancy. The use of electronic fetal heart rate and uterine activity monitoring in pregnant trauma victims may aid in the detection of abruptio placentae. Most cases of abruptio placentae associated with trauma become manifest within 24 hours. In the presence of uterine activity, at least 24 hours of continuous uterine activity monitoring is recommended. In the absence of uterine contractions and with a reassuring fetal heart rate pattern, monitoring for 4–6 hours is probably sufficient. In women who experienced uterine contraction frequency of more than one every 10 minutes in the first 4 hours, 20% had abruptio placentae. Presence of nonreassuring fetal heart rate patterns, persistent vaginal bleeding, significant uterine tenderness, or irritability indicates a high probability of abruptio placentae.

Ultrasonography is useful in excluding placenta previa, but it is not a sensitive method of diagnosing abruptio placentae. A large retroplacental clot is identified by ultrasonography as a hyperechogenic or isoechogenic mass. This echogenicity may be misinterpreted as a thick placenta. Resolving retroplacental clots appear hyperechogenic within 1 week and are sonolucent in 2 weeks. In general, by the time ultrasonographic findings are diagnostic, the clinical presentation is impressive and ultrasonography is not required to make the diagnosis. Ultrasonography can be useful in following high-risk or suspicious cases expectantly.

The Kleihauer–Betke test is used to differentiate fetal erythrocytes from maternal erythrocytes and to quantify fetal–maternal hemorrhage. A recent study showed that the incidence of a positive Kleihauer–Betke test result did not differ between low-risk patients and trauma patients and nor did it correlate with abruptio placentae. Thus, a positive Kleihauer–Betke test result does not necessarily indicate pathologic fetal–maternal hemorrhage.

D-dimer levels have been used to exclude venous thromboembolism in nonpregnant patients. Some have used D-dimer to assess pregnancy complications that may be associated with activation of the coagulation system. However, during pregnancy there is a progressive increase as well as interindividual variations of D-dimer, which makes its use in pregnancy difficult.

Abruptio placentae is still largely a clinical diagnosis. Classical findings of abruptio placentae are vaginal bleeding, increased uterine tone, uterine tenderness, nonreassuring fetal heart rate patterns, hypovolemia, and disseminated intravascular coagulation. Although vaginal bleeding is the major distinguishing feature of abruptio placentae, in approximately 10% of patients, such bleeding may be concealed with retroplacental separation occurring close to the center of the placenta. Table 80-1 shows grading of abruptio placentae.

Vasa previa, marginal placenta previa, uterine rupture, and preterm labor may be associated with vaginal bleeding but do not fit this clinical presentation. Bleeding from vasa previa is associated with nonreassuring fetal heart rate changes and occurs after membranes have ruptured. Placenta previa should be diagnosed by ultrasonography. Uterine rupture is likely to be associated with maternal and fetal deterioration. Preterm labor will be associated with cervical changes.

TABLE 80-1. Grading of Abruptio Placentae

Grade	Description
0	Asymptomatic patient with a small retroplacental clot
1	Vaginal bleeding; uterine tetany and tenderness may be present; no signs of maternal shock or nonreassuring fetal status
2	Vaginal bleeding possible; signs of nonreassuring fetal status; no signs of maternal shock
3	Vaginal bleeding possible; marked uterine tetany, yielding a board-like consistency on palpation; persistent abdominal pain, with maternal shock and fetal demise; coagulopathy may be evident in 30% of cases

Konje JC, Taylor DJ. Bleeding in late pregnancy. In: James DK, Steer PJ, Weiner CP, Gonik B, editors. High risk pregnancy. 3rd ed. London: Saunders Elsevier; 2005. p. 1267. Copyright 2005 by Elsevier.

American College of Obstetricians and Gynecologists. Obstetric aspects of trauma management. ACOG Educational Bulletin 251. Washington, DC: ACOG; 1998.

Clark SL. Placenta previa and abruptio placentae. In: Creasy RK, Resnik R, Iams JD, editors. Maternal–fetal medicine: principles and practice. 5th ed. Philadelphia (PA): WB Saunders Co.; 2004. p. 707–22.

Dhanraj D. Lambers D. The incidences of positive Kleihauer-Betke test in low-risk pregnancies and maternal trauma patients. Am J Obstet Gynecol 2004;190:1461–3.

Epiney M, Boehlen F, Boulvain M, Reber G, Antonelli E, Morales M, et al. D-dimer levels during delivery and the postpartum. J Thromb Haemost 2005;3:268–71.

Kline JA, Williams GW, Hernandez-Nino J. D-dimer concentrations in normal pregnancy: new diagnostic thresholds are needed. Clin Chem 2005;51:825–9.

Konje JC, Taylor DJ. Bleeding in late pregnancy. In: James DK, Steer PJ, Weiner CP, Gonik B, editors. High risk pregnancy. 3rd ed. London: Saunders Elsevier; 2005. p. 1259–72.

81

Shoulder dystocia

A 25-year-old healthy woman has a normal labor and a spontaneous delivery of the fetal head. On expulsion of the head, a shoulder dystocia is recognized. Before instituting maneuvers, the next step is to

* (A) tell the patient not to push
* (B) apply fundal pressure
* (C) increase or initiate oxytocin administration
* (D) cut a large episiotomy

Shoulder dystocia occurs in approximately 0.5–2.0% of vaginal deliveries. Almost always, the anterior shoulder is impacted above the pubic symphysis and the posterior shoulder has passed through the inlet of the pelvis and is situated in the concavity of the sacrum. Rarely are both shoulders impacted above the inlet.

The vast majority are successfully resolved without injury to mother or neonate; however, fatalities, central nervous system injuries, and brachial plexus injuries may occur. The goal for these deliveries should be a timely and deft resolution of a shoulder dystocia that does not add irreversible stress or injury to the mother or fetus. The training and experience of the clinician should dictate the sequence of maneuvers that will be used; however, initially, it is best to do nothing to further impact the anterior shoulder above the pubic symphysis. The simplest way to avoid further impaction is to ask the patient to stop pushing.

Although practiced widely in the past, it is currently empirically believed that pushing forcefully on the maternal fundus simply duplicates a directional expulsive force that has already failed to deliver the fetal shoulder(s) and serves only to further impact the anterior shoulder behind the symphysis pubis. If significantly too much force is exerted, there is a risk of maternal trauma, including uterine rupture. In the modern management of a shoulder dystocia, this maneuver should not be used.

Similarly, increasing the frequency, duration, or intensity of uterine contraction with oxytocin (Pitocin) agents is not helpful, because the second stage forces of labor have already resulted in the expulsion of the head and the impaction of the shoulder(s). Continuing or intensifying these forces will, at this point, be counterproductive.

The decision to do an episiotomy or to enlarge an already existing episiotomy must be based on the clinician's judgment as to the laxness of the vaginal introitus in relationship to the clinician's ability to insert his or her hand into the vagina to execute maneuvers to resolve the shoulder dystocia. In many cases, such procedures will be unnecessary. It may not be necessary to routinely cut an episiotomy immediately upon recognizing a shoulder dystocia until the patient stops pushing and an assessment of the perineal anatomy is made.

Once the patient has stopped pushing, a variety of classically described maneuvers are available, ie, McRoberts maneuver (hyperflexion of legs) with suprapubic pressure; Rubin maneuver (anterior rotation of shoulder); delivery of the posterior arm; and Woods screw maneuver. When appropriately done, such maneuvers usually will suffice to resolve this emergency.

Gherman RB, Chauhan S, Ouzounian JG, Lerner H, Gonik B, Goodwin TM. Shoulder dystocia: the unpreventable obstetric emergency with empiric management guidelines. Am J Obstet Gynecol 2006;195: 657–72.

Gurewitsch ED, Kim EJ, Yang JH, Outland KE, McDonald MK, Allen RH. Comparing McRoberts' and Rubin's maneuvers for initial management of shoulder dystocia: an objective evaluation [published erratum appears in Am J Obstet Gynecol 2005;192:662]. Am J Obstet Gynecol 2005;192:153–60.

Poggi SH, Spong CY, Allen RH. Prioritizing posterior arm delivery during severe shoulder dystocia. Obstet Gynecol 2003;101:1068–72.

Shoulder dystocia. ACOG Practice Bulletin No. 40. American College of Obstetricians and Gynecologists. Obstet Gynecol 2002;100: 1045–50.

82

Diabetes mellitus

A 25-year-old woman with pregestational diabetes mellitus had elevated antepartum glucose levels despite insulin therapy. She gave birth to a 5,000-g neonate at 39 weeks of gestation. The most likely adverse effect to the infant of poorly controlled maternal diabetes mellitus is

    (A) neonatal hyperglycemia
    (B) childhood thyroid dysfunction
    (C) neonatal anemia
    (D) neonatal hypercalcemia
*   (E) childhood type 2 diabetes mellitus

Maternal hyperglycemia results in fetal hyperglycemia because glucose crosses the placenta by facilitated diffusion. This stimulates fetal pancreatic islet cell hypertrophy with corresponding fetal hyperinsulinemia. Insulin acts as a growth hormone in the fetus resulting in fetal macrosomia. The newborn of the uncontrolled diabetic mother undergoes a sudden interruption of glucose delivery with the clamping of the umbilical cord at birth. This event in association with high insulin levels causes neonatal hypoglycemia. Significant hypoglycemia is present in up to 50% of infants of diabetic mothers and is more common in macrosomic or growth-restricted infants than in appropriate-size infants of women with diabetes.

Fetal hyperglycemia and fetal hyperinsulinemia increase fetal total body oxygen consumption by as much as 30%. The placenta has limited ability in increasing oxygen delivery in the presence of increased fetal demand, which may be further compromised in women with diabetes and vascular disease. The resultant relative fetal hypoxemia is associated with metabolic acidosis, erythropoiesis, altered iron distribution, and fetal death. Increased erythropoietin production as a result of the hypoxemia causes polycythemia and the fetal red cell mass expands by up to 30%. This expanded red cell mass also increases the risk for hyperbilirubinemia.

Hypocalcemia and hypomagnesemia occur within the first 72 hours in up to 50% of infants of women with diabetes. Newborns who have respiratory distress or birth asphyxia are at greater risk. The symptoms are similar to those of hypoglycemia and include jitteriness, sweating, tachypnea, irritability, and seizures. Clinical presentation occurs approximately 24–72 hours after delivery, later than for hypoglycemia, which usually occurs at 1–3 hours of life. In utero, the fetal parathyroid glands are relatively inactive because of the high transplacental influx of cal-

cium. The neonatal parathyroid hormone system becomes active in early neonatal life. Abnormalities in calcium and magnesium metabolism in infants of diabetic mothers are thought to represent a delay in the postnatal parathyroid hormone response.

The contribution of intrauterine and early postnatal environment to the development of disease in later life has been acknowledged (the Barker hypothesis). Underweight at birth in particular has been shown to lead to increased risk of metabolic syndrome in later life. This early epigenetic conditioning has been described as "nutritional programming." Larger birth weight also has been associated with programming. Studies in offspring of women with diabetes have contributed to this hypothesis. Elevated insulin concentrations during critical perinatal periods of development may contribute to a lasting malprogramming of neuroendocrine systems regulating body weight and metabolism. Although diabetes can be transmitted genetically, studies in Pima Indians attributed 40% of type 2 diabetes mellitus among 5- to 19-year-old children to maternal diabetes mellitus in pregnancy. Breastfeeding was noted to be protective. Clinical and epidemiologic evidence support the observation that offspring of diabetic mothers are programmed to develop obesity, diabetes mellitus, and metabolic syndrome in later life. Such metabolic problems of later life have been shown to be acquired independent of the genetic predisposition and depend on perinatal hyperinsulinism. This supports a possibility of primary prevention of obesity and diabetes by the treatment of maternal diabetes during pregnancy and lactation.

Maternal diabetes mellitus is not a known risk factor for childhood thyroid disease. Figure 82-1 shows an algorithm of fetal and neonatal events attributable to fetal hyperglycemia.

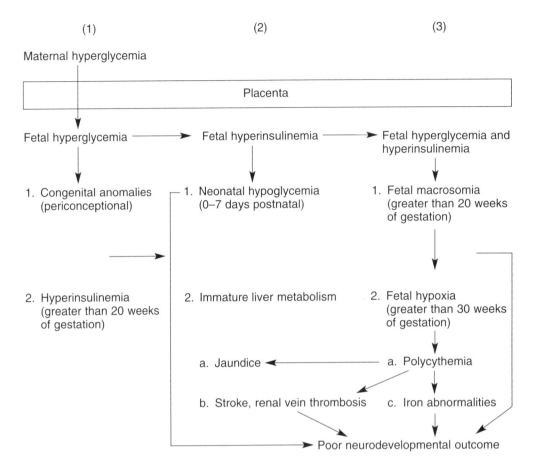

FIG. 82-1. Fetal and neonatal events attributable to fetal hyperglycemia (column 1), fetal hyperinsulinemia (column 2), or both in synergy (column 3). Time to risk is denoted in parentheses. RVT, renal vein thrombosis; TTN, transient tachypnea. (Modified from Nold JL, Georgieff MK. Infants of diabetic mothers. Pediatr Clin North Am 2004;51:620. Copyright 2004 by Elsevier.)

Catalano PM, Kirwan JP, Haugel-de Mouzon S, King J. Gestational diabetes and insulin resistance: role in short- and long-term implications for mother and fetus. J Nutr 2003;133(suppl):1674s–83s.

Nold JL, Georgieff MK. Infants of diabetic mothers. Pediatr Clin North Am 2004;51:619–37, viii.

Plagemann A. Perinatal programming and functional teratogenesis: impact on body weight regulation and obesity. Physiol Behav 2005;86:661–8.

Young TK, Martens PJ, Taback SP, Sellers EA, Dean HJ, Cheang M, et al. Type 2 diabetes mellitus in children: prenatal and early infancy risk factors among native Canadians. Arch Pediatr Adolesc Med 2002;156:651–5.

83

Uterine inversion

A 22-year-old woman, gravida 1, para 0, presents in active labor. She has had an uncomplicated prenatal course. Her labor progresses normally and she gives birth to a healthy 3,400-g newborn. Traction is applied to the umbilical cord to facilitate delivery of the placenta when a large globular mass, with the placenta attached, is noted at the perineum. The diagnosis of uterine inversion is made. The most appropriate management is

* (A) an immediate attempt to replace the uterus
(B) administration of oxytocin to decrease blood loss
(C) laparotomy
(D) administration of nitroglycerine

Acute uterine inversion occurs in approximately 1 in 3,000 vaginal births and 1 in 1,800 cesarean deliveries. Postpartum hemorrhage complicates 65% of cases with 48% requiring blood transfusion. Classification systems for uterine inversion have been described, and the most commonly used system divides uterine inversion by timing:

- Acute (less than 24 hours after delivery)
- Subacute (between 24 hours and 4 weeks after delivery)
- Chronic (greater than 4 weeks after delivery)

The severity of the uterine inversion can be further classified into first degree (inversion to the cervical ring, but not through the ring), second degree (through the cervical ring), third degree (complete inversion to the perineum), and total (inversion of the vagina).

The occurrence of uterine inversion appears to be higher in primiparous women. Furthermore, it appears more likely with fundal attachment of the placenta, which may be more common in primiparas. The use of oxytocin and magnesium sulfate has been attributed to a higher risk of uterine inversion, but this remains controversial. The most commonly held belief is that uterine inversion is the result of excessive traction on the umbilical cord or fundal pressure in the third stage of labor, but this has been recently challenged. The recurrence risk is low.

The diagnosis of uterine inversion, especially first-degree uterine inversion, can be challenging, and, in stable patients, imaging techniques such as magnetic resonance imaging may be needed to make the diagnosis. Although, in the past, it was commonly believed that maternal shock out of proportion to blood loss was one of the cardinal signs of uterine inversion, this view has been challenged. A globular mass in the vagina or at the perineum is a common presenting sign of uterine inversion. However, the most common presenting sign of uterine inversion is postpartum hemorrhage, which may lead to shock.

The key to a successful outcome in patients with uterine inversion is quick recognition with immediate uterine replacement and the treatment of hypovolemia or shock.

Large-bore intravenous access, availability of blood products, and securing the presence of support personnel are the cornerstones to success. Close surveillance of the maternal vital signs and laboratory studies, such as blood count and coagulation profile, are essential. All oxytocic agents should be avoided until reposition of the uterus has occurred. Immediate attempt at replacement of the uterus should be the first step. If the placenta is attached, it should not be removed for fear of facilitating hemorrhage. The manual replacement involves grasping the fundus of the uterus and pushing towards the maternal umbilicus through the cervix. If the uterus is successfully replaced, the operator's hand should not be removed. Oxytocic agents should be started. After the uterus contracts, the operator's hand can be removed and packing may be placed to decrease the chances of recurrence.

If manual replacement cannot be facilitated, consideration should be given to the use of uterine relaxing agents, such as intravenous or subcutaneous terbutaline, halothane-based inhaled anesthetics, and nitroglycerine. If these strategies prove unsuccessful, an operative strategy must be initiated. After a laparotomy incision, the inverted uterus and the round ligaments are isolated, and distorted anatomy is common. Careful attention should be paid to the anatomy before placement of an Allis or Babcock clamp on the round ligaments. Traction is used to return the uterus to the abdominal cavity. If this is not successful, an incision should be made through the uterine or cervical contraction ring in order to facilitate return of the uterus to its normal position.

Baskett TF. Acute uterine inversion: a review of 40 cases. J Obstet Gynecol Can 2002;24:953–6.

Brar HS, Greenspoon JS, Platt LD, Paul RH. Acute puerperal uterine inversion. New approaches to management. J Reprod Med 1989; 34:173–7.

Kochenour NK. Diagnosis and management of uterine inversion. In: Hankins GDV, Clark SL, Cunningham FG, Gilstrap LC, editors. Operative obstetrics. Norwalk (CT): Appleton & Lange; 1995. p. 273–81.

Shah-Hosseini R, Evrard JR. Puerperal uterine inversion. Obstet Gynecol 1989;73:567–70.

84

Severe preeclampsia

A 38-year-old primigravid woman at 29 weeks of gestation has elevated blood pressures of 166/108 mm Hg and 150/110 mm Hg on two occasions 8 hours apart. A 24-hour urine analysis shows 7.2 g protein, and the peripheral blood culture and liver function test results are normal. She reports no headache, scotomata, or abdominal pain. An ultrasonogram shows a size-appropriate fetus, and the amniotic fluid appears to be normal. The fetal heart rate is reassuring. The next step in care is

    (A) immediate cesarean delivery
    (B) outpatient monitoring
    (C) immediate induction of labor
*   (D) inpatient expectant management

Preeclampsia occurs in approximately 4–6% of pregnancies and is an important contributor to maternal and fetal outcomes. Diagnostic criteria include blood pressure of 140/90 mm Hg or higher on two separate occasions after 20 weeks of gestation, and 300 mg of protein or more on a 24-hour urine collection in women with no history of hypertension. Preeclampsia is categorized as mild or severe. Severe preeclampsia is defined by the presence of any additional criteria (Box 84-1). The management of preeclampsia varies by gestational age and severity of the disease.

At term, severe preeclampsia is an indication for delivery. However, when present remote from term, the management is more difficult, and inpatient management is desired. If and when the patient is stable, transfer to a tertiary care facility should be a priority, and the involvement of specialists in maternal–fetal medicine and neonatology is optimal. The approach to women with severe preeclampsia at less than 24 weeks of gestation is controversial, but because of poor perinatal outcomes (even with some delay in delivery) and the potential for adverse maternal outcomes, it has been suggested that termination be offered.

Women who present with severe preeclampsia between 24 and 32 weeks of gestation should be offered expectant management. The evidence from both observational and randomized trials comparing delivery with expectant management has shown improved outcomes, including perinatal survival, in women who were managed expectantly versus immediate delivery or delivery after antenatal corticosteroid administration. Delivery, at presentation or during the course of expectant management, is indicated for any of the following conditions:

- Eclampsia
- Abruptio placentae
- Hemolysis, elevated liver enzymes, and low platelets (HELLP) syndrome or a platelet count of less than 100,000/mm^3

- Uncontrolled severe hypertension (blood pressure higher than 160/110 mm Hg) despite maximum doses of at least two antihypertensive agents
- Pulmonary edema
- Persistent severe headache
- Persistent visual disturbances
- Persistent epigastric or right upper quadrant pain
- Evidence of poor fetal well-being (eg, nonreassuring fetal heart rate pattern)
- A deterioration in renal function (serum creatinine level greater than 1.4 mg/dL)
- Gestational age of 34 weeks or more

BOX 84-1

Diagnosis of Severe Preeclampsia

One or more of the following criteria must be present to meet the diagnosis

- Blood pressure 160 mm Hg systolic or higher or 110 mm Hg diastolic or higher on two occasions at least 6 hours apart while the patient is on bed rest
- Proteinuria of 5 g or higher in a 24-hour urine specimen or 3 g or greater on two random urine samples at least 4 hours apart
- Oliguria of less than 500 mL in 24 hours
- Cerebral or visual disturbances
- Pulmonary edema or cyanosis
- Epigastric or right upper quadrant pain
- Impaired liver function
- Thrombocytopenia
- Intrauterine growth restriction

Diagnosis and management of preeclampsia and eclampsia. ACOG Practice Bulletin No. 33. American College of Obstetricians and Gynecologists. Obstet Gynecol 2002;99:159–67.

The amount of proteinuria is rarely a sole indication for delivery. Women with severe preeclampsia who are before 34 weeks of gestation do not appear to benefit from expectant management and delivery should be initiated. Women between 32 and 34 weeks of gestation with severe preeclampsia may be cared for expectantly, but management is dictated by the individual situation.

Inpatient management should be provided at a tertiary care hospital. The patient should be observed at least initially in the labor and delivery suite, where corticosteroids for pulmonary maturity should be administered and close fetal and maternal surveillance can be performed. Antihypertensive medications should be used to control severe hypertension. Intravenous access should be maintained. Laboratory tests to assess kidney and liver function as well as platelet count should be performed, along with a complete blood count. Ultrasonography to assess fetal size and amniotic fluid volume should be performed along with Doppler flow studies. If the patient and fetus remain stable, the patient can be managed in an antepartum unit with daily assessment for signs of imminent eclampsia, blood pressure assessment every 4 hours if they are treated with antihypertensive medication, and daily laboratory assessment of liver function and platelet count. Furthermore, daily fetal assessment is warranted with either nonstress testing or biophysical profiles. If nonstress testing is used, amniotic fluid volume also should be assessed weekly.

Once the patient meets the criteria for delivery, the optimal delivery route is controversial. Some recommend a cesarean delivery if the patient has an unfavorable cervix and is at less than 30 weeks of gestation. After that time, attempted vaginal delivery seems prudent.

Diagnosis and management of preeclampsia and eclampsia. ACOG Practice Bulletin No. 33. American College of Obstetricians and Gynecologists. Obstet Gynecol 2002;99:159–67.

Haddad B, Deis S, Goffinet F, Paniel BJ, Cabrol D, Sibai BM. Maternal and perinatal outcomes during expectant management of 239 severe preeclamptic women between 24 and 33 weeks gestation. Am J Obstet Gynecol 2004;190:1590–5; discussion 1595-7.

Haddad B, Sibai BM. Expectant management of severe preeclampsia: proper candidates and pregnancy outcome. Clin Obstet Gynecol 2005; 48:430–40.

Sibai BM, Mercer BM, Schiff E, Friedman SA. Aggressive versus expectant management of severe preeclampsia at 28 to 32 weeks' gestation: a randomized controlled trial. Am J Obstet Gynecol 1994;171: 818–22.

85

Down syndrome

A 26-year-old woman comes to the office for her first prenatal visit at 10 weeks of gestation. She inquires about her options for Down syndrome screening. You inform her that, given her current gestational age, the option with the greatest sensitivity and lowest false-positive rate to detect Down syndrome is the

    (A) first-trimester screen
    (B) second-trimester ultrasound examination
*   (C) first- and second-trimester integrated screen
    (D) second-trimester triple marker screen
    (E) first- and second-trimester independent sequential screen

Down syndrome is the most frequent chromosomal disorder among liveborn children, with an expected prevalence of 1 in every 600–800 live births. It is the most common identifiable cause of mental retardation and is associated with high rates of structural congenital anomalies, such as congenital heart defects. Several strategies for Down syndrome screening are currently available, with varying degrees of sensitivity. All women should be offered aneuploidy screening, regardless of maternal age. Which test to offer will depend on which test is available, gestational age at presentation, and which strategy best meets the needs of the patient. Table 85-1 describes currently available techniques and testing necessary for each approach.

First-trimester screening, which includes ultrasonographic nuchal translucency measurement as well as serum analyte testing (beta subunit of human chorionic gonadotropin [β-hCG] and a pregnancy-associated plasma protein A [PAPP-A] level), is performed between 11 and 13 6/7 weeks of gestation. This approach has been demonstrated to provide efficient Down syndrome risk assessment with a detection rate of 84% (95% confidence

interval [CI], 80–87%), at a fixed false-positive rate of 5%. The utility of first-trimester screening is limited by the small time frame in which the test can be performed and the specific training and certification required for nuchal translucency measurement. It is imperative that nuchal translucency and first-trimester aneuploidy screening be carried out only at certified centers. In the United States, the Fetal Medicine Foundation and the Society of Maternal–Fetal Medicine certify individuals and prenatal diagnosis centers, and maintain annual quality assurance programs for nuchal translucency and first-trimester screening. Box 85-1 shows the requirements for measuring nuchal translucency. Figure 85-1 shows an ultrasonographic image of a normal nuchal translucency. If a first-trimester screen is performed, a second-trimester maternal serum alpha-fetoprotein (MSAFP) level should be offered in the second trimester to screen for open neural tube defects. Care should be taken to ensure that only the MSAFP is performed at this time as opposed to the complete second-trimester triple or quadruple aneuploidy screens.

The triple and quadruple marker analytes can be assessed between 14 and 22 weeks of gestation. The triple

TABLE 85-1. Down Syndrome Risk Assessment Approaches and Detection Rates (5% Positive Screen Rate)

Down Syndrome Risk Assessment	Tests Performed	Detection Rate (%)
First-trimester screen	Nuchal translucency, PAPP-A, β-hCG	82–87
Second-trimester triple screen	MSAFP, β-hCG, unconjugated estriol	69
Second-trimester quadruple screen	MSAFP, β-hCG, unconjugated estriol, inhibin A	81
Integrated screen (nondisclosure of first-trimester results)	First-trimester nuchal translucency and PAPP-A Second-trimester quadruple screen	94–96

β-hCG, beta subunit of human chorionic gonadotropin; MSAFP, maternal serum alpha-fetoprotein; PAPP-A, pregnancy-associated plasma protein A.

Nuchal Translucency Ultrasonographic Technique

1. Nuchal translucency ultrasonography should be performed only by ultrasonographers or sonologists trained and experienced in the technique.
2. Transabdominal or transvaginal approach should be left to the ultrasonographer's discretion, based on maternal body habitus, gestational age, and fetal position.
3. Gestation should be limited between 10 weeks 3 days and 13 weeks 6 days (approximate fetal crown–rump length, 36–79 mm).
4. Fetus should be examined in a mid-sagittal plane.
5. Fetal neck should be in a neutral position.
6. Fetal image should occupy at least 75% of the viewable screen.
7. Fetal movement should be awaited to distinguish between amnion and overlying fetal skin.
8. Calipers should be placed on the inner borders of the nuchal fold.
9. Calipers should be placed perpendicular to the long axis of the fetal body.
10. At least 20 minutes may need to be dedicated to the nuchal translucency measurement before abandoning the effort as failed.

Malone FD. Nuchal translucency-based Down syndrome screening: barriers to implementation. Semin Perinatol 2005;29:273.

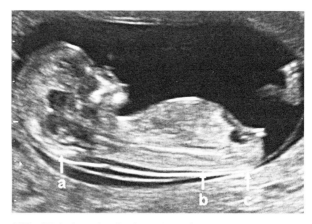

FIG. 85-1. Longitudinal section of a 12-week-old fetus demonstrating the measurement of the fetal nuchal translucency length, between the occiput **(A)** and the lower end of the sonolucency **(B)** and the spinal length, between the occiput **(A)** and the sacral tip **(C)**. (Molina FS, Avgidou K, Kagan KO, Poggi S, Nicolaides KH. Cystic hygromas, nuchal edema, and nuchal translucency at 11–14 weeks of gestation. Obstet Gynecol 2006;107:680.)

marker screen measures the levels of maternal serum alpha-fetoprotein (MSAFP), β-hCG, and unconjugated estriol. It has a detection rate of approximately 65–69% for the Down syndrome, with a 5% false-positive rate. The quadruple marker screen tests inhibin A level in addition to the serum analytes measured in the triple marker screen, and has a higher sensitivity for Down syndrome detection than triple marker screening. Estimates from two of the most recent large studies, the Serum, Urine, and Ultrasound Screening Study (SURUSS) and the First- and Second-Trimester Evaluation of Risk (FASTER) for aneuploidy trial have yielded similar detection rates of approximately 80% with a 5% false-positive rate for the quadruple screen.

Several ultrasonographic markers have been associated with Down syndrome; however, identification of individual ultrasonographic markers, such as echogenic bowel, intracardiac echogenic focus, and dilated renal pelvis yield a low sensitivity and specificity of Down syndrome, particularly when used to screen a low-risk population. Even in combination with gross anomalies such as thickened nuchal fold or cardiac defects, Down syndrome detection rates approach only 50–75% with high false-positive rates (4.8–17%).

The integrated screen provides the highest sensitivity with the lowest false-positive rate. This integrated approach to screening uses both first- and second-trimester markers to calculate a single risk that is reported to the patient in the second trimester. Measurement of nuchal translucency and PAPP-A are performed in the first trimester; however, the results are not disclosed to the patient at that time. Patients return at 15 weeks of gestation, when the quadruple markers are obtained (Table 85-1), and the results of the first- and second-trimester tests are combined to provide a single Down syndrome risk assessment in the second trimester. Of the Down syndrome screening options currently available, integrated screening yields the highest detection rate with the lowest false-positive rate. In the FASTER and SURUSS trials, an integrated screening program had a sensitivity of 95% and 94%, with false-positive rates of 4.0% and 4.9%, respectively.

Independent sequential testing involves the independent interpretation of first- and second-trimester tests. The first-trimester test results are disclosed as soon as they are available so the patient can act on these results. Second-trimester testing is offered unless the patient has undergone chorionic villus sampling (CVS). However, the second-trimester test is interpreted without taking into account the first-trimester test results (ie, maternal age is used as the a priori risk for second-trimester testing). Although the sensitivity is high, this is the least efficient risk assessment strategy because the additive false-positive rate is unacceptably high and, therefore, should not be offered for Down syndrome screening assessment.

Malone FD, Canick JA, Ball RH, Nyberg DA, Comstock CH, Bukowski R, et al. First-trimester or second-trimester screening, or both, for Down's syndrome. First- and Second-Trimester Evaluation of Risk (FASTER) Research Consortium. N Engl J Med 2005;353:2001–11.

Reddy UM, Mennuti MT. Incorporating first-trimester Down syndrome studies into prenatal screening: executive summary of the National Institute of Child Health and Human Development workshop. Obstet Gynecol 2006;107:167–73.

Screening for fetal chromosomal abnormalities. ACOG Practice Bulletin No. 77. American College of Obstetricians and Gynecologists. Obstet Gynecol 2007;109:217–27.

Wald NJ, Rodeck C, Hackshaw AK, Walters J, Chitty L, Mackinson AM. First and second trimester antenatal screening for Down's syndrome: the results of the Serum, Urine, and Ultrasound Screening Study (SURUSS). SURUSS Research Group. Health Technol Assess 2003;7:1–77.

Wald NJ, Watt HC, Hackshaw AK. Integrated screening for Down's syndrome on the basis of tests performed during the first and second trimesters. N Engl J Med 1999;341:461–7.

Wapner R, Thom E, Simpson JL, Pergament E, Silver R, Filkins K, et al. First-trimester screening for trisomies 21 and 18. First Trimester Maternal Serum Biochemistry and Fetal Nuchal Translucency Screening (BUN) Study Group. N Engl J Med 2003;349:1405–13.

86

Antiphospholipid syndrome

A 29-year-old woman, gravida 4, comes to the office for a prenatal visit. She has had an unexplained 21-week intrauterine fetal demise and two unexplained first-trimester losses. Her anti-β_2-glycoprotein I antibody test results, drawn on two occasions 12 weeks apart, exceed the 99th percentile. She is currently taking low-dose aspirin. The other medication that should be added for appropriate therapy for her pregnancy is

    (A) clopidogrel (Plavix)
    (B) prednisone
    (C) intravenous immunoglobulin
*   (D) heparin

Antiphospholipid syndrome is an autoimmune syndrome characterized by thrombosis and recurrent pregnancy loss. The diagnosis requires both clinical and laboratory components. The laboratory component includes anticardiolipin antibodies, lupus anticoagulant, and anti-β_2-glycoprotein I antibodies. The clinical component includes vascular thrombosis and pregnancy morbidity. The pregnancy morbidity includes an unexplained fetal death, three or more consecutive unexplained spontaneous abortions, or an indicated preterm birth before 34 weeks of gestation caused by severe preeclampsia or placental insufficiency (Appendix I).

The treatment for antiphospholipid syndrome is heparin and aspirin. The combination of these medications can reduce recurrent pregnancy loss by 54%. The medications are started in the first trimester when there is documentation of a viable embryo. The regimen will depend on whether the woman's clinical criteria comprise pregnancy morbidity or vascular thrombosis. In the case of women with pregnancy morbidity, a prophylactic heparin regimen is appropriate. For women with vascular thrombosis, a therapeutic heparin regimen should be used. Evidence suggests that the combination of unfractionated heparin and aspirin significantly reduces recurrent pregnancy loss. Low molecular weight heparin is currently used interchangeably with unfractionated heparin. However, more randomized control trials need to be performed to demonstrate its efficacy in this situation. For all patients with antiphospholipid syndrome, this treatment regimen should be continued through at least 6 weeks postpartum, when the risk for vascular thrombosis is highest.

In women with antiphospholipid syndrome, aspirin therapy alone did not reduce the rate of pregnancy loss. Clopidogrel is not used as a therapy for women with this condition. The combination of aspirin and prednisone increased the rate of premature birth and gestational diabetes mellitus without significant benefit to the women taking these medications. Similarly, intravenous immunoglobulin increased the rate of pregnancy loss and premature birth when compared with heparin and aspirin therapy.

Women with antiphospholipid syndrome are also at increased risk for pregnancy complications associated with uteroplacental insufficiency. As a result, their antenatal management should include careful assessment of fetal growth. If there is evidence of intrauterine growth restriction, antenatal testing should be initiated. If the fetus is appropriately grown, antenatal testing is initiated at 32 weeks of gestation. A pregnant woman with this condition should be delivered by her estimated date of confinement.

Derksen RH, Khamashta MA, Branch DW. Management of the obstetric antiphospholipid syndrome. Arthritis Rheum 2004;50:1028–39.

Empson M, Lassere M, Craig JC, Scott JR. Recurrent pregnancy loss with antiphospholipid antibody: a systematic review of therapeutic trials. Obstet Gynecol 2002;99:135–44.

Empson M, Lassere M, Craig J, Scott J. Prevention of recurrent miscarriage for women with antiphospholipid antibody or lupus anticoagulant.

Cochrane Database of Systematic Reviews 2005, Issue 2. Art. No.: CD002859. DOI: 10.1002/14651858.CD002859.pub2.

Rai R, Cohen H, Dave M, Regan L. Randomised controlled trial of aspirin and aspirin plus heparin in pregnant women with recurrent miscarriage associated with phospholipid antibodies (or antiphospholipid antibodies). BMJ 1997;314:253–7.

87

Pyelonephritis

Your partner admits a 37-year-old woman, gravida 3, para 2, to the hospital at 24 weeks of gestation with a temperature of 38.3°C (101°F), right flank pain, and 200 white blood cells per high power field on urine microscopy. He orders intravenous fluids and intravenous ceftriaxone. When you make rounds the next morning, the patient has a respiratory rate of 30 breaths per minute and an oxygen saturation by pulse oximetry of 88% while breathing room air. The most likely cause of her respiratory distress is

    (A) intravenous fluid overload with pulmonary edema
    (B) community-acquired pneumonia
*   (C) sepsis-induced acute lung injury
    (D) pulmonary embolism
    (E) unrecognized heart disease with pulmonary edema

Pyelonephritis is a common cause of antepartum hospital admission. It is usually caused by *Escherichia coli* or another gram-negative organism and responds to appropriate intravenous antibiotic therapy. However, serious complications may occur, including acute lung injury, acute respiratory distress syndrome (ARDS), septic shock, preterm delivery, and stillbirth. Approximately 1% of patients with pyelonephritis develop pulmonary complications. The pathophysiology is thought to involve gram-negative organisms that invade the bloodstream and the bactericidal action of antibiotics that releases cell wall endotoxin. The interaction of microbes and microbial structural components with neutrophils, monocytes, macrophages, and endothelial cells causes release of numerous mediators, including cytokines, proteolytic enzymes, oxygen-free radicals, complement components, and coagulation factors. This results in injury to endothelial cells that cause a capillary leak, a form of nonhydrostatic pulmonary edema. If the leak is not too severe, the physiologic consequence is acute lung injury; if the leak is severe, it is ARDS. The recommended criteria for acute lung injury are acute onset, bilateral infiltrates on chest X-ray, pulmonary artery wedge pressure of 18 mm Hg or less, or no clinical evidence of left atrial hypertension, and a ratio of partial pressure of oxygen in arterial blood to fraction of inspired oxygen (Pao_2/Fio_2) of 300 or less.

The criteria for ARDS are the same for timing, chest X-ray, and pulmonary artery wedge pressure, but ARDS requires a Pao_2/Fio_2 of 200 or less. Therapy for acute lung injury and ARDS involves treatment of the underlying cause and maintenance of oxygenation by nasal cannula, face mask, or mechanical ventilation with positive end-expiratory pressure.

Intravenous fluid overload would be unlikely in a healthy woman such as the patient described. Careful review of previous intake and output should identify this problem. Underlying heart disease would be uncommon and diagnosed by history, cardiac examination, chest X-ray, and echocardiogram. There was no cough or sputum production to indicate pneumonia. Pulmonary embolism is uncommon in pregnancy, particularly in the absence of other predisposing factors.

Bernard GR, Artigas A, Brigham KL, Carlet J, Falke K, Hudson L, et al. The American–European Consensus Conference on ARDS. Definitions, mechanisms, relevant outcomes, and clinical trial coordination. Am J Respir Crit Care Med 1994;149:818–24.

Cunningham FG, Lucas MJ, Hankins GD. Pulmonary injury complicating antepartum pyelonephritis. Am J Obstet Gynecol 1987;156:797–807.

Mabie WC, Barton JR, Sibai BM. Septic shock in pregnancy. Obstet Gynecol 1997;90:553–61.

Parrillo JE. Pathogenetic mechanisms of septic shock. N Engl J Med 1993;328:1471–7.

88

Maternal age counseling

A 44-year-old primigravid woman comes to the office for her first prenatal visit at 8 weeks of gestation and inquires about risks to her pregnancy. You tell her that there are genetic risks associated with advanced maternal age. You inform her that in addition to the increased risk of cesarean delivery, preeclampsia, gestational diabetes mellitus, and placenta previa, her age puts her at increased risk for

    (A) midtrimester loss
    (B) postterm pregnancy
* (C) stillbirth
    (D) postpartum depression

As an increasing number of women older than 40 years contemplate pregnancy or become pregnant, preconception and prenatal counseling of these older women has become more common and important. In 2002, the birth rate in women aged 40–44 years increased to 9.0 per 1,000 women. There are likely many reasons for the increased rate of pregnancy in older women, including delayed childbearing, second marriages, and better contraceptive options. In the past, counseling for patients with advanced maternal age was focused on the genetic risks, such as an increased likelihood of Down syndrome and other chromosomal abnormalities. However, recent information has suggested that older women also may be at increased risk for certain nongenetic complications of pregnancy. This body of literature is somewhat confounded because older women have higher rates of medical complications, such as chronic hypertension and diabetes mellitus, that can directly increase risk of adverse pregnancy outcomes. Thus, it can be difficult to differentiate the independent effect of age from the effects of other age-associated medical complications on adverse pregnancy outcomes.

Several recent studies have attempted to assess these issues by using observational study designs and controlling for relevant confounding factors. These studies suggest that women older than 40 years have an increased risk of preterm birth and growth restriction (see Table 88-1). Several studies have assessed the relationship between maternal age and fetal death, and the risk appears to be 1.5–2.5-fold higher in women older than 40 years. In addition, placenta previa is more common in these women. One study suggested a 10-fold increase in the risk of placenta previa in nulliparous women older than 40 years compared to nulliparous women younger than 29 years. It is less clear whether maternal age is independently associated with abruptio placentae. Some studies have suggested that, after controlling for parity, there

TABLE 88-1. Risk of Pregnancy Complications in Older Women

Complication	Risk (%)
Preeclampsia	5–10
Gestational diabetes mellitus	7–12
Placenta previa	3
Stillbirth	0.6
Cesarean delivery	30

is no association between maternal age and abruptio placentae. Increasing age is associated with an increased risk of preeclampsia and diabetes. It is important to communicate to patients that although these risks are increased relative to younger women, the absolute risk of such complications is quite low and does not constitute a contraindication to pregnancy. Increasing maternal age has not been associated with midtrimester pregnancy loss.

Because of these risks, patients older than 40 years ideally should be offered preconception counseling. At such a visit, women can be counseled about likely reproductive outcomes and make informed choices. If preconception counseling is not an option, then the patient should be counseled early in pregnancy. During pregnancy, these women should be monitored closely for signs and symptoms of preeclampsia and screened for gestational diabetes mellitus. Although not based on level I evidence, a recommendation to monitor such patients for fetal growth disturbances and to initiate antepartum surveillance seems reasonable.

Fretts RC, Elkin EB, Myers ER, Heffner LJ. Should older women have antepartum testing to prevent unexplained stillbirth? Obstet Gynecol 2004;104:56–64.

Fretts RC, Usher RH. Fetal death in women in the older reproductive age group. Contemp Rev Obstet Gynecol 1997;9:173–7.

Fretts RC. Effect of advanced age on fertility and pregnancy in women. UpToDate http://patients.uptodate.com/topic.asp?file=antenatl/14857.

89

Maternal human immunodeficiency virus

A 22-year-old primigravid woman comes to the office for preconception counseling. She is infected with the human immunodeficiency virus (HIV) and has a normal CD4 count, a viral load of less than 1,000 copies, and negative serology for syphilis, hepatitis B, and hepatitis C. In regard to her risk of infectious disease complications, you advise her the most likely outcome of a pregnancy would be

    (A) congenital toxoplasmosis
*   (B) no acceleration of HIV disease
    (C) *Pneumocystis carinii* pneumonia (PCP)
    (D) congenital cytomegalovirus

Acquired immunodeficiency syndrome (AIDS) was first recognized as a disease entity in 1981, and by 1985 an enzyme-linked immunosorbent assay (ELISA) test became available to diagnose infection with HIV, an RNA retrovirus. The term retrovirus refers to the feature of this class of viruses that allows them to transcribe genomic RNA to DNA using the enzyme reverse transcriptase. The replication cycle of this virus begins with binding of the gp120 protein to its receptor on the host cell surface, the CD4 molecule. Once this step has occurred, a series of steps ensue that allow for entry of the virus into the cell.

The management of HIV in pregnancy has been relatively successful over the past 20 years. Before introduction of antiretroviral therapy, vertical transmission rates were in the range of 30–40%. Intrapartum zidovudine (AZT) therapy reduced transmission rates to less than 10%. With the advent of tests to determine viral load, drug regimens that kept viral load levels under 1,000 copies, and increased use of elective cesarean delivery, rates have been reduced to less than 2%.

Epidemiologic data accumulated over the past two decades demonstrate that women with HIV infection during pregnancy do have some elevated obstetric risks. Rates of preterm delivery, premature rupture of membranes, and postpartum endometritis are all increased in HIV-positive women. The reasons for these increased risks are varied and may not refer entirely to a cause–effect relationship, because many other factors associated with HIV seropositivity also are associated with these same adverse events. There is no evidence, however, to link the occurrence of pregnancy to acceleration of HIV infection progression as long as antiretroviral therapy is given appropriately for the disease state. In the patient described, the presence of a normal CD4 count, a low viral load, and absent infectious comorbidities (syphilis, hepatitis B, and hepatitis C) suggests immunocompetence and, thus, the fetus would not be expected to be at increased risk for congenital infections like toxoplasmosis or cytomegalovirus, nor would the patient described be at increased risk for opportunistic infection like PCP.

Barbieri RL, Repke JT. Medical disorders during pregnancy. In: Kasper DL, Braunwald E, Fauci AS, Hauser SL, Longo DL, Jameson JH, editors. Harrison's principles of internal medicine. 16th ed. New York (NY): McGraw-Hill; 2005. p. 32–8.

Duff P. Maternal and perinatal infections. In: Gabbe SG, Niebyl JR, Simpson JL, editors. Obstetrics: normal and problem pregnancies. 4th ed. New York (NY): Churchill Livingstone; 2002. p. 1320–5.

90

Management of postterm pregnancy

A 21-year-old primigravid woman is seen for the first time at 41 weeks of gestation based on a known last menstrual period and corroboration with first-trimester ultrasonography. The current pregnancy has been uncomplicated. Cervical examination demonstrates an undilated, uneffaced cervix with the vertex at –2 station. The clinical estimate of fetal weight is 3,700 g. A limited ultrasonographic scan reveals an amniotic fluid index (AFI) of 4. The next step in this patient's care should be

     (A) ultrasonography to confirm gestational age
     (B) cesarean delivery within the next week
*   (C) immediate labor induction
     (D) return office visit in 1 week
     (E) repeat AFI in 3–4 days

Postterm pregnancy is defined as pregnancy that has extended to or beyond 42 weeks of gestation. Postterm pregnancy has been associated with an increased incidence of stillbirth and an increased rate of neonatal morbidity and mortality. There is also an increased incidence of large-for-gestational-age fetuses and macrosomia, a higher rate of cesarean delivery, and a 20% incidence of dysmaturity syndrome. Shoulder dystocia, obstetric trauma, fetal distress in labor, and obstetric hemorrhage have been described as occurring at a higher rate in association with postterm gestation. Few data support elective labor induction as a strategy to prevent postterm pregnancy and thereby lessen these complications. To minimize the risk of adverse outcome, several strategies are available. Accurate dating of gestational age in early pregnancy can be useful to help develop a management strategy as term approaches.

In the patient described, ultrasonography would not be useful to confirm gestational age. The error rate for ultrasonography carried out to assess gestational age at her stage of pregnancy has been reported to be as high as plus or minus 3 weeks.

Based on the clinical data provided, there would be no reason to schedule an elective cesarean delivery. The combination of cervical ripening and labor induction should yield a favorable likelihood of vaginal delivery. Although some additional fetal surveillance and delay of delivery for another week could be entertained, in these circumstances the AFI of 4 suggests oligohydramnios and possible fetal compromise. In these circumstances, immediate labor induction should be carried out.

If the patient described had a normal AFI then it would be appropriate to continue expectant management of the pregnancy until the pregnancy became postterm at 42 weeks. A woman with a postterm gestation and an unfavorable cervix may undergo labor induction or continue with expectant management. Although it is acceptable to begin antenatal surveillance at 41 weeks of gestation, there is insufficient evidence to indicate whether routine antenatal surveillance of low-risk patients between 40 and 42 weeks of gestation improves perinatal outcome.

American College of Obstetricians and Gynecologists. Management of postterm pregnancy. ACOG Practice Bulletin 55. Washington, DC: ACOG; 2004.

Divon MY. Prolonged pregnancy. In: Gabbe SG, Niebyl JR, Simpson JL, editors. Obstetrics: normal and problem pregnancies. 4th ed. New York (NY): Churchill Livingstone; 2002. p. 931–42.

91

Macrosomia

A woman, gravida 1, para 0, at 40 weeks of gestation, confirmed by first-trimester ultrasonography, reports a decrease in fetal movement. She is 1.6 m (5 ft 4 in.) tall and weighs 74.8 kg (165 lb). An ultrasonogram reveals a biophysical profile of 8/8 and an estimated fetal weight of 4,600 g. Her glucose loading test result was reported as normal. The cervix is long, closed, and thick. She is not having uterine contractions. The next step in her care is to

      (A)   arrange for a cesarean delivery now
      (B)   repeat ultrasonography in 1 week
      (C)   initiate cervical ripening procedures
*   (D)   await onset of labor

The delivery of a macrosomic fetus (defined as a fetus of birth weight of 4,500 g or more) is associated with prolonged labor, an increased likelihood of operative delivery, shoulder dystocia, and brachial plexus injury. Newborn infants with a weight greater than 4,500 g are at increased risk for neonatal morbidity, which includes assisted ventilation and meconium aspiration. Infants who weigh at least 5,000 g have greater infant mortality rates than do infants who weigh between 4,000 and 4,499 g. Maternal complications that are associated with the delivery of macrosomic infants include operative delivery, postpartum hemorrhage, laceration of the anal sphincter, and postpartum infection.

Because clinicians would prefer to avoid these complications, it is intuitively appealing to intervene with labor induction if a fetus is suspected of being macrosomic. However, reviews of such protocols consistently have failed to show a reduction in these complications when labor induction has been used.

Since its inception more than 30 years ago, ultrasonographic fetal biometry has been assumed to be more accurate than clinical methods to estimate fetal weight. However, when the ability of 20 different ultrasonographic fetal biometric algorithms to predict term fetal weight to within 15% of actual birth weight was studied, results ranged from 44% to 89%. For those neonates with birth weight greater than 4,000 g, the positive predictive value ranged from 20% to 48%. Years of experience of the examiners did not enhance the accuracy of estimating birth weight. The estimated fetal weight determined during labor by residents was as accurate as the estimated fetal weight reported in the literature when performed by ultrasonographers. Therefore, the initial ultrasonogram estimated fetal weight in the described case needs to be looked on with circumspection, and surgical decisions should not be made based solely on this value.

A study evaluated 138 patients with singleton pregnancies who had ultrasonography between 34.0 and 36.9 weeks of gestation and again at 37 or more weeks of gestation and found that the earlier ultrasonograms were more accurate in the assessment of birth weight. Therefore, repeat ultrasonography in 1 week would not be beneficial as the next step in management.

In an effort to avoid continued fetal weight gain and the corresponding increase in cesarean deliveries and fetal injury that may be expected to occur, some have advocated labor induction when the fetus exceeds a given weight. However, there is no evidence from either observational or randomized trials that the induction of labor for macrosomia prevents shoulder dystocia, brachial plexus injury, or other adverse neonatal outcome. Based on this information, there is no evidence to support preemptory inductions for macrosomia or impending macrosomia, especially in the face of an unripe cervix.

In the case described, active intervention might appear to offer the most attractive option. However, evidence-based obstetrics indicates that to await the onset of labor is the wisest course.

American College of Obstetricians and Gynecologists. Fetal macrosomia. ACOG Practice Bulletin 22. Washington, DC: ACOG; 2000.

Chauhan SP, Grobman WA, Gherman RA, Chauhan VB, Chang G, Magann EF, et al. Suspicion and treatment of the macrosomic fetus: a review. Am J Obstet Gynecol 2005;193:332–46.

Chien PF, Owen P, Khan KS. Validity of ultrasound estimation of fetal weight. Obstet Gynecol 2000;95:856–60.

Nahum GG, Stanislaw H. Ultrasonographic prediction of term birth weight: how accurate is it? Am J Obstet Gynecol 2003;188:566–74.

Noumi G, Collado-Khoury F, Bombard A, Julliard K, Weiner Z. Clinical and sonographic estimation of fetal weight performed during labor by residents. Am J Obstet Gynecol 2005;192:1407–9.

Pressman EK, Bienstock JL, Blakemore KJ, Martin SA, Callan NA. Prediction of birth weight by ultrasound in the third trimester. Obstet Gynecol 2000;95:502–6.

92

Use of biophysical profile to manage pregnancy

A 32-year-old woman at 36 weeks of gestation was referred for a biophysical profile (BPP) because of decreased fetal movements over the past 12 hours. The cardiotocograph reveals a fetal heart rate of 155 beats per minute, with two accelerations of 15 beats per minute and lasting 25 seconds. Ultrasonography shows one episode of opening and closing of the hand; one fetal breathing episode lasting 30 seconds; three fetal body and limb movements; and maximum vertical amniotic fluid pocket of 3.5 cm. In view of these findings, the most appropriate care for this patient is

(A) repeat the BPP in 24 hours
(B) repeat the BPP in 1 week
(C) admit for induction of labor
(D) admit for prolonged monitoring
* (E) no further testing

The BPP is a frequently used noninvasive test for antenatal fetal surveillance. The BPP combines information from two sources: ultrasonography and cardiotocography. Ultrasonography allows real-time evaluation of fetal breathing, fetal body movements, and fetal tone as well as an estimation of the amount of amniotic fluid. The length of the ultrasonographic observation is 30 minutes; however, if the fetus demonstrates all variables in less than 30 minutes, the study can be terminated. A BPP cannot be deemed abnormal unless the 30 minutes have elapsed. The cardiotocograph records the fetal heart rate in a nonstress test (NST) as the rate changes in response to fetal moments. The order in which ultrasonography and the NST are performed is not important. However, if all four of the ultrasonographic variables are normal, the NST may be omitted without compromising the validity of the BPP (Table 92-1).

Multiple articles discuss which technique should be used to assess the amount of amniotic fluid: amniotic fluid index (AFI) or the largest (deepest) single amniotic fluid pocket. Several recent studies have shown that, if reassuring, the AFI offers no advantage over the single largest pocket of amniotic fluid. The AFI is obtained by visually dividing the abdomen into four equal quadrants and measuring the deepest pocket (devoid of fetal parts or cord) and then adding them together. With the use of the AFI, oligohydramnios is defined as the sum of the quadrants equalling 5 cm or less; in contrast, when using the single deepest pocket, oligohydramnios is defined as a pocket of fluid of 2 cm or less. When using the AFI to assess fluid volume, a significantly greater number of pregnancies are labeled as having oligohydramnios than when the single deepest pocket is used.

Interpretation of the BPP scores is as follows:

• Normal (score 8/10 or 10/10)

• Equivocal (score of 6/10)

• Abnormal (score of 4/10 or less)

When findings are normal, the BPP is a reliable predictor of normal tissue oxygenation and, therefore, absence of fetal asphyxia. However, regardless of the score in the presence of oligohydramnios, further evaluation or delivery is warranted. In cases when the BPP score is 6/10 or equivocal, multiple factors need to be taken into consideration, such as fetal age, score composition by individual parameters, and the presence of other fetal and maternal factors. In approximately two thirds of the equivocal BPPs, if repeated within 24 hours, the results will be normal, especially if the missing variables are fetal breathing movements and a nonreactive NST. However, in term pregnancies, a BPP score of 6/10 or less generally is an indication for delivery (Table 92-2).

A study in which cordocentesis was performed immediately following a BPP demonstrated that there is a linear relationship between the BPP score and the pH level of the antepartum fetal umbilical venous cord. Essentially, a normal BPP is a predictor of a good outcome and in essence excludes the possibility of acidemia; an equivocal BPP score is a poor predictor of an abnormal outcome; and an abnormal score (especially when the BPP is 0/10) is a powerful predictor of an abnormal outcome.

The modified BPP refers to an NST plus an amniotic fluid volume only. The modified BPP, if reassuring, much like the BPP, is indicative of fetal well-being and low risk of an intrauterine fetal death.

In the case presented, the BPP scores were 2 points for the NST; 2 points for opening and closing of the hand (fetal tone); 2 points for fetal breathing episode of 30 seconds; 2 points for fetal body and limb movements; and 2 points for an amniotic fluid pocket of 3.5 cm. The overall score in this case was 10/10 or a normal score. The interpretation is that the fetus is not asphyxiated, and conservative management with no further testing is an appropriate next step. However, if the patient continues to have

TABLE 92-1. Criteria for Coding of Fetal Biophysical Variables as Normal or Abnormal

Biophysical Variable	Score = 2 (Normal or Present)	Score = 0 (Abnormal, Absent, or Insufficient)
Fetal breathing movements	One or more episodes of 30 seconds or more duration within 30 minutes	Absent or no episode of 30 seconds or more duration in 30 minutes
Gross body movements	Three or more discrete body or limb movements within 30 minutes	Fewer than three episodes of body or limb movements within 30 minutes
Fetal tone	One or more episodes of extension of a fetal extremity with return to flexion, or opening or closing of a hand	Slow extension with return to partial flexion, movement of limb in full extension, absent fetal movement, or partially open fetal hand
Amniotic fluid volume	A single vertical pocket of amniotic fluid exceeding 2 cm	Either no pockets or largest pocket is less than 2 cm in vertical axis
Reactive fetal heart rate (FHR)	Two or more episodes of acceleration of 15 beats per minute or greater and of 15 seconds or greater associated with fetal movement within 20 minutes	0–1 episodes of acceleration of fetal heart rate or acceleration of less than 15 beats per minute within 20 minutes

Modified from Manning FA. Fetal biophysical profile. Obstet Gynecol Clin North Am 1999;26:557–77, v. Copyright 1999 by Elsevier.

TABLE 92-2. Recommended Fetal Management by Biophysical Profile Score

Result	Interpretation	% Risk of Asphyxia*	Risk of Fetal Death (per 1,000/week)	Recommended Management
10/10	Nonasphyxiated	0	0.565	Conservative management
8/10 (normal AFV)	Nonasphyxiated	0	0.565	Conservative management
8/8 (NST not done)	Nonasphyxiated	0	0.565	Conservative management
8/10 (decreased AFV)	Chronic compensated asphyxia	5–10 (estimate)	20–30	If mature (37 weeks or more), deliver; serial testing (twice weekly in the immature fetus)
6/10 (normal AFV)	Acute asphyxia possible	0	50	If mature (37 weeks or more), deliver; repeat test in 24 hours in immature fetus; if 6/10 or less, deliver
6/10 (decreased AFV)	Chronic asphyxia with possible acute asphyxia	Greater than 10	Greater than 50	Factor in gestational age; if mature (32 weeks or more), deliver; if less than 32 weeks, test daily
4/10 (normal AFV)	Acute asphyxia likely	36	115	Factor in gestational age; if 32 weeks or more, deliver; if less than 32 weeks, test daily
4/10 (decreased AFV)	Chronic asphyxia with acute asphyxia likely	Greater than 36	Greater than 115	If 26 weeks or more, deliver
2/10 (normal AFV)	Acute asphyxia nearly certain	73	220	If 26 weeks or more, deliver
0/10	Gross severe asphyxia	100	550	If 26 weeks or more, deliver

AFV, amniotic fluid volume; NST, nonstress test.

*Umbilical venous blood pH less than 7.25.

Modified from Manning FA. Fetal biophysical profile. Obstet Gynecol Clin North Am 1999;26:557–77, v. Copyright 1999 by Elsevier.

decreased fetal movement, further antenatal surveillance may be warranted.

American College of Obstetricians and Gynecologists. Antepartum fetal surveillance. ACOG Practice Bulletin 9. Washington, DC: ACOG; 1999.

Chauhan SP, Doherty DD, Magann EF, Chahanding F, Moreno F, Klausen JH. Amniotic fluid index vs. single deepest pocket technique during modified biophysical profile: a randomized clinical trial. Am J Obstet Gynecol 2004;191:661–7; discussion 667–8.

Magann EF, Doherty DA, Field K, Chauhan SP, Muffley PE, Morrison JC. Biophysical profile with amniotic fluid volume assessments. Obstet Gynecol 2004;104:5–10.

Manning FA. Fetal biophysical profile. Obstet Gynecol Clin North Am 1999;26:557–77, v.

Manning FA, Snijders R, Harman CR, Nicolaides K, Menticoglou S, Morrison I. Fetal biophysical profile score. VI. Correlation with antepartum umbilical venous fetal pH. Am J Obstet Gynecol 1993;169:755–63.

93

Mastitis

A 19-year-old woman, gravida 1, para 1, presents at 3 weeks postpartum with a temperature of 38.3°C (101°F) and redness and nipple pain in her right breast. She had an uncomplicated vaginal delivery. She has been breastfeeding exclusively. The breast is significantly swollen, and the neonate is fussy and having difficulty feeding. The patient is considering discontinuing breastfeeding. The most appropriate next step is to

* (A) begin empiric outpatient antibiotics
  (B) admit to the hospital for systemic antibiotics
  (C) culture milk and begin antibiotics after identification of organism
  (D) obtain breast ultrasonography
  (E) feed from unaffected breast only

Numerous studies indicate that breastfeeding is beneficial to both infant and mother. Human milk provides age-specific nutrients for the infant and supplies immunoglobulin A and other substances with antimicrobial properties that protect against infection. Research on the protective effects of human milk reveal that the incidence or severity of diarrhea, lower respiratory infection, otitis media, bacterial meningitis, botulism, urinary tract infection, and necrotizing enterocolitis are decreased by feeding with human milk. Maternal benefits of breastfeeding include decreased blood loss, decreased risk of developing ovarian and premenopausal breast cancer, suppression of ovulation allowing for birth spacing, and the psychologic benefits of nurturing and bonding. Information for 2005 showed that 72.9% of women in the United States initiate breastfeeding in the early postpartum period, and 36% of women surveyed breastfeed to some degree at 6 months postpartum.

Mastitis is an infectious process of the parenchymal tissues of the mammary glands that affects approximately 2–33% of breastfeeding mothers at least once during the first 12 months postpartum. Its onset is most frequently in the first 2–4 weeks postpartum. The differential diagnosis includes marked breast engorgement, clogged milk duct, breast abscess, or, rarely, inflammatory breast carcinoma.

Usually, the infection is unilateral with localized erythema, induration, and tenderness. Often chills, high fever (39–40°C), nausea, vomiting, and malaise accompany mastitis. Bacteria from the infant's nose and throat may enter the breast through a nipple abrasion or fissure. The most commonly isolated organism is *Staphylococcus aureus*, which is also the most common cause of abscess formation. Other frequently isolated organisms are *Haemophilus influenzae* and *H parainfluenzae, Escherichia coli, Enterococcus faecalis, Klebsiella pneumoniae, Enterobacter cloacae, Serratia marcescens,* and *Pseudomonas pickettii.* Initial treatment is prompt antibiotic therapy begun empirically with dicloxacillin. Alternative medications include cephalexin for penicillin-sensitive women who can tolerate cephalosporins or erythromycin or clindamycin for women with severe penicillin allergies. Resolution can be facilitated by supportive care such as increased fluid intake, analgesics such as ibuprofen, breast support, assessment of nursing technique, and emptying both breasts either by feeding or pumping.

Approximately 3–11% of women with mastitis develop a breast abscess. Management of a breast abscess typically requires surgical drainage or ultrasonographic-guided needle aspiration in addition to antibiotic therapy. An abscess may develop because of inadequate or delayed treatment, or if resistant organisms such as methicillin-resistant *S aureus* are encountered.

Treatment of uncomplicated mastitis should begin with prompt antibiotic therapy and supportive care. Because of resistant strains of staphylococcus at various institutions or in the case of a patient with multiple drug allergies limiting antibiotic choices, sometimes breast milk may need to be expressed for culture. In such cases, antibiotic therapy should be initiated before culture results are available and altered if organism identification and sensitivities warrant. Hospital admission and systemic antibiotics usually are not necessary with an uncomplicated mastitis. Breast ultrasonography may be beneficial if an abscess is suspected. The patient with mastitis should continue to feed or express milk from both breasts so that the affected breast is emptied.

Healthy People 2010 has set a goal to increase the proportion of mothers who breastfeed their babies to 75% in the early postpartum period, 50% at 6 months, and 25% at 12 months.

Barbosa-Cesnik C, Schwartz K, Foxman B. Lactation mastitis. JAMA 2003;289:1609–12.

Breastfeeding: maternal and infant aspects. ACOG Committee Opinion No. 361. American College of Obstetricians and Gynecologists. Obstet Gynecol 2007;109:279–80.

Breastfeeding: maternal and infant aspects. ACOG Committee on Health Care for Underserved Women and ACOG Committee on Obstetric Practice. American College of Obstetricians and Gynecologists. ACOG Clin Rev 2007;12(suppl):1S–16S.

Centers for Disease Control and Prevention. Breastfeeding: data and statistics: breastfeeding practices—results from the 2005 National Immunization Survey. Available at: http://www.cdc.gov/breastfeeding/data/NIS_data/data_2005.htm. Retrieved March 26, 2007.

Mattar CN, Chong YS, Chan YS, Chew A, Tan P, Chan YH, et al. Simple antenatal preparation to improve breastfeeding practice: a randomized controlled trial. Obstet Gynecol 2007;109:73–80.

Newton ER. Physiology of lactation and breast-feeding. In: Gabbe SG, Niebyl JR, Simpson JL, editors. Obstetrics: normal and problem pregnancies. 4th ed. New York (NY): Churchill Livingstone; 2002. p. 105–36.

The puerperium. In: Cunningham FG, Leveno KJ, Bloom SL, Hauth JC, Gilstrap L 3rd, Wenstrom KD, editors. Williams obstetrics. 22nd ed. New York (NY): McGraw-Hill; 2005. p. 695–710.

94

Stillbirth management in subsequent pregnancies

A 32-year-old woman, gravida 5, para 3, at 18 weeks of gestation comes to the office for her first prenatal visit. She had an unexplained fetal death at 33 weeks in her last pregnancy, and the workup included a finding of a normal fetal karyotype. Her blood pressure is normal. Her glucose challenge test result, thyroid-stimulating hormone (TSH) level, and free thyroxine level are all normal. Ultrasonography shows normal fetal anatomy and fetal growth with adequate amniotic fluid compatible with 18 weeks of gestation. Anticardiolipin antibodies and lupus anticoagulant test results are negative. The most appropriate management is

   (A)   amniocentesis for fetal karyotype
   (B)   low-dose heparin
* (C)   serial fetal testing from 32 weeks of gestation
   (D)   cytomegalovirus (CMV) and toxoplasmosis titers
   (E)   ultrasonography at 38 weeks of gestation

Assessment of stillbirths should include clinical examination with maternal and fetal evaluation. Box 94-1 shows different types of tests for stillbirth. Fetal autopsy should be encouraged and the placenta should always be sent for histopathology. The frequency of chromosomal abnormalities in unselected stillbirths is approximately 5–10%. Amniocentesis for culture of amniocytes is the best method for a successful cytogenetic analysis, because failure increases with duration from time of fetal death. However, amniocentesis is not indicated in the subsequent pregnancy unless a genetic condition was detected which is amenable to prenatal diagnosis.

Toxoplasmosis, rubella, cytomegalovirus, and herpes simplex (TORCH) titers have not been included routinely in protocols. This is especially true if there are no placental or autopsy findings of congenital infections.

Comprehensive postpartum assessment of stillbirths has been shown to have a diagnostic yield of 40–70%. The Wisconsin Stillbirth Service Program studied 1,477 stillborns and showed that when comprehensive, nonselective analysis was performed, new information was discovered relevant to recurrence risk estimation, prenatal diagnosis recommendation, and future treatment in 51% of the cases.

The risk of recurrent stillbirth in a subsequent pregnancy is estimated to be increased up to threefold. A history of stillbirth is recognized as an indication for fetal monitoring. To date, there has been no adequate study to

BOX 94-1

Types of Tests for Stillbirth

Maternal testing
- Review of prenatal records and laboratory testing
- Hemoglobin (Hb) A_{1C} and fasting glucose
- Complete blood count with platelet count
- Antibody screen
- VDRL
- Kleihauer–Betke test
- Urine toxicology screen
- Thyroid function tests
- Antiphospholipid antibodies

Testing for selected cases
- Cytomegalovirus, toxoplasmosis, parvovirus, or other viral testing
- Listeria, other bacterial cultures
- Ultrasonography
- Inherited thrombophilia

Fetal testing
- Clinical examination
- Genetic analysis
- Amniotic fluid (best method), fetal blood, skin, or fascia lata or placenta
- Postmortem photographs
- Autopsy
- Placenta, umbilical cord, and membranes histopathology

Additional studies
- X-rays
- Magnetic resonance imaging

VDRL, Venereal Disease Research Laboratory testing.

determine the best time to start fetal testing in pregnancies with previous stillbirth. A retrospective cohort study suggested that fetal testing should be initiated in patients with a history of stillbirth as the only indication for testing at 32 weeks of gestation. The investigators noted that there was no intervention for abnormal tests in 300 women with previous stillbirth before 32 weeks of gestation. Additionally, they found no correlation with gestational age of the previous stillbirth, although that finding could possibly have resulted from ascertainment bias. Nevertheless, many clinicians arbitrarily choose to start fetal monitoring a few weeks before the gestational age of the previous stillbirth.

Routine fetal movement counting may reduce the occurrence of stillbirth. Decreased fetal movements have been associated with a higher risk of fetal distress in labor, growth restriction, and increased stillbirth risk. A biophysical profile or modified biophysical profile (nonstress test [NST] and amniotic fluid index [AFI]) can be used as a primary means of fetal testing. Failure to diagnose and adequately manage intrauterine growth restriction has been noted as the most common error of potentially preventable deaths. Ultrasonography should be considered to detect intrauterine growth restriction in high-risk groups. Doppler velocimetry has been accepted to be useful in the management of growth restriction.

Older women are at increased risk for unexplained stillbirths. A decision analysis study showed that a strategy of antepartum testing between 37 weeks and 41 weeks of gestation would reduce the number of unexplained stillbirths at term and would result in fewer labor inductions and cesarean deliveries per fetal death averted than a strategy of no antepartum testing but induction at 41 weeks of gestation.

Few data are available to guide the timing of delivery in patients with previous stillbirth. Data from a large population study not restricted to women with a prior stillbirth showed that the fetal death rate is lowest from 38 to 41 weeks of gestation. Most clinicians, however, will initiate delivery by 39–40 weeks of gestation in a patient with a previous stillbirth.

In selected cases, antiphospholipid antibodies and inherited thrombophilias have been associated with fetal demise. The most commonly used treatment is heparin and aspirin. However, in the absence of thrombophilia diagnosis, anticoagulant therapy has not been found to be beneficial and may cause harm such as bleeding or osteoporosis.

Carp H. Antiphospholipid syndrome in pregnancy. Curr Opin Obstet Gynecol 2004;16:129–35.

Fretts RC. Etiology and prevention of stillbirth. Am J Obstet Gynecol 2005;193:1923–35.

Fretts RC, Elkin EB, Myers ER, Heffner LJ. Should older women have antepartum testing to prevent unexplained stillbirth? Obstet Gynecol 2004;104:56–64.

Frias AE Jr, Luikenaar RA, Sullivan AE, Lee RM, Porter TF, Branch W, et al. Poor obstetrical outcome in subsequent pregnancies in women with prior fetal death. Obstet Gynecol 2004;104:521–6.

Michalski ST, Porter J, Pauli RM. Costs and consequences of comprehensive stillbirth assessment. Am J Obstet Gynecol 2002;186:1027–34.

Smulian JC, Ananth CV, Vintzileos AM, Scorza WE, Knuppel RA. Fetal deaths in the United States. Influence of high-risk conditions and implications for management. Obstet Gynecol 2002;100:1183–9.

Weeks JW, Asrat T, Morgan MA, Nageotte M, Thomas SJ, Freeman RK. Antepartum surveillance for a history of stillbirth: when to begin? Am J Obstet Gynecol 1995;172:486–92.

95

Vulvar hematoma

A 24-year-old woman, gravida 1, para 1, is postpartum following an uncomplicated delivery. You are called for severe perineal pain and vaginal bleeding. Examination reveals a 4-cm tense mass lateral to the labia that does not appear to be expanding. A diagnosis of a vulvar hematoma is made. The most appropriate initial management is

* (A) observation
  (B) a vaginal pack
  (C) needle aspiration
  (D) incision and evacuation of the hematoma
  (E) interventional radiologic embolization

Puerperal hematomas are a common complication and occur in approximately 1 in 500 vaginal deliveries. Puerperal hematomas can be located in the vulvar, vulvo-vaginal, paravaginal, and subperitoneal areas. Vulvar hematomas can be further divided into those in the anterior or posterior triangles of the perineum. This distinction is important because hematomas in the posterior triangle may dissect into the larger ischiorectal space, which can accumulate large amounts of blood quickly. The most common vessel involved in the formation of puerperal hematomas is the pudendal artery.

Several factors predispose a patient to vulvar hematomas, including blood dyscrasias, preeclampsia, instrument delivery, pudendal anesthesia, episiotomy, primiparity, breech presentation, and multifetal pregnancies. The most common presenting sign is severe perineal pain in the postpartum period. Commonly, women with vulvar hematomas receive additional analgesic medication without proper pelvic examination, which may result in delayed diagnosis. Hematomas often are diagnosed when a mass is discovered or if the woman has hemodynamic instability. The hematomas usually appear as a tense, discolored mass. Some women may experience rectal pain depending on the position and size of the hematoma.

Management of puerperal hematoma usually is based on the size of the hematoma and whether it is expanding. If a hematoma is less than 5 cm in size and not expanding, it should be observed and the mother given analgesia. The size of the hematoma should be measured, recorded, and marked to identify expansion on a subsequent examination. Frequent examinations, at least initially, should be performed. Ice packs can help to reduce edema and pain. If the hematoma is greater than 5 cm or expanding, surgical drainage should be considered.

Surgical drainage should be performed in the operating room with proper anesthesia provided by an anesthesiologist. Hemodynamic status should be monitored carefully because approximately 50% of women who have hema-

tomas that require drainage will require a transfusion. An indwelling catheter in the bladder will facilitate identification of proper anatomic landmarks and will help to monitor maternal volume status.

A 2–4-cm incision usually is made in the area with the greatest distension. However, if an incision can be easily made in the vagina that provides good visualization and space for evacuation, such an incision can be considered. An incision also helps reduce the risk of perineal scarring associated with spontaneous rupture. Once the hematoma is evacuated, the source of the bleeding should be identified, clamped, and ligated. Often no specific vessel can be isolated, but if generalized oozing is noted, placement of several figure-of-eight sutures can decrease such bleeding. Draining the space should be considered, especially if there is continued oozing uncontrolled with sutures. Vaginal packing may be of use especially in vulvovaginal hematomas. However, packing is not effective in vulvar hematomas.

Interventional radiologic procedures that interrupt the blood supply have been shown to be an effective method of treating these types of hematomas. The criteria are the same as that for surgical drainage. Although this can be a very effective treatment option, interventional radiology is not always available and the procedure still leaves a hematoma, which has the potential to become infected.

Benrubi G, Neuman C, Nuss RC, Thompson RJ. Vulvar and vaginal hematomas: a retrospective study of conservative versus operative management. South Med J 1987;80:991–4.

Hankins GDV. Puerperal hematomas and lower genital tract lacerations. In: Hankins GD, Clark SL, Cunningham FG, Gilstrap LC 3rd, editors. Operative obstetrics. Norwalk (CT): Appleton & Lange; 1995. p. 257–71.

Sheikh GN. Perinatal genital hematomas. Obstet Gynecol 1971;38:571–5.

Zahn CM, Hankins GD, Yeomans ER. Vulvovaginal hematomas complicating delivery. Rationale for drainage of the hematomas cavity. J Reprod Med 1996;41:569–74.

Zahn CM, Yeomans ER. Postpartum hemorrhage: placenta accreta, uterine inversion, and puerperal hematomas. Clin Obstet Gynecol 1990;33:422–31.

96

Screening for fetal Down syndrome in older women

A 37-year-old woman, gravida 1, para 0, at 10 weeks of gestation comes to your office to discuss her options regarding noninvasive screening tests for the detection of fetal Down syndrome. She would like to avoid a chorionic villus sampling (CVS) or an amniocentesis. You inform her that the noninvasive screening test for the detection of fetal Down syndrome with highest detection rate and lowest false-positive rate is

   (A) triple screen: alpha-fetoprotein (AFP) + total human chorionic gonadotropin (hCG) + unconjugated estriol
   (B) quadruple screen: AFP + total hCG + unconjugated estriol + inhibin A
   (C) nuchal translucency screen only
   (D) first-trimester combined screen: nuchal translucency + pregnancy-associated plasma protein A (PAPP-A) + free β-hCG
 * (E) integrated screen: nuchal translucency + PAPP-A + free β-hCG + AFP + total hCG + unconjugated estriol + inhibin A

All pregnant women, regardless of age, should be offered aneuploidy screening or diagnostic testing before 20 weeks of gestation. Some women are using this information to choose whether or not to undergo an invasive test (CVS or amniocentesis). In one study that assessed the rates of invasive testing in 1991–2002, the authors found that the rates of CVS and amniocentesis declined by approximately 50% with a statistically nonsignificant increase in the number of abnormal fetal karyotypes detected. They attributed the decrease in the rates of invasive testing to the fact that second-trimester serum screening and ultrasonography have substantially contributed to the more effective use of invasive testing.

When nuchal translucency screening alone is used, the detection rates of Down syndrome vary widely from 29% to 100%, with false-positive rates in the range of 0.3–11.6% and positive predictive values in the range of 1.6–50%. Therefore, in the absence of serum screening, nuchal translucency screening alone has low specificity and is not recommended for screening in singleton pregnancies.

The triple screen can detect approximately 75% of the cases of Down syndrome with a false-positive rate of 5% in women aged 35 years or older. In women younger than 35 years, the detection rate of the triple screen for Down syndrome is 60–75% with a false-positive rate of 5%. Using the quadruple test, one group of authors reported a 92% detection rate of Down syndrome with a 13% false-positive rate in women age 35 years or older. In contrast, for women younger than 35 years, the detection rate was 77% with a 2.3% false-positive rate.

Recently, two large U.S. multicenter studies have examined screening for Down syndrome. The First Trimester Maternal Serum Biochemistry and Ultrasound Fetal Nuchal Translucency Screening Study (BUN study) screened 8,514 women with a singleton pregnancy between days 74–97 (approximately 11–14 weeks) of gestation, using nuchal translucency screening combined with the first-trimester serum markers, PAPP-A, and free β-hCG. Among women aged 35 years and older, the detection rate for trisomy 21 was 89.9% with a false-positive rate of 15.2%, and for trisomy 18, the detection rate was 100%. In this population of women older than 35 years, first-trimester detection rates for Down syndrome were comparable to the reported rates using second-trimester serum markers.

The First and Second Trimester Evaluation of Risk (FASTER) study addressed how best to screen women for the presence of fetal Down syndrome during the first trimester, during the second trimester, or incorporating results from both trimesters. Screening was performed in 38,167 women with singleton pregnancies using first-trimester combined screening (ie, nuchal translucency, PAPP-A, and free β-hCG) between 10 3/7 weeks of gestation to 13 6/7 weeks of gestation, and quadruple screening (ie, AFP, total hCG, unconjugated estriol, and inhibin A) between 15 and 18 weeks of gestation. A subgroup analysis was performed in women younger than 35 years and women older than 35 years. The first-trimester combined screening detected 95% of the cases of Down syndrome with a 22% false-positive rate in women aged 35 years and older. However, when the results of the first-trimester screen were combined or integrated with the second-trimester results (ie, integrated screening), the detection rate for Down syndrome was 91% with a false-positive test result of 2% (Table 96-1).

TABLE 96-1. First-Trimester Detection of Down Syndrome Using Serum Markers

Study	Screening Test	Age Younger Than 35 Years		Age 35 Years or More	
		Detection Rate (%)	False-positive Rate (%)	Detection Rate (%)	False-positive Rate (%)
Wapner 2003*	First-trimester combined	78.7	5	89.8	15.2
Malone 2005†	First-trimester combined	75	5	95	22
	Integrated	77	0.4	91	2

*Wapner R, Thom E, Simpson JL, Pergament E, Silver R, Filkins K, et al. First-trimester screening for trisomies 21 and 18. First-Trimester Maternal Serum Biochemistry and Fetal Nuchal Translucency Screening (BUN) Study Group. N Engl J Med 2003;349:1405–13.

†Malone FD, Canick JA, Ball RH, Nyberg DA, Comstock CH, Bukowski R, et al. First-trimester or second-trimester screening, or both, for Down's syndrome. First- and Second-Trimester Evaluation of Risk (FASTER) Research Consortium. N Engl J Med 2005;353:2001–11.

A major advantage of the first-trimester combined screen is that the results become available early in pregnancy when CVS can be performed. If CVS is normal, safer and earlier termination of pregnancy is available. The major disadvantage of integrated screening is that in the group of patients with highest risk of Down syndrome, the results only become available after 15–18 weeks of gestation.

Sequential screening obviates some of the disadvantages of the integrated screen. When using sequential screening, the patients at highest risk for aneuploidy are informed about the first-trimester screening results and may opt for an early diagnostic procedure. Patients at lower risk can still take advantage of the higher detection rate achieved with additional second-trimester screening.

Screening for fetal chromosomal abnormalities. ACOG Practice Bulletin No. 77. American College of Obstetricians and Gynecologists. Obstet Gynecol 2007;109:217–27.

Benn PA, Egan JF, Fang M, Smith-Bindman R. Changes in the utilization of prenatal diagnosis. Obstet Gynecol 2004;103:1255–60.

Chasen ST, McCullough LB, Chervenak FA. Is nuchal translucency screening associated with different rates of invasive testing in an older obstetric population? Am J Obstet Gynecol 2004;190:769–74.

Malone FD, Canick JA, Ball RH, Nyberg DA, Comstock CH, Bukowski R, et al. First-trimester or second-trimester screening, or both, for Down's syndrome. First- and Second-Trimester Evaluation of Risk (FASTER) Research Consortium. N Engl J Med 2005;353:2001–11.

Malone FD, D'Alton ME. First-trimester sonographic screening for Down syndrome. Society for Maternal-Fetal Medicine. Obstet Gynecol 2003;102:1066–79.

Wapner R, Thom E, Simpson JL, Pergament E, Silver R, Filkins K, et al. First-trimester screening for trisomies 21 and 18. First-Trimester Maternal Serum Biochemistry and Fetal Nuchal Translucency Screening (BUN) Study Group. N Engl J Med 2003;349:1405–13.

97

Labor dystocia

A 22-year-old primigravid woman with a fetus estimated to weigh 3,400 g receives epidural anesthesia at 6 cm cervical dilation. An arrest of dilation ensues and is treated with oxytocin (Pitocin) augmentation. At full dilation, the fetal position is occiput posterior and the station is −1. Oxytocin is continued. The patient has uterine contractions that are firm by palpation, occur every 2 minutes, and last 1 minute in duration. She is pushing with every contraction. The fetal monitor tracing is reassuring. Three hours later, the presentation and station are unchanged, but caput and molding of the fetal head is at +2 station. The next step in management is

(A) instruct the patient to continue to push
(B) insert an intrauterine pressure catheter
(C) arrange for an operative vaginal delivery
* (D) arrange for a cesarean delivery

The graphic assessment of labor progress initially allowed various aberrations of dilation and descent to be diagnosed and studied retrospectively. Among the factors that influence progress in the second stage of labor are:

• The size and shape of the pelvis, which may be related to the mother's ethnicity and body habitus
• Neonatal birth weight
• Quality of uterine contractions: frequency; intensity; duration
• Maternal soft-tissue resistance
• Maternal effort
• Cephalic position and degree of flexion, caput, and molding

All of these factors may be clinically encapsulated into the end result of quality of contraction, descent, and rotation, which allows simplified assessment and resolution of abnormal labors.

Descent in the second stage of labor usually is accompanied by rotation of the presenting part as it negotiates the pelvis. Arrest of descent frequently is associated with fetal malpositions such as occiput posterior and occiput transverse positions. Numerous investigators have suggested that abnormalities of rotation from these positions are an important prognostic factor in the second stage. Studies have assessed the effects of such malpositions and absence of rotation on maternal and neonatal morbidity and found higher rates of cesarean delivery, higher estimated blood loss, and a higher incidence of third- or fourth-degree perineal tears.

In spite of these observations and the recognition of these risks, the optimal strategy of management for the second stage of labor that would allow the greatest probability of safe delivery with the least risk of maternal and neonatal morbidity is not well clarified.

A study to evaluate progress in the second stage of labor and subsequent uncomplicated vaginal delivery reported

that a station 1+ or higher at the beginning of the second stage predicted a spontaneous vaginal delivery rate of only 36.7%. Malposition coupled with a high station was predictive of longer time spent in the second stage. In the case described, the fetus is in a persistent occiput posterior position, the labor curve documents an arrest of descent in the face of oxytocin administration and an adequate quality of uterine contractions by clinical evaluation. This situation is unlikely to result in a successful and atraumatic vaginal delivery in any reasonable amount of time. Continued pushing would therefore be inadvisable. Nor is it likely that more precise measurement of uterine contraction force would provide truly more relevant information than clinical assessment by physical examination. Insertion of the intrauterine pressure catheter is therefore not necessary.

Some intervention needs to occur to deliver this fetus. It would not be appropriate, however, to confuse station of the bony presenting part with depth of caput to influence the decision for the next step in management. In this patient, the station is too high for an instrumental delivery. Cesarean delivery is the next appropriate step in management.

Bofill JA, Rust OA, Perry KG, Roberts WE, Martin RW, Morrison JC. Operative vaginal delivery: a survey of fellows of ACOG. Obstet Gynecol 1996;88:1007–10.

Plunkett BA, Lin A, Wong CA, Grobman WA, Peaceman AM. Management of the second stage of labor in nulliparas with continuous epidural analgesia. Obstet Gynecol 2003;102:109–14.

Ponkey SE, Cohen AP, Heffner LJ, Lieberman E. Persistent fetal occiput posterior position: obstetric outcomes. Obstet Gynecol 2003; 101:915–20.

Senecal J, Xiong X, Fraser WD. Effect of fetal position on second-stage duration and labor outcome. Pushing Early Or Pushing Late with Epidural study group. Obstet Gynecol 2005;105:763–72.

Sizer AR, Evans J, Bailey SM, Wiener J. A second-stage partogram. Obstet Gynecol 2000;96:678–83.

Yancey MK, Pierce B, Schweitzer D, Daniels D. Observations on labor epidural analgesia and operative delivery rates. Am J Obstet Gynecol 1999;180:353–9.

98

Forceps- versus vacuum-assisted delivery

A 40-year-old primigravid woman has been pushing adequately in the second stage for 3 hours. The vertex is at +3/+5 station, in a direct occiput anterior position. The fetus is estimated to weigh 3,629 g (8 lb) and the pelvis is estimated to be adequate. The woman is exhausted and accepts operative vaginal delivery. In counseling her regarding complications of forceps or vacuum, you advise her that, compared to vacuum-assisted delivery, forceps delivery is associated with a higher incidence of

* * (A) maternal perineal lacerations
  (B) neonatal retinal hemorrhages
  (C) shoulder dystocia
  (D) postpartum hemorrhage
  (E) cephalohematoma

Rates of operative vaginal deliveries have been decreasing since 1996. The 2002 rate for delivery by forceps or vacuum extraction was 5.9% compared with the 1994 rate of 9.5%. Vacuum-assisted delivery accounted for 68% of all operative deliveries in 2000, an increase of 41% since 1990.

Vacuum and forceps are the two approaches for assisted or operative vaginal delivery. The indications for either approach are the same and include inefficient maternal effort (eg, exhaustion or underlying medical condition precluding pushing) and nonreassuring fetal heart rate tracing. Prolonged second stage, defined as 2 or more hours without regional anesthesia or 3 or more hours with regional anesthesia in nulliparous women, and 1 or more hours without regional anesthesia or 2 or more hours with regional anesthesia in multiparous women, is another criterion used for offering operative delivery.

No indication for operative vaginal delivery is absolute. Alternatives, including allowing the patient to labor longer, oxytocin augmentation, and cesarean delivery should always be considered.

When used by experienced operators, operative vaginal delivery is safe for both mother and baby and effective in obtaining vaginal delivery, with forceps having slightly higher success rates.

Complication rates differ between vacuum and forceps, with neonatal injuries more common with vacuum-assisted delivery and maternal perineal or vaginal injuries more common with forceps-assisted delivery. The incidences of retinal hemorrhages and hyperbilirubinemia are significantly higher with vacuum extraction than with forceps delivery. Failed vaginal delivery, as well as shoulder dys-

tocia and postpartum hemorrhage, also is significantly more common with vacuum extraction, based on randomized trial results.

The choice of instrument is decided after appropriate counseling, and it depends also on operator experience. Insufficient evidence exists to compare different types of forceps. Soft vacuum cups fail to attain vaginal delivery more often than rigid cups but have a lower rate of significant scalp trauma. Rigid cups may be better for occiput posterior and other more difficult deliveries, and soft cups may be better suited for less complicated, routine deliveries.

If vacuum application is attempted, discontinuation should be considered if the vacuum cup pops off the fetal head three times. Attempts to use a different extraction instrument after failing with one should be avoided, as cephalopelvic disproportion may be present, and the incidence of neonatal intracranial hemorrhage, as well as other neonatal injuries, is highest among infants delivered using forceps and vacuum extraction sequentially.

Johanson R, Menon V. Soft versus rigid vacuum extractor cups for assisted vaginal delivery. Cochrane Database of Systematic Reviews 2000, Issue 2. Art. No.: CD000446. DOI: 10.1002/14651858. CD000446.

Johanson RB, Menon V. Vacuum extraction versus forceps for assisted vaginal delivery. Cochrane Database of Systematic Reviews 1999, Issue 2. Art. No.: CD000224. DOI: 10.1002/14651858.CD000224.

Towner D, Castro MA, Eby-Wilkens E, Gilbert WM. Effect of mode of delivery in nulliparous women on neonatal intracranial injury. N Engl J Med 1999;341:1709–14.

Williams MC, Knuppel RA, O'Brien WF, Weiss A, Kanarek KS. A randomized comparison of assisted vaginal delivery by obstetric forceps and polyethylene vacuum cup. Obstet Gynecol 1991;78:789–94.

99

Intraamniotic infection

A 23-year-old woman, gravida 2, with a history of good prenatal care is in preterm labor at 25 weeks of gestation. Her cervix is 2 cm dilated and 80% effaced. She is having regular uterine contractions, and the fetus is in vertex presentation. She has a temperature of 38°C (100.4°F) and a suggestion of fundal tenderness on abdominal palpation. Amniocentesis results show glucose 25 mg/dL, few white blood cells, and no bacteria on Gram stain. Besides a rapid test for group B streptococci, the best next step in management is to

(A) perform a cesarean delivery
(B) induce labor
* (C) administer tocolytic therapy and corticosteroids
(D) administer antibiotics

In the described scenario, despite the maternal fever and presentation with preterm labor, the amniocentesis results are reassuring and do not indicate intraamniotic infection as an etiology of preterm labor. Thus, it would be reasonable to proceed with tocolysis and steroids after a thorough evaluation for other sources of infection.

Intraamniotic infection is associated with preterm labor, preterm premature rupture of membranes, and preterm birth. An inverse relationship exists between the gestational age at preterm labor and the risk of intraamniotic infection. The rate of infection has been estimated to be as high as 10–20% in women who present in preterm labor.

Signs and symptoms of intraamniotic infection that should be assessed in women who are in preterm labor include fever, fundal tenderness, leukocytosis, and fetal tachycardia. None of these signs or symptoms alone is sufficiently sensitive and specific to guide clinical management. Thus, if clinical suspicion for intraamniotic infection in a woman with preterm labor is high, consideration should be given to direct assessment of amniotic fluid for infection using amniocentesis.

The criterion standard for the diagnosis of intraamniotic infection is a positive amniotic fluid culture. However, because culture results may not be available for 24–48 hours, clinical decisions must be made using rapid tests such as amniotic fluid glucose levels and Gram stain. The presence of bacteria on Gram stain is strongly correlated with culture results and therefore can be used alone for clinical management of suspected intraamniotic infection.

Amniotic fluid glucose levels are reported as a continuous variable. The cutoff for a normal amniotic fluid glucose is above 10–20 mcg/mL. Amniotic fluid glucose tests are less well correlated with culture results, with a false-positive rate of almost 10% (Table 99-1). Thus, amniotic fluid glucose levels should seldom be used in isolation in clinical decision making. Interleukin-6 levels in amniotic fluid have been tested as a marker for intraamniotic infection. Despite high sensitivity, testing of interleukin-6 levels in amniotic fluid is not widely available for clinical use.

Delivery is not indicated because the amniocentesis results are normal. No role exists for antibiotics and expectant management in cases with confirmed intraamniotic infection; antibiotics in the setting of preterm labor should be reserved for group B streptococcal prophylaxis or chorioamnionitis.

If the Gram stain result had been positive for bacteria, there would be no role for tocolysis. Intraamniotic infection is not a contraindication to labor induction or vaginal delivery.

Hussey MJ, Levy ES, Pombar X, Meyer P, Strassner HT. Evaluating rapid diagnostic tests of intra-amniotic infection: Gram stain, amniotic fluid glucose level, and amniotic fluid to serum glucose level ratio. Am J Obstet Gynecol 1998;179:650–6.

Management of preterm labor. ACOG Practice Bulletin No. 43. American College of Obstetricians and Gynecologists. Obstet Gynecol 2003;101:1039–47.

Romero R, Sibai B, Caritis S, Paul R, Depp R, Rosen M, et al. Antibiotic treatment of preterm labor with intact membranes: a multicenter, randomized double-blinded, placebo controlled trial. Am J Obstet Gynecol 1993;169:764–74.

TABLE 98-1. Diagnostic Indexes of Amniotic Fluid Tests in Detection of Positive Amniotic Fluid Culture in Patients With Preterm Labor and Intact Membranes

Test	Sensitivity	Specificity	Positive Predictive Value	Negative Predictive Value
Gram stain	7/11 (63.6%)	108/109 (99.1%)	7/8 (87.5%)	108/112 (96.4%)
IL-6 (greater than 11.30 ng/mL)	11/11 (100%)	90/109 (82.6%)	11/30 (36.7%)	90/90 (100%)
White blood cell count (greater than 50 cells/mm^3)	7/11 (63.6%)	103/109 (94.5%)	7/13 (53.9%)	103/107 (96.3%)
Glucose (less than 14 mg/dL)	9/11 (81.8%)	89/109 (81.7%)	9/29 (31.0%)	89/91 (97.8%)
Gram stain plus white blood cell count (greater than 50 cells/mm^3)	10/11 (90.9%)	102/109 (93.6%)	10/17 (58.8%)	102/103 (99.0%)
Gram stain plus glucose (less than 14 mg/dL)	10/11 (90.9%)	88/109 (80.7%)	10/31 (32.3%)	88/89 (98.9%)
Gram stain plus IL-6 (greater than 11.30 ng/mL)	11/11 (100%)	89/109 (81.7%)	11/31 (35.5%)	89/89 (100%)
Gram stain plus glucose (less than 14 mg/dL) plus white blood cell count (greater than 50 cells/mm^3)	10/11 (90.9%)	85/109 (78.0%)	10/34 (29.4%)	85/86 (98.8%)
Gram stain plus white blood cell count (greater than 50 cells/mm^3) plus IL-6 (greater than 11.30 ng/mL)	11/11 (100%)	87/109 (79.8%)	11/33 (33.3%)	87/87 (100%)
Gram stain plus glucose (less than 14 mg/dL) plus IL-6 (greater than 11.30 ng/mL)	11/11 (100%)	78/109 (71.6%)	11/42 (26.2%)	78/78 (100%)
Gram stain plus white blood cell count (greater than 50 cells/mm^3) plus IL-6 (greater than 11.30 ng/mL) plus glucose (less than 14 mg/dL)	11/11 (100%)	76/109 (69.7%)	11/44 (25.0%)	76/76 (100%)

IL-6, interleukin-6.

Romero R, Yoon BH, Mazor M, Gomez R, Diamond MP, Kenney JS, et al. The diagnostic and prognostic value of amniotic fluid white blood cell count, glucose, interleukin-6, and gram stain in patients with preterm labor and intact membranes. Am J Obstet Gynecol 1993;169:812. Copyright 1993 by Elsevier.

100
Preterm birth

An 18-year-old woman, gravida 3, para 0, presents at 35 weeks of gestation with abdominal cramping. Monitoring reveals that her uterus is contracting every 3 minutes, with reassuring fetal testing. Physical examination reveals that her cervix is 2 cm dilated, 80% effaced, and the fetal presentation is vertex at –2 station. One hour later, her cervix is 3 cm dilated, 90% effaced, with no further descent of the fetus. Her group B streptococci (GBS) status is unknown. The most appropriate management is

        (A) steroids for fetal maturity
        (B) tocolysis
*   (C) GBS prophylaxis
        (D) artificial rupture of membranes

Preterm labor leading to preterm birth occurs in approximately 6% of pregnancies in the United States, and accounts for 50% of cases of preterm births. Preterm labor usually is defined by the presence of uterine contractions (four or more in 20 minutes, or eight or more in 1 hour) and documented cervical change with intact membranes or advanced cervical dilation at 20–36 6/7 weeks of gestation. The neonatal morbidity and mortality associated with preterm birth occurs mostly in women who deliver before 34 weeks of gestation, especially before 32 weeks. At 34 weeks of gestation and beyond, the neonate has less than 1% risk of death, and less than 1% risk of intraventricular hemorrhage or of necrotizing enterocolitis.

Given the very low incidence of neonatal mortality and morbidity, efforts to prevent preterm birth are not justified for the care of women with preterm labor or preterm premature rupture of membranes at 35 weeks of gestation. The only morbidity or outcome significantly more common at 35 weeks that at 37 or more weeks of gestation is hypothermia. Tocolysis can be associated with significant morbidity and mortality and usually is not indicated later than 34 weeks. Contraindications to tocolysis also include:

• Maternal chorioamnionitis

• Severe vaginal bleeding or abruptio placentae

• Preeclampsia

• Medical contraindications to specific tocolytic agents

• Other maternal medical conditions that make continuing the pregnancy inadvisable

• Fetal death

• Lethal fetal anomaly or chromosome abnormality

• Other fetal conditions in which prolongation of pregnancy is inadvisable

• Documented fetal maturity

Betamethasone valerate and dexamethasone are the only two corticosteroids that reliably cross the placenta. The proposed mechanism of action for these drugs is that they enhance changes in lung architecture and induction of lung enzymes resulting in biochemical maturation. The benefits of decreased neonatal mortality and morbidity apply to gestational ages of 24–33 6/7 weeks.

Asymptomatic GBS colonization in the mother is associated with an incidence of neonatal GBS disease of approximately 1–2% without intervention. Early or late onset of neonatal disease may occur, with such possible complications as sepsis, pneumonia, and meningitis. Less frequently, focal infections or death can occur. Major risk factors for neonatal GBS sepsis are prolonged rupture of membranes (18 or more hours), preterm delivery, and maternal temperature 38.0°C (100.4°F) or higher. Given the imminent preterm delivery at 35 weeks of gestation, with unknown status, GBS prophylaxis is indicated in this patient. Universal prenatal maternal screening and intrapartum antibiotic treatment are the most efficacious of the current strategies for prevention of early-onset disease, and 50% more effective than a risk-factor-based strategy. There is no prevention of late-onset GBS sepsis. Screening involves collecting an anovaginal specimen at 35–37 weeks (labeled "penicillin allergy" if appropriate). Women who are GBS positive are treated with penicillin in labor. Ampicillin is a reasonable alternative. If the patient is allergic to penicillin, but not at high risk for anaphylaxis, cefazolin sodium (Ancef, Kefzol) is the agent of choice. When chorioamnionitis is diagnosed, intrapartum treatment is recommended regardless of GBS maternal status.

Routine early amniotomy is associated with a significant reduction in labor duration of approximately 53 minutes, primarily due to a shorter first stage, and with a decrease in the use of oxytocin, and upwards of a 25%

increase in the risk of cesarean delivery. Early amniotomy is not associated with an increase or decrease in nonreassuring fetal heart testing overall, but there was such association in one large trial. There is no evidence that use of amniotomy has any effect on the mother's satisfaction with labor. The data suggest that early amniotomy should not be routinely used in women in normal labor. It can possibly be reserved for women with slow labor progress.

Roberts D, Dalziel S. Antenatal corticosteroids for accelerating fetal lung maturation for women at risk of preterm birth. Cochrane Database of Systematic Reviews 2006, Issue 3. Art. No.: CD004454. DOI: 10.1002/14651858.CD004454.pub2.

Schrag S, Gorwitz R, Fultz-Butts K, Schuchat A. Prevention of perinatal group B streptococcal disease. Revised guidelines from CDC. MMWR Recomm Rep 2002;51(RR-11):1–22.

Seubert DE, Stetzer BP, Wolfe HM, Treadwell MC. Delivery of the marginally preterm infant: what are the minor morbidities? Am J Obstet Gynecol 1999;181:1087–91.

101

Multiple sclerosis

A 32-year-old woman, gravida 2, para 2, with known relapsing multiple sclerosis for 4 years, was treated with natalizumab (Tysabri) 1 year before her pregnancy and high-dose prednisone during the antenatal period to reduce the incidence of relapses. Acute stress corticosteroids and epidural analgesia were administered. On postpartum day 4, she reported gait instability, bladder incontinence, fatigue, and double vision. Her vital signs were normal and her laboratory evaluation revealed normal electrolytes and a normal complete blood count. The most likely diagnosis is

  (A) epidural toxicity
  (B) postpartum psychosis
  (C) natalizumab-induced progressive multifocal leukoencephalopathy
* (D) multiple sclerosis flare
  (E) adrenal insufficiency

Multiple sclerosis often strikes women during their childbearing years, and the effect of pregnancy on the disease is poorly understood. For patients who present a constellation of neurologic symptoms subsequent to delivery, medical history and recent intrapartum and delivery interventions may result in confounding elements that may confuse the evaluation.

Controversy and concern continue to surround the role of regional analgesia and the precipitation of postpartum exacerbations of multiple sclerosis. There are no modern data to support such concerns. Epidural analgesia has been used successfully in patients with multiple sclerosis, and no association between epidural analgesia and relapse-rate has been noted.

Postpartum psychosis represents a psychiatric emergency that requires immediate intervention because of the risk of infanticide and suicide. Onset usually occurs within the first 2 weeks after giving birth. This disorder differs from other psychotic episodes because it usually involves extreme disorganization of thought; bizarre behavior; unusual hallucinations, which may be visual, olfactory, or tactile; and delusions, all of which suggest an organic cause. Positive responses to the following questions necessitate psychiatric referral:

- "Have you ever had 4 continuous days when you were feeling so excited that other people thought you were not your normal self or you got into trouble?"

  or

- "Have you experienced 4 continuous days when you were so irritable that you found yourself shouting at people or starting fights or arguments?"

The signs and physical symptoms presented by this patient are not those of psychosis.

Progressive multifocal leukoencephalopathy is a demyelinating disease of the central nervous system that is encountered most frequently in the setting of immunodeficiency. The disease is caused by the human polyomavirus, Jakob-Creutzfeldt virus, a common and widespread infection in humans. The disease has been reported in a very few patients who received natalizumab (Tysabri), a recombinant antibody directed to the α_4 integrins. Natalizumab was recently approved by the U.S. Food and Drug Administration for the treatment of relapsing forms of multiple sclerosis. More than 3,000 patients received natalizumab while participating in clinical trials. Of these, 44 patients were referred to the expert panel because of clinical findings of possible progressive multifocal leukoencephalopathy; it was ruled out in 43 of the 44 patients, but it could not be ruled out in one patient. Therefore, although deterioration of neurologic signs might make a clinician suspicious of this complication, it is unlikely that remote exposure to natalizumab, as described in the previous case, would relate to the current signs and symptoms.

Multiple sclerosis flares are common in the postpartum interval. In a study of 254 women during 269 pregnancies complicated with multiple sclerosis, followed during their pregnancies and for up to 12 months after delivery, the relapse rate in each trimester was compared with the rate during the year before the pregnancy. The effects of epidural analgesia and breastfeeding on the frequency of relapse during the first 3 months postpartum and at 12 months postpartum also were determined. The mean (plus or minus standard deviation) rate of relapse declined during pregnancy. It was 0.7 plus or minus 0.9 per woman per year in the year before pregnancy; 0.5 plus or minus 1.3 during the first trimester ($P = .03$), 0.6 plus or minus 1.6 during the second trimester ($P = .17$), and 0.2 plus or minus 1.0 during the third ($P < .001$). This decline was followed by an increase to 1.2 plus or minus 2.0 during the first 3 months postpartum ($P < .001$) and then the relapse rate returned to the prepregnancy rate. Neither breastfeeding nor epidural analgesia had an adverse effect on the rate of relapse or on the progression of disability in multiple sclerosis. A multiple sclerosis flare is the most likely diagnosis in the described patient.

Adrenal insufficiency is a rare complication of pregnancy characterized by hypotension and hyponatremia. Additional abnormalities, such as hyperkalemia, hypoglycemia, acidosis, and hypercalcemia (rare), encountered in some patients with adrenal insufficiency, can lead to the diagnosis or rule it out. There is no laboratory indication of adrenal insufficiency in this patient.

Confavreux C, Hutchinson M, Hours MM, Cortinovis-Tourniaire P, Moreau T. Rate of pregnancy-related relapse in multiple sclerosis. Pregnancy in Multiple Sclerosis Group. N Engl J Med 1998;339: 285–91.

Ferrero S, Pretta S, Ragni N. Multiple sclerosis: management issues during pregnancy. Eur J Obstet Gynecol Rep Bio 2004;115:3–9.

Oelkers W. Adrenal insufficiency. N Engl J Med 1996;335:1206–12.

Wisner KL, Parry BL, Pointex CK. Clinical practice. Postpartum depression. N Engl J Med 2002;347:194–9.

Yousry TA, Major EO, Ryschkewitsch C, Fahle G, Fischer S, Hou J, et al. Evaluation of patients treated with natalizumab for progressive multifocal leukoencephalopathy. N Engl J Med 2006;354:924–33.

102

Congenital malformations caused by isotretinoin

A 28-year-old woman has been taking isotretinoin (Accutane) for nodular acne for the past year. She was using oral contraceptives (OCs) and condoms for contraception. She recently got married and stopped taking OCs. She accidentally conceived while using a condom. The risks to the fetus include

* (A) craniofacial malformations
* (B) abdominal wall defects
* (C) genitourinary malformation
* (D) neural tube defects
* (E) limb reduction defects

Isotretinoin is a metabolite of vitamin A and is used to treat severe, recalcitrant, nodular acne. Isotretinoin ingestion during pregnancy causes significant teratogenesis. Characteristic malformations caused by inadvertent exposure to isotretinoin during pregnancy include craniofacial, cardiac, thymic, and central nervous system (CNS) malformations, as well as mental retardation. Box 102-1 shows the most common specific malformations caused by isotretinoin.

Because of the significant teratogenic effect of isotretinoin, the American Academy of Dermatology recommends an initial negative pregnancy test result with the initiation of two separate effective forms of contraception before initiating isotretinoin. After 1 month of two forms of contraception, another pregnancy test is performed on the second day of the next menstrual cycle. With the assurance of two negative pregnancy tests and two forms of contraception, a 1-month supply of isotretinoin is given. Concurrently, information regarding emergency contraception is provided. Women on isotretinoin who wish to conceive need to discontinue the medication for at least 1 month before having unprotected intercourse.

Isotretinoin is a derivative of vitamin A. Preformed vitamin A in the diet comes from dairy products, liver, and fortified foods. Ingestion of greater than 10,000 international units of preformed vitamin A also can be teratogenic with an increase in cranial neural crest defects. As a result, the maximum daily allowance of vitamin A in pregnancy is 3,000 international units. Beta carotene and other carotenoids are plant-synthesized precursors and are converted to retinol during or after absorption. Beta carotene is not associated with an increased risk of congenital malformation. Topical tretinoin has not been shown to be associated with congenital malformations.

Omphalocele is not caused by medication ingestion during organogenesis, although gastroschisis has been associated with vasoactive medication exposure in the first trimester. Neural tube defects have been associated with antiepileptic medications, especially valproic acid but not isotretinoin. Genitourinary malformations have not been associated with isotretinoin, but second-trimester exposure to an angiotensin-converting enzyme (ACE) inhibitor can cause fetal renal failure. Limb reduction defects are not associated with the use of isotretinoin. However, chorionic villus sampling before 10 weeks of gestation has been shown to be associated with limb reduction defects. Cardiac malformations have been associated with antiepileptic medications and lithium ingestion in the first trimester. A recent study has linked first-trimester exposure to ACE inhibitors with cardiac malformations. In addition to isotretinoin and high-dose vitamin A, warfarin therapy in the first trimester is associated with nasal hypoplasia and ophthalmologic abnormalities.

Cooper WO, Hernandez-Diaz S, Arbogast PG, Dudley JA, Dyer S, Gideon PS, et al. Major congenital malformations after first-trimester exposure to ACE inhibitors. N Engl J Med 2006;354:2443–51.

Goldsmith LA, Bolognia JL, Callen JP, Chen SC, Feldman SR, Lim HW, et al. American Academy of Dermatology Consensus Conference on the safe and optimal use of isotretinoin: summary and recommenda-

---

BOX 102-1

Common Malformations Caused by Isotretinoin (Accutane)

* Microtia or anotia
* Micrognathia
* Cleft palate
* Facial dysmorphy
* Heart defects
* Thymic hypoplasia
* Microcephaly
* Hydrocephaly
* Retina and optic nerve abnormalities

tions. American Academy of Dermatology [published erratum appears in J Am Acad Dermatol 2004;51:348. dosage error in text]. J Am Acad Dermatol 2004;50:900–6.

Mills JL, Simpson JL. Cunningham GC, Conley MR, Rhoads GC. Vitamin A and birth defects. Am J Obstet Gynecol 1997;177:31–6.

Nau H. Teratogenicity of isotretinoin revisited: species variation and the role of all-trans-retinoic acid. J Am Acad Dermatol 2001;45:S183–7.

Rothman KJ, Moore LL, Singer MR, Nguyen US, Mannino S, Milunsky A. Teratogenicity of high vitamin A intake. N Engl J Med 1995;333:1369–73.

103

Fetal death

A 28-year-old woman, gravida 2, para 1, comes to your office at 20 weeks of gestation with a report of spotting. She has not felt fetal movement. Her previous pregnancy was normal, except that she had a low transverse caesarean delivery for failure to progress. On evaluation, you are unable to find fetal heart tones. You send her for an ultrasonographic examination, which confirms an intrauterine fetal demise. Fetal biometry is consistent with 20 weeks of gestation. You counsel the patient about these findings and, because the cause of the demise is unknown, you suggest, and the patient agrees, that an autopsy would be desirable. When she asks about her options for terminating the pregnancy, you tell her that her best option is

    (A) to await spontaneous labor
    (B) intravaginal dinoprostone suppository
*   (C) misoprostol induction of labor
    (D) hysterotomy
    (E) induction of labor with oxytocin (Pitocin)

A second-trimester termination of pregnancy may be performed either surgically or medically. Surgical approaches include hysterotomy and dilation and evacuation.

Hysterotomy is a major abdominal surgical procedure that leaves a classical scar on the uterus, which requires a cesarean delivery in future pregnancies. Hysterotomy is associated with the highest rates of adverse outcomes, such as need for blood transfusion, longer hospitalization, and infection.

Dilation and evacuation (D&E) is widely considered the safest route for a second-trimester termination in patients with an unscarred uterus. Studies have shown only slightly higher risks in patients with a previous cesarean delivery than in those with an unscarred uterus. No studies have compared D&E to induction of labor in patients with previous cesarean deliveries. In patients who desire an autopsy, D&E has been considered a relative contraindication to the procedure because it may make the autopsy difficult to perform. In addition, D&E is operator dependent and may not be available in all hospitals in the country.

Medical treatment of a second-trimester intrauterine fetal demise consists of induction of labor or expectant management. In general, expectant management will result in an increased complication rate, including infection, patient dissatisfaction, and prolonged diagnosis to delivery time. Delay also may interfere with interpretation of autopsy findings.

Induction of labor has been attempted with oxytocin alone or after intraamniotic infusion of hypertonic saline or urea, before the widespread availability of prostaglandins. Oxytocin alone is the least effective option.

Prostaglandins were first infused intraamniotically, but more recently are given vaginally or orally in much higher doses than with full-term cervical ripening or labor induction. The effectiveness of these medications is clear, but safety in patients with a prior cesarean delivery is less well studied. A few small case series exist, none of which are randomized. Unlike in the third trimester, there is no apparent increase in uterine rupture in any of the induction of labor methods, including misoprostol, mifepristone, and oxytocin. Although most studies are underpowered, the reported rate of rupture is less than 1%. This rate compares with a rate of uterine rupture with an unscarred uterus of less than 0.5%. In general, this is similar to the rate of complications from D&E. For this patient, complications of D&E and induction of labor with misoprostol are similar with a better chance for autopsy with an induction of labor. Dinoprostone is associated with a much higher rate of unpleasant side effects than misoprostol, including diarrhea and pyrexia, and its use has been largely discontinued.

Autry AM, Hayes EC, Jacobson GF, Kirby RS. A comparison of medical induction and dilation and evacuation for second-trimester abortion. Am J Obstet Gynecol 2002;187:393–7.

Chasen ST, Kalish RB, Gupta M, Kaufman J, Chervenak FA. Obstetric outcomes after surgical abortion at 20 weeks' gestation. Am J Obstet Gynecol 2005;193:1161–4.

Dickinson JE. Misoprostol for second-trimester pregnancy termination in women with a prior cesarean delivery. Obstet Gynecol 2005;105: 352–6.

Scioscia M, Pontrelli G, Vimercati A, Santamato S, Selvaggi L. A short-scheme protocol of gemeprost for midtrimester termination of pregnancy with uterine scar. Contraception 2005;71:193–6.

104

Cervical insufficiency

A 34-year-old woman, gravida 6, reports two prior first-trimester elective terminations, followed by two spontaneous preterm births at 34 and 26 weeks of gestation, and most recently a 22-week pregnancy loss. For the last two deliveries, she presented with painless, advanced dilation, with no palpable contractions. The diagnosis that is most consistent with her medical history is

      (A) uterine anomaly

      (B) preterm labor

      (C) chronic uterine infection

*   (D) cervical insufficiency

      (E) recurrent sexually transmitted disease

Preterm birth can occur spontaneously, following preterm labor (50%) or preterm premature rupture of membranes (preterm PROM) (30%), or it can occur as a result of maternal or fetal factors (20%). Preterm birth is defined as birth between 20 weeks and 36 6/7 weeks of gestation. Cervical insufficiency, previously called cervical incompetence, usually is defined as painless cervical dilation leading to recurrent second-trimester pregnancy losses. Cervical insufficiency may comprise about 1% of spontaneous preterm births. Cervical insufficiency represents one extreme of spontaneous preterm birth.

The risk factors for spontaneous preterm birth preceded by preterm labor and preterm PROM are similar, but the particular risk factors for cervical insufficiency are multiple induced abortions, other surgery to the cervix (eg, multiple dilation and curettage procedures, cone biopsies), with only a very small minority not associated with a risk factor. The scenario that the described patient has had multiple preterm births and second-trimester pregnancy losses, two with painless dilation, is consistent with a diagnosis of cervical insufficiency.

Uterine anomalies are associated with increased risks of pregnancy loss and preterm birth. The diagnosis of uterine anomaly cannot be based on history alone, but necessitates a uterine study. Sonohysterography, hysterosalpingography, magnetic resonance imaging (MRI), and hysteroscopy, with or without laparoscopy, are modalities used to diagnose uterine anomalies. Given the clinical situation described, uterine anomaly cannot be assumed to be present without a diagnostic study. This woman with

multiple prior preterm births should have such a study before attempting another pregnancy. Recurrent preterm birth can be prevented by resection of a uterine septum.

Preterm labor is defined by the presence of contractions and cervical change. The last two deliveries of this patient were characterized by painless dilation. Because the patient has a history of painless cervical dilation leading to recurrent second-trimester pregnancy losses, with no record of contractions being palpable, this clinical scenario is most consistent with cervical insufficiency, not preterm labor. No study has been published that demonstrates diagnosis of cervical insufficiency between pregnancies.

Uterine infection is associated with preterm birth, and the earlier the preterm birth, the higher the association with uterine infection. Uterine infection cannot be diagnosed by history alone. Some physicians have postulated that a chronic uterine infection can be treated after a preterm birth, in the interval between pregnancies, to prevent a future preterm birth. In women with a prior spontaneous preterm birth before 34 weeks of gestation, administration of oral azithromycin and metronidazole every 4 months after the preterm birth and before the next conception does not significantly reduce subsequent preterm birth. This antibiotic therapy is in fact associated with trends for earlier gestational age at delivery and lower birth weight. Given the lack of proven benefit of therapy, routine screening for chronic infection in women with prior preterm birth may not be justified.

Sexually transmitted diseases (STDs), including gonorrhea, chlamydia, syphilis, and trichomonas, have been associated with preterm birth. A history of recurrent preterm births cannot be assumed to be due to STDs, but needs to be confirmed by specific diagnostic tests. For chlamydia and gonorrhea, prevention strategies shown to be effective include condoms, screening to identify asymptomatic cases in high-risk populations, early diagnosis, treatment, and partner notification and treatment. Treatment of some STDs may not reduce the incidence of preterm birth. For example, metronidazole does not prevent preterm birth in asymptomatic women with *Trichomonas vaginalis* infection. In fact, in this population, metronidazole is associated with 78% higher incidence of preterm birth before 37 weeks of gestation, and similar incidences of preterm birth before 32 weeks of gestation and perinatal mortality. Even in women with a prior preterm birth, metronidazole is associated with an 84% higher risk of preterm birth. Metronidazole does eradicate *T vaginalis* in greater than 90% of pregnant women with this infection. Therefore, at least for the purpose of decreasing preterm birth, asymptomatic women, even with high-risk factors for preterm birth, should not be screened for *T vaginalis* and treated with metronidazole if their test results are positive for this infection. Symptomatic women with *T vaginalis* should still be adequately treated.

Andrews WW, Goldenberg RL, Hauth JC, Cliver SP, Copper R, Conner M. Interconceptional antibiotics to prevent spontaneous preterm birth: a randomized clinical trial. Am J Obstet Gynecol 2006;194:617–23.

Cervical insufficiency. ACOG Practice Bulletin No. 48. The American College of Obstetricians and Gynecologists. Obstet Gynecol 2003;102:1091–9.

Henriet L, Kaminski M. Impact of induced abortions on subsequent pregnancy outcome: the 1995 French national perinatal survey. BJOG 2001;108:1036–42.

Klebanoff MA, Carey JC, Hauth JC, Hillier SL, Nugent RP, Thom EA, et al. Failure of metronidazole to prevent preterm delivery among pregnant women with asymptomatic Trichomonas vaginalis infection. National Institute of Child Health and Human Development Maternal-Fetal Medicine Units Network. N Engl J Med 2001;345:487–93.

105

Preterm premature rupture of membranes

A 26-year-old woman, gravida 4, at 28 6/7 weeks of gestation, presents with leakage of amniotic fluid. A diagnosis of preterm premature rupture of membranes (preterm PROM) is made based on a positive nitrazine test result, ferning, pooling of fluid in the vagina, and pH greater than 4.5. The most effective management to decrease neonatal morbidity and mortality is

      (A) immediate delivery
*   (B) intramuscular betamethasone
      (C) periodic fetal testing
      (D) tocolytic therapy with magnesium sulfate
      (E) antibiotic prophylaxis with amoxicillin plus clavulanic acid

Preterm premature rupture of membranes complicates approximately 4% of pregnancies in the United States. The risk factors associated with preterm PROM are similar to the ones associated with preterm birth in general (see Appendix E). Maternal and fetal complications are inversely correlated with gestational age at the time of preterm PROM. Preterm delivery and complications of prematurity are the most important causes of perinatal mortality and morbidity. Complications decrease with advancing gestational age. The most common neonatal morbidities are respiratory distress syndrome (RDS), intraventricular hemorrhage, periventricular leukomalacia (PVL), infection, and necrotizing enterocolitis. Major neonatal infections occur in 5% of preterm PROM cases.

The mother is at risk for chorioamnionitis (incidence, 15–20%), endometritis, and sepsis. Serious maternal consequences are uncommon. Other complications that are most common with very early preterm PROM (eg, less than 28 weeks of gestation) are abruptio placentae, cord prolapse, perinatal death, pulmonary hypoplasia, compression syndrome, long-term infant morbidities, increased need for cesarean delivery, and retained placenta.

Antenatal corticosteroid therapy should be administered to women with preterm PROM at 24–32 weeks of gestation, because this therapy is associated with lower neonatal complications: 44% less RDS, 53% less intraventricular hemorrhage, 79% less necrotizing enterocolitis, and a trend for a 32% lower incidence in neonatal death, without any increase in maternal or neonatal infection. Antenatal corticosteroid therapy should not be repeated routinely in patients with preterm PROM. Weekly administration improves severe RDS and results in less composite neonatal morbidity among neonates delivered at 24–27 weeks of gestation, but is associated with shorter latency, higher risks of chorioamnionitis and neonatal sepsis, and no improvement in overall composite neonatal morbidity.

Delivery before 30 weeks of gestation is recommended only in cases of intrauterine infection, labor after 48 hours of steroids, or nonreassuring fetal heart test results. Expectant management in cases of preterm PROM at less than 32 weeks of gestation, in the absence of these complications, is recommended. The role is limited for expectant management in women at or beyond 34 weeks of gestation; there are no fetal or neonatal benefits, and in all studies, maternal infection is increased with expectant management.

Fetal testing in cases of preterm PROM to assess fetal well-being is controversial. The two most common types of fetal surveillance are the nonstress test (NST) and the biophysical profile (BPP). Abnormalities of these test results can be somewhat predictive of fetal infection and umbilical cord compression related to oligohydramnios. Insufficient evidence exists, however, to prove that fetal testing improves neonatal outcome, or to assess the optimal type or frequency of these tests. The NST or BPP performed daily has poor sensitivity for infection (39% and 25%, respectively). One trial has shown no improvement in perinatal outcome using these tests.

Insufficient evidence is available to recommend the routine use of tocolytic therapy in women with preterm PROM. In fact, the evidence shows no improvements with the use of this therapy in this particular patient population. The randomized trials on this subject are small, with all eight trials showing no significant benefits in maternal or neonatal outcomes. Most trials evaluated rito-

drine, a β-mimetic agent, as a tocolytic. This agent is no longer available.

The largest randomized trial to assess the effect of antibiotic prophylaxis in women with preterm PROM showed that amoxicillin plus clavulanic acid is associated with a significantly higher rate of necrotizing enterocolitis, and therefore should not be used in this population. Instead, ampicillin and erythromycin or erythromycin alone are associated with significant benefits in neonatal outcomes, and should be used routinely in women with preterm PROM at 24–34 weeks. Compared with placebo, these antibiotics for women with preterm PROM are associated with reductions in chorioamnionitis; preterm birth within 48 hours; preterm birth within 7 days; neonatal infection; and abnormal cerebral ultrasound scan (including intraventricular hemorrhage) before discharge from hospital. It has also been observed that RDS and necrotizing enterocolitis decreased with ampicillin and erythromycin treatment.

Harding JE, Pang JM, Knight DB, Liggins GC. Do antenatal corticosteroids help in the setting of preterm rupture of membranes? Am J Obstet Gynecol 2001;184:131–9.

Kenyon S, Boulvain M, Neilson J. Antibiotics for preterm rupture of membranes. Cochrane Database of Systematic Reviews 2003, Issue 2. Art. No.: CD001058. DOI: 10.1002/14651858.CD001058.

Kenyon SL, Taylor DJ, Tarnow-Mordi W. Broad-spectrum antibiotics for preterm, prelabour rupture of fetal membranes: the ORACLE I randomised trial. ORACLE Collaborative Group [published erratum appears in Lancet 2001;358:156]. Lancet 2001;357:979–88.

Lewis DF, Adair CD, Weeks JW, Barrilleaux PS, Edwards MS, Garite TJ. A randomized clinical trial of daily nonstress testing versus biophysical profile in the management of preterm premature rupture of membranes. Am J Obstet Gynecol 1999;181:1495–9.

Mercer BM, Miodovnik M, Thurnau GR, Goldenberg RL, Das AF, Ramsey RD, et al. Antibiotic therapy for reduction of infant morbidity after preterm premature rupture of the membranes. A randomized controlled trial. National Institute of Child Health and Human Development Maternal–Fetal Medicine Units Network. JAMA 1997;278:989–95.

Naef RW 3rd, Allbert JR, Ross EL, Weber BM, Martin RW, Morrison JC. Premature rupture of membranes at 34 to 37 weeks' gestation: aggressive versus conservative management. Am J Obstet Gynecol 1998;178:126–30.

106

Maternal hypothyroidism

A 28-year-old woman comes to the office for her first prenatal visit at 15 weeks of gestation. She informs you that she has hypothyroidism, which was diagnosed a few months ago, and she was given a prescription for a "thyroid medication," which she did not take because she found out she was pregnant. To further evaluate her condition, you perform laboratory measurements of thyroid-stimulating hormone (TSH), thyroid-stimulating immunoglobulin, free thyroxine index, and free thyroxine (T_4). The set of findings that would confirm the diagnosis of primary hypothyroidism is

(A) decreased TSH and increased thyroid-stimulating immunoglobulin levels
* (B) increased TSH and decreased free T_4 levels
(C) decreased thyroid-stimulating immunoglobulin and increased free T_4 levels
(D) decreased TSH and decreased thyroid-stimulating immunoglobulin levels
(E) increased thyroid-stimulating immunoglobulin and increased free thyroxine index levels

Maternal hypothyroidism is almost always primary in nature, often due to autoimmune thyroiditis or destruction of the gland by radioactive iodine or surgical removal. In rare cases, it may be caused by a pituitary or hypothalamic disorder. Inadequately treated maternal hypothyroidism in pregnancy is associated with increased rates of miscarriage, preeclampsia, abruptio placentae, growth restriction, prematurity, and stillbirth. Untreated maternal hypothyroidism also can affect fetal neurologic development, resulting in cretinism in the most severe cases (eg, growth failure, mental retardation, and other neuropsychologic deficits).

The single most important diagnostic test is measurement of the serum TSH, which is increased in patients with primary hypothyroidism. Serum total and free T_4 will be decreased in all forms of hypothyroidism. The American Association of Clinical Endocrinologists and the American Thyroid Association recommend an initial TSH test to screen for and evaluate symptomatic disease. The free component of TSH is the biologically active portion and is not subject to change, even in conditions such as pregnancy that alter thyroid-binding globulin (Table 106-1).

During early pregnancy, serum TSH levels are suppressed due to thyroid stimulation by the structurally similar placental human chorionic gonadotropin (hCG). These physiologic changes may confound the diagnosis of thyroid disease in the first trimester. As such, in a pregnant patient with known or suspected hypothyroidism, both a TSH level and a free T_4 level should be assessed initially and repeated every 4 weeks if dosage is adjusted to keep the TSH at the lower end of normal and free T_4 within normal levels. The free thyroxine index also can be calculated if direct free T_4 levels are not available. In a recent prospective study, the required levothyroxine dose increased in subjects with hypothyroidism on replacement therapy during the first 16–20 weeks of gestation but plateaued thereafter, confirming the need for regular testing of thyroxine levels during pregnancy to assess the need for dose adjustments. These investigators propose that women with hypothyroidism should have a 30% increase in their levothyroxine dose once pregnancy is confirmed.

An increased incidence of neonatal Graves disease has been associated with high maternal thyroid-stimulating immunoglobulin levels. However, the presence or absence of these antibodies is not necessary for the diagnosis or

TABLE 106-1. Changes in Thyroid Function Test Results in Normal Pregnancy and in Thyroid Disease

Maternal Status	TSH	Free T_4	FTI	Total T_4	Total T_3	RT_3U
Pregnancy	No change	No change	No change	Increase	Increase	Decrease
Hypothyroidism	Increase	Decrease	Decrease	Decrease	Decrease or no change	Decrease

TSH, thyroid-stimulating hormone; T_4, thyroxine; FTI, free thyroxine index; T_3, triiodothyronine; RT_3U, resin T_3 uptake.

Modified from Thyroid disease in pregnancy. ACOG Practice Bulletin No. 37. American College of Obstetricians and Gynecologists. Obstet Gynecol 2002;100:387–96.

treatment of hypothyroidism in pregnancy, and their clinical usefulness in management of thyroid disease in pregnancy is controversial.

Alexander EK, Marquese E, Lawrence J, Jarolim P, Fischer GA, Larsen PR. Timing and magnitude of increases in levothyroxine requirements during pregnancy in women with hypothyroidism. N Engl J Med 2004;351:241–9.

Neale D, Burrow G. Thyroid disease in pregnancy. Obstet Gynecol Clin North Am 2004;31:893–905, xi.

Thyroid disease in pregnancy. ACOG Practice Bulletin No. 37. American College of Obstetricians and Gynecologists. Obstet Gynecol 2002;100:387–96.

Tan GH, Gharib H, Goellner JR, van Heerden JA, Bahn RS. Management of thyroid nodules in pregnancy. Arch Intern Med 1996; 156:2317–20.

107

Preeclampsia

A 24-year-old woman, gravida 2, para 1, comes to the office for prenatal care at 20 weeks of gestation. She reports that in her prior pregnancy she gave birth to a healthy 3,459 g (7 lb 10 oz) infant at term. She recalls being told that she had developed preeclampsia during her labor but does not recall any special treatment being required. The best treatment for this patient after 16 weeks of gestation is

      (A) daily low-dose aspirin
      (B) daily elemental calcium
      (C) daily vitamins C and E
*   (D) no additional treatment
      (E) daily omega-3 fatty acids (fish oil)

Preeclampsia is a disorder that complicates approximately 5–7% of all pregnancies, is the most important cause of maternal mortality worldwide, and is one of the leading causes of perinatal morbidity and mortality. The etiology of preeclampsia remains unknown although a number of theories have been proposed. Preeclampsia has been associated with alterations in prostaglandin metabolism. One hypothesis suggests that in a normal pregnancy there is a balance between vasodilating (prostacyclin) and vasoconstricting (thromboxane) prostaglandins and that in preeclampsia this balance is disrupted by a predominance of vasoconstricting prostaglandins. Alternative theories have suggested that intracellular calcium may be increased in patients with preeclampsia, that oxidative stress may result in release of metabolites that cause damage to the endothelium, or that thrombophilias may be an underlying cause of the disorder. Although it is clear that such hypotheses can account for some part of preeclampsia's manifestations, there remains the lack of a unifying theory to explain preeclampsia.

A number of preventive strategies have been proposed based on the findings of various studies:

- Low-dose aspirin therapy to reestablish the prostaglandin balance
- Calcium supplementation to restore to the normal balance between intracellular and extracellular calcium

- Antioxidant therapy to prevent the endothelial damage that might occur as a result of oxidative stress

An initial small series investigation had suggested that low-dose aspirin had been associated with a reduced incidence of preeclampsia. Two large clinical trials undertaken by the National Institute of Child Health and Human Development Network of Maternal–Fetal Medicine Units failed to demonstrate that 60 mg of aspirin taken daily after 16 weeks of gestation would prevent preeclampsia in either low-risk or high-risk women. Likewise, early trials of calcium supplementation appeared very promising but when subjected to a larger randomized clinical trial format also failed to significantly reduce the incidence of preeclampsia. Most recently, the use of antioxidant therapy, specifically supplemental vitamin C and vitamin E, has been proposed as a means to prevent or reduce endothelial cell damage and, therefore, reduce the incidence of preeclampsia. One early clinical trial of this antioxidant therapy appeared promising, but a recently published larger trial again failed to establish the efficacy of this approach. Likewise, supplementation with fish oil, a source of antioxidant omega-3 fatty acids, failed to demonstrate a reduction in the rate of hypertensive disorders of pregnancy. Given these findings, the most reasonable recommendation for the patient described would be no additional treatment other than standard prenatal health and nutrition.

Caritis S, Sibai B, Hauth J, Lindheimer MD, Klebanoff M, Thom E, et al. Low-dose aspirin to prevent preeclampsia in women at high risk. National Institute of Child Health and Human Development Network of Maternal–Fetal Medicine Units. N Engl J Med 1998;338:701–5.

Chappell LC, Seed PT, Briley AL, Kelly FJ, Lee R, Hunt BJ, et al. Effect of antioxidants on the occurrence of pre-eclampsia in women at increased risk: a randomised trial. Lancet 1999;354:810–6.

Levine RJ, Hauth JC, Curet LB, Sibai BM, Catalano PM, Morris CD, et al. Trial of calcium to prevent preeclampsia. N Engl J Med 1997;337: 69–76.

Olafsdottir AS, Skuladottir GV, Thorsdottir I, Hanksson A, Thorgeirsdottir H, Steingrimsdottir L. Relationship between high con-

sumption of marine fatty acids in early pregnancy and hypertensive disorders of pregnancy. BJOG 2006;113:301–9.

Rumbold AR, Crowther CA, Haslam RR, Dekker GA, Robinson JS. Vitamins C and E and the risks of preeclampsia and perinatal complications. ACTS Study Group. N Engl J Med 2006;354:1796–806.

Sibai BM, Caritis SN, Thom E, Klebanoff M, McNellis D, Rocco L, et al. Prevention of preeclampsia with low-dose aspirin in healthy nulliparous pregnant women. National Institute of Child Health and Human Development Network of Maternal–Fetal Medicine Units. N Engl J Med 1993;329:1213–8.

108

Labor induction

A 26-year-old primigravid woman comes to the office at 39 weeks of gestation for a routine prenatal visit. Her pregnancy has been uncomplicated and a recent ultrasonogram reveals a normal fetal weight. Her cervix is long, uneffaced, undilated, and firm. The fetal head is floating. Due to a recent change in her home situation, she requests to have her labor induced in the next 2 days. In counseling the patient regarding the risk of cesarean delivery, you advise her that

* (A) elective induction increases her risk
  (B) pharmacologic methods of labor induction reduce her risk
  (C) mechanical methods of cervical ripening reduce her risk
  (D) her risk would be similar if she presented in spontaneous labor

Induction of labor in the United States has reached an all-time high: almost 20% of women receive induction of labor. Elective induction of labor is an important contributor to this increasing rate. Some centers report induction rates of 40–50% with a rate of elective induction of labor of 71%.

Elective induction of labor, that is, labor induced without a medical cause, is most often due to patient or physician convenience. Although it has been shown that elective induction of labor does result in more daytime deliveries, it appears to come at a significant cost.

The risk of cesarean delivery has consistently increased in nulliparous women who have electively induced labor. Risks associated with elective induction are varied but are approximately twice the risk of women who present in spontaneous labor. The reason for this is not completely clear but it appears that there is an increase in first stage dystocia in nulliparous women who had elective induction of labor.

A recent report found that nulliparous women who are electively induced had substantially slower latent and early active phases of labor. However, these women were noted to have faster labor progression from 4 cm dilated to 10 cm. Women who had elective induced labor had an increased risk of operative delivery, shoulder dystocia,

longer labor, and higher health care costs. The neonates of women who had elective induction of labor appeared to be more likely to be admitted to the neonatal intensive care unit, although this may have been a result of the higher cesarean delivery rate in this population.

The risk for cesarean delivery in multiparous women who have elective labor induction is less clear. Some studies have reported a higher cesarean delivery rate and others show no difference compared with women who have spontaneous labor. This finding may be related to the condition of the cervix when elective induction is begun rather than multiparity.

Preinduction cervical ripening can be performed by either mechanical methods or pharmacologic methods. Mechanical methods do not usually result in labor, and another agent such as oxytocin must be administered after preinduction cervical ripening is complete. However, patients who receive pharmacologic methods, particularly those that are prostaglandin based, often enter labor during or soon after the preinduction cervical ripening process.

One of the most commonly used mechanical methods of preinduction cervical ripening is the Foley catheter. The Foley catheter has been shown to be as effective as prostaglandin-based agents while causing fewer contractile abnormalities. The Foley catheter works by gradual mechanical stretching of the cervix and by the release of prostaglandins. After the catheter is placed in the cervix, the balloon is inflated at or above the internal os. The Foley catheter is then placed on gentle traction by taping the end of the tube to the inside of the woman's thigh. Most women are 3–4 cm dilated after extrusion of the Foley catheter, although they are not commonly in labor. Intravenous oxytocin is then administered followed by artificial rupture of membranes.

The most common forms of prostaglandin for preinduction cervical ripening are intravaginal misoprostol, intracervical or vaginal prostaglandin E$_2$ (PGE$_2$) gel, and a slow-release PGE$_2$ vaginal insert. Prostaglandin-based preparations have been shown to be superior to placebo for cervical ripening, but there is no consensus about whether some preparations are more effective than others.

Despite numerous methods and preparations for preinduction cervical ripening and the induction of labor, women with unfavorable cervices who receive preinduc-

tion cervical ripening, regardless of the method, have not been shown to be at a decreased risk for cesarean delivery. However, women who have a Bishop score greater than 8 who undergo induction of labor have a rate of vaginal delivery that is comparable to that of women who enter labor spontaneously.

Cammu H, Martens G, Ruyssinck G, Amy JJ. Outcome after elective labor induction in nulliparous women: a matched cohort study. Am J Obstet Gynecol 2002;186:240–4.

Dublin S, Lydon-Rochelle M, Kaplan RC, Watts DH, Critchlow CW. Maternal and neonatal outcomes after induction of labor without an identified indication. Am J Obstet Gynecol 2000;183:986–94.

Maslow AS, Sweeny AL. Elective induction of labor as a risk factor for cesarean delivery among low-risk women at term. Obstet Gynecol 2000;95:917–22.

Seyb ST, Berka RJ, Socol M, Dooley SL. Risk of cesarean delivery with elective induction of labor at term in nulliparous women. Obstet Gynecol 1999;94:600–7.

Vahratian A, Zhang J, Troendle JF, Sciscione A, Hoffman MK. Labor progression and risk of cesarean delivery in electively induced nulliparas. Obstet Gynecol 2005;105:698–704.

109

Asthma medications

A 28-year-old woman with a history of mild intermittent asthma presents at 24 weeks of gestation with increasing shortness of breath over the past 3 weeks. She currently needs to use her albuterol metered dose inhaler two or three times per day. On further questioning, she reports no associated fever, productive cough, or malaise. The best treatment strategy for improving her asthma control is to

        (A) increase the albuterol dose
*   (B) change to a low-dose inhaled corticosteroid
        (C) add inhaled cromolyn sodium
        (D) add a leukotriene receptor antagonist
        (E) add theophylline

Asthma is reported to affect approximately 4–8% of pregnant women, making it the most common potentially serious medical complication of pregnancy. Two recent, large prospective studies to assess the effects of maternal asthma on perinatal outcomes suggest that maternal asthma increases the risk of perinatal mortality, preeclampsia, preterm birth, and low birth weight infants. Mothers with more severe disease are at a higher risk, whereas disease that is well controlled is associated with decreased risks. Because maintaining adequate control of asthma during pregnancy is important for the health and well-being of both the woman and the fetus, asthma exacerbations during pregnancy should be managed aggressively. The ultimate goal of asthma therapy during pregnancy is to

prevent hypoxic episodes in the mother, thereby maintaining adequate oxygenation of the fetus. Preferred and alternative medication options are available for the treatment of asthma, depending on the severity of disease (Table 109-1).

Short-acting bronchodilators, particularly short-acting inhaled β$_2$-agonists, are recommended as quick relief medication for the treatment of symptoms in patients with mild intermittent asthma. Albuterol is the preferred short-acting inhaled β$_2$-agonist because, in addition to its excellent general safety profile, it is the subject of the largest pool of data related to safety during pregnancy of any currently available inhaled β$_2$-agonist. However, if a patient's symptoms require the use of short-acting bronchodilators

TABLE 109-1. Recommended Preferred and Alternative Therapy for Patients With Asthma

Category	Therapy	
	Preferred	**Alternative**
Mild intermittent	Inhaled β_2-agonist as needed	
Mild persistent	Low-dose inhaled corticosteroids	Cromolyn, leukotriene receptor antagonist, or theophylline
Moderate persistent	Inhaled corticosteroids and salmeterol	Inhaled corticosteroid and either leukotriene receptor antagonist or theophylline
Severe persistent	High-dose inhaled corticosteroid and salmeterol and oral corticosteroid if needed	High-dose inhaled corticosteroid and theophylline and oral corticosteroid if needed

Adapted from National Asthma Education and Prevention Program. Working group report on managing asthma during pregnancy: recommendations for pharmacologic treatment—update 2004. Bethesda (MD): U.S. Department of Health and Human Services; National Institutes of Health; National Heart, Lung, and Blood Institute; 2004.

more than twice per week, consideration should be given to initiating an alternative regimen for better long-term control.

In the current scenario, this patient's asthma has progressed to mild persistent disease. The preferred treatment for long-term control in mild persistent asthma is a daily low-dose inhaled corticosteroid (Table 109-1). This preference is based on the strong effectiveness data in nonpregnant women, as well as studies demonstrating the effectiveness and safety of this treatment in pregnant women with no increased risk of adverse perinatal outcomes. Budesonide is the preferred inhaled corticosteroid because it has a larger body of reassuring evidence on the safety of its use during pregnancy than any other inhaled corticosteroid available. However, if asthma is well controlled by a different inhaled corticosteroid before pregnancy, it may be reasonable to continue that medication during pregnancy.

Cromolyn, leukotriene receptor antagonists, and theophylline are treatment alternatives, but they are not preferred therapies. Cromolyn has an excellent safety profile, but it has limited effectiveness compared with inhaled corticosteroids. Leukotriene receptor antagonists provide statistically significant but modest improvements in children and nonpregnant adults with asthma, although in studies comparing the overall efficacy of the two classes of drugs, most outcomes clearly favor inhaled corticosteroids. Published data are minimal regarding the use of leukotriene receptor antagonists during pregnancy; however, animal safety data submitted to the U.S. Food and Drug Administration are reassuring. Thus, leukotriene receptor antagonists can be considered as a second-choice option for treatment in pregnant women, and they are most appropriate for women whose asthma was successfully controlled with this class of medication before pregnancy.

The use of theophylline has demonstrated clinical effectiveness in some studies and has been used for years in pregnant women with asthma. However, it too has the potential for serious toxicity resulting from excessive use or certain drug–drug interactions (eg, with erythromycin). The use of theophylline during pregnancy requires careful titration of the dose and regular monitoring to maintain the recommended serum theophylline concentration range of 5–12 mcg/mL.

Bracken MB, Triche EW, Belanger K, Saftlas A, Beckett WS, Leaderer BP. Asthma symptoms, severity, and drug therapy: a prospective study of effects on 2205 pregnancies. Obstet Gynecol 2003;102:739–52.

Dombrowski MP, Schatz M, Wise R, Momirova V, Landon M, Mabie W, et al. Asthma during pregnancy. National Institute of Child Health and Human Development Maternal–Fetal Medicine Units Network and the National Heart, Lung, and Blood Institute. Obstet Gynecol 2004;103:5–12.

National Asthma Education and Prevention Program. Expert panel report: guidelines for the diagnosis and management of asthma—update on selected topics 2002. Bethesda (MD): U.S. Department of Health and Human Services; National Institutes of Health; National Heart, Lung, and Blood Institute; 2003.

National Asthma Education and Prevention Program. Working group report on managing asthma during pregnancy: recommendations for pharmacologic treatment—update 2004. Bethesda (MD): U.S. Department of Health and Human Services; National Institutes of Health; National Heart, Lung, and Blood Institute; 2004.

The use of newer asthma and allergy medications during pregnancy. American College of Obstetricians and Gynecologists and the American College of Allergy, Asthma and Immunology. Ann Allergy Asthma Immunol 2000;84:475–80.

110

Folic acid supplementation during pregnancy

A 20-year-old woman, gravida 1, para 1, is seen postpartum after the delivery of a fetus with a meningomyelocele. You advise her that the best recommendation to reduce the risk of a future neural tube defect is to start folic acid

- (A) 4 mg in the 12th week of gestation
- (B) 0.4 mg after she conceives
- (C) 4 mg after she conceives
- *   (D) 4 mg at least 1 month before planned conception
- (E) 0.4 mg at least 1 month before planned conception

In the United States, the incidence of neural tube defects (NTDs) is approximately 1.4–2 per 1,000 pregnancies; however, this risk increases appreciably if there is a family history of an NTD. If one of the parents has an NTD, the risk to the children is as high as 4.5%. If a previous sibling is affected, the recurrence risk is approximately 4% and, if two previous siblings are affected, the risk increases to 10%.

A decrease in folate intake has been shown to be associated with an increased risk of NTDs. It has been shown that women whose pregnancies are complicated by a fetal NTD have lower levels of vitamin B_{12} and folate than do women whose pregnancies are unaffected. Folic acid can help prevent 50–70% of cases of NTDs. Most studies suggest that folic acid works by correcting a nutritional deficiency. Folic acid is involved in the conversion of homocysteine to methionine; this pathway is implicated in the development of the NTDs.

The Centers for Disease Control and Prevention have recommended that all women of childbearing age should consume 0.4 mg folic acid for the prevention of NTDs. It is important to note that not all NTDs will be eliminated with the use of folic acid. Therefore, it is imperative to continue to screen women for these defects with maternal serum alpha-fetoprotein and ultrasonography. For women who have had a child with an NTD, the recommended dose of folic acid is 4 mg per day, much higher than that present in prenatal vitamins. The folic acid supplementation needs to be taken at least a month before conception and continued for the first 12 weeks of pregnancy. Preconception use is critical because the neural tube forms during the first 28 days of gestation, before the first period is missed. The risks of higher doses of folic acid are considered to be minimal. Folic acid is not toxic even in high doses and is rapidly excreted in the urine. However, higher doses of folic acid must be taken under the supervision of a physician in order not to mask an underlying condition such as pernicious anemia (vitamin B_{12} deficiency).

The current recommendations for folic acid supplementation in the United States are based on two large European studies. The first study, conducted in Great Britain in 1991, was a randomized double-blind prevention trial, in which women with a child with an NTD were allocated at random to one of four groups: folic acid, multivitamins, both, or neither. The study results showed a 72% reduction in pregnancies with NTDs (relative risk = 0.28) in both groups of women that received folic acid versus no reduction in the groups that did not receive folic acid supplementation. In a randomized, controlled trial of periconceptional multivitamin supplementation in Hungary reported in 1992, low-risk women were divided into two groups; one group was given 0.8 mg folic acid daily and the second group was the control group. In the group of women that received folic acid supplementation, there were no NTDs compared with six NTDs in the untreated group. In addition, the treated women had a statistically significant lower number of births with major anomalies than did the untreated women.

In 1998, the U.S. Food and Drug Administration required the fortification of cereals, breads, and pasta with folic acid. Since this program began, the rate of NTDs in newborns has decreased by approximately 25%. However, the amount of folic acid in these foods is small and women of childbearing age still need to continue to supplement their diet with folic acid. Women with a child with an NTD need 10 times the recommended dose of folic acid to minimize the risk of recurrence.

Czeizel AE, Dudas I. Prevention of the first occurrence of neural tube defects by periconceptional vitamin supplementation. N Engl J Med 1992;327:1832–5.

Prevention of neural tube defects: results of the Medical Research Council Vitamin Study. MRC Vitamin Study Research Group. Lancet 1991;338:131–7.

Neural tube defects. ACOG Practice Bulletin No. 44. American College of Obstetricians and Gynecologists. Obstet Gynecol 2003;102:203–13.

Recommendations for the use of folic acid to reduce the number of cases of spina bifida and other neural tube defects. MMWR Recomm Rep 1992;41(RR-14):1–7.

Spina bifida and anencephaly before and after folic acid mandate— United States, 1995–1996 and 1999–2000. Centers for Disease Control and Prevention. MMWR Morb Mortal Wkly Rep 2004;53:362–5.

111

Tocolysis contraindications

A 22-year-old woman at 27 weeks of gestation with a twin pregnancy is receiving magnesium sulfate tocolysis to manage preterm labor. She complains of chest tightness and dyspnea. Her oxygen saturation by pulse oximetry is 89%. Crackles are auscultated at both lung bases, and her respiratory rate is 28 breaths per minute. In addition to ordering an arterial blood gas and chest radiograph, the most appropriate next step in care is to

    (A) administer heparin
    (B) order a spiral computed tomography (CT)
    (C) order a maternal echocardiogram
*   (D) discontinue tocolysis
    (E) order a magnesium level

Preterm birth is the leading cause of neonatal morbidity in the United States and developed countries and is responsible for a substantial percentage of long-term neurologic impairment in surviving children. Despite improvements in obstetric care, the rate of prematurity has not declined in the past four decades. About half of all preterm births are preceded by preterm labor, defined as regular uterine contractions with associated cervical change between 20 and 37 weeks of gestation. The exact cause of preterm labor is poorly understood, although many pathways have been investigated. Even though the efficacy of tocolytics is unclear, intervention with tocolytic agents may prolong gestation for 48 hours or more, allowing time for antenatal corticosteroid administration and possible maternal transport to a tertiary care facility. Several tocolytic agents are available for use in the United States with the goal of inhibiting or reducing the strength and frequency of uterine contractions. Tocolytic agents must be individualized to the particular clinical scenario and maternal condition. The potentially serious maternal and fetal side effects of the various tocolytic agents are listed in Table 111-1.

Additionally, there are absolute, general, and relative contraindications to tocolysis. General contraindications to tocolysis may include the following:

- Severe preeclampsia or eclampsia
- Intraamniotic infection
- Fetal demise of a singleton gestation
- Lethal congenital or chromosomal abnormality
- Hydrops fetalis
- Nonreassuring fetal heart rate tracing

- Advanced cervical dilatation
- Fetal pulmonary maturity
- Maternal hemodynamic instability, such as hemorrhage or disseminated intravascular coagulopathy

Box 111-1 lists contraindications for specific tocolytic agents. Magnesium sulfate is one of the most frequently used tocolytics, and its mechanism of action is calcium antagonism. Absolute contraindications to magnesium sulfate use are myasthenia gravis and heart block.

The described patient has a twin gestation, and tocolysis was accomplished with magnesium sulfate. A well-recognized complication of magnesium sulfate tocolysis is pulmonary edema, especially with multiple gestations. Many of these patients will have received aggressive intravenous hydration in an attempt to abate uterine contractions. Often the patient will complain of chest tightness and dyspnea. Low oxygenation saturation, tachypnea, and findings on the chest examination point to the correct diagnosis of pulmonary edema.

Because the most likely diagnosis is pulmonary edema, initial efforts include discontinuation of tocolysis, judicious fluid management, and treatment with furosemide. If the patient does not respond appropriately to initial measures, a spiral computed tomography scan and maternal echocardiogram may be necessary to further evaluate the chest and cardiac function. Heparin therapy would be a therapeutic option if pulmonary embolism was strongly suspected. The need to obtain magnesium levels may cause delay in an emergency situation and could place the patient at additional risk.

TABLE 111-1. Potential Maternal and Fetal Complications of Tocolytic Agents

Agent	Maternal	Fetal
β-adrenergic agents	Hyperglycemia Hypokalemia Hypotension Tremor Palpitations Nervousness Pulmonary edema Cardiac insufficiency Arrhythmias Tachycardia Myocardial ischemia Maternal death	Tachycardia Hyperinsulinemia Fetal hyperglycemia Neonatal hypoglycemia Hypocalcemia Hypotension Ileus Myocardial and septal hypertrophy Myocardial ischemia
Magnesium sulfate	Pulmonary edema Respiratory depression Cardiac arrest Maternal tetany Muscular paralysis Hypotension Muscle weakness Flushing Lethargy Headache	Hypotonia Lethargy Respiratory depression Bone demineralization (prolonged use)

Prostaglandin synthetase inhibitors	Gastrointestinal
	  bleeding
	Nausea
	Heartburn
	Gastritis
		Oligohydramnios
		Constriction of fetal ductus
		  arteriosis
		Pulmonary hypertension
		Intraventricular hemorrhage
		Hyperbilirubinemia
		Necrotizing enterocolitis

Calcium channel blockers	Flushing Headache Dizziness Nausea Transient hypotension	None known

Modified from Management of preterm labor. ACOG Practice Bulletin No. 43. American College of Obstetricians and Gynecologists. Obstet Gynecol 2003;101:1039–47.

> **BOX 111-1**
>
> ### Contraindications for Specific Tocolytic Agents
>
> **β-adrenergic agents**
> - Maternal cardiac arrhythmias
> - Maternal cardiac disease
> - Poorly controlled diabetes
> - Poorly controlled thyroid disease
>
> **Magnesium sulfate**
> - Myasthenia gravis
> - Heart block
>
> **Prostaglandin synthetase inhibitors**
> - NSAID-sensitive asthma
> - Active peptic ulcer disease
> - Significant renal or hepatic impairment
> - Coagulation disorders or thromobocytopenia
> - Sensitivity to NSAIDs
> - Oligohydramnios
> - Congenital fetal heart disease (ductal dependent)
>
> **Calcium channel blockers**
> - Cardiac disease
> - Renal disease (use caution)
> - Maternal hypotension (blood pressure less than 90/50 mm Hg)
> - Magnesium sulfate (avoid concomitant use)
>
> ---
>
> NSAIDs, nonsteroidal antiinflammatory drugs
>
> Management of preterm labor. ACOG Practice Bulletin No. 43. American College of Obstetricians and Gynecologists. Obstet Gynecol 2003;101:1039–47.

Ables AZ, Romero AM, Chauhan SP. Use of calcium channel antagonists for preterm labor. Obstet Gynecol Clin North Am 2005;32: 519–25.

Goldenberg RL. The management of preterm labor. Obstet Gynecol 2002;100:1020–37.

Management of preterm labor. ACOG Practice Bulletin No. 43. American College of Obstetricians and Gynecologists. Obstet Gynecol 2003;101:1039–47.

Preterm birth. Cunningham FG, Leveno KJ, Bloom SL, Hauth JC, Gilstrap L 3rd, Wenstrom KD, editors. Williams obstetrics. 22nd ed. New York (NY): McGraw-Hill; 2005. p. 855–80.

112

Community-acquired pneumonia

A 33-year-old woman, gravida 4, para 3, at 22 weeks of gestation presents with a 4-day history of fever, shaking chills, and cough productive of yellow sputum. She has a 12-pack-per-year smoking history and has chronic active hepatitis C. A chest X-ray shows scattered bibasilar infiltrates. The patient is admitted to the hospital. The initial antibiotic treatment should be intravenous

* *   (A)   ceftriaxone and azithromycin
* (B)   levofloxacin
* (C)   doxycycline
* (D)   clindamycin and vancomycin
* (E)   ampicillin

Community-acquired pneumonia occurs in approximately 0.78–2.7 per 1,000 pregnancies, a rate similar to the nonpregnant population. Even with extensive diagnostic investigation, the responsible pathogen is unknown in greater than 50% of cases. Causative agents include *Streptococcus pneumoniae, Haemophilus influenzae, Mycoplasma pneumoniae, Chlamydia pneumoniae, Legionella* species, respiratory viruses, *Mycobacterium tuberculosis*, and endemic fungi. The organism that is more likely to occur in smokers than in nonsmokers is *H influenzae*. Recommended testing includes complete blood count, serum electrolytes, hepatic enzymes, tests of renal function, chest X-ray, pulse oximetry, sputum Gram stain and culture, and two sets of blood cultures. Treatment is empiric, and antibiotics should be started within 8 hours of arrival at the hospital. Most studies show that the etiologic agents of community-acquired pneumonia in pregnancy are the same as in the nonpregnant population; therefore, the same treatment guidelines are used in pregnancy. Particular care is given to select antibiotics that are safe for the fetus.

According to the American Thoracic Society guidelines for community-acquired pneumonia, patients are stratified by place of therapy, comorbidity, and modifying factors. Place of therapy (outpatient, hospital ward, or intensive care unit) is a reflection of severity of illness. Comorbidity is the presence of coexisting illness such as chronic obstructive pulmonary disease, congestive heart failure, diabetes mellitus, renal insufficiency, or chronic liver disease. Modifying factors include risk factors for drug-resistant pneumococcus (eg, exposure to child in day care center, corticosteroid therapy), risk factors for Gram-negative infection (eg, residence in a nursing home), or risk factors for *Pseudomonas aeruginosa* (eg, bronchiec-tasis, broad-spectrum antibiotic therapy in the past month). These three discriminating features affect the likelihood of particular etiologic agents, and should therefore affect the initial choice of antimicrobial therapy.

The patient described has community-acquired pneumonia with coexisting chronic liver disease. Such patients may be treated with either a β-lactam and macrolide combination or monotherapy with an antipneumococcal fluoroquinolone. Fluoroquinolones, such as levofloxacin, are relatively contraindicated in pregnancy because of concern about effects on fetal cartilage; therefore, the appropriate initial antibiotic treatment for this patient should be intravenous ceftriaxone and azithromycin. Doxycycline, a tetracycline, has a role in the treatment of community-acquired pneumonia, but it is contraindicated in pregnancy because of adverse effects on fetal teeth and bones and concern about maternal liver toxicity. Clindamycin and vancomycin do not provide coverage for enteric gram-negative organisms or atypical agents such as *C pneumoniae* and *M pneumoniae*. Ampicillin is not recommended because of organism resistance to this antibiotic and lack of coverage of atypical agents.

Briggs GG, Freeman RK, Yaffe SJ. Drugs in pregnancy and lactation. 7th ed. Philadelphia (PA): Lippincott Williams & Wilkins; 2005. p. 912–14, 1549–53.

Goodnight WH, Soper DE. Pneumonia in pregnancy. Crit Care Med 2005;33:S390–7.

Mandel J, Weinberger SE. Pulmonary diseases. In: Burrow GN, Duffy TP, Copel JA, editors. Medical complications during pregnancy. 6th ed. Philadelphia (PA): Elsevier Saunders; 2004. p. 375–414.

Niederman MS, Mandell LA, Anzueto A, Bass JB, Broughton WA, Campbell GD, et al. Guidelines for the management of adults with community-acquired pneumonia. Diagnosis, assessment of severity, antimicrobial therapy and prevention. American Thoracic Society. Am J Respir Crit Care Med 2001;163:1730–54.

113

Mitral valve prolapse

A 23-year-old primigravid woman with mitral valve prolapse (MVP) is in active labor. An echocardiogram in the first trimester confirmed the diagnosis of MVP but showed no evidence of mitral regurgitation or leaflet thickening. The appropriate management for this patient is

    (A) ampicillin and gentamicin sulfate
    (B) vancomycin hydrochloride and gentamicin sulfate
    (C) cefazolin sodium (Ancef, Kefzol)
*   (D) no prophylaxis

Mitral valve prolapse occurs in 2–6% of the population. It can occur as an isolated finding without any mitral regurgitation; however, MVP is the most common cause of significant mitral regurgitation. Normally, the mitral valve leaflets close at or below the mitral annulus. Dehydration and tachycardia are common causes of intermittent MVP. As a result, MVP is often an abnormality of volume status or adrenergic state and not an abnormality of valve structure or function. Abnormal valve motion is not responsible for an increased risk of endocarditis; however, mitral regurgitation creates the shearing force and flow abnormalities that increase the risk of bacterial adherence to an abnormal valve. The echocardiographic findings of the mitral valve that warrant antibiotic therapy during bacteremia-producing procedures include mitral regurgitation, leaflet thickening, elongated chordae, left atrial enlargement, or left ventricular dilatation.

In 1997, the American Heart Association (AHA) revised its guidelines for the prevention of bacterial endocarditis. The AHA guidelines state that vaginal and cesarean deliveries are not procedures that cause significant bacteremia, and, as a result, endocarditis prophylaxis usually is not recommended. However, in high-risk patients, antibiotic prophylaxis may be considered during a vaginal delivery. High-risk patients include women with prosthetic heart valves, complex cyanotic congenital heart disease, or surgically constructed systemic pulmonary shunts or conduits. Since the publication of these recommendations, some evidence suggests that the rate of bacteremia in parturient women is higher than previously believed. The rates of bacteremia can be as high as 14% in laboring women who require a cesarean delivery. As a result, it would be reasonable to consider antibiotic prophylaxis for labor and delivery for women with moderate risk conditions (Table 113-1).

The antibiotic regimen recommended by the AHA is ampicillin plus gentamicin sulfate followed by ampicillin or amoxicillin 6 hours after the procedure. If the patient is allergic to penicillin, vancomycin is recommended as a replacement.

The patient described has uncomplicated MVP and, as a result, no antibiotic prophylaxis is recommended. If the woman has complicated MVP, identified by mitral regurgitation, leaflet thickening, left atrial enlargement, or left ventricular dilatation, endocarditis prophylaxis can be considered. In a patient who is not allergic to penicillin, the ampicillin and gentamicin sulfate regimen is appropriate. However, if the patient is allergic to penicillin, the vancomycin and gentamicin sulfate regimen is warranted. Cefazolin sodium (Ancef, Kefzol) is not recommended as endocarditis prophylaxis.

Boggess KA, Watts DH, Hillier SL, Krohn MA, Benedetti TJ, Eschenbach DA. Bacteremia shortly after placental separation during cesarean delivery. Obstet Gynecol 1996;87:779–84.

Bonow RO, Carabello B, de Leon AC Jr, Edmunds LJ Jr, Fedderly BJ, Freed MD, et al. Guidelines for the management of patients with valvular heart disease: executive summary. A report of the American College of Cardiology/American Hearth Association Task Force on Practice Guidelines (Committee on Management of Patients with Valvular Heart Disease). Circulation 1998;98:1949–84.

Dajani A, Taubert KA, Wilson W, Bolger AF, Bayer A, Ferrieri P, et al. Prevention of bacterial endocarditis. Recommendations by the American Heart Association. JAMA 1997;277:1794–801.

Elkayam U, Bitar F. Valvular heart disease and pregnancy part I: native valves. J Am Coll Cardiol 2005;46:223–30.

Petanovic M, Zagar Z. The significance of asyptomatic bacteremia for the newborn. Acta Obstet Gynecol Scand 2001;80:813–7.

TABLE 113-1. American College of Cardiology/American Heart Association Recommendations for Antibiotic Prophylaxis to Prevent Bacterial Endocarditis

Cardiac Lesion	Prophylaxis for Uncomplicated Delivery	Prophylaxis for Suspected Bacteremia*
High-Risk Category		
Prosthetic cardiac valves (both homograft and bioprosthetic)	Optional	Recommended
Prior bacterial endocarditis	Optional	Recommended
Complex cyanotic congenital cardiac malformations	Optional	Recommended
Surgically constructed systemic pulmonary shunts or conduits	Optional	Recommended
Moderate-Risk Category		
Congenital cardiac malformations (except repaired atrial septal defect, ventricular septal defect, or patent ductus arteriosus, or isolated secundum atrial septal defect)	Not recommended	Recommended
Acquired valvular dysfunction (most commonly rheumatic heart disease)	Not recommended	Recommended
Hypertrophic cardiomyopathy	Not recommended	Recommended
Mitral valve prolapse with valvar regurgitation or thickened leaflets or both	Not recommended	Recommended
Negligible-Risk Category†		
Mitral valve prolapse without valvar regurgitation	Not recommended	Not recommended
Physiologic, functional, or innocent heart murmurs	Not recommended	Not recommended
Previous Kawasaki disease without valvar dysfunction	Not recommended	Not recommended
Previous rheumatic fever without valvar dysfunction	Not recommended	Not recommended
Cardiac pacemakers and implanted defibrillators	Not recommended	Not recommended
Prior coronary bypass graft surgery	Not recommended	Not recommended

*Eg, intraamniotic infection.

†Risk for developing endocarditis is not higher than that of the general population.

Data from Bonow RO, Carabello B, de Leon AC Jr, Edmunds LH Jr, Fedderly BJ, Freed MD, et al. Guidelines for the management of patients with valvular heart disease: executive summary. A report of the American College of Cardiology/American Heart Association Task Force on Practice Guidelines (Committee on Management of Patients with Valvular Heart Disease). Circulation 1998;98:1949–84. Dajani AS, Taubert KA, Wilson W, Bolger AF, Bayer A, Ferrieri P, et al. Prevention of bacterial endocarditis: recommendations by the American Heart Association. JAMA 1997;277:1794–801.

114

Operative complications in the obese patient

A 34-year-old woman with a body mass index (weight in kilograms divided by height in meters squared [kg/m²]) of 41 is having a scheduled elective repeat cesarean delivery. In addition to preoperative antibiotic treatment, the approach most likely to reduce her risk of postoperative wound infection is

 (A) interrupted Smead–Jones closure
 (B) drain placement through the surgical site
 (C) closure of the peritoneum
* (D) subcutaneous tissue closure
 (E) continuation of antibiotics postoperatively

The prevalence of obesity in the United States has increased dramatically over the past 20 years. The obese gravid woman is prone to more frequent wound complications even with the use of prophylactic antibiotics. Obese women who have a cesarean delivery are at markedly increased risk for postpartum endometritis and wound complications such as infection, seromas, hematomas, and dehiscence.

The technique used for closure of the abdominal wound is thought by many to be an important factor in both early and late wound complications. Most agree that decreasing operative time will optimize outcome; as such, closure of the abdominal wall should be fast and easy. When closing a transverse incision, usually the peritoneum need not be closed because this does not add strength to the wound and spontaneous closure will occur in 24–48 hours. However, peritoneal closure may decrease adhesions to the abdominal wall and this has no effect on wound infection. With a vertical incision, single-layer mass closure techniques in which the fascia and peritoneum are closed together, like the Smead–Jones technique, provides a strong closure in patients at high risk for infection. Studies have demonstrated no difference in postoperative complications, including infection and dehiscence, between interrupted Smead–Jones closure and running mass closure. However, most favor using a continuous suture over an interrupted closure because it is easier and faster and so decreases operating time, reducing the risk of morbidity secondary to infection.

The use of a drain in the subcutaneous fat layer at the time of cesarean delivery was evaluated in a Cochrane review. There was no evidence in this review to suggest that the routine use of a drain confers any benefit. Additionally, drain placement through the surgical site increases the risk of surgical-site infection. For this reason, if a drain is used, placement should be accomplished through a separate stab wound.

Investigators have demonstrated that suture closure of the subcutaneous layer after cesarean delivery in obese patients may lead to a significant reduction in the incidence of postoperative wound disruption. In one study, the wound disruption rate increased significantly with thickened subcutaneous tissue. Women with subcutaneous tissue greater than 2 cm had a wound disruption rate of 27.2% compared with 18.7% of controls. Other studies have confirmed that using a subcutaneous suture in all patients with greater than 2-cm subcutaneous depth significantly reduces the risk of wound disruption and seroma formation.

Several well-designed studies have documented the efficacy of prophylactic, preoperative antibiotics in reducing the rates of postpartum endometritis and wound infection in women undergoing elective or nonelective cesarean delivery, and standard antibiotic prophylaxis at the time of cesarean delivery is recommended for all women. Compared with placebo, the use of antibiotic prophylaxis generally reduces the rate of febrile morbidity and postpartum endometritis from an average of 35–40% to 15% or less. However, despite having a larger volume of distribution, larger doses or continued antibiotic administration in obese women have not been studied or reported to decrease postpartum morbidity secondary to infection.

Brockmeyer AD, Mutch DG. Wound infection: a review of risk factors and prevention. Postgraduate Obstet Gynecol 2005;25(15):1–7; quiz 8.

Cetin A, Cetin M. Superficial wound disruption after cesarean delivery: effect of depth and closure of subcutaneous tissue. Int J Gynaecol Obstet 1997;57:17–21.

Chelmow D, Rodriguez EJ, Sabatini MM. Suture closure of subcutaneous fat and wound disruption after cesarean delivery: a meta-analysis. Obstet Gynecol 2004;103:974–80.

Gates S, Anderson ER. Wound drainage for caesarean section. Cochrane Database of Systematic Reviews 2005, Issue 1. Art. No.: CD004549. DOI: 10.1002/14651858.CD004549.pub2.

Obesity in pregnancy. ACOG Committee Opinion No. 315. American College of Obstetricians and Gynecologists. Obstet Gynecol 2005; 106:671–5.

115

Decreased fetal movement

A 31-year-old primigravid woman at 34 weeks of gestation comes to the office for routine prenatal care. She has had an uncomplicated pregnancy. She tells you that she has noted decreased fetal movement over the past 24 hours. The most appropriate approach to management is

    (A) patient reassurance
    (B) placing the patient on a fetal movement program
*   (C) immediately performing a nonstress test
    (D) increasing oral hydration
    (E) immediate delivery

Fetal movement is established early in pregnancy. The perception of fetal movement by the mother or "quickening" usually is perceived by 18–22 weeks of gestation. The maternal perception of normal fetal movement as a sign of fetal well-being dates to antiquity, and diminished fetal movement often precedes fetal demise.

Because of the association between a decrease in the maternal perception of fetal movement and fetal demise, fetal counting protocols were designed. These protocols vary but generally define adequate fetal movement, and movement counts less than adequate constitutes an alarm. An abnormal result is followed by further evaluation with a nonstress test, biophysical profile, or contraction stress test, depending on the preference of the practitioner.

The "count to 10" method is a commonly employed method and appears to decrease the risk of fetal demise in a high-risk population. The mother is asked to lie down or sit in a quiet area and count the number of distinct fetal movements during a specified period of time daily. If 10 movements are not perceived in 2 hours, further testing is warranted. Once the mother has detected 10 movements, the count can be discontinued. Cumulatively, multiple studies have shown a decrease in the perinatal mortality rate using fetal movement counting.

The perception of fetal movement can be decreased by several factors, including maternal smoking, fetal abnormality, anterior placenta, and maternal medication use. The reliability of fetal movement counting has been varied, most likely due to various methods, poor instructions, varied abilities to perceive fetal movements among mothers, and poor maternal compliance. The rate of poor maternal compliance is disturbing, with up to 20% of women not performing the testing or falsifying records. Although the rate of false-positive results appears to be high, the simplicity, cost, and potential benefits appear to outweigh those risks, especially in pregnancies at high risk for stillbirth. The complete cessation of fetal movements is compelling and warrants immediate evaluation. Multiple reports of decreased fetal movement prompt continued fetal assessment.

American College of Obstetricians and Gynecologists. Antepartum fetal surveillance. ACOG Practice Bulletin 9. Washington, DC: ACOG; 1999.

Grant A, Elbourne D, Valentin L, Alexander S. Routine formal fetal movement counting and risk of antepartum late death in normally formed singletons. Lancet 1989;2:345–9.

Miller DA. Antepartum testing. Clin Obstet Gynecol 1998;41:647–53.

Moore T, Piacquadio K. A prospective evaluation of fetal movement screening to reduce the incidence of antepartum death. Am J Obstet Gynecol 1989;160:1075–80.

116

Eisenmenger syndrome

A 41-year-old primigravid woman comes to the office for her first prenatal visit. Ultrasonography performed a week earlier reveals a single live intrauterine pregnancy at 18 weeks of gestation. She feels well and her vital signs are normal. Her medical history reveals Eisenmenger syndrome found after evaluation for episodes of dyspnea on exertion. A maternal echocardiogram revealed a ventricular septal defect with a right-to-left shunt and marked pulmonary hypertension. The most likely time of acute worsening of right-to-left shunt is

    (A) in the first trimester
    (B) in the second stage of labor
*   (C) with epidural placement
    (D) in the first stage of labor
    (E) in the third stage of labor

Eisenmenger syndrome is a congenital heart defect that results from a long-standing uncorrected congenital heart defect, such as ventricular septal defect, atrial septal defect, or patent ductus arteriosus. As a result of the communication between the higher pressure system of the left and right sides of the heart, there is a left-to-right shunt of blood toward the pulmonary vasculature. The increase in pulmonary vasculature pressure leads to pulmonary hypertension and hypertrophy. Over time, pulmonary vascular hypertrophy worsens and increased right-sided ventricular pressure is necessary for perfusion. Increasing right-sided pressure will ultimately lead to shunt reversal to a right-to-left shunt, which results in the diagnosis of Eisenmenger syndrome. Most defects are detected and corrected in infancy and result in few of these women presenting with the condition at reproductive age. However, if the correction is late, pulmonary hypertension and irreversible vascular damage can still be present despite the repair.

Although successful pregnancies occur in women with Eisenmenger syndrome, the risk to the mother and fetus is substantial with maternal mortality rates reported to be as high as 70%. The physiologic changes associated with pregnancy can pose a significant risk to the mother and fetus. The normal decrease in systemic vascular resistance associated with pregnancy can create a worsening of the right-to-left shunt. This results in decreased pulmonary blood flow and a concomitant decrease in oxygenation. Women with Eisenmenger syndrome may tolerate the antepartum period relatively well.

Women with Eisenmenger syndrome tolerate acute systemic vascular hypotension poorly. This leads to a substantial right-to-left shunt and a profound decrease in pulmonary blood flow with resultant hypoxia that can lead to maternal cardiopulmonary arrest and death. The first and second stages of labor are tolerated fairly well. The greatest risk of hypotension is at the time of epidural anesthesia or blood loss at delivery. Epidural anesthesia can be used in women with Eisenmenger syndrome, but great care must be paid to appropriate hydration and to avoid hypotension. Women with the condition can tolerate the normal blood loss at delivery despite the potential decrease in plasma volume. However, postpartum hemorrhage and resultant hypotension is tolerated poorly. Efforts to avoid and treat postpartum hemorrhage are well spent. Because of these potential problems in women with Eisenmenger syndrome, the intrapartum period is the time of highest maternal mortality. Administration of oxygen, which acts as a pulmonary vascular dilator, and continuous electrocardiographic monitoring during labor should be considered for women with Eisenmenger syndrome. Some studies have reported benefits from administration of L-arginine, sildenafil, inhaled nitric oxide, and prostacyclin in pregnant women with the syndrome.

Antepartum, intrapartum, and postpartum management should be performed with a team of health care providers familiar with the challenges of Eisenmenger syndrome in pregnant women. Cesarean delivery is reserved for obstetric reasons, and elective induction of labor is often performed to assure that proper personnel are available. Intrauterine growth restriction, stillbirth, and premature birth occur at higher rates in women with Eisenmenger syndrome. Antepartum fetal monitoring, including serial ultrasonography and antenatal testing, should be used in caring for these patients.

Elkayam U, Gleicher N, editors. Cardiac problems in pregnancy. New York (NY): Wiley Liss; 1998. p. 49–50.

Gleicher N, Midwall J, Hochberger D, Jaffin H. Eisenmenger's syndrome and pregnancy. Obstet Gynecol Surv 1979;34:721–4.

Sciscione AC, Callan NA. Pregnancy and contraception. In: Skorton DJ, Garson A, editors. Cardiology clinics: congenital heart disease in adolescents and adults. Philadelphia (PA): WB Saunders; 1993. p. 701–9.

Yentis SM, Steer PJ, Plaat F. Eisenmenger's syndrome in pregnancy: maternal and fetal mortality in the 1990's. Br J Obstet Gynaecol 1998;105:921–2.

117

Ultrasonography to date pregnancy

A 28-year-old woman, gravida 2, para 1, comes to the office for her first prenatal visit. She gave birth to a healthy male infant 11 months ago and is still breastfeeding. Her gestational age based on her last menstrual period (LMP), which was heavier than usual, is consistent with 18 weeks of gestation. The bimanual pelvic examination revealed a 20-week irregularly shaped uterus. Your office ultrasound dating is consistent with 15 weeks and 2 days of gestation. Given the size and dates discrepancy between the LMP, ultrasound examination, and bimanual examination, the estimated day of delivery (EDD) should be based on

*   (A) ultrasonographic findings
      (B) last menstrual period
      (C) bimanual examination
      (D) average using the three findings
      (E) a scan in 3 weeks, then change dates if needed

Correct estimation of the gestational age is important for the optimal antenatal management of pregnancy. Ultrasonographic dating of the pregnancy has been shown to decrease the incidence of postdates inductions and the administration of tocolytics. The pregnancy is commonly dated using three different methods:

• The menstrual history, ie, the LMP

• The size of the uterus estimated during the clinical examination

• By ultrasonography

Estimating the gestational age based on LMP and clinical examination results in significant errors in assessing an accurate EDD. In many countries pregnancies are routinely dated by ultrasonography. Relying on the LMP to date the pregnancy often results in dating errors due to variation in the length of the cycle and day of ovulation. Moreover, it has been reported that 10–45% of the women cannot provide a reliable LMP due to many factors such as inability to recall the dates, irregular cycles, use of oral contraceptives, and bleeding during pregnancy. As many as 18% of women with a certain LMP have significant differences between LMP and ultrasound dating. A rate of postterm pregnancy of 5–14% has been reported when the LMP is used to calculate the EDD compared with 2.2–3.0% when ultrasound dating is used. Estimating the gestational age based on clinical examination is highly subjective and factors such as maternal body habitus, multiple pregnancy, leiomyomata, and a full bladder may result in wrong estimation of the dates.

The most accurate method to estimate gestational age is based on crown–rump length (CRL), which is measured during the first trimester of the pregnancy. The CRL dates the pregnancy within plus or minus 3–5 days. Second-trimester ultrasonography, routinely performed in many countries, has been found to be more accurate than the LMP (plus or minus 7–14 days) for predicting delivery date. During the third trimester, ultrasonographic estimation of the gestational age is highly variable because of individual variation in fetal size. The estimates of gestational age during the third trimester have confidence intervals of plus or minus 3 weeks. First-trimester ultrasonographic dating is the most accurate. As the pregnancy advances, the variability of gestational estimates increases using ultrasonography.

In a prospective study of a nonselected population of 15,241 women, ultrasonographic measurement of the biparietal diameter (BPD) between 15 and 22 weeks of gestation was significantly better than the LMP for predicting the EDD. In women with a reliable LMP and spontaneous onset of labor, the ultrasonographic estimate was a significantly better predictor of the day of delivery in 52% versus 46% for the LMP. Sixty-one percent of the women gave birth within 7 days of the predicted ultrasound EDD compared with 56% for the LMP. The proportion of postterm pregnancies was 4% when using ultrasound-derived EDD and 10% when using the LMP dating. In patients with a discrepancy between the LMP and ultrasound dating, ultrasonography was a better predictor of the day of delivery in the majority of the cases. When the discrepancy was 7 days or less, both ultrasonography and LMP were equally good. Investigators concluded that, in this situation, either method can be used. However, as the difference between the ultrasound dating and the LMP dating increased, ultrasonography performed better in predicting the EDD.

Bennett KA, Crane JM, O'Shea P, Lacelle J, Hutchens D, Copel JA. First trimester ultrasound screening is effective in reducing postterm labor induction rates: a randomized controlled trial. Am J Obstet Gynecol 2004;190:1077–81.

Chervenak FA, Skupski DW, Romero R, Myers MK, Smith-Levitin M, Rosenwaks Z, et al. How accurate is fetal biometry in the assessment of fetal age? Am J Obstet Gynecol 1998;178:678–87.

Geirsson RT. Ultrasound instead of last menstrual period as the basis of gestational age assignment. Ultrasound Obstet Gynecol 1991;1:212–9.

Jeanty P. Fetal biometry. In: Fleischer AC, Manning FA, Jeanty P, Romero R, editors. Sonography in obstetrics and gynecology: principles and practice. 6th ed. New York (NY): McGraw Hill; 2001. p. 139–56.

Mongelli M, Wilcox M, Gardosi J. Estimating the date of confinement: ultrasonographic biometry versus certain menstrual dates. Am J Obstet Gynecol 1996;174:278–81.

Tunon K, Eik-Nes SH, Grottum P. A comparison between ultrasound and a reliable last menstrual period as predictors of the day of delivery in 15,000 examinations. Ultrasound Obstet Gynecol 1996;8:178–85.

118

Elevated maternal serum alpha-fetoprotein level

A 35-year-old woman, gravida 2, para 1, is seen in your office for a visit at 20 weeks of gestation for routine prenatal care. Her antenatal course has been remarkable for a maternal serum alpha-fetoprotein level of 4.2 multiples of the median (MoM). A fetal anatomic survey showed a single live fetus at 20 weeks of gestation with no evidence of a neural tube defect or other gross structural anomalies. Results of an amniocentesis showed a normal fetal karyotype with normal amniotic fluid alpha-fetoprotein and no acetylcholinesterase. The condition for which this patient is most at risk is

* (A) intrauterine growth restriction
  (B) gestational diabetes mellitus
  (C) postterm pregnancy
  (D) hydramnios
  (E) breech presentation

In the United States, all pregnant women are routinely offered screening with maternal serum alpha fetoprotein (MSAFP) for neural tube defects (NTDs) at 15–20 weeks of gestation, unless they are planning to have an amniocentesis, in which case the amniotic fluid AFP will be tested. An abnormal or elevated value is defined as one that exceeds 2–2.5 MoM. Elevated levels of MSAFP occur in approximately 3% of pregnant women. In approximately two thirds of women, an etiology for the elevated level can be found during ultrasonography. For the rest of the patients, or approximately 1% of the overall obstetric patient population, the elevated level of MSAFP will remain unexplained. The mechanism of action of the increased levels appears to be related to placental "malfunction" or a disruption at the fetal maternal interface, and thus allowing a transfer of AFP into the maternal circulation.

Alpha-fetoprotein is a glycoprotein that is initially synthesized in the embryonic yolk sac and subsequently by the fetal liver and gastrointestinal tract. The molecule enters the amniotic fluid via fetal urination, gastrointestinal tract secretions, and transudation from exposed blood vessels. It enters the maternal circulation by either diffusion across the placenta or by diffusion across the amnion.

Neural tube defects (NTDs) and other structural anomalies are associated with elevated MSAFP. Among low-risk women, MSAFP screening results in the detection of 80–90% of cases of fetal open NTDs. However, wrong dates and multiple pregnancies are the most common etiologies for the elevated value.

The initial workup for an elevated MSAFP is genetic counseling and ultrasonography. The purpose of the ultrasonographic scan is to document fetal life and number of fetuses, confirm gestational age, and exclude fetal structural defects such as NTDs (anencephaly, encephalocele, and spina bifida) or abdominal wall defects (omphalocele, gastroschisis). The sensitivity for the ultrasonographic diagnosis of NTDs in experienced hands is excellent. For example, the sensitivity for anencephaly has been reported to be 100% and the overall sensitivity for the detection of NTDs to be 97% with a specificity of 100%. The role of amniocentesis in these cases needs to be individualized and the risks and benefits discussed with the patient. Elevated levels of amniotic fluid AFP together with elevated acetylcholinesterase are considered to be diagnostic for open fetal NTD. Acetylcholinesterase has been reported to be positive in 100% of cases of anencephaly and open spina bifida and in 20%

of cases of ventral wall defects, with a false-positive rate of 2.2 in 1,000 amniocenteses. In general, amniocentesis is reserved for use when key structures are inadequate.

Researchers have documented the association between unexplained elevated levels of MSAFP and poor obstetric outcomes, such as intrauterine fetal death, low birth weight, growth restriction, preterm birth, preeclampsia, oligohydramnios, and abruptio placentae. Generally, the higher the level of MSAFP, the higher the risk of pregnancy complications. In a recent study of 14,374 high- and low-risk women screened with both MSAFP and hCG, the results showed that unexplained elevated levels of MSAFP are associated with an increased risk of pregnancy complications in both high- and low-risk women (Table 118-1).

TABLE 118-1. Univariate Analysis of Unexplained Elevated Alpha Fetoprotein* and the Risk of Adverse Outcomes[†]

Outcomes	Relative Risk
Pregnancy-induced hypertension	1.4
Abruptio placentae	3.5
Intrauterine growth restriction	3.1
Fetal death	9.1
Preterm birth	4.5
Spontaneous preterm birth or premature rupture of the membranes	3.6

*Greater than 4.2 multiples of the median (MoM).

[†]Study group, 5,789 high-risk women and 8,585 low-risk women.

Modified from Chandra S, Scott H, Dodds L, Watts C, Blight C, Van Den Hof M. Unexplained elevated maternal serum alpha fetoprotein and/or human chorionic gonadotropin and the risk of adverse outcomes. Am J Obstet Gynecol 2003;189:777.

At present, the need for antenatal surveillance as well as the optimal time for initiating the testing remains controversial. Elevated MSAFP is not associated with gestational diabetes mellitus, postterm pregnancy, hydramnios, and breech presentation.

Alkazaleh F, Chaddha V, Viero S, Malik A, Anastasiades C, Sroka H, et al. Second-trimester prediction of severe placental complications in women with combined elevations in alpha fetoprotein and human chorionic gonadotrophin. Am J Obstet Gynecol 2006;194:821–7.

Chandra S, Scott H, Dodds L, Watts C, Blight C, Van Den Hof M. Unexplained elevated maternal serum alpha fetoprotein and/or human chorionic gonadotropin and the risk of adverse outcomes. Am J Obstet Gynecol 2003;189:775–81.

Neural tube defects. ACOG Practice Bulletin No. 44. American College of Obstetricians and Gynecologists. Obstet Gynecol 2003;102:203–13.

Wilkins-Haug L. Unexplained elevated maternal serum alpha fetoprotein: what is the appropriate follow-up? Curr Opin Obstet Gynecol 1998;10:469–74.

119

Pulmonary embolism

A healthy primigravid woman complains of the acute onset of chest pain. An imaging study has confirmed the presence of a pulmonary embolism. Unfractionated heparin is chosen for treatment. The most important benefit of shortening the interval of time from diagnosis to achieving a therapeutic anticoagulation level is avoidance of

* (A) recurrent embolization
* (B) thrombocytopenia
* (C) osteoporosis
* (D) formation of retroplacental hematoma

Thromboembolic complications of pregnancy remain among the top three causes of maternal mortality. A high index of suspicion and the use of appropriate diagnostic procedures often leads to the correct diagnosis. The challenge for the clinician, after making the diagnosis, is to prevent the occurrence of another embolism by timely and prompt establishment of appropriate anticoagulation.

The importance of achieving the therapeutic range within 24 hours according to the activated partial thromboplastin time (aPTT) is well documented. Failure to promptly achieve a therapeutic aPTT level in patients with venous thromboembolism treated with unfractionated heparin was associated with a statistically significant and clinically important increase in the risk of subsequent recurrent thromboembolism. The rate of recurrence was three times lower in patients who achieved the therapeutic aPTT threshold within the first 24 hours of therapy than in those who did not.

Heparin constitutes the cornerstone of management. It accelerates the action of antithrombin III, thereby preventing an additional thrombus from forming and permitting endogenous fibrinolysis to dissolve some of the clot. Initial therapy with an oral anticoagulant and no heparin may paradoxically intensify hypercoagulability and increase the frequency of recurrent venous thromboembolism. In the absence of overt contraindications, such as active gastrointestinal hemorrhage, patients with a moderate or high clinical likelihood of pulmonary embolism should receive intensive anticoagulation with heparin during the diagnostic workup. The use of heparin nomograms facilitates proper dosing.

Heparin-induced thrombocytopenia is a syndrome of antibody-mediated thrombocytopenia that paradoxically is often associated with thrombosis. Most patients with this disorder produce immunoglobulin G (IgG) antibodies against complexes of platelet factor 4 and heparin. Typically, heparin-induced thrombocytopenia begins with the appearance of thrombocytopenia about a week after the start of heparin therapy. Occasionally, a more rapid decrease in the platelet count occurs if the patient has previously been treated with heparin. The rapidity of achieving full anticoagulation is not associated with more rapid onset of thrombocytopenia.

Heparin causes bone loss in some patients after long-term use in pregnancy. Both the phalangeal-cortical area ratio and spine and hip X-ray studies have been reported to be statistically significantly altered by long-term therapy (more than 25 weeks) in pregnant patients who receive 20,000 U per day versus those who receive less than 7 weeks of therapy. Nearly half the women were reexamined 6–12 months postpartum, and the changes were reversible in most cases. No correlation was found between degree of bone loss and rapidity of heparin dosing. Unfractionated heparin has a high molecular weight, which precludes transplacental transfer. It will not cause a retroplacental hematoma.

Barbour LA, Kick SD, Steiner JF, LoVerde ME, Heddleston LN, Lear JL, et al. A prospective study of heparin-induced osteoporosis in pregnancy using bone densitometry. Am J Obstet Gynecol 1994;170:862–9.

Goldhaber SZ. Pulmonary embolism. N Engl J Med 1998;339:93–104.

Hull RD, Raskob GE, Brant RF, Pineo GF, Valentine KA. The importance of initial heparin treatment on long-term clinical outcomes of antithrombotic therapy. The emerging scene of delayed recurrence. Arch Intern Med 1997;157:2317–21.

Hull RD, Raskob GE, Brant RF, Pineo GF, Valentine KA. Relation between the time to achieve the lower limit of APTT therapeutic range and recurrent venous thromboembolism during heparin treatment for deep vein thrombosis. Arch Intern Med 1997;157:2562–8.

Warkentin TE, Kelton JG. Temporal aspects of heparin-induced thrombocytopenia. N Engl J Med 2001;344:1286–92.

120

Syphilis

A 19-year-old asymptomatic woman at 9 weeks of gestation had an initial obstetric examination and prenatal laboratory panel 1 week ago. The nonspecific antitreponemal antibody test result was reactive with a titer of 1:2. The specific antitreponemal antibody test was reactive. The remainder of the laboratory panel test results was normal, and a human immunodeficiency virus (HIV) test result was negative. The patient has no systemic complaints, has no prior testing for syphilis, and has normal physical and pelvic examinations. The next step in management is

* (A) benzathine penicillin for three doses
   (B) ceftriaxone
   (C) tetracycline
   (D) erythromycin

Although the incidence of syphilis in the United States has decreased, this infection remains a public health problem. Increased rates of syphilis are linked to substance abuse and inadequate prenatal care. Syphilis is a systemic infection caused by *Treponema pallidum*, a spirochete that can readily cross the placenta and result in congenital syphilis. Several adverse outcomes are associated with congenital syphilis infection, including preterm labor, preterm birth, fetal death, and neonatal infection by transplacental or perinatal infection. The fetus usually does not manifest an inflammatory response before 18 weeks of gestation. Ultrasonographic findings of a progressive congenital infection follow a continuous course with hepatic involvement, followed by anemia, thrombocytopenia, and then ascites and hydrops fetalis.

Syphilis is a disease that progresses to different stages if untreated. Stages of early syphilis include primary (painless chancre), secondary (generalized maculopapular rash on palms and soles and mucocutaneous lesions), and early latent syphilis of less than 1 year's duration (asymptomatic). Latent syphilis exhibits no pertinent findings on physical examination but shows serology consistent with the diagnosis. Late latent syphilis is the classification applied to infection occurring more than 1 year after initial infection or if the time of initial infection is unknown. Tertiary syphilis typically presents with signs of cardiovascular system involvement (aortitis, gumma). Patients with neurosyphilis have clinical evidence of central nervous system involvement, which may include cognitive dysfunction, motor or sensory deficits, ophthalmic (iritis, uveitis) or auditory symptoms, cranial nerve palsies, and symptoms of meningitis.

Screening for syphilis usually is performed at the first prenatal visit and repeated at the time of delivery. In high-risk groups, a third test may be performed in the third trimester. Nonspecific tests for syphilis include the Venereal Disease Research Laboratory (VDRL) test, rapid

plasma reagin (RPR) test, or automated reagin test (ART). Results of the nonspecific tests are reported as a quantitative titer reflecting disease activity. False-positive results often accompany autoimmune disorders such as with the presence of anticardiolipin antibodies. Specific treponemal tests include the fluorescent treponemal antibody absorption test, microhemagglutination assay for antibodies to *T pallidum* (MHA-TP), and *T pallidum* passive particle agglutination test. A positive result from any of these tests almost always confirms the diagnosis of syphilis.

Penicillin G, administered parenterally, is the treatment of choice for all stages of syphilis. The type of penicillin (ie, benzathine, procaine, or aqueous crystalline), the dosage, and the length of therapy are determined by the stage and clinical manifestations of the disease. Other options exist for treatment of syphilis in the nonpregnant population, but penicillin G is the only proven therapy for the prevention of congenital syphilis. Medications such as erythromycin adequately treat the mother but may not adequately treat the fetus. Ceftriaxone and azithromycin have been used in penicillin-sensitive adults, but their efficacy in pregnancy has not been adequately evaluated. Tetracyclines are effective in treating syphilis but are not recommended in pregnancy because of the risk of tooth discoloration in the fetus. For patients with a reported allergy to penicillin, skin testing should be performed to confirm an allergy. If an allergy is confirmed, oral penicillin desensitization followed by administration of penicillin is the recommended treatment (Table 120-1).

A recommended treatment regimen for pregnant women with syphilis is shown in Table 120-2. One dose of benzathine penicillin G is recommended for early syphilis if the infection can be documented to have occurred within the past year. Treatment failures may occur more frequently in pregnant patients with secondary syphilis, and a second dose of benzathine penicillin G 1 week after the initial dose is recommended by some

TABLE 120-1. Oral Penicillin Desensitization Protocol

Dose*	Penicillin V Suspension (units/mL)	Amount† (mL)	Amount (units)	Cumulative Dose (units)
1	1,000	0.1	100	100
2	1,000	0.2	200	300
3	1,000	0.4	400	700
4	1,000	0.8	800	1,500
5	1,000	1.6	1,600	3,100
6	1,000	3.2	3,200	6,300
7	1,000	6.4	6,400	12,700
8	10,000	1.2	12,000	24,700
9	10,000	2.4	24,700	48,700
10	10,000	4.8	48,000	96,700
11	80,000	1.0	80,000	176,000
12	80,000	2.4	164,000	336,700
13	80,000	4.8	320,000	656,700
14	80,000	8.0	640,000	1,296,700

After desensitization, patients are observed for 30 minutes before parenteral injection of benzathine penicillin. Patients who have been desensitized previously, have received benzathine intramuscularly, and are returning for their second shot do not require additional desensitization. Although desensitization is usually lost within 2 days of terminating the penicillin therapy, long-acting benzathine penicillin will sustain the sensitized state for periods of up to 3 weeks.

*Interval between doses: 15 minutes; elapsed time: 3 hours and 45 minutes; cumulative dose: 1.3 million units.

†The specific amount of drug is diluted in approximately 30 mL of water and then given orally.

Modified from Wendel GD Jr, Stark BJ, Jamison RB, Molina RD, Sullivan TJ. Penicillin allergy and desensitization in serious infections during pregnancy. N Engl J Med 1985;312:1229–32. Copyright 1985 by the Massachusetts Medical Society.

TABLE 120-2. Recommended Treatment for Pregnant Women With Syphilis

Category	Treatment
Early syphilis*	Benzathine penicillin G, 2.4 million units intramuscularly as a single injection; some recommend a second dose 1 week later
More than 1 year's duration†	Benzathine penicillin G, 2.4 million units intramuscularly weekly for three doses
Neurosyphilis‡	Aqueous crystalline penicillin G, 18 million–24 million units per day, administered as 3–4 million units intravenously every 4 hours or continuous infusion, for 10–14 days
	Or
	Procaine penicillin, 2.4 million units intramuscularly once daily, plus Probenecid 500 mg orally four times daily, both for 10–14 days

*Primary, secondary, and latent syphilis of less than 1 year duration.

†Latent syphilis of unknown or more than 1 year duration; tertiary syphilis.

‡Some recommend benzathine penicillin, 2.4 million units intramuscularly after completion of the neurosyphilis treatment regimens.

Workowski KA, Berman SM. Sexually transmitted disease treatment guidelines 2006. Centers for Disease Control and Prevention. MMWR Recomm Rep 2006;55(RR-11):26–7.

experts. A second dose is also considered for women initially treated in the third trimester. Syphilis infection of more that 1 year's duration or of unknown duration is treated with benzathine penicillin G given in weekly injections for 3 weeks. Antibody titers correlate with disease activity, and therapeutic response is documented by serial titers that should fall fourfold or decrease by two dilutions (eg, 1:16 to 1:4) within 6 months. If titers rise fourfold or do not fall appropriately, a new infection or treatment failure should be suspected. Pregnant women with diagnosed syphilis should be tested for HIV infection and other sexually transmitted diseases.

The patient in this scenario has latent syphilis of unknown duration and requires weekly injections of benzathine penicillin G for adequate treatment. Ceftriaxone would not provide adequate coverage. Intravenous aqueous crystalline penicillin G for 10 to 14 days is the treatment for neurosyphilis. Daily injections of procaine penicillin is an alternate treatment for neurosyphilis and

is administered with oral probenecid for 10 to 14 days course. Erythromycin may adequately treat the maternal infection, but it may not prevent congenital syphilis because it does not adequately cross the placenta and is not recommended as an alternative to penicillin treatment in pregnancy.

American Academy of Pediatrics and American College of Obstetricians and Gynecologists. Guidelines for perinatal care. 6th ed. Elk Grove Village (IL): AAP; Washington, DC: ACOG; 2007. p. 339–343.

Hollier LM, Workowski K. Treatment of sexually transmitted infections in pregnancy. Clin Perinatol 2005;32:629–56.

Workowski KA, Berman SM. Sexually transmitted disease treatment guidelines 2006. Centers for Disease Control and Prevention [published erratum appears in MMWR Morb Mortal Wkly Rep 2006;55:997]. MMWR Recomm Rep 2006;55(RR-11):1–94.

Wendel GD Jr, Stark BJ, Jamison RB, Molina RD, Sullivan TJ. Penicillin allergy and desensitization in serious infections during pregnancy. N Engl J Med 1985;312:1229–32.

Sexually transmitted diseases. In: Cunningham FG, Leveno KJ, Bloom SL, Hauth JC, Gilstrap LC 3rd, Wenstrom KD, editors. Williams obstetrics. 22nd ed. New York (NY): McGraw-Hill; 2005. p. 1301–25.

121

Postpartum hemorrhage

A 24-year-old primigravid woman experiences heavy vaginal bleeding secondary to uterine atony after a vaginal delivery. She is given intravenous oxytocin, intramuscular methylergonovine maleate (Methergine), rectal misoprostol, and intramyometrial 15-methyl-prostaglandin alpha. Bimanual compression has been attempted with no success. The best next step in her care is

   (A) bilateral uterine artery ligation
   (B) selective arterial embolization
   (C) B-Lynch suture
   (D) abdominal hysterectomy
 * (E) uterine packing or tamponade

This patient has persistent postpartum hemorrhage and medical therapy has failed to stop it. Uterine hemorrhage is one of the major causes of maternal mortality worldwide, and uterine atony is the most common cause. Irreversible hemorrhagic shock can occur with intractable bleeding; thus, urgent intervention is required. Surgical management is indicated when medical therapy fails. Abdominal hysterectomy is expeditious and definitive therapy, and it should be reserved for failed conservative measures or for patients rapidly deteriorating with hemodynamic instability.

In urgent situations, especially when a laparotomy has not been performed, intrauterine tamponade may be useful and is associated with good results. Intrauterine tamponade can be achieved by packing the uterine cavity

with gauze or by inflating saline-filled balloons inside the uterine cavity (ie, Rusch balloon or the SOS Bakri tamponade balloon [Fig. 121-1]). It should be considered in patients who are poor risks for surgery, for whom other methods are not available, or when there is a strong desire to conserve the uterus. For the patient described who has a vaginal delivery, if successful, uterine packing may eliminate the need for an operative procedure. Intrauterine tamponade may be left in place until the patient is stable or requires further therapeutic measures. It is important to monitor the patient for symptoms and signs of continuous bleeding or decompensation and to proceed to an operative procedure if indicated.

Bilateral internal iliac (hypogastric) artery ligation (Fig. 121-2) is useful in the management of intraoperative

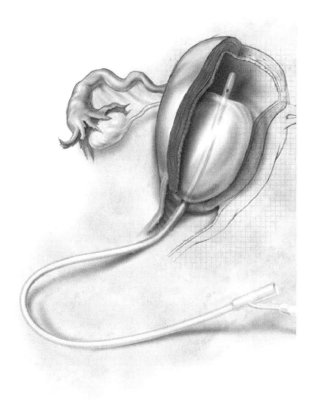

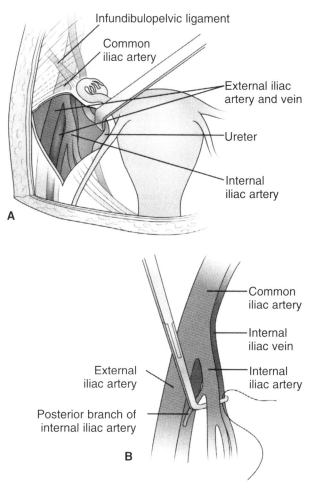

FIG. 121-1. Tamponade balloon SOS Bakri. (Illustration courtesy of Cook Medical, Bloomington, IN.)

FIG. 121-2. Operative technique of internal iliac ligation. **A.** The retroperitoneal space over the right internal and external iliac vessels has been opened and the ureter retracted medially. **B.** A right-angled clamp is passed between the iliac artery and vein to receive a ligature of number 0 silk. The vessel should be doubly ligated. (Rogers MS, Chang AM. Postpartum hemorrhage and other problems of the third stage. In: James DK, Steer PJ, Weiner CP, Gonik B, editors. High risk pregnancy. 3rd ed. Saunders Elsevier; 2005. p. 1568. Copyright 2005 by Elsevier.)

intractable bleeding during pelvic surgery and obstetric hemorrhage. It can be lifesaving and may preserve the uterus. Full-term pregnancies have been reported after bilateral internal iliac artery ligation. Bleeding from the uterus decreases because the ligation ensures that there is no arterial pressure or pulsation in the arteries. There are both vertical and horizontal anastomoses in the pelvic cavity. The vertical anastomoses, which comprise the iliolumbar, lateral sacral, uterine, and middle rectal arteries, is activated on bilateral internal iliac artery ligation. Injury to the ureters (in as high as 20% of patients) and other structures can occur. The procedure should be performed by those who have the necessary expertise, is technically more difficult in pregnancy and has a poor success rate (less than 50% success). In a recent review of 37 obstetric cases, the uterus was saved in 13 cases (35%).

Bilateral uterine artery ligation (Appendix J) was proposed as an alternative to bilateral internal iliac artery ligation. Reported success rates for this procedure vary between 80% and 100%. Bilateral uterine artery ligation is technically easier and safer to perform than internal iliac artery ligation. Uterine artery ligation may be used to control persistent severe hemorrhage after failed medical therapy. In cases in which bilateral uterine artery ligation is unsuccessful, proceeding to ligation of the uterine–ovarian anastomosis medial to the ovary (Fig. 121-3) is

recommended. A stepwise procedure with progressive ligation of the uterine and ovarian arteries may be an alternative to embolization and hysterectomy.

Arterial embolization requires fluoroscopy, correct arterial catheters, embolic materials, and a radiologist experienced in angiographic and interventional skills. It is usually performed in the angiography suite and requires 1–2 hours. Femoral artery puncture and bilateral internal iliac artery catheterization is performed. Angiography is used to identify bleeding sites. Embolization is usually performed with the use of gelatin pads (Gelfoam pledgets), which cause temporary occlusion for approximately 4 weeks. Uterine artery embolization is indicated in postpartum hemorrhage refractory to medication. Before elective cesarean delivery in cases in which profuse bleeding is anticipated, catheters may be placed to facilitate subsequent embolization. Limited data have yielded a success rate of 80–95% with 50% of failed cases caused by abnormal placentation. The overall complication rate reported in the literature is approximately 6–9%. Complications may occur as a result of inadvertent embolization of adjacent vessels. Bladder, rectum, genital tract, and lower limb necroses have been reported and are more common if permanent vascular occlusion (polyvinyl alcohol) particles are used. Ovarian failure, as a possible sequela of ovarian vascular compromise, also has been reported. For ongoing hemorrhage, arterial embolization may take too long and is likely to increase net blood loss.

Uterine compression sutures running through the full thickness of both uterine walls have been used for the sur-

gical management of postpartum hemorrhage due to atony. The B-Lynch suture (Fig. 121-4), introduced in 1997, is one of a number of uterine compression techniques that have been described. The suture exerts continuous vertical vascular compression. Cessation of bleeding by bimanual uterine compression predicts a high likelihood that application of the suture will stop the hemorrhage. The procedure is simple and inexpensive and has a high success rate. No major complications have been noted, but recently uterine necrosis that required hysterectomy has been reported.

Recombinant factor VIIa has been found to be an effective hemostatic agent in patients with life-threatening postpartum hemorrhage unresponsive to conventional methods.

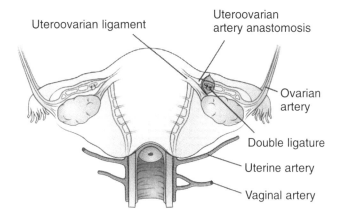

FIG. 121-3. Area for ovarian artery ligation. The vesicouterine fold of peritoneum has been incised transversely and the bladder mobilized inferiorly. A number 1 chromic catgut suture on a large smooth needle has been placed through the avascular space of the broad ligament and through the uterus. The suture includes the uterine vessels and several centimeters of myometrium. (Rogers MS, Chang AM. Postpartum hemorrhage and other problems of the third stage. In: James DK, Steer PJ, Weiner CP, Gonik B, editors. High risk pregnancy. 3rd ed. Saunders Elsevier; 2005. p. 1568. Copyright 2005 by Elsevier.)

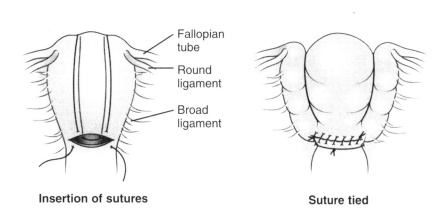

FIG. 121-4. B-Lynch suture for the control of massive postpartum hemorrhage. (Rogers MS, Chang AM. Postpartum hemorrhage and other problems of the third stage. In: James DK, Steer PJ, Weiner CP, Gonik B, editors. High risk pregnancy. 3rd ed. Saunders Elsevier; 2005. p. 1568. Copyright 2005 by Elsevier. Reproduced by permission of Christopher B-Lynch, MD)

Allam MS, B-Lynch C. The B-Lynch and other uterine compression suture techniques. Int J Gynaecol Obstet 2005;89:236–41.

Bouwmeester FW, Jonkhoff AR, Verheijen RH, van Geijn HP. Successful treatment of life threatening postpartum hemorrhage with recombinant activated factor VII. Obstet Gynecol 2003;101:1174–6.

Chou YJ, Cheng YF, Shen CC, Hsu TY, Chang AY, Kung FT. Failure of uterine arterial embolization: placenta accreta with profuse postpartum hemorrhage. Acta Obstet Gynecol Scand 2004;83:688–90.

Ojala K, Perala J, Kariniemi J, Ranta, Raudaskoski T, Tekay A. Arterial embolization and prophylactic catheterization for the treatment of severe obstetric hemorrhage. Acta Obstet Gynecol Scand 2005;84: 1075–80.

Papp Z, Toth-Pal E, Papp C, Sziller I, Gavai M, Silhavy M, et al. Hypogastric artery ligation for intractable pelvic hemorrhage. Int J Gynaecol Obstet 2006;92:27–31.

Treloar EJ, Anderson RS, Andrew HS, Bailey JL. Uterine necrosis following B-Lynch suture for primary postpartum haemorrhage. BJOG 2006;113:486–8.

Verspyck E, Resch B, Sergent F, Marpeau L. Surgical uterine devascularization for placenta accreta: immediate and long term follow-up. Acta Obstet Gynecol Scand 2005;84:444–7.

122

Amnioinfusion

A 25-year-old woman, gravida 1, at 39 weeks of gestation, presents in labor. Her cervix is 4 cm dilated and she has regular uterine contractions every 2 minutes. Two hours after admission, she has spontaneous rupture of membranes, and thick meconium staining is noticed. Transcervical amnioinfusion may be effective in the management of

      (A) early decelerations

*   (B) variable decelerations

      (C) late decelerations

      (D) bradycardia

      (E) absence of variability

Fetal passage of meconium is common (12%) and usually happens after 34 weeks of gestation. In a minority of cases, the association of meconium with fetal hypoxia may be secondary to fetal hypoxic stress, which may stimulate colonic activity and fetal gasping leading to meconium aspiration. Therefore, meconium may not be causative but only associated with fetal hypoxia and its complications.

Transcervical amnioinfusion has been advocated as a technique to reduce the incidence of meconium aspiration and to improve neonatal outcome. In a meta-analysis, amnioinfusion for meconium is associated with a 38% decrease in meconium aspiration syndrome and a trend for a 49% decrease in perinatal mortality. However, these cumulative beneficial results stem from many small studies. The largest trial, larger than all other studies combined, did not show any benefit or detriment from this intervention. This may be because meconium passage may predate labor. Because of this cumulative evidence, routine prophylactic use of transcervical amnioinfusion for the dilution of meconium-stained amniotic fluid is not recommended.

In the presence of a fetal heart rate abnormality, such as recurrent variable decelerations (usually with preceding oligohydramnios), transcervical amnioinfusion to relieve cord compression may be effective. Randomized trials have shown that transcervical amnioinfusion in women with variable decelerations, with or without meconium staining of amniotic fluid, significantly reduces the rate of persistent variable decelerations, cesarean delivery for suspected nonreassuring fetal heart rate, and overall cesarean delivery, compared to no treatment. The incidences of both umbilical arterial pH less than 7.20 and postpartum endometritis are decreased.

Amnioinfusion has not been shown to be beneficial in pregnancies with early decelerations, late decelerations, bradycardia, or absent variability. It is important to be able to recognize these patterns in fetal heart monitoring. Appendix B shows the National Institute of Child Health and Human Development Research Planning definitions of fetal heart rate patterns. Late decelerations and absent variability represent nonreassuring fetal status, and amnioinfusion not only has not been shown to be effective but would also delay effective interventions.

Numerous variations of the amnioinfusion technique exist, but a "typical" protocol calls for infusion via an intrauterine pressure catheter in a woman with dilated cervix and ruptured membranes by bolus or continuous infusion technique, with similar ability to relieve recurrent variable decelerations. Neither pumps nor warmers are necessary with amnioinfusion. In fact, the use of an infusion pump during amnioinfusion significantly increases the risk of fetal nonreassuring status. Either lactated Ringer's solution or normal saline can be used to place a crystalloid solution into the uterus without altering the neonatal electrolyte balance. Amnioinfusion has been associated with several complications, but these can be minimized with proper technique.

Oropharyngeal and nasopharyngeal suctioning before delivery of the shoulder does not decrease the incidence of meconium aspiration syndrome, the need for mechanical ventilation for meconium aspiration syndrome, other associated morbidities, or neonatal mortality. Therefore, suctioning of meconium before delivery of the shoulder is no longer recommended.

Fraser WD, Hofmeyr J, Lede R, Faron G, Alexander S, Goffinet F, et al. Amnioinfusion for the prevention of the meconium aspiration syndrome. Amnioinfusion Trial Group. N Engl J Med 2005;353:909–17.

Hofmeyr GJ. Amnioinfusion for meconium-stained liquor in labour. Cochrane Database of Systematic Reviews 2002, Issue 1. Art. No.: CD000014. DOI: 10.1002/14651858.CD000014.

Hofmeyr GJ. Amnioinfusion for potential or suspected umbilical cord compression in labour. Cochrane Database of Systematic Reviews 1998, Issue 1. Art. No.: CD000013. DOI: 10.1002/14651858. CD000013.

Electronic fetal heart rate monitoring: research guidelines for interpretation. National Institute of Child Health and Human Development Research Planning Workshop. Am J Obstet Gynecol 1997;177:1385–90.

Vain NE, Szyld EG, Prudent LM, Wiswell TE, Aguilar AM, Vivas NI. Oropharyngeal and nasopharyngeal suctioning of meconium-stained neonates before delivery of their shoulders: multicentre, randomised controlled trial. Lancet 2004;364:597–602.

123

Immunization in pregnancy

A pregnant patient at 15 weeks of gestation informs you that she must travel to Venezuela to care for her dying mother. She inquires what vaccinations she may need and their safety in pregnancy. You learn that Venezuela is within the yellow fever endemic zone. You inform her that the use of this live-attenuated vaccination in pregnancy is

(A) absolutely contraindicated
(B) safe only in the third trimester
(C) indicated only in the immunocompromised patient
* (D) indicated when traveling to a known endemic area
(E) associated with a high risk of fetal malformations

Yellow fever is a mosquito-transmitted viral infection that occurs only in Africa and South America. Infected individuals will demonstrate symptoms ranging from that of an influenzalike syndrome to severe hepatitis and hemorrhagic fever. The risk of acquiring yellow fever is determined by factors such as immunization status, location of travel, season, duration of exposure, and the local rate of yellow fever virus transmission at the time of travel. The risk of death due to yellow fever in an unvaccinated traveler in endemic areas in Africa is estimated to be 1 in 5,000 per month. Although this risk is reported to be 10 times lower for South American travelers, four of the five fatalities reported among travelers from the United States and Europe in 1996–2002 were in travelers exposed in South America. All five cases occurred among unvaccinated travelers. With the ever-growing immigrant population in the United States, travel to endemic disease areas during pregnancy will likely continue to increase. Close attention to and compliance with vaccination requirements for travel to endemic areas are critical. Updated health information for international travelers and listings for authorized U.S. vaccination centers is available from the Centers for Disease Control and Prevention (CDC) through their web site, http://www.cdc.gov/travel/yb.

The yellow fever vaccine is a live, attenuated virus preparation made from the 17D yellow fever virus strain. Historically, the YF17D vaccine, manufactured under approval by the World Health Organization to meet international vaccination criteria, has been considered one of the safest and most effective live virus vaccines ever developed. The risks to a fetus of immunization with any live, attenuated virus vaccine such as the vaccine for measles, mumps, rubella, poliomyelitis, varicella, and yellow fever are essentially unknown. As such, most live virus vaccines are relatively but not absolutely contraindicated in pregnancy. If the risk of exposure to the disease is high, the benefits of immunization to the pregnant woman and her neonate usually outweigh the theoretic risks of adverse effects.

There are two reported studies cited by the CDC with a combined total of 81 infants born to mothers vaccinated during pregnancy with YF17D. Of the fetuses exposed to the YF17D vaccine, infection occurred in 1 of 81, and there were no associated congenital anomalies reported. Another case–control study reported a relative risk for spontaneous abortion of 2.3 (95% confidence interval 0.65–8.03, not significant) among women vaccinated with YF17D during early pregnancy. Information from limited clinical trials in Africa and Europe indicates that the risk from vaccination for pregnant women who cannot avoid mosquito exposure in yellow fever endemic areas is outweighed by the risk for yellow fever infection.

The CDC recommends that the yellow fever vaccine be administered during pregnancy only if travel to an endemic area is unavoidable and if an increased risk for exposure exists. Therefore, pregnant women who must travel to areas where the risk for yellow fever infection is high should be vaccinated. Because the seroconversion rate after vaccination of a pregnant woman may be significantly lower than that in other healthy nonpregnant adults, serologic testing to document an appropriate immune response should be considered when used in pregnancy. If possible, postponement of travel is preferable to vaccination because of the unknown risk. However, vaccination of infants younger than 9 months is not recommended because of the risk for encephalitis.

Therefore, although postponement of the trip to avoid vaccination during pregnancy may be theoretically safer for the fetus, travel with a newborn to such endemic areas would potentially be more dangerous in light of the vaccine being contraindicated during this time. Despite the apparent safety of this vaccine, because so little is known about its effects in pregnancy, infants born to women vaccinated during pregnancy should be monitored closely for evidence of congenital infection and other possible adverse effects resulting from yellow fever vaccination.

Administration of a live-attenuated vaccine in pregnancy when indicated can be performed in any trimester. Administration during pregnancy is not an indication for pregnancy termination. The safety profile of the yellow fever vaccination on the basis of gestational age of pregnancy is not known. Administration of a live-attenuated virus vaccine like the yellow fever vaccine generally is contraindicated in the immunocompromised patient.

Centers for Disease Control and Prevention. Health information for international travel, 2005–2006. Atlanta (GA): U.S. Department of Health and Human Services, Public Health Service; 2005.

Cetron MS, Marfin AA, Julian KG, Gubler DJ, Sharp DJ, Barwick RS, et al. Yellow fever vaccine. Recommendations of the Advisory Committee on Immunization Practices (ACIP), 2002. MMWR Recomm Rep 2002;51(RR-17):1–11; quiz CE1–4.

Immunization during pregnancy. ACOG Committee Opinion No. 282. American College of Obstetricians and Gynecologists. Obstet Gynecol 2003;101:207–12.

Nasidi A, Monath TP, Vandenberg J, Tomori O, Calisher CH, Hurtgen X, et al. Yellow fever vaccination and pregnancy: a four-year prospective study. Trans R Soc Trop Med Hyg 1993;87:337–9.

Nishioka Sde A, Nunes-Araujo FR, Pires WP, Silva FA, Costa HL. Yellow fever vaccination during pregnancy and spontaneous abortion: a case-control study. Trop Med Int Health 1998;3:29–33.

Tsai TF, Paul R, Lynberg MC, Letson GW. Congenital yellow fever virus infection after immunization in pregnancy. J Infect Dis 1993;168:1520–3.

124

Glucose-6-phosphate dehydrogenase deficiency

One week after treatment for a urinary tract infection with nitrofurantoin, a 19-year-old woman of Mediterranean descent returns to your office because she has been feeling weak, dizzy, and light headed, and she has back pain. She is at 22 weeks of gestation, and, on questioning, she recalls that she was instructed as a child to avoid eating fava beans. A complete blood count was sent, and the hemoglobin level was 6.0 g/dL. The test that is most diagnostic is to obtain a

* (A) glucose-6-phosphate dehydrogenase enzyme activity level
  (B) reticulocyte count
  (C) prothrombin time
  (D) ferritin
  (E) hemoglobin electrophoresis

Glucose-6-phosphate dehydrogenase (G6PD) deficiency is the most common enzyme deficiency and is estimated to affect more than 400 million people worldwide. The deficiency occurs most commonly in regions in Africa, Asia, the Middle East, and the Mediterranean and causes episodic hemolytic anemia. The G6PD enzyme aids red blood cell (RBC) anaerobic glucose use in the pentose phosphate pathway. The function of the G6PD pathway is to protect RBCs against oxidative damage. A deficiency in this enzyme results in increased susceptibility of RBCs to oxidative stressors such as certain drugs (Box 124-1), viral or bacterial infections, or fava beans, which can trigger erythrocyte destruction and anemia. The deficiency has more than 400 variants, and the amount of enzyme activity varies with the particular gene mutation. Likewise, the degree of hemolysis in response to an oxidative stressor depends on the amount of enzyme activity present.

BOX 124-1

Drugs That Cause Hemolysis in Subjects Deficient in Glucose-6-Phosphate Dehydrogenase

- Antimalarials: Primaquine, pamaquine, dapsone
- Sulfonamides: Sulfamethoxazole
- Nitrofurantoin
- Analgesics: Acetanilid
- Miscellaneous: Vitamin K (water-soluble form), doxorubicin, methylene blue, nalidixic acid, furazolidone, niridazole, phenazopyridine

Bunn HF, Rosse W. Hemolytic anemias and acute blood loss. In: Kasper DL, Braunwald E, Fauci AS, Hauser SL, Longo DL, Jameson JL, editors. Harrison's principles of internal medicine. 16th ed. New York (NY): McGraw-Hill; 2005. p. 611.

The G6PD deficiency is an X-linked recessive disorder. Homozygous G6PD deficiency affects both X chromosomes, resulting in markedly deficient enzyme activity. Only one X chromosome is affected in the heterozygous individual, and they usually are only mildly anemic. The two most recognized forms of G6PD deficiency are the Mediterranean form, which results in severe hemolysis after an oxidative stress, and the African-American form, which usually results in mild hemolysis following an oxidative stress. The Mediterranean variant is clinically more severe due to a much lower enzyme activity. After an oxidative stress, the older enzyme-deficient RBCs are replaced by new RBCs (reticulocytes) with normal G6PD activity, which decreases over time. The in vivo half-life of RBCs is normally 62 days. With an oxidative stress, RBCs with the African-American form of G6PD deficiency have a half-life of 13 days, and mild hemolysis is noted. With the Mediterranean form, deficient RBCs have a half-life of hours leading to severe hemolysis after exposure to an oxidative stress. The G6PD deficiency variants have been classified according to their enzyme activity and degree of hemolysis by the World Health Organization (Box 124-2).

Patients with a G6PD deficiency are usually healthy with hemolysis occurring after an oxidative stress. Laboratory findings may include anemia, elevated reticulocytes, elevated indirect bilirubin, Heinz bodies, and "bite" cells on a peripheral culture. The anemia is self-limited because the older RBCs with lower enzyme activity are cleared from the system and replaced with new RBCs. Diagnosis of G6PD deficiency is made by documentation of a decreased level of enzyme activity in RBCs.

In this scenario, the patient is of Mediterranean ancestry and has been advised to avoid fava beans. Fava or broad beans (*Vicia faba*) are part of the eastern Mediterranean diet and contain oxidants that can induce hemolytic anemia in patients deficient in G6PD. This

BOX 124-2

World Health Organization Classification of Glucose-6-Phosphate Dehydrogenase Deficiency Variants

- Class I: severe enzyme deficiency (less than 10% of normal); chronic nonspherocytic hemolytic anemia
- Class II: severe enzyme deficiency (less than 10% of normal); intermittent hemolysis
- Class III: moderate enzyme deficiency (10–60% of normal); intermittent hemolysis
- Class IV: mild to no deficiency (60–150% of normal); no hemolysis
- Class V: no deficiency (increased enzyme activity, greater than 150% of normal)

patient presents with signs and symptoms of anemia after treatment with nitrofurantoin. Certain drugs, most commonly sulfonamides, antimalarials, and nitrofurantoin, may induce hemolysis in susceptible individuals with G6PD deficiency. The best diagnostic test to determine the etiology of her hemolytic anemia is to assess the G6PD enzyme activity level.

Reticulocytes are RBCs recently released from the bone marrow following hemolytic anemia. The reticulocyte count may be elevated in response to anemia but would not differentiate the etiology. Prothrombin time is a measure of coagulation and would not delineate the cause of anemia in this patient. Ferritin levels correlate with total body iron stores and are used clinically in diagnosing iron-deficiency anemia, but they are not useful in cases of hemolytic anemia. A hemoglobin electrophoresis identifies hemoglobinopathies, but would not be the optimal diagnostic test in this case.

Beutler E. G6PD deficiency. Blood 1994;84:3613–36.

Bunn HF, Rosse W. Hemolytic anemias and acute blood loss. In: Kasper DL, Braunwald E, Fauci AS, Hauser SL, Longo DL, Jameson JL, editors. Harrison's principles of internal medicine. 16th ed. New York (NY): McGraw-Hill; 2005. p. 607–17.

Chinevere TD, Murray CK, Grant E Jr, Johnson GA, Duelm F, Hospenthal DR. Prevalence of glucose-6-phosphate dehydrogenase deficiency in U.S. Army personnel. Mil Med 2006;171:905–7.

Frank JE. Diagnosis and management of G6PD deficiency. Am Fam Physician 2005;72:1277–82.

Hematologic disorders. In: Cunningham FG, Leveno KJ, Bloom SL, Hauth JC, Gilstrap L 3rd, Wenstrom KD, editors. Williams obstetrics. 22nd ed. New York (NY): McGraw-Hill; 2005. p. 1143–67.

Strong J. Anemia and white blood cell disorders. In: James DK, Steer PJ, Weiner CP, Gonik B, editors. High-risk pregnancy management options. 3rd ed. Philadelphia (PA): Elsevier Saunders; 2006. p. 865–88.

125
Cholelithiasis

A 35-year-old woman at 18 weeks of gestation, with body mass index (weight in kilograms divided by height in meters squared [kg/m²]) of 35, complains of unremitting right upper quadrant abdominal pain. The pain has been unresponsive to her physician's appropriate conservative treatments. Ultrasonography reveals a normal fetus and maternal gallstones. The most appropriate next step in management is

  * (A) a laparoscopic cholecystectomy
     (B) an open cholecystectomy
     (C) continuation of conservative measures
     (D) extracorporeal shock wave lithotripsy

Pregnancy is associated with an increased incidence of cholelithiasis. Most women are asymptomatic; however, biliary colic does occur in approximately 0.05–0.1% of pregnant women. Ultrasonography has greatly enhanced the ability to diagnose gallbladder disease safely and accurately in pregnancy. Accuracies higher than 90% have been regularly reported. The incidence of gallbladder disease during pregnancy ranges from 0.02% to 0.3%.

Often, gallstones are discovered incidentally by radiography or ultrasonography during the investigation of other symptoms. In such circumstances, neither open nor laparoscopic cholecystectomy is recommended because patients with asymptomatic gallstones seldom develop complications.

Patients with obstructive jaundice, signs and symptoms unresponsive to medical management, or peritonitis should undergo prompt operative intervention in any trimester. The second trimester is the safest time to perform surgery. In addition, the rates of preterm labor are very low during the second trimester, compared with the potential risk of 40% for premature delivery in the third trimester. Finally, the potential risk of teratogenesis during the second trimester is very small and the uterus is still of such proportion that it does not obliterate the operative field as might occur during the third trimester.

Cholecystectomy is the optimal management for cholelithiasis because it removes both the gallstones and the gallbladder, preventing recurrent disease. The only common consequence of removing the gallbladder is an increase in stool frequency, which is clinically important in less than 5% of patients and responds well to standard antidiarrheal drugs when necessary.

Laparoscopic cholecystectomy has been adopted rapidly since its introduction in 1987, and most cholecystectomies are now carried out in this way. The only specific contraindications to laparoscopic cholecystectomy are coagulopathy and the later stages of pregnancy. Acute cholecystitis and previous gastroduodenal surgery are no longer contraindications but are associated with a higher rate of conversion to open cholecystectomy. The major advantages of laparoscopic surgery during pregnancy are small abdominal incisions, rapid postoperative recovery, minimized increase in risk of thromboembolism, early return of gastrointestinal activity, fewer incisional hernias, decreased rate of fetal depression due to decreased pain and less narcotic use, shorter hospitalization time, and prompt return to regular life.

In a retrospective case–control study, 16 pregnant patients who underwent laparoscopic surgery were compared with 18 control pregnant patients who underwent open laparotomy during their first or second trimester. There was no difference between laparotomy and laparoscopy outcomes in their series, suggesting that laparoscopic surgery can be performed safely in the pregnant patient during both the first and second trimester. In practice, management often depends on local availability and skills of surgical consultants and hospital facilities; however, laparoscopic cholecystectomy should be the favored operation.

Continued conservative management in the face of unremitting and nonresolving signs and symptoms places the patient in danger of significant morbid and mortal complications and is unwarranted. Several nonsurgical techniques have been used to treat gallstones in nonpregnant patients: oral dissolution therapy (chenodeoxycholic and ursodeoxycholic acid); contact dissolution (direct instillation of methyltetrabutyl ether or monooctanoin); and stone shattering with extracorporeal shockwave lithotripsy. These treatments should be used only in patients who refuse surgery and are not pregnant because there are insufficient studies showing data.

Carringer M, Swartz R, Johansson JE. Management of ureteric calculi during pregnancy by ureteroscopy and laser lithotripsy. J Urolog 1998;159:1781–2.

Fatum M, Rojansky N. Laparoscopic surgery during pregnancy. Obstet Gynecol Surv 2001;56:50–9.

Ghumman E, Barry M, Grace PA. Management of gallstones in pregnancy. Brit J Surg 1997;84:1646–50.

Simmons DC, Tarnasky PR, Rivera-Alsina ME, Lopez JF, Edman CD. Endoscopic retrograde cholangiopancreatography (ERCP) in pregnancy without the use of radiation. Am J Obstet Gynecol 2004;190:1467–9.

126

Episiotomy

A primiparous patient in labor with a fetus at an estimated weight of 3,600 g (8 lb 4 oz) has been pushing for 3 hours. She has received adequate epidural analgesia. Her bony pelvis is felt to be adequate. She has brought the leading bony part of the vertex to 4+ station. The position is occiput anterior. The fetal heart tracing, which previously showed no decelerations and moderate variability, has begun to show significant variable decelerations and minimal variability. The major reason to perform an episiotomy in this patient is

      (A) it is routine intrapartum care
      (B) to avoid a third- or fourth-degree laceration
      (C) to reduce the incidence of urinary or fecal incontinence
*   (D) to expedite delivery

Episiotomy is one of the most commonly performed surgical procedures in the United States. Although frequency of use of the procedure is decreasing, use remains higher than many systematic reviews conclude is warranted. When the procedure was first introduced, indications for episiotomy included facilitating difficult births; saving fetal lives; preventing severe perineal tears; avoiding fetal hypoxia and intracranial hemorrhage; reducing postpartum urinary and fecal incontinence; and encouraging earlier return to (and better) sexual function. In the early years of the 20th century, the use of episiotomy shifted from prophylactic indications to preventive or routine, particularly in primigravid patients, reaching a rate of 65.1% in 1979. In the middle to late 1980s, however, investigators sought evidence to support or refute the use of episiotomy. Randomized clinical trials found that routine episiotomy compared with restrictive use was associated with a higher risk of anal sphincter and rectal injuries and precluded a woman from giving birth with an intact or minimally damaged perineum. Larger trials in more varied populations followed in the 1990s, with similar results. Recent randomized trials that compared routine with restrictive episiotomy use concluded that restrictive episiotomy use was associated with less posterior perineal trauma, less suturing, fewer healing complications, decreased maternal blood loss, and earlier return to sexual intercourse, but with greater anterior perineal trauma, which was usually minor. No differences were noted in severe vaginal or perineal trauma including anal sphincter lacerations, dyspareunia, urinary incontinence, or long-term pain. A reasonable conclusion should be that routine use of episiotomy should be abandoned.

Several observational studies have shown that episiotomy is associated with an increased risk of anal sphincter laceration (third- or fourth-degree). The adjusted odds ratios for such complications range from 4.0 to 12.0. After primary repair of anal sphincter lacerations, 20–50% of women have anal incontinence symptoms. Anal sphincter lacerations resulting from birth trauma are the leading cause of fecal incontinence in young women. Long-term sequelae such as perineal pain, fecal incontinence, urgency, or sexual dysfunction may occur years later. Several follow-up studies on the outcome of perineal trauma involving the external sphincter indicate that fecal incontinence may develop in 29–57% of patients. Therefore, neither avoidance of lacerations nor reduction in short- or long-term incontinence would be an appropriate indication for use of episiotomy in this patient.

In the case described, episiotomy may be used to expedite delivery due to the low station because episiotomy shortens the second stage and because the previously reassuring fetal heart rate pattern has changed to one in which there is the potential for hypoxemia.

Clemons JT, Towers GD, McClure GB, O'Boyle AL. Decreased anal sphincter lacerations associated with restrictive episiotomy use. Am J Obstet Gynecol 2005;192:1620–5.

Episiotomy. ACOG Practice Bulletin No. 71. American College of Obstetricians and Gynecologists. Obstet Gynecol 2006;107:957–62.

Hartmann K, Viswanathan M, Palmieri R, Gartlehner G, Thorp J Jr, Lohr KN. Outcomes of routine episiotomy: a systematic review. JAMA 2005;293:2141–8.

Hudelist G, Gelle'n J, Singer C, Ruecklinger E, Czerwenka K, Kandolf O, et al. Factors predicting severe perineal trauma during childbirth: role of forceps delivery routinely combined with mediolateral episiotomy. Am J Obstet Gynecol 2005;192:875–81.

Schoon P. Episiotomy: yea or nay [editorial]. Obstet Gynecol Surv 2001;56:667–9.

127

Genital herpes

A 25-year-old woman with a history of genital herpes comes to the office at 28 weeks of gestation for a routine prenatal visit. She reports herpes outbreaks one or two times per year. Her most recent outbreak was approximately 3 months ago. The best strategy to reduce the risk of recurrence of genital herpes during labor is to administer

    (A) valacyclovir starting immediately
    (B) famciclovir at 32 weeks of gestation
*   (C) acyclovir at 36 weeks of gestation
    (D) valacyclovir at 40 weeks of gestation
    (E) acyclovir at the onset of labor

Herpes simplex virus (HSV) infection of the genital tract is one of the most common viral sexually transmitted diseases (STDs). Based on positive serology test results for HSV-2 and estimates of genital HSV-1 infection, it is estimated that approximately 50 million adolescent and adult Americans are infected with genital herpes. Up to 25% of women with known genital herpes will have an HSV outbreak in the last month of pregnancy. Neonatal HSV infection, though rare, can result in disseminated or central nervous system (CNS) disease. Most cases of neonatal HSV infection are the consequence of vaginal delivery of a neonate through an infected birth canal.

Because 85% of neonatal herpes results from viral transmission near delivery, it is currently recommended that a cesarean delivery be offered to any woman with an active genital herpes lesion who presents in labor. However, more than 70% of neonatal herpes will occur in infants of women who asymptomatically shed virus near delivery. This being the case, in order to try to decrease both neonatal transmission and the need for cesarean delivery, strategies to decrease not only HSV outbreaks before the onset of labor but also asymptomatic viral shedding near term have been studied.

A randomized trial of acyclovir given after 36 weeks of gestation in women with recurrent genital herpes infection demonstrated a significant decrease in maternal clinical recurrences. The trial also showed a reduction in the number of cesarean deliveries performed for active infection, although this finding was not statistically significant. Another recent randomized trial to assess the efficacy and safety of valacyclovir prophylaxis after 36 weeks of gestation showed similar efficacy in reducing recurrent outbreaks, viral shedding, and cesarean deliveries, with no increased morbidities noted.

All three agents, acyclovir, valacyclovir, and famciclovir, are approved by the U.S. Food and Drug Administration for the treatment of primary genital herpes, the treatment of episodes of recurrent disease, and the daily treatment for suppression of outbreaks of recurrent genital herpes (Appendix D). Numerous studies have demonstrated the safety of acyclovir when used during pregnancy. Acyclovir, valacyclovir, and famciclovir are pregnancy risk category B medications. Because of potential clear beneficial effects of suppressive therapy in decreasing viral shedding and decreasing cesarean birth rates in women with HSV, the American College of Obstetricians and Gynecologists recommends consideration of antiviral therapy for women at or beyond 36 weeks of gestation with either primary or recurrent HSV. The decision of which agent is used will depend on cost, availability, and physician preference.

Whether it would be beneficial to initiate prophylaxis earlier than 36 weeks of gestation in patients with significant risk of preterm delivery is not known. The decision should be made on a case-by-case basis in order to optimize outcome. In the described scenario, there is no indication for immediate initiation of prophylaxis because the patient is at only 28 weeks of gestation. Similarly, initiating prophylaxis at 32 weeks of gestation has not been evaluated to assess for any additional benefits. Postponement of prophylaxis until 40 weeks of gestation or until the onset of labor would likely not be beneficial in decreasing asymptomatic viral shedding or HSV outbreaks in labor.

American College of Obstetricians and Gynecologists. Management of herpes in pregnancy. ACOG Practice Bulletin 8. Washington, DC: ACOG; 1999.

Brown ZA, Gardella C, Wald A, Morrow RA, Corey L. Genital herpes complicating pregnancy [published errata appear in Obstet Gynecol 2006;107:428; Obstet Gynecol 2007;109:207]. Obstet Gynecol 2005;106:845–56.

Scott LL, Hollier LM, McIntire D, Sanchez PJ, Jackson GL, Wendel GD Jr. Acyclovir suppression to prevent recurrent genital herpes at delivery. Infect Dis Obstet Gynecol 2002;10:71–7.

Sheffield JS, Hill JB, Hollier LM, Laibl VR, Roberts SW, Sanchez PJ, et al. Valacyclovir prophylaxis to prevent recurrent herpes at delivery; a randomized clinical trial [published erratum appears in Obstet Gynecol 2006;108;695]. Obstet Gynecol 2006;108:141–7.

Sheffield JS, Hollier LM, Hill JB, Stuart GS, Wendel GD. Acyclovir prophylaxis to prevent herpes simplex virus recurrence at delivery: a systematic review. Obstet Gynecol 2003;102:1396–403.

Watts DH, Brown ZA, Money D, Selke S, Huang ML, Sacks SL, et al. A double-blind, randomized, placebo-controlled trial of acyclovir in late pregnancy for the reduction of herpes simplex virus shedding and cesarean delivery. Am J Obstet Gynecol 2003;188:836–43.

Xu F, Sternberg MR, Kottiri BJ, McQuillan GM, Lee FK, Nahmias AJ, et al. Trends in herpes simplex virus type 1 and type 2 seroprevalence in the United States. JAMA 2006;296:964–73.

128

Fetal risks of maternal cholestasis

A 29-year-old woman, gravida 2, para 1, is seen at 34 weeks of gestation for unrelenting itching on her palms, soles, trunk, and extremities. Laboratory findings reveal normal liver function test results and elevated fasting serum bile acid levels. She is concerned about how this may affect her fetus and asks that delivery be initiated. The next step in management is

       (A) administration of antenatal corticosteroids

*   (B) weekly fetal nonstress tests

       (C) immediate delivery

       (D) induction of labor if delivery has not occurred by 41 weeks

The clinical picture of this patient is most consistent with intrahepatic cholestasis of pregnancy. Cholestasis of pregnancy is a disorder specific to pregnancy that is characterized by generalized pruritus without a rash. Pruritus usually occurs in the second half of pregnancy, may be mild to incapacitating, is worse at night, and is most prevalent on the palms and soles. Some affected individuals develop clinical jaundice. The maternal course is self-limited with symptoms disappearing shortly after delivery. However, intrahepatic cholestasis of pregnancy is associated with increased perinatal morbidity and mortality. Specifically, it carries significant risk for spontaneous preterm birth, intrapartum nonreassuring fetal heart rate tracing (including both abnormal fetal heart rate patterns and meconium-stained amniotic fluid), and intrauterine fetal demise.

Although intrahepatic cholestasis of pregnancy has been described in most ethnic groups, it is seen more frequently in Chile, especially in the native Araucanian Indian population, and in Scandinavia. The incidence of intrahepatic cholestasis of pregnancy is much lower in the United States, affecting only approximately 0.1% of pregnancies. The precise cause of the condition is not known, but endocrine, genetic, and environmental factors are thought to be involved. Cholestasis may result from a predisposition to the cholestatic effects of increased estrogens, which are higher in the third trimester and are increased in multiple gestations. Cholestasis is five times more common in twin pregnancies than in singleton gestations. Progesterone or its metabolites also have been suggested to be causally related to the condition. Family history of intrahepatic cholestasis of pregnancy and a personal history of hepatitis C are also associated with an increased incidence of cholestasis.

The diagnosis of intrahepatic cholestasis of pregnancy is based on clinical findings of pruritus without a skin rash and confirmed with laboratory findings of elevated fasting serum bile acid levels. Elevated aminotransferases and bilirubin levels also may be present. Pruritus usually precedes laboratory findings by days to several weeks. A prolonged prothrombin time also may be observed in women with cholestasis due to liver involvement, placing them at risk for postpartum hemorrhage. Daily oral vitamin K should be considered in these cases. Cholestasis is a diagnosis of exclusion, and other diseases affecting the liver, such as hepatitis and preeclampsia, must be excluded. Management involves reduction of maternal symptoms with medications, but the only definitive treatment is delivery.

Adverse fetal effects of intrahepatic cholestasis of pregnancy include preterm delivery before 37 weeks, nonreassuring fetal heart rate pattern in labor, meconium-stained amniotic fluid, and intrauterine demise. In this scenario, some form of fetal surveillance should be considered with the diagnosis of cholestasis. There is no ideal method of antepartum surveillance that ensures a favorable perinatal outcome, and it is impossible to predict which affected pregnancies are at risk for fetal complications. Weekly nonstress tests or biophysical profiles may be initiated at diagnosis. Daily maternal perception of fetal activity is another form of noninvasive surveillance.

One large study suggested following total serum bile acid levels and expectantly managing those women with low levels, thereby decreasing overall medical costs. Fetal risks were not increased if bile acid levels remained below 40 micromole per liter. However, not all women with intrahepatic cholestasis of pregnancy have elevated bile acid levels.

Antenatal corticosteroids are used to enhance fetal lung maturity in fetuses at risk for preterm delivery between 24 weeks and 34 weeks of gestation; however, antenatal corticosteroids are not suggested in the present case because the fetus has reached a gestational age of 34 weeks.

Immediate delivery would put the fetus at risk for complications of prematurity including neonatal respiratory distress syndrome, feeding problems, and risk for infection. Delivery is suggested at 37–38 weeks of gestation to decrease the incidence of adverse fetal outcomes, specifically third-trimester fetal demise. Timing of delivery may be influenced by the severity of maternal symptoms and by how favorable is the cervix.

Amniocentesis to assess fetal lung maturity, followed by delivery if the lungs are mature, is another option to be considered at 36 weeks of gestation. Because intrauterine fetal demise associated with intrahepatic cholestasis of pregnancy occurs more frequently after 37 weeks of gestation, delaying induction of labor until 41 weeks is risky and is not recommended. Antepartum surveillance often is instituted in cases of intrahepatic cholestasis of pregnancy in an effort to decrease perinatal morbidity and mortality, and its use must be weighed against more invasive interventions.

Egerman RS, Riely CA. Predicting fetal outcome in intrahepatic cholestasis of pregnancy: is the bile acid level sufficient? Hepatol 2004;40:287–8.

Germain AM, Carcajal JA, Glasinovic JC, Kato S, Williamson CD. Intrahepatic cholestasis of pregnancy: an intriguing pregnancy-specific disorder. J Soc Gynecol Investig 2002;9:10–4.

Glantz A, Marschall H, Mattsson L. Intrahepatic cholestasis of pregnancy: relationships between bile acid levels and fetal complication rates. Hepatol 2004;40:467–74.

Kenyon AP, Piercy CN, Williamson C, Tribe RM, Shennan AH. Obstetric cholestasis, outcome with active management: a series of 70 cases. BJOG 2002;109:282–8.

Williamson C, Hems LM, Goulis DG, Walker I, Chambers J, Donaldson O, et al. Clinical outcome in a series of cases of obstetric cholestasis identified via a patient support group. BJOG 2004;111:67–81.

129

Twin–twin transfusion syndrome

Ultrasonographic evaluation of a 27-year-old primigravid woman at 22 weeks of gestation shows a twin gestation with one fetus measuring 35% larger than the other. Both fetuses are female. The dividing membrane is thin. Hydramnios surrounds the larger twin, and the smaller twin has severe oligohydramnios and no bladder visualized. No other anatomic abnormalities are noted. The most likely diagnosis is

* (A) twin–twin transfusion syndrome
  (B) growth restriction of the smaller twin
  (C) placental chorioangioma
  (D) congenital infection
  (E) renal agenesis of the smaller twin

Twenty percent of all twin pregnancies are monochorionic and diamniotic, and such twin pregnancies are associated with a higher risk of perinatal mortality than dichorionic pregnancies. Ultrasonographic determination of chorionicity should be attempted on all multiple gestations ideally in the first trimester because it is most easily accomplished at this time. Determination of monochorionicity requires diligence at the time of ultrasonography, but it can be confirmed in most cases. The presence of one placenta is a supportive but unreliable indicator of monochorionicity, having a positive predictive value of only 42%. More reliable indicators include the absence of triangular projection between the layers of the membranes where they meet the placenta (lambda or twin peak sign) and a membrane thickness of less than 2 mm. No single indicator is sufficiently predictive to use alone. However, a composite assessment of the presence of four factors (ie, concordance of fetal sex, a thin dividing membrane, a single placenta, and absence of the lambda sign) can accurately detect more than 90% of monochorionic pregnancies.

Approximately 15–20% of all monochorionic, diamniotic pregnancies will be complicated by twin–twin transfusion syndrome. The etiology of the syndrome has not yet been fully elucidated, but it appears to be related to the imbalance in blood flow through a common placenta. Unidirectional flow takes precedence, resulting in one twin becoming a "donor" twin and the other a "recipient" twin. The recipient twin becomes plethoric, and the donor becomes growth restricted. Given these underlying physiologic adaptations, the diagnosis of twin–twin transfusion syndrome is based on the presence of all of the following ultrasonographic findings:

- A single placenta
- Concordance of sex
- Discordant amniotic fluid volumes (hydramnios and oligohydramnios)
- A 20% or greater discrepancy in estimated fetal weights

Because there are different severities of twin–twin transfusion syndrome, a grading system of 1–5, with 5 being the most severe, has been used to help guide therapy and prognosis (Table 129-1). If untreated, the perinatal mortality rate associated with twin–twin transfusion syndrome is approximately 90%, with 30% of survivors having a neurologic handicap.

Treatment can improve outcomes significantly. The two most common treatment modalities are serial amnioreduction and laser photocoagulation. Serial amnioreduction, the most common form of therapy, is achieved by performing serial amniocenteses and withdrawing 1–2 liters of amniotic fluid from the sac of the recipient twin. The survival rates for fetuses treated with serial amnioreduction vary dramatically, with reports between 37% and 83% survival. Neurologic morbidity following serial amnioreduction is as high as 58%. Recently, laser photocoagulation has been shown to be an effective treatment for twin–twin transfusion syndrome. Laser photocoagulation is performed by placing a fetoscope into the uterus and using a laser to coagulate placental surface vascular anastomoses. The survival rates are approximately 60%, and the risk of a neurologic handicap is approximately 8%.

TABLE 129-1. Grading System for Twin–Twin Transfusion Syndrome

Stage	Findings
1	Bladder of the donor twin is visible and Doppler studies are normal.
2	Bladder of the donor twin is not visible and Doppler studies are abnormal but not critically.
3	Doppler studies are critically abnormal.
4	Ascites, pericardial effusion, pleural effusion, overt hydrops, or scalp edema are present.
5	One or both twins are dead.

In the case described, congenital infection is unlikely due to the apparently normal fetal anatomy. Placental chorioangiomas are rare and most often present with a normally grown fetus with a vascular placental mass. These fetuses are at risk for hydrops and fetal death. Ultrasonographic evidence of bilateral renal agenesis includes oligohydramnios, lack of a fetal bladder, and absence of fetal kidneys in a normally grown fetus.

Duncan KR. Twin–to–twin transfusion: update on management options and outcomes. Curr Opin Obstet Gynecol 2005;17:618–22.

Mari G, Roberts A, Detti L, Kovanci E, Stefos T, Bahado-Singh RO, et al. Perinatal morbidity and mortality rates in severe twin–twin transfusion syndrome: results of the International Amnioreduction Registry. Am J Obstet Gynecol 2001;185:708–15.

Quintero RA, Dickinson JE, Morales W, Bornick P, Bermudez C, Cincotta R, et al. Stage-based treatment of twin–twin transfusion syndrome. Am J Obstet Gynecol 2003;188:1333–40.

Senat MV, Deprest J, Boulvain M, Paupe A, Winer N, Ville Y. Endoscopic laser surgery versus serial amnioreduction for severe twin–to–twin transfusion syndrome. N Engl J Med 2004;351:136–44.

130

Statins and drug exposure during pregnancy

A 41-year-old hypertensive woman, gravida 3, para 2, with a history of a myocardial infarction 4 years ago, comes to the office for prenatal care at 8 weeks of gestation. A recent maternal echocardiogram and cardiac stress test result are both normal. An ultrasonogram reveals a live intrauterine pregnancy. She currently takes simvastatin (Zocor) for hypercholesterolemia and labetalol for her hypertension. The most appropriate management is to

*   (A)   discontinue simvastatin
         (B)   check serum cholesterol in each trimester
         (C)   initiate an angiotensin-converting enzyme (ACE) inhibitor
         (D)   order fetal echocardiogram

Statins, or 3-hydroxy-3-methylglutaryl coenzyme A (HMG-CoA) reductase inhibitors, are primarily used to lower cholesterol and to decrease the risk of death and ischemic cardiac events. Because HMG-CoA reductase is the rate limiting step for the formation of cholesterol in the liver and other tissues, HMG-CoA reductase inhibitors decrease both the formation of cholesterol and total serum cholesterol levels. Other beneficial effects of HMG-CoA reductase inhibitors include reduction in low-density lipoprotein (LDL), increase in high-density lipoprotein (HDL), antiatherothrombotic effects, and a reduction in triglycerides. Several types of HMG-CoA reductase inhibitors are available in the United States. These agents have similar mechanisms of action, but the degree of effect on the different types of cholesterol varies among the agents. The most common side effect is myopathy. This appears to be related to the decrease in myocyte cholesterol.

Clinically, HMG-CoA reductase inhibitors have shown a benefit in many situations. Perhaps the most significant potential benefit is in patients with stable coronary artery disease and acute coronary syndromes. Investigators of multiple trials have found that the use of HMG-CoA reductase inhibitors is associated with a reduction in mortality, myocardial infarction, stroke, readmission to the

hospital, and unstable angina. These drugs also appear to have beneficial effects in patients with medical conditions such as diabetes mellitus and hypertension. Treatment with HMG-CoA reductase inhibitors is becoming standard therapy in patients with atherosclerotic vascular disease, and emerging evidence continues to provide support for their use for other disorders.

With an aging maternal population, myocardial infarction and other vascular diseases are becoming more common in pregnant women. As additional studies suggest a beneficial effect of HMG-CoA reductase inhibitors on diseases that complicate pregnancy, obstetricians are likely to encounter women who are taking HMG-CoA reductase inhibitors and seeking guidance about the safety of these drugs in pregnancy.

Based on premarketing animal studies that demonstrated teratogenicity, the U.S. Food and Drug Administration classified HMG-CoA reductase inhibitors in pregnancy risk category X. Case reports of fetuses who were exposed to HMG-CoA reductase inhibitors in the first trimester have found evidence of congenital anomalies including vertebral anomalies, anal atresia, cardiac defects, tracheoesophageal fistula, renal anomalies, and limb anomalies (VACTERL), as well as growth restriction, cleft lip and palate, hypospadias, and polydactyly.

However, the frequency of these anomalies is unlikely to be higher than is seen in the general population. Nevertheless, because interruption of HMG-CoA reductase inhibitor therapy does not likely affect the long-term treatment of women who are taking these drugs, it is recommended to discontinue these drugs before a planned pregnancy or as soon as pregnancy is confirmed. The use of statin drugs is not recommended during breastfeeding.

It is not recommended to discontinue antihypertensive therapy in the pregnant patient with hypertension. Changing to a different antihypertensive agent is useful when a patient's antihypertensive agent is an ACE inhibitor. Although beta-blockers have been associated with untoward fetal effects such as growth restriction, maternal benefits outweigh those small risks. In this patient with a history of a myocardial infarction, antihypertensive therapy provides further maternal benefit. Total cholesterol normally increases during pregnancy and does not require monitoring in patients with a history of hypercholesterolemia.

Briggs GG, Freeman RK, Yaffe SJ. Drugs in pregnancy and lactation. 6th ed. New York (NY): Lippincott Williams & Wilkins; 2005. p. 1258–60.

Colli S, Werba JP, Tremoli E. Statins in atherothrombosis. Semin Vasc Med 2004;4:407–15.

Lee JW. Statins and cardiovascular risks. Int Anesthesiol Clin 2005;43: 55–68.

Patel C, Edgerton L, Flake D, Smits A. Clinical inquiries. What precautions should we use with statins for women of childbearing age? J Fam Pract 2006;55:75–7.

Vaughan CJ, Gotto AM Jr. Update on statins: 2003. Circulation 2004; 110:886–92.

131

Aspiration pneumonia

A 26-year-old woman, gravida 2, para 1, at 37 weeks of gestation reported decreased fetal movement. An external fetal monitor was applied and showed a fetal heart rate of 80 beats per minute, which was confirmed by ultrasonography. The patient was counseled and underwent an emergency cesarean delivery under general anesthesia. Uterine atony was treated with intramuscular methylergonovine maleate (Methergine). In the recovery room, the patient became dyspneic, oxygen saturation was 85% while she was breathing room air, and chest X-ray showed bilateral lower lobe infiltrates. The most likely predisposing factor in the development of this clinical picture is

    (A) preoperative oral administration of sodium citrate (Bicitra)

    (B) rapid sequence induction of anesthesia

    (C) cricoid pressure during intubation

    (D) intraoperative administration of intramuscular methylergonovine maleate

*   (E) extubation before full emergence from the anesthetic

The patient probably has aspirated gastric contents into her lungs. This syndrome was first described by Mendelson, an obstetrician, in 1946. The pathogenesis involves airway obstruction by particulate matter and chemical injury if the pH of gastric contents is below 2.5. The particulate matter causes variable obstruction, even asphyxia, depending on its size and consistency. Orotracheal suctioning or bronchoscopy may be necessary to remove aspirated food. Chemical injury produces an inflammatory pneumonitis with noncardiogenic pulmonary edema or the acute respiratory distress syndrome. Treatment of this aspect involves maintenance of adequate oxygenation and antibiotic therapy if gram-negative or anaerobic superinfection develops.

Because treatment is problematic, attempts have been made to prevent aspiration. The pregnant woman is at greatest risk for aspiration during delivery, although antepartum epileptic seizures and eclampsia are other predisposing factors. The described patient is at high risk for aspiration because of an emergency cesarean delivery under general anesthesia. Precautions taken to prevent aspiration during cesarean delivery are shown in Box 131-1. Intraoperative administration of methylergonovine maleate for uterine bleeding should not predispose to aspiration. The other three procedures help to prevent aspiration during cesarean delivery.

Cunningham FG, Leveno KJ, Bloom SL, Hauth JC, Gilstrap LC 3rd, Wenstrom KD, editors. Williams obstetrics. 22nd ed. New York (NY): McGraw-Hill; 2005. P. 488–91.

BOX 131-1

Precautions to Prevent Aspiration During Cesarean Delivery

- Use of regional anesthesia when possible
- Preoperative anesthesia consult for difficult airway
- Personnel and equipment available to deal with failed intubation
- Modest intake of clear liquids during normal labor
- Fasting for 8 hours before elective cesarean delivery
- Oral administration of sodium citrate to neutralize gastric contents when the decision is made to perform cesarean delivery
- Lateral uterine displacement
- Preoxygenation
- Rapid sequence induction with cricoid pressure
- Extubation only after patient is conscious enough to follow commands and to maintain oxygen saturation with spontaneous breathing

---

Mandel J, Weinberger SE. Pulmonary diseases. In: Burrow GN, Duffy TP, Copel JA, editors. Medical complications during pregnancy. 6th ed. Philadelphia (PA): Elsevier Saunders; 2004. p. 375–414.

Obstetric analgesia and anesthesia. ACOG Practice Bulletin No. 36. American College of Obstetricians and Gynecologists. Obstet Gynecol 2002;100:177–91.

132

Management of labor in patient with human immunodeficiency virus infection

A 27-year-old primigravid woman, at 38 weeks of gestation, presents in active labor. She has human immunodeficiency virus (HIV) infection and is taking a highly active antiretroviral therapy (HAART) regimen. Her last viral load measurement 2 weeks ago was undetectable. In addition to her HAART regimen, the best labor management plan for this patient is

       (A) oral zidovudine (Retrovir) and vaginal delivery
*   (B) intravenous zidovudine and vaginal delivery
       (C) no additional therapy and vaginal delivery
       (D) no additional therapy and cesarean delivery

Without intervention, the risk of perinatal transmission from women who are HIV-positive to their infants is approximately 25%. Risk factors for mother–to–child transmission include a high plasma viral load, choriodecidual inflammation, preterm delivery, clinical herpes simplex virus infection, prolonged rupture of membranes, and vaginal delivery. With the use of HAART regimens and the subsequent reduction in plasma viral loads, mother–to–child transmission has decreased to less than 2%.

Initially, the Pediatric AIDS Clinical Trials Group conducted a study and found that zidovudine therapy during pregnancy, labor, and delivery could reduce perinatal transmission from 25% to 8%. Cesarean delivery before labor could reduce the perinatal transmission rate even further to 2%. As antiviral therapy regimens became more successful in reducing plasma viral loads to undetectable levels, vaginal delivery for women with HIV infection became a more acceptable option.

A pregnant woman with HIV infection and a viral load less than 1,000 copies/mL is a candidate for vaginal delivery. No consistent evidence has been produced to suggest that a cesarean delivery would decrease the perinatal transmission rate further. Intrapartum therapy for either mode of delivery is intravenous zidovudine; the regimen is based on previous trials. For a woman who elects labor and a vaginal delivery, the zidovudine is continued until delivery of the infant. A woman who gives birth by cesarean delivery will require 3 hours of intravenous zidovudine before beginning her operative delivery. The maternal antenatal antiretroviral regimen should be continued on schedule during labor to provide maximal virologic effect and to minimize drug resistance.

Further reduction in the perinatal HIV transmission rate depends on correct identification of all pregnant women with HIV infection before labor and delivery. The Centers for Disease Control and Prevention and the American College of Obstetricians and Gynecologists believe that every pregnant woman should have a prenatal HIV test and that high-risk women should be retested in the third trimester. If no documented HIV test result is on a woman's prenatal record when she is admitted to labor and delivery, a rapid HIV test should be offered. A rapid HIV test has sensitivity and specificity of 99%. Women who are identified as HIV positive and given zidovudine prophylaxis during labor and delivery can reduce the perinatal transmission rate from 25% to approximately 10%. Women who are identified as HIV positive by a rapid HIV test require a confirmatory Western blot test because the positive predictive value of rapid HIV test results varies between 50% and 95% depending on the prevalence of HIV infection in the community.

Bulterys M, Jamieson DJ, O'Sullivan MJ, Cohen MH, Maupin R, Nesheim S, et al. Rapid HIV-1 testing during labor: a multicenter study. Mother-Infant Rapid Intervention at Delivery (MIRIAD) Study Group. JAMA 2004;292:219–23.

Minkoff H. Human immunodeficiency virus infection in pregnancy. Obstet Gynecol 2003;101:797–810.

Prenatal and perinatal human immunodeficiency virus testing: expanded recommendations. ACOG Committee Opinion No. 304. American College of Obstetricians and Gynecologists. Obstet Gynecol 2004;104:1119–24.

Public Health Service Task Force. Recommendations for use of antiretroviral drugs in pregnant HIV-1-infected women for maternal health and interventions to reduce perinatal HIV-1 transmission in the United States. October 12, 2006. Available at: http://aidsinfo.nih.gov/content-files/PerinatalGL.pdf. Retrieved March 27, 2007.

133

Ultrasonographic markers of Down syndrome

A 33-year-old woman, gravida 1, para 0, at 18 weeks of gestation is scheduled to undergo genetic ultrasonography. The ultrasonographic marker of Down syndrome, seen during the second trimester as an isolated finding, that has the highest likelihood ratio for Down syndrome is

    (A) echogenic intracardiac focus
    (B) echogenic bowel
    (C) pyelectasis
    (D) short femur
*   (E) thick nuchal fold

Genetic ultrasonography during the second trimester of the pregnancy enables a detailed anatomic evaluation of the fetus to exclude structural malformations and to search for ultrasonographic markers that increase the likelihood of fetal Down syndrome. This needs to be performed with experienced personnel. An ultrasonographically recognizable major malformation is present in approximately 25% of fetuses with Down syndrome. Therefore, most of the fetuses with Down syndrome will be missed if the presence of a major malformation is the primary method of detection. Ultrasonographic markers of Down syndrome are more common than structural abnormalities and, in the presence of multiple markers or structural abnormalities, the risk of Down syndrome increases. Ultrasonographic markers are nonspecific, may be transient (ie, they resolve with advancing gestational age), and are often seen in fetuses without chromosomal abnormalities.

Genetic ultrasonography can be combined with the second-trimester maternal serum screen, to provide an a priori risk for each patient. Likelihood ratios are used to adjust the a priori risk by using Bayes' theorem to determine a patient's specific risk of carrying a fetus with Down syndrome. Clinically, the calculation of likelihood ratios can be useful because it allows couples to consider their individual risk of having a fetus with Down syndrome. Such risk estimates can assist them in deciding whether or not to pursue invasive testing (amniocentesis) (Table 133-1).

Classically, an amniocentesis has been offered to patients in whom the risk of Down syndrome was 1 in 270 or greater based on age, serum screening, or both. In the presence of normal genetic ultrasonography, the risk of Down syndrome can be significantly reduced regardless of the indication for the testing. Therefore patients may reasonably undergo a genetic sonogram before deciding about an amniocentesis.

Intracardiac echogenic focus denotes a calcification of the papillary muscle of the fetal heart, which has been associated with Down syndrome. The intracardiac echogenic focus is most commonly seen in the left ven-

tricle of the heart. Ethnic variability in the incidence of intracardiac echogenic focus has been described. New evidence suggests that the presence of an isolated intracardiac echogenic focus in a low-risk woman younger than age 35 years with normal serum biochemistry (triple or quadruple screen) may not warrant an amniocentesis. This is because in this scenario, the intracardiac echogenic focus may represent a benign variant and may not be a marker for Down syndrome.

Echogenic or hyperechoic bowel refers to bowel that is as bright as bone when viewed with ultrasonography. Echogenic bowel when present increases the likelihood of fetal Down syndrome. However, most fetuses with echogenic bowel will be chromosomally normal. Echogenic bowel can be seen as a result of fetal swallowing of blood after maternal bleeding; in cases of in utero infection with cytomegalovirus or toxoplasmosis, fetal cystic fibrosis, or gastrointestinal malformation as well as being associated with intrauterine growth restriction.

Pyelectasis, ie, dilatation of the fetal renal pelvis, is measured in a transverse section of the fetal abdomen. An anterior–posterior measurement of 4 mm or more, during the second trimester, is the cut-off point used for pyelectasis. Approximately 17–25% of fetuses with Down syndrome will have pyelectasis; however, most fetuses with renal pyelectasis are chromosomally normal.

A short femur can be seen in fetuses with Down syndrome. However, in clinical practice, the usefulness of this marker to identify fetuses with Down syndrome is controversial because there are inherent differences in the size of the fetal femur in different ethnic populations.

The nuchal fold was the first ultrasonographic marker suggested for the detection of Down syndrome during the second trimester (ie, 15–20 weeks of gestation). This marker continues to have the highest likelihood ratio for the diagnosis of fetal Down syndrome during the second trimester. The measurement is obtained in a transverse section of the fetal head to include the posterior fossa and the occipital bone. Only the skinfold is measured, from

TABLE 133-1. Likelihood Ratios for Down Syndrome Using Isolated Markers

Isolated Marker	Nyberg et al., 1998*	Nyberg et al., 2001†	Smith-Bindman et al., 2001‡	Bromley et al., 2002§
Major anomaly	25	ND	ND	3.3
Nuchal fold	18.6	11	17	ND
Short humerus	2.5	5.1	7.5	5.8
Short femur	2.2	1.5	2.7	1.2
Hyperechoic bowel	5.5	6.7	6.1	ND
Pyelectasis	1.6	1.5	1.9	1.5
Echogenic intracardiac focus	2	1.8	2.8	1.4

ND, not determined.

*Nyberg DA, Luthy DA, Resta RG, Nyberg BC, Williams MA. Age-adjusted ultrasound risk assessment for fetal Down's syndrome during the second trimester: description of the method and analysis of 142 cases. Ultrasound Obstet Gynecol 1998;12:8–14.

†Nyberg DA, Souter VL, El-Bastawissi A, Young S, Luthhardt F, Luthy DA. Isolated sonographic markers for detection of fetal Down syndrome in the second trimester of pregnancy. J Ultrasound Med 2001;20:1053–63.

‡Smith-Bindman R, Feldstein VA, Goldberg JD. The genetic sonogram in screening for Down syndrome. J Ultrasound Med 2001;20:1153–8.

§Bromley B, Lieberman E, Shipp TD, Benacerraf BR. The genetic sonogram. A method of risk assessment for Down syndrome in the second trimester. J Ultrasound Med 2002;21:1087–96; quiz 1097–8.

the outer edge of the occipital bone to the outer skin edge. A measurement of 5–6 mm or greater is considered to be abnormal.

Benacerraf BR. The role of the second trimester genetic sonogram in screening for fetal Down syndrome. Semin Perinatol 2005;29:386–94.

Bradley KE, Santulli TS, Gregory KD, Herbert W, Carlson DE, Platt LD. An isolated intracardiac echogenic focus as a marker for aneuploidy. Am J Obstet Gynecol 2005;192:2021–6; discussion 2026-8.

Bromley B, Lieberman E, Shipp TD, Benacerraf BR. The genetic sonogram: a method of risk assessment for Down syndrome in the second trimester. J Ultrasound Med 2002;21:1087–96; quiz 1097–8.

Nyberg DA, Souter VL, El-Bastawissi A, Young S, Luthhardt F, Luthy DA. Isolated sonographic markers for detection of fetal Down syndrome in the second trimester of pregnancy. J Ultrasound Med 2001; 20:1053–63.

Vintzileos AM, Guzman ER, Smulian JC, Yeo L, Scorza WE, Knuppel RA. Down syndrome risk estimation after normal genetic sonography. Am J Obstet Gynecol 2002;187:1226–9.

134
Thrombophilia

A 25-year-old woman, gravida 2, para 1, has a history of an unexplained 34-week intrauterine fetal demise. Titers were negative in serologic tests for toxoplasmosis, other agents, rubella, cytomegalovirus, and herpes simplex (TORCH tests). The fetal karyotype was 46,XY. The fetus had no congenital malformations. The patient has no evidence of antiphospholipid syndrome. She is homozygous for factor V Leiden. The best medical therapy during this pregnancy is

    (A) no medical therapy
    (B) warfarin sodium (Coumadin)
    (C) aspirin
    (D) vitamin C and vitamin E
*   (E) heparin

Inherited thrombophilias are a heterogeneous group of disorders associated with a predisposition to thrombotic events. As a result of thrombosis in the uteroplacental circulation, they also are associated with many adverse pregnancy outcomes, such as intrauterine growth restriction (IUGR), intrauterine fetal demise, severe preeclampsia remote from term, abruptio placentae, and (possibly) recurrent pregnancy loss. The most common inherited thrombophilias are factor V Leiden mutation, prothrombin G20210A mutation, and methylenetetrahydrofolate reductase C677T (*MTHFR*) mutation. Antithrombin III (ATIII) deficiency, protein C deficiency, and protein S deficiency are rare causes.

As a group, inherited thrombophilias are associated with adverse pregnancy outcomes and thromboembolic disease. For most of the conditions, the risk of thromboembolism during pregnancy can be calculated. Factor V Leiden and prothrombin mutation are inherited in an autosomal dominant fashion. The risk of thromboembolism in an asymptomatic pregnant carrier is 0.2% for factor V Leiden and 0.5% for prothrombin mutation. This risk is significantly increased for homozygosity of either mutation or compound heterozygosity of both mutations. The most common thrombogenic thrombophilia is ATIII deficiency, with a 70–90% lifetime risk of thromboembolism. Pregnant women with ATIII deficiency have a 60% risk of thrombosis in the antenatal period and a 33% risk of thrombosis in the puerperium. Protein C and protein S deficiency in pregnant women carries a 5–20% risk of thromboembolism. The *MTHFR* mutation is associated with hyperhomocysteinemia. Hyperhomocysteinemia is associated with thromboembolism, atherosclerosis, and fetal neural tube defects. In addition, it has a weak association with recurrent pregnancy loss.

If a pregnant woman has a history of a thromboembolic event and has a thrombophilia, heparin therapy is indicated. If the pregnant woman has ATIII deficiency, homozygosity for factor V Leiden or prothrombin gene mutation, or compound heterozygosity for factor V Leiden and prothrombin gene mutation, she will need therapeutic anticoagulation during pregnancy and for at least 6 weeks postpartum. If the pregnant woman has a history of a venous thromboembolism and protein C deficiency, protein S deficiency, heterozygosity for factor V Leiden, or prothrombin gene mutation, she will need prophylactic anticoagulation during pregnancy and for at least 4–6 weeks postpartum. The postpartum therapy can be accomplished with either heparin or warfarin sodium, which is compatible with breastfeeding.

No randomized controlled trials have been carried out to assess medical intervention for women with an inherited thrombophilia and an adverse pregnancy outcome. A series of observational nonrandomized studies have demonstrated an improved live birth rate and a decrease in other adverse pregnancy outcomes with prophylactic low molecular weight heparin. In the absence of prospective trials, the efficacy of heparin in improving pregnancy outcome is uncertain.

This pregnant woman is homozygous for factor V Leiden and she had an unexplained intrauterine fetal demise. Therefore, anticoagulation is warranted in a subsequent pregnancy. Coumadin can be used in the postpartum period; however, in the first trimester, Coumadin is a teratogen and is contraindicated. Coumadin embryopathy occurs in 5% of exposed pregnancies in the first trimester. This syndrome includes nasal hypoplasia, bone stippling, ophthalmologic abnormalities, and mental retardation. Aspirin therapy has not been as successful in improving the live birth rate as it is when combined with heparin; as a result, aspirin should not be used alone in this patient's regimen. Vitamin C and vitamin E would not be appropriate to prescribe for her. Antioxidants have been used in an attempt to reduce preeclampsia. However, there is some evidence to suggest that antenatal therapy with these vitamins may cause low birth weight. In this clinical scenario, no medical therapy is not a reasonable option, because of an elevated thrombosis risk.

Gris JC, Mercier E, Quere I, Lavigne-Lissalde G, Cochery-Nouvellon E, Hoffet M, et al. Low-molecular-weight heparin versus low-dose aspirin in women with one fetal loss and a constitutional thrombophilic disorder. Blood 2004;103:3695–9.

Lockwood CJ. Inherited thrombophilias in pregnant patients: detection and treatment paradigm. Obstet Gynecol 2002;99:333–41.

Paidas MJ, Ku DH, Langhoff-Roos J, Arkel YS. Inherited thrombophilias and adverse pregnancy outcome: screening and management. Semin Perinatol 2005;29:150–63.

Poston L, Briley AL, Seed PT, Kelly FJ, Shennan AH. Vitamin C and vitamin E in pregnant women at risk for pre-eclampsia (VIP trial): randomised placebo-controlled trial. Vitamins in Pre-eclampsia (VIP) Trial Consortium. Lancet 2006;367:1145–54.

135

Risk of toxoplasmosis during pregnancy

A 31-year-old woman, gravida 2, para 1, at 18 weeks of gestation informs you that her cat has toxoplasmosis. Serologic testing (titers) for toxoplasma-specific immunoglobin M (IgM) and IgG are ordered. While waiting for the serologic testing, you ask her to undergo ultrasonography. The ultrasonographic finding that will be most suggestive of severe congenital toxoplasmosis is

* (A) hydrocephaly
  (B) echogenic intracardiac focus
  (C) double bubble
  (D) oligohydramnios
  (E) dolichocephaly

It has been estimated that annually in the United States per year approximately 400 to 4,000 infants are born with congenital toxoplasmosis—a rate of 1 in 10,000 births. Primary infection in a healthy nonimmunocompromised individual is asymptomatic approximately 90% of the time. Symptomatic infection resembles a mononucleosis type illness with low-grade fever, malaise, headache, and cervical lymphadenopathy.

Maternal–fetal transmission increases with advancing gestational age. During the first trimester, the transmission rate is approximately 10–15%; during the second trimester, approximately 25%; and during the third trimester, more than 60%. The severity of the infection also depends on what point in the pregnancy the infection occurred. The earlier the infection takes place, the more severe is the fetal infection. Box 135-1 shows general sanitation and food handling recommendations for pregnant women to reduce the risk of toxoplasmosis during pregnancy.

The diagnosis of toxoplasmosis is based on clinical symptoms and serologic test results. During pregnancy, the main objective is to determine when the infection occurred. Infection before conception does not pose a substantial risk to the fetus; in contrast, infection during the pregnancy poses a significant risk to the fetus. Thus, IgG and IgM toxoplasma serologic testing constitutes the first line of tests and are usually done within the first

2 weeks, during the acute infection. If IgG is detected alone, this signifies a previous infection. Antibody from such a previous infection will persist in the body indefinitely and the fetus is not at risk for infection. Therefore, no further testing is suggested. However, if both IgG and IgM are present, further serologic testing in a reference laboratory is indicated because IgM may be detected up to 18 months after an acute infection. The IgG avidity test is another test that can help time the infection by distinguishing between a recent and a distant infection. A high IgG avidity test suggests that the infection occurred at least 3–5 months earlier. Therefore, a high IgG avidity test result during the first 12–16 weeks of gestation essentially rules out an infection acquired during pregnancy. A low IgG avidity test is not helpful because the low avidity antibodies may persist for months after the infection.

If primary maternal infection is documented, the most sensitive way to diagnose in utero fetal infection is using a polymerase chain reaction test performed on amniotic fluid. Fetal blood sampling is not indicated because it carries a higher fetal risk and the results are less sensitive.

The ultrasonographic findings seen in cases of fetal toxoplasmosis include liver calcifications or echogenic foci within the liver parenchyma, hydrops fetalis, intracranial calcifications, and hydrocephaly. Echogenic intracardiac foci have been associated with fetal Down

BOX 135-1

Recommendations for Lowering the Risk of Primary Toxoplasmosis Among Pregnant Women

1. Avoid consumption of undercooked meat. Cook all meat until it is no longer pink and the juices run clear.
2. Always use gloves while handling raw meat and wash hands thoroughly afterward.
3. Thoroughly wash all utensils that are in contact with undercooked meat.
4. Wash all uncooked vegetables thoroughly.
5. Wear gloves when gardening or working in soil. Wash hands immediately after contact with soil.
6. If possible, keep cats indoors throughout pregnancy and do not feed cats uncooked meat.
7. Use gloves while changing cat litter. Immediately after changing cat litter, be sure to wash hands thoroughly.

Modified from Kravetz JD, Federman DG. Toxoplasmosis in pregnancy. Am J Med 2005;118:214. Copyright 2005 by Elsevier.

than 5 cm; this is not a feature of fetal toxoplasmosis. Dolichocephaly refers to an elongated shape of the fetal head that can be seen in breech presentations, in the presence of oligohydramnios, or as a result of premature closure of the sagittal suture of the fetal head.

If results are positive, ultrasonographic follow-up is indicated. Signs such as intracranial calcifications, microcephaly, hydrocephaly, and severe intrauterine growth restriction strongly suggest in utero infection in the presence of documented maternal infection.

Clinical manifestations of toxoplasmosis in fetuses and neonates vary. The typical triad of hydrocephaly, chorioretinitis, and intracranial calcifications is not always observed. Although most infected infants do not have clinical symptoms at birth, approximately 55–85% will develop sequelae, such as deafness, mental retardation, and learning difficulties, later in life.

American College of Obstetricians and Gynecologists. Perinatal viral and parasitic infections. ACOG Practice Bulletin 20. Washington, DC: ACOG; 2000.

Gras L, Wallon M, Pollak A, Cortina-Borja M, Evengard B, Hayde M, et al. Association between prenatal treatment and clinical manifestations of congenital toxoplasmosis in infancy: a cohort study in 13 European centres. Acta Paediatr 2005;94:1721–31.

Hohlfeld P, Daffos F, Costa JM, Thulliez P, Forestier F, Vidaud M. Prenatal diagnosis of congenital toxoplasmosis with a polymerase-chain-reaction test on amniotic fluid. N Engl J Med 1994;331:695–9.

Kravetz JD, Federman DG. Toxoplasmosis in pregnancy. Am J Med 2005;118:212–6.

Lopez A, Dietz VJ, Wilson M, Navin TR, Jones JL. Preventing congenital toxoplasmosis. MMWR Recomm Rep 2000;49(RR-2):59–68.

Rorman E, Zamir CS, Rilkis I, Ben-David H. Congenital toxoplasmosis—prenatal aspects of Toxoplasma gondii infection. Reprod Toxicol 2006;21:458–72.

syndrome, although they are most commonly seen in chromosomally normal fetuses. The double bubble represents the fluid-filled stomach and duodenum seen in fetuses with duodenal atresia. Approximately 30–40% of fetuses with duodenal atresia have Down syndrome. Oligohydramnios is defined as a pocket of fluid measuring less than 2 cm or an amniotic fluid index (AFI) of less

136

Oligohydramnios

A 16-year-old primigravid obese adolescent comes to the office at 18 weeks of gestation for ultrasonography. The anatomy ultrasonogram was limited by maternal obesity but did reveal oligohydramnios and the absence of a fetal bladder. A previous ultrasonogram at 14 weeks of gestation revealed normal amniotic fluid volume. A speculum examination is performed and the results of the examination are negative for pooling, ferning, and nitrazine testing. The most likely diagnosis is

    (A) maternal dehydration
    (B) rupture of membranes
* (C) bilateral renal agenesis
    (D) posterior urethral valves

Amniotic fluid is an essential part of fetal well-being. An understanding of amniotic fluid dynamics is important to understand the potential causes and outcomes of pregnancies complicated by oligohydramnios.

Amniotic fluid is derived from many sources, including fetal tracheal secretions, maternal fluid crossing the fetal membranes, maternal fluid crossing the placenta and umbilical cord, fetal skin, and fetal urine production. Before the early second trimester, the fetal kidneys do not function fully, and the first four sources of amniotic fluid take precedence. However, from the mid-second trimester until delivery, fetal urine production is the primary source of amniotic fluid. Daily fetal urine output is approximately 30% of the fetal weight.

In this patient, the lack of amniotic fluid at 18 weeks of gestation coupled with the absence of a fetal bladder is compelling evidence in support of bilateral renal agenesis. Repeat ultrasonogram with color Doppler studies of the renal arteries can be further confirmation. Because fetal well-being and normal development depend on amniotic fluid, the outcome of fetuses with bilateral renal agenesis is bleak. Most infants with bilateral renal agenesis die from in utero cord entrapment before birth or pulmonary hypoplasia at birth. In contrast, fetuses with early onset posterior urethral valves most often have ultrasonographic findings of an enlarged bladder, oligohydramnios, and dysplastic kidneys, although the prognosis is equally bleak.

In cases of oligohydramnios, especially in the third trimester, maternal rehydration has been used as a strategy to increase the amniotic fluid volume in nonanomalous fetuses. Maternal rehydration is achieved by either increased oral fluid intake or intravenous hydration over 12–24 hours. The results have been mixed, but it appears that maternal hydration does mildly increase the amniotic fluid level. Unfortunately, more clinically relevant outcomes such as neonatal death have not been studied.

Renal dysplasia usually is characterized by echogenic, enlarged kidneys with multiple cysts. Possible etiologies include urinary obstruction, inherited disorders, tumors, syndromes, or hematomas. Prognosis depends on the cause and extent of the problem.

Premature rupture of membranes is a common cause of oligohydramnios and should always be considered when oligohydramnios is discovered. In this scenario, the lack of definitive evidence of rupture of membranes such as fluid arborization, vaginal pooling, or a positive nitrazine test result should prompt the clinician to look for other possible causes of oligohydramnios.

Hill LM. Oligohydramnios: sonographic diagnosis and clinical implications. Clin Obstet Gynecol 1997;40:314–27.

Hofmeyr GJ, Gulmezoglu AM. Maternal hydration for increasing amniotic fluid volume in oligohydramnios and normal amniotic fluid volume. Cochrane Database of Systematic Reviews 2002, Issue 1. Art. No.: CD000134. DOI: 10.1002/14651858.CD000134.

Sepulveda W, Stagiannis KD, Flack NJ, Fisk NM. Accuracy of prenatal diagnosis of renal agenesis with color flow imaging in severe second trimester oligohydramnios. Am J Obstet Gynecol 1995;173:1788–92.

Sherer DM. A review of amniotic fluid dynamics and the enigma of isolated oligohydramnios. Am J Perinatol 2002;19:253–66.

137

Antiphospholipid syndrome

A 38-year-old woman, gravida 2, comes to the office for a preconception consultation. She has had two first-trimester spontaneous abortions. Karyotypes on the products of conception were normal. She has a normal uterine cavity by hysterosalpingogram. She has a normal karyotype. She has an anticardiolipin antibody of 80 immunoglobulin G (IgG) phospholipid units two times 12 weeks apart. For a diagnosis of antiphospholipid syndrome, the outcome of her next pregnancy needs to be

    (A) severe preeclampsia at term
*   (B) first-trimester spontaneous abortion
    (C) preterm premature rupture of membranes (preterm PROM)
    (D) growth restriction at term with normal umbilical artery Doppler velocimetry

Antiphospholipid syndrome is an autoimmune condition characterized by vascular thrombosis and pregnancy complications. To confirm the diagnosis, a woman must have met clinical and laboratory criteria. The diagnosis has been redefined by the Eleventh International Congress on Antiphospholipid Antibodies, which revised the 1999 Sapporo classification.

The clinical features include vascular thrombosis and first-, second-, or third-trimester pregnancy complications (Appendix I). The vascular complications comprise one or more clinical episodes of arterial, venous, or small vessel thrombosis in any tissue or organ. The thrombosis must be confirmed by an imaging study or histopathology. The pregnancy morbidity includes one or more unexplained deaths of a morphologically normal fetus at or beyond the 10th week of gestation, an indicated preterm birth before 34 weeks of gestation caused by severe preeclampsia or placental insufficiency, or three or more consecutive spontaneous abortions before the 10th week of gestation with normal maternal, anatomic, and hormonal studies and normal maternal and paternal karyotypes.

The laboratory features include a lupus anticoagulant, anticardiolipin antibodies, or anti-β_2-glycoprotein I antibodies on two separate occasions at least 12 weeks apart.

The anticardiolipin antibodies can be either the immunoglobulin M (IgM) or IgG isotype present in medium or high titers. The anti-β_2-glycoprotein I antibodies can be either the IgM or IgG isotype in a titer greater than the 99th percentile.

The described patient meets the laboratory criteria for antiphospholipid syndrome. However, she does not meet the clinical criteria for the condition. She needs an additional unexplained first-trimester spontaneous abortion to fulfill the criteria for recurrent pregnancy loss. Severe preeclampsia at term is not part of the clinical definition of antiphospholipid syndrome; however, severe preeclampsia before 34 weeks of gestation is one of the clinical criteria for the diagnosis. Intrauterine growth restriction with normal Doppler velocimetry is not indicative of placental insufficiency, and therefore not one of the clinical criteria for the diagnosis. Finally, preterm PROM is not a clinical characteristic of antiphospholipid syndrome.

Branch DW. Summary of the 11th International Congress on antiphospholipid autoantibodies, Australia, November 2004. J Reprod Immunol 2005;66:85–90.

Miyakis S, Lockshin MD, Atsumi T, Branch DW, Brey RL, Cervera R, et al. International consensus statement on an update of the classification criteria for definite antiphospholipid syndrome (APS). J Thromb Haemost 2006;4:295–306.

138
Placenta accreta

A 28-year-old primigravid woman has an in vitro fertilization singleton pregnancy complicated by placenta previa and is admitted for a cesarean delivery at term. After delivery of the infant and the placenta, diffuse bleeding occurs from the uterine incision and the placental bed. A second intravenous line is started. Uterotonics are administered. With the loss of 1,500 mL of blood, a transfusion of packed red blood cells is begun. If bleeding persists, the next step in surgical management would be

      (A) hysterectomy
      (B) bilateral hypogastric artery ligation
      (C) bilateral uterine artery embolization
      (D) compression sutures
 *   (E) bilateral uterine artery ligation

The incidence of placenta accreta has increased dramatically in the past 80 years from less than 1 in 30,000 from 1930 to the 1950s, 1 in 2,500 in 1980, to 1 in 533 at the present time. The increase in the incidence of this serious condition is closely tied to the rising cesarean delivery rate. The risk factors for placenta accreta include placenta previa, advanced maternal age, previous cesarean delivery, grand multiparity, previous myomectomy, Asherman syndrome, and submucous myoma.

Women with placenta previa have about a 4–5% incidence of placenta accreta. The described patient has clinical signs suggestive of a placenta accreta. In this circumstance, where the possible clinical diagnosis of placenta accreta is being aggressively managed, it is reasonable to proceed with conservative therapy, especially in a primigravid woman. The first step in conservative management in this patient would include bilateral uterine artery ligation (Appendix J) to decrease pulse pressure. This procedure is easily performed and commonly results in reduced bleeding. Care should be taken to avoid injury to the ureters.

Multiple case series have documented different variations of compression sutures that have been used for conservative management of postpartum hemorrhage. These techniques include B-Lynch suture, parallel vertical compression sutures, and interrupted circular sutures. One of these procedures may be used as the next line in therapy if bilateral uterine artery ligation is unsuccessful.

If compression sutures are unsuccessful, there is persistent hemorrhage, and the patient is being adequately resuscitated and hemodynamically stable, bilateral uterine artery embolization would be the next intervention. Bilateral hypogastric artery ligation reduces the pulse

pressure to the uterus and is effective in promoting clot formation. However, the surgical technique is very difficult and most obstetrician–gynecologists are inexperienced in operating in the retroperitoneal space. In addition, there is a significant complication rate associated with the procedure. If the institution does not offer interventional radiology, and a gynecologic oncologist or a vascular surgeon can assist in the management of the patient, a bilateral hypogastric artery ligation could be considered in a patient who wanted to preserve her fertility. If the obstetrician–gynecologist is adequately trained in the procedure, then they can proceed with a bilateral hypogastric artery ligation during severe postpartum hemorrhage.

If the conservative measures fail or the patient becomes hemodynamically unstable, a hysterectomy is recommended. Some patients with a placenta accreta may not respond to conservative measures, in which case a hysterectomy would need to be performed. If the patient has a placenta previa and a placenta accreta, a supracervical hysterectomy may not resolve the hemorrhage, and a total abdominal hysterectomy should be considered.

Bennett MJ, Sen RC. "Conservative" management of placenta praevia percreta: report of two cases and discussion of current management options. Aust N Z J Obstet Gynaecol 2003;43:249–51.

Harma M, Gungen N, Ozturk A. B-Lynch uterine compression suture for postpartum haemorrhage due to placenta praevia accreta. Aust N Z J Obstet Gynaecol 2005;45:93–5.

Ornan D, White R, Pollak J, Tal M. Pelvic embolization for intractable postpartum hemorrhage: long-term follow-up and implications for fertility. Obstet Gynecol 2003;102:904–10.

Usta IM, Hobeika EM, Musa AA, Gabriel GE, Nassar AH. Placenta previa–accreta: risk factors and complications. Am J Obstet Gynecol 2005;193:1045–9.

139–143

Maternal and fetal side effects of antihypertensives

Match the maternal and fetal side effect (139–143) with the corresponding antihypertensive agent (A–E).

(A) Atenolol (Tenormin)
(B) Labetalol hydrochloride (Normodyne, Trandate)
(C) Alpha-methyldopa (Aldomet)
(D) Enalapril (Vasotec)
(E) Hydralazine hydrochloride

D **139.** Neonatal renal failure

A **140.** Intrauterine growth restriction

E **141.** Maternal tachycardia

E **142.** Maternal lupuslike reaction

C. **143.** Positive maternal Coombs test

Chronic hypertension in pregnancy is defined as hypertension (blood pressure greater than 140/90 mm Hg) either preceding pregnancy or diagnosed before 20 weeks of gestation. Debate exists about the relative merits and risks associated with the pharmacologic treatment of mild hypertension during pregnancy. To date, no conclusive evidence supports the hypothesis that pharmacologic treatment of mild hypertension during pregnancy improves perinatal outcome. When pharmacologic therapy is indicated, decisions must be made relative to the best choice of agent or combination of agents.

Alpha-methyldopa is frequently cited as the agent of choice for the treatment of hypertension during pregnancy. It is a centrally acting α-adrenergic agonist that acts by reducing sympathetic outflow to effect a generalized decrease in vascular tone resulting in decreased peripheral vascular resistance without significantly altering heart rate or cardiac output. Longevity of experience with this drug in pregnancy has documented its safety. Side effects include sedation and postural hypotension. With prolonged therapy, patients may develop elevations in serum transaminases and a positive Coombs test result.

Labetalol hydrochloride (Normodyne, Trandate) is a frequently used agent and is a combined α- and β-blocker. Labetalol also may be considered a first-line agent in the management of hypertension during pregnancy, and may be superior to pure β-blocking agents, one of which, atenolol, has been associated with intrauterine growth restriction. Beta-blocking drugs should be used with caution in patients with diabetes mellitus or asthma due to the sympathetic nervous system response to hypoglycemia in patients with diabetes and the potential for bronchial constriction in patients with asthma. These drugs have not been associated with an increased incidence of premature uterine contractions.

Hydralazine hydrochloride is a peripheral vasodilator and is best used in the acute setting of hypertensive crisis, but it has some use in the management of chronic hypertension. As with all peripheral vasodilating agents, the use of hydralazine may be associated with maternal tachycardia, and with sodium and free water retention. Long-term use of hydralazine has been associated with a lupuslike reaction. Side effects may include headache, tachycardia, and postural hypotension.

Enalapril (Vasotec) belongs to a class of drugs referred to as angiotensin-converting enzyme (ACE) inhibitors. These drugs, as well as angiotensin-receptor blocking agents, are better avoided during pregnancy, particularly in the second and third trimesters when they have been associated with fetal and neonatal renal failure. Recent data suggest that ACE inhibitors also may be linked to an increased risk of congenital malformations when used in the first trimester of pregnancy. Therefore, complete avoidance of both ACE inhibitors and angiotensin-receptor blockers during the course of pregnancy is recommended.

Table 139–143-1 shows antihypertensive drugs by class, mechanism of action, cardiac output, renal blood flow, and maternal and fetal side effects.

Chronic hypertension in pregnancy. ACOG Practice Bulletin No. 29. American College of Obstetricians and Gynecologists. Obstet Gynecol 2001;98:177–85.

Cooper WO, Hernandez-Diaz S, Arbogast PG, Dudley JA, Dyer S, Gideon PS, et al. Major congenital malformations after first trimester exposure to ACE inhibitors. N Engl J Med 2006;354:2443–51.

TABLE 139–143-1. Antihypertensive Drugs

Class	Drugs	Mechanism of Action	Cardiac Output	Renal Blood Flow	Side Effects Maternal	Side Effects Fetal
Diuretic	Hydrochloro-thiazide	Initial: decreased plasma volume and cardiac output	Decreased	Decreased	Potassium depletion, hyperglycemia, hyperuricemia, hypercholesterolemia, dermatitis, purpura, depression, hypercalcemia, thrombocytopenia, hemorrhagic pancreatitis	Thrombocytopenia
		Later: decreased peripheral vascular resistance	Unchanged	Unchanged or increased		
Central anti-adrenergic agents	Methyldopa	Central false neurotransmitter, CNS effect	Unchanged	Unchanged	Lethargy, fever, hepatitis, dry mouth, hemolytic anemia, positive Coombs test	
	Clonidine	CNS effect	Unchanged or increased	Unchanged	Drowsiness, dry mouth, rebound hypertension after abrupt withdrawal, insomnia	
Vasodilators	Hydralazine hydrochloride	Acts directly on smooth muscle to cause vasodilatation	Increased	Unchanged or increased	Headaches, flushing, lupuslike syndrome	Thrombocytopenia
Peripheral antiadrenergic-agents	Propranolol hydrochloride (Inderal, Inderide)	Blocks β_1 and β_2 receptors	Decreased	Decreased	Dizziness, depression, bronchospasm, nausea, vomiting, diarrhea, constipation, heart failure, fatigue, Raynaud phenomenon, hallucinations, hypertriglyceridemia, hypercholesterolemia, psoriasis	Neonatal bradycardia, hypoglycemia, hyperbilirubinemia, intrauterine growth restriction, respiratory depression, blocking of tachycardic response to hypoxia
β-blocker	Metoprolol tartrate	Blocks β_1 receptors				
	Atenolol (Tenormin)	Blocks β_1 receptors				
Calcium channel antagonists	Nifedipine	Calcium channel antagonists	Unchanged	Unchanged	Tachycardia, flushing, palpitations, gastrointestinal disturbances, hyperkalemia, edema, headache	
	Felodipine					

TABLE 139–143-1. Antihypertensive Drugs (*continued*)

Class	Drugs	Mechanism of Action	Cardiac Output	Renal Blood Flow	Side Effects	
					Maternal	**Fetal**
Peripheral antiadrenergic agents α- and β-receptor blocker	Labetalol hydrochloride (Normodyne, Trandate)	Blocks β- and α-receptors	Unchanged	Unchanged	Headache, tremulousness, heart block, dry mouth	Small for gestational age, hypoglycemia
Angiotensin-converting enzyme inhibitors	Captopril (Capoten, Capozide) Enalapril (Vasotec)	Angiotensin-converting enzyme inhibitors	Unchanged	Unchanged	Hypotension, cough, angioedema, urticarial rash, fever, loss of taste, acute renal failure inbilateral renal artery stenosis, hyperkalemia	Renal dysplasia, oligohydramnios, pulmonary hypoplasia, limb abnormalities and craniofacial defects

144–147

Cervical length

Match the clinical scenario (144–147) with the predictive accuracy for preterm birth of a cervical length of less than 25 mm on transvaginal ultrasonography (A–D).

    (A) High sensitivity, high positive predictive value
    (B) Low sensitivity, low positive predictive value
    (C) Low sensitivity, high positive predictive value
    (D) High sensitivity, low positive predictive value

B   **144.** Singleton gestation in a low-risk patient

A   **145.** Singleton gestation in a woman with a prior spontaneous preterm birth

A   **146.** Singleton gestation in a woman with active preterm labor

C   **147.** Twin gestation

Assessment of cervical length by transvaginal ultrasonography has been studied in a variety of settings and different patient populations and has been shown to be one of the most accurate predictors of preterm birth when used in the appropriate population. Transvaginal ultrasonography of the cervix has been found to be safe and acceptable to patients. A cervical length of less than 25 mm between 16 and 24 weeks of gestation has been shown to be the most reliable threshold for an increased risk of preterm birth. The shorter the cervical length, the higher the risk of preterm birth, and the earlier in gestational age the shortening occurs, the higher the risk.

Prediction of preterm birth by transvaginal ultrasonography of the cervix is markedly dependent on the patient population studied (Appendix C). In women with a singleton gestation and no risk factors, with a low prevalence of preterm birth, both the sensitivity and positive predictive value of this screening test are low, as in patient 144. Even with a cervical length less than 25 mm before 24 weeks of gestation, the chance of preterm birth before 35 weeks of gestation in terms of positive predictive value is less than 20–30%.

In women such as patient 145, with a prior preterm birth and therefore a high prevalence of recurrent preterm birth, the sensitivity and positive predictive value are both greater than 50%, making this screening test more predictive in this population. Women with a singleton gestation and a prior preterm birth, who have a cervical length by transvaginal ultrasonography of less than 25 mm at 16–23 6/7 weeks of gestation, are the group that may benefit from cerclage to prevent preterm birth. Cervical length is also predictive of preterm birth in other women at high-risk for preterm birth, such as those with a prior cone biopsy, müllerian anomalies, and multiple induced abortions.

The finding of a short cervical length less than 25 mm by transvaginal ultrasonography has sensitivity and positive predictive value greater than 50% also in women with preterm labor, as in patient 146 (Appendix C). The high positive predictive value may be due to the fact that women with active preterm labor have a higher prevalence of preterm birth than asymptomatic women. Interventions proven to decrease preterm birth must be confirmed by prospective trials before screening women with preterm labor with cervical length by transvaginal ultrasonography can be recommended.

In multiple gestations, such as in patient 147, transvaginal ultrasonography measurement of cervical length has a low sensitivity and a positive predictive value greater than 50%. The high positive predictive value is probably secondary to the high prevalence of preterm birth in multiple gestations, not to the accuracy of the test. Preterm birth in multiple gestations may follow contractions caused by uterine overdistention, and may not be related to cervical insufficiency. In fact, cerclage for a short cervical length in twin pregnancies may increase, rather than ameliorate, the incidence of preterm birth in these pregnancies. This may be due to the fact that the presence of a foreign body such as cerclage, especially when placed in a normal cervix such as that of most multiple gestations, can be associated with increased inflammation and uterine contractions.

Screening frequency should depend on obstetric history, with serial ultrasonographic examinations of the cervix having a better predictive accuracy than an isolated examination, especially in high-risk populations. Accumulating evidence shows that transvaginal ultrasonography can be used to safely avoid cerclage placement until cervical change occurs, but this management also needs to be confirmed by appropriate prospective trials.

Berghella V, Obido AO, To MS, Rust OA, Althiusius SM. Cerclage for short cervix on ultrasound: meta-analysis of trials using individual patient-level data. Obstet Gynecol 2005;106:181–9.

Goldenberg RL, Iams J, Miodovnik M, Van Dorsten PJ, Thurnau G, Bottoms S, et al. The preterm prediction study: risk factors in twin gestation. Am J Obstet Gynecol 1996;175:1047–53.

Iams JD, Goldenberg RL, Meis PJ, Mercer BM, Moawad A, Das A, et al. The length of the cervix and the risk of spontaneous premature delivery. N Engl J Med 1996;334:567–72.

Murakawa H, Utumi T, Hasegawa I, Tanaka K, Fuzimori R. Evaluation of threatened preterm delivery by transvaginal ultrasonographic measurement of cervical length. Obstet Gynecol 1993;82:829–32.

Owen J, Yost N, Berghella V, Thom E, Swain M, Dildy GA, et al. Midtrimester endovaginal sonography in women at high risk for spontaneous preterm birth. JAMA 2001;286:1340–8.

148–151

Counseling for a woman with a prior cesarean delivery

For each case scenario (148–151), select the most appropriate mode of delivery (A–B).

(A) Vaginal birth after cesarean delivery (VBAC)
(B) Repeat cesarean delivery

A **148.** A 23-year-old woman, gravida 2, para 1, at 36 weeks of gestation underwent one prior low-transverse cesarean delivery 2 years ago for a breech presentation. She strongly desires a trial of labor and presents to triage in early labor.

A **149.** A 42-year-old woman, gravida 3, para 1, at 41 weeks of gestation with one prior low-transverse cesarean delivery returns to discuss delivery options. A recent biophysical profile was reassuring, but the amniotic fluid index was 3.2 cm, and her cervix is 3 cm dilated and completely effaced.

B **150.** A 26-year-old woman, gravida 4, para 1, presents to triage at 39 weeks of gestation for delivery. Her initial cesarean delivery was performed at 25 weeks of gestation in another country, and the operative report is not available.

B **151.** A 39-year-old nulliparous woman underwent a multiple myomectomy last year as part of infertility treatment. She strongly desires a vaginal delivery.

The cesarean delivery rate has steadily increased in the United States over the past two decades, reaching a record high of 29.1% in 2004. Obstetricians have the responsibility of counseling an increasing number of pregnant women with one or more prior cesarean scars about the mode of delivery. A trial of labor after prior cesarean delivery is one way to decrease the overall cesarean delivery rate. Initial enthusiasm for vaginal birth after cesarean delivery (VBAC) led to a decrease in the cesarean delivery rate in the United States in the mid-1990s. Subsequently, the safety of VBAC was questioned when a number of reports were published detailing complications of VBAC, including uterine rupture, with associated maternal and perinatal morbidity. Physician and patient perceptions about the management of women with a prior cesarean delivery vary and have contributed to the current increasing cesarean delivery rate and reluctance to undergo a labor trial. In 1999, the American College of Obstetricians and Gynecologists first issued a statement that a physician must be immediately available throughout active labor capable of monitoring labor and performing an emergency cesarean delivery in women undergoing a trial of labor. This caused some physicians and hospitals to not offer VBACs due to safety concerns or limitations of the facility.

Appropriate candidates for a trial of labor are women with a low-transverse uterine incision and no contraindications to vaginal delivery. Boxes 148–151-1 and 148–151-2 list selection criteria for appropriate VBAC candidates and contraindications for VBAC. Approximately 60–80% of women with a previous cesarean delivery who attempt a trial of labor will give birth vaginally. Certain factors that may influence the likelihood of successful vaginal delivery after cesarean include previous vaginal delivery, previous VBAC, or an initial cesarean delivery performed for a nonrecurring indication such as malpresentation. Lower VBAC success rates are seen in women who require labor induction, those with a body

BOX 148–151-1

Conditions for Vaginal Birth After Cesarean Delivery

- One previous low-transverse cesarean delivery
- Clinically adequate pelvis
- No other uterine scars or previous rupture
- Physician immediately available throughout active labor capable of monitoring labor and performing an emergency cesarean delivery
- Availability of anesthesia and personnel for emergency cesarean delivery

Vaginal birth after previous cesarean delivery. ACOG Practice Bulletin No. 54. American College of Obstetricians and Gynecologists. Obstet Gynecol 2004;104: 203–12.

BOX 148–151-2

Contraindications for Vaginal Birth After Cesarean Delivery

- Previous classical or T-shaped incision or extensive transfundal uterine surgery
- Previous uterine rupture
- Medical or obstetric complication that precludes vaginal delivery
- Inability to perform emergency cesarean delivery because of unavailable surgeon, anesthesia, sufficient staff, or facility
- Two prior uterine scars and no vaginal deliveries

Vaginal birth after previous cesarean delivery. ACOG Practice Bulletin No. 54. American College of Obstetricians and Gynecologists. Obstet Gynecol 2004;104: 203–12.

mass index (weight in kilograms divided by height in meters squared [kg/m^2]) of 30 or more, and those whose prior indication for cesarean delivery was dystocia. Neither elective repeat cesarean delivery nor VBAC is risk free. A failed labor trial may have significant maternal complications including uterine rupture, hysterectomy, operative injury, endometritis, and need for blood product transfusion. Hypoxic–ischemic encephalopathy may occur in infants following uterine rupture. Maternal risks of placenta previa and accreta, operative injury, duration of operative time, and need for blood products increase with the number of prior cesarean deliveries.

In counseling women with a prior cesarean delivery, an honest appraisal must be given. Reasons for the initial cesarean delivery should be evaluated, and an approximate success rate should be discussed with the patient. The safety of VBAC for suitable candidates in a setting equipped with personnel capable of managing potential complications of VBAC should be discussed. Concerns about safety necessitate a discussion about possible com-

plications associated with VBAC. The absolute risk of uterine rupture with a prior low-transverse uterine incision is less than 1%. Estimated risk of uterine rupture in women with a prior cesarean delivery are as follows:

- Previous classical incisions: 4–9%
- T-shaped incisions: 4–9%
- Low-vertical incision: 1–7%
- Low-transverse incision: 0.2–0.5%

Induction of labor occasionally is necessary in women with a prior cesarean delivery for either a maternal or fetal indication and remains a reasonable option. The induction of labor with and without prostaglandins (specifically prostaglandin E_2) sparks controversy because of the potentially increased risk of uterine rupture. Cervical ripening with misoprostol (prostaglandin E_1) in women with prior cesarean deliveries has been shown to be associated with a significant risk of uterine rupture and is not recommended. Selection of appropriate VBAC candidates that will likely give birth vaginally and avoiding sequential use of prostaglandins and oxytocin appear to offer the lowest risk of uterine rupture.

In patient 148, since the initial cesarean delivery was performed for a nonrecurring indication, her chance for a successful VBAC when admitted in early labor is at least 80%, and a trial of labor is a reasonable option. Patient 149 may undergo a trial of labor avoiding the sequential use of prostaglandins and oxytocin. A labor trial in a woman with an unfavorable cervix is unlikely to be successful and may increase the maternal and fetal morbidity and mortality; a repeat cesarean delivery is a better option. A repeat cesarean delivery is the best choice for the patient with a preterm cesarean delivery with an unknown scar (patient 150). It also offers the best option for the woman with a prior multiple myomectomy because the active segment of the uterus was probably involved (patient 151). Allowing labor in these cases places the patient at increased risk for uterine scar rupture.

The absolute risk of adverse outcomes when undergoing a trial of labor after one prior low-transverse cesarean delivery remains low. Appropriate candidates should be counseled and given the option of a labor trial.

Induction of labor for vaginal birth after cesarean delivery. ACOG Committee Opinion No. 342. American College of Obstetricians and Gynecologists. Obstet Gynecol 2006;108:465–7.

Landon MB, Hauth JC, Leveno KJ, Spong CY, Leindecker S, Varner MW, et al. Maternal and perinatal outcomes associated with a trial of labor after a prior cesarean delivery. National Institute of Child Health and Human Development Maternal-Fetal Medicine Units Network. N Engl J Med 2004;351:2581–9.

Landon MB, Leindecker S, Spong CY, Hauth JC, Bloom S, Varner MW, et al. The MFMU cesarean registry: factors affecting the success of trial of labor after previous cesarean delivery. National Institute of Child Health and Human Development Maternal-Fetal Medicine Units Network. Am J Obstet Gynecol 2005;193:1016–23.

Macones GA, Cahill A, Pare E, Stamilio DM, Ratcliffe S, Stevens E, et al. Obstetric outcomes in women with two prior cesarean deliveries: is vaginal birth after cesarean delivery a viable option? Am J Obstet Gynecol 2005;192:1223–8; discussion 1228–9.

Silver RM, Landon MB, Rouse DJ, Leveno KJ, Spong CY, Thom EA, et al. Maternal morbidity associated with multiple repeat cesarean deliveries. National Institute of Child Health and Human Development Maternal-Fetal Medicine Units Network. Obstet Gynecol 2006; 107:1226–32.

Vaginal birth after previous cesarean delivery. ACOG Practice Bulletin No. 54. American College of Obstetricians and Gynecologists. Obstet Gynecol 2004;104:203–12.

Yeh J, Wactawski-Wende J, Shelton JA, Reschke J. Temporal trends in the rates of trial of labor in low-risk pregnancies and their impact on the rates and success of vaginal birth after cesarean delivery. Am J Obstet Gynecol 2006;194:144.

152–156

Maternal and fetal side effects of tocolysis

Match the maternal and fetal side effect (152–156) with the corresponding tocolytic agent (A–D).

(A) Indomethacin (Indocin)
(B) Terbutaline sulfate
(C) Nifedipine (Adalat, Procardia)
(D) Magnesium sulfate

B   **152.** Maternal hypokalemia

A   **153.** Oligohydramnios

A   **154.** Fetal ductus arteriosus constriction

D   **155.** Maternal respiratory depression

D   **156.** Neonatal hypotonia

Obstetric tocolytic use remains a therapeutic modality that is under discussion. Issues of efficacy, duration of prolongation of pregnancy, and ultimate perinatal outcome are largely unresolved. Nonetheless, tocolytics remain in common use for the management of premature labor, and these agents bring with them unique and potentially adverse side effects.

Indomethacin (Indocin) is the most widely used antiprostaglandin tocolytic in the United States. Because of its effects on renal blood flow and fetal cardiovascular dynamics, indomethacin may be associated with premature constriction of the ductus arteriosus, fetal tricuspid regurgitation, and fetal pulmonary vascular changes. With prolonged use, such changes could result in neonatal pulmonary hypertension and persistent patent ductus arteriosus. The effect of indomethacin on renal blood flow also has been linked with oligohydramnios.

Magnesium sulfate is a nonspecific calcium channel blocker. It may be associated with maternal muscle weakness and respiratory depression that may limit its use and therefore its efficacy. Magnesium ions also cross the placenta freely, and neonatal hypermagnesemia may result in neonatal hypotonia and in some cases respiratory depression. Limited data suggest an increase in total pediatric mortality, although these data are highly controversial.

Terbutaline sulfate is predominantly a β_2-agonist, and relaxes smooth muscle. Its effects on β-receptors result in hyperglycemia and hyperinsulinemia, the combination of which tends to move potassium from the extracellular to the intracellular compartment with resultant maternal hypokalemia.

Nifedipine (Adalat, Procardia) is a dihydropyridine class calcium channel blocker and has been used as a tocolytic. It is more selective than magnesium sulfate with respect to which calcium channels are blocked, and therefore would not be expected to be as efficacious, although the data on this point are unclear. Perhaps because of its more selective calcium channel blocking nature or dosage differences, nifedipine generally is well tolerated with very few maternal or fetal side effects. Side effects may be more apparent if this agent is used in combination with other tocolytics.

Iams JD. Preterm birth. In: Gabbe SG, Niebyl JR, Simpson JL, editors. Obstetrics: normal and problem pregnancies. 4th ed. New York (NY): Churchill Livingstone; 2002. p. 755–826.

Management of preterm labor. ACOG Practice Bulletin No. 43. American College of Obstetricians and Gynecologists. Obstet Gynecol 2003;101:1039–47.

157–160
Cardiovascular physiology

For the hemodynamic parameter (157–160), select the effect (A–C) that occurs during pregnancy.

(A) Increased
(B) Decreased
(C) Unchanged

C   **157.** Pulmonary artery occlusion pressure (wedge pressure)

C   **158.** Central venous pressure

B   **159.** Systemic vascular resistance

B   **160.** Pulmonary vascular resistance

Prospective, randomized, clinical trials have failed to show a survival benefit from use of the pulmonary artery catheter. In addition, discoveries about the pathophysiology of obstetric complications through use of pulmonary artery catheter monitoring over the years have lessened the need for such monitoring in current obstetric practice. All the same, pulmonary artery catheter hemodynamic monitoring is still used in some critically ill obstetric patients with complex problems such as severe mitral stenosis, septic shock, and acute respiratory failure. When pulmonary artery catheter monitoring is used, the normal values for pregnancy should be known so that the hemodynamic data may be properly interpreted.

One landmark study provided normal values for pulmonary artery catheter hemodynamic monitoring. Ten nulliparous women had pulmonary artery catheters and radial artery catheters inserted at 36–38 weeks of gestation and central hemodynamic values were obtained. The 10 patients had repeat studies performed at 11–13 weeks postpartum (Table 157–160-1). Although blood volume increased 40–50% during pregnancy, mean arterial pressure was unchanged. Right ventricular filling pressure (central venous pressure) and left ventricular filling pressure (pulmonary artery occlusion pressure) were unchanged during pregnancy. Cardiac output increased because of an increase in both heart rate and stroke volume. Systemic and pulmonary vascular resistances fell. There was no change in left ventricular contractility as measured by left ventricular stroke work index.

Maternal adaptations to pregnancy such as dilation of the venous capacitance system, refractoriness to angiotensin II and norepinephrine, and vascular changes in the

TABLE 157–160-1. Central Hemodynamic Changes in Pregnancy

Measure	Nonpregnant	Pregnant	Significant Change
Mean arterial pressure (mm Hg)	86.4 ± 7.5	90.3 ± 5.8	None
Central venous pressure (mm Hg)	3.7 ± 2.6	3.6 ± 2.5	None
Pulmonary artery occlusion pressure (mm Hg)	6.3 ± 2.1	7.5 ± 1.8	None
Cardiac output (L/minute)	4.3 ± 0.9	6.2 ± 1.0	+43%
Heart rate (beats/minute)	71 ±10	83 ± 10	+17%
Systemic vascular resistance (dynes/cm/sec^{-5})	1,530 ± 520	1,210 ± 266	−21%
Pulmonary vascular resistance (dynes/cm/sec^{-5})	119 ± 47	78 ± 22	−34%
Left ventricular work index (g/m/m^{-2})	41 ± 8	48 ± 6	None

Modified from Clark SL, Cotton DB, Lee W, Bishop C, Hill T, Southwick J, et al. Central hemodynamic assessment of normal term pregnancy. Am J Obstet Gynecol 1989;161:1441.

uterus and renal circulations are thought to be mediated by nitric oxide (endothelium-derived relaxing factor), prostaglandins, endothelin, relaxin, and other substances. The mechanisms for the reduction in vascular resistance and the relative importance of the various mediators are not fully understood.

Carbillon L, Uzan M, Uzan S. Pregnancy, vascular tone, and maternal hemodynamics: a crucial adaptation. Obstet Gynecol Surv 2000;55: 574–81.

Clark SL, Cotton DB, Lee W, Bishop C, Hill T, Southwick J, et al. Central hemodynamic assessment of normal term pregnancy. Am J Obstet Gynecol 1989;161:1439–42.

Cunningham FG, Leveno KJ, Bloom SL, Hauth JC, Gilstrap LC 3rd, Wenstrom KD, editors. Williams obstetrics. 22nd ed. New York (NY): McGraw-Hill; 2005. p. 989–96.

Wheeler AP, Bernard GP, Thompson BT, Schoenfeld D, Wiedemann HP, deBoisblanc B, et al. Pulmonary-artery versus central venous catheter to guide treatment of acute lung injury. The National Heart, Lung, and Blood Institute Acute Respiratory Distress Syndrome (ARDS) Clinical Trials Network. N Engl J Med 2006;354:2213–24.

161–164

Evaluation of embryonic and extraembryonic fetal structures

Match the embryonic structure (161–164) with the gestational age in weeks (A–E) from the last menstrual period at which the structure is seen by ultrasonography.

- (A) 4 weeks
- (B) 5 weeks
- (C) 6 weeks
- (D) 8 weeks
- (E) 11 weeks

C **161.** Cardiac activity

A **162.** Chorionic sac

E **163.** Physiologic midgut rotation

B **164.** Yolk sac

Transabdominal ultrasonography and transvaginal ultrasonography both allow early visualization of the pregnancy. However, with transvaginal ultrasonography, structures can be seen about 7–10 days earlier than with transabdominal ultrasonography, because it uses higher ultrasound frequencies, 5–7 MHz, which results in better resolution of the early pregnancy. Another advantage of transvaginal ultrasonography is that the probe can be placed close to the uterus. Therefore, maternal body factors such as obesity or abdominal scars do not preclude adequate imaging of the uterus and embryo.

At approximately 4 weeks from the last menstrual period (LMP) or 2 weeks from conception or embryo transfer, the chorionic sac can be seen to one side of the cavity line within the thick decidual reaction of the endometrium. If free serum β-hCG is available, this would correspond to an approximate value of 1,000 mIU/mL. To differentiate between a fluid collection in the endometrium and a true chorionic sac is important for careful evaluation of the trophoblastic-decidual reaction. The true chorionic sac can be identified by its round shape and its brightly echogenic outer rim within the thick decidual reaction of the endometrium.

At approximately 5 weeks from the LMP or 3 weeks from embryo transfer or conception, the yolk sac should be seen within the sonolucent chorionic sac. By a mean chorionic sac size of 6 mm, a yolk sac should be present. A chorionic sac greater than 8 mm without a yolk sac is suggestive of a pregnancy failure. However, care must be exercised and the physician should always repeat the scan in 5–7 days to confirm the findings.

The embryo can be clearly imaged by transvaginal ultrasonography by 6 weeks of gestation when it measures approximately 2–3 mm. The embryo at this gestational age appears as a linear structure in very close proximity to the yolk sac. Cardiac activity begins at approximately 36 days from the LMP or a crown–rump length (CRL) of approximately 1.5–3 mm. All embryos by the time they reach 5 mm or a gestational age of 6 weeks and 4 days should have cardiac activity visible on ultrasonographic examination.

A number of factors may preclude visualization of the chorionic sac, yolk sac, and embryo early in pregnancy:

- Frequency of the transducer (transabdominal ultrasonography versus transvaginal ultrasonography)
- Position of the uterus
- Presence of leiomyomata
- Experience of the observer
- Degree of magnification of the image

When scanning at this early gestational age, the image should be magnified to encompass most of the ultrasound screen.

By the time the embryo reaches the eighth week of gestation or a CRL of approximately 20 mm, the head can be seen as a separate entity from the torso and the upper and lower limb buds can be clearly imaged. In addition, fetal body movements can be detected for the first time.

The fetal period begins at approximately 70 days from the LMP or the 9th week of gestation. Beyond this point, the fetus clearly resembles a baby and can be easily recognized as such.

Physiologic midgut herniation refers to temporary herniation of the fetal bowel into the residual extraembryonic coelom at the base of the umbilical cord. The physiologic midgut herniation is ultrasonographically evident between 9 and 11 weeks of gestation. Reduction of this hernia occurs by 12 weeks of gestation; at this time, the CRL is 53–66 mm. Bowel present at the base of the cord beyond 12 weeks is consistent with an omphalocele.

Fleischer AC, Kepple DM. Transvaginal sonography of early pregnancy. In: Fleischer AC, Manning FA, Jeanty P, Romero R, editors. Sonography in obstetrics and gynecology: principles and practice. 6th ed. New York (NY): McGraw Hill; 2001. p. 61–88.

Goldstein SR, Timor-Tritsch EI. Early pregnancy. In: Tritsch IE, Goldstein SR, editors. Ultrasound in gynecology. 2nd ed. New York (NY): Churchill Livingstone, Elsevier; 2007. p. 139–50.

Monteagudo A, Timor-Tritsch IE. First trimester anatomy scan: pushing the limits. What can we see now? Curr Opin Obstet Gynecol 2003;15:131–41.

165–168

Acute fatty liver of pregnancy

Match the case presentation (165–168) with the most likely diagnosis (A-F).

(A) Acute fatty liver of pregnancy
(B) Hemolysis, elevated liver enzymes, and low platelets (HELLP) syndrome
(C) Acute viral hepatitis
(D) Thrombotic thrombocytopenic purpura
(E) Cholelithiasis
(F) Cholestasis of pregnancy

A **165.** A 26-year-old primigravid woman presents at 33 weeks of gestation with a 3-day history of nausea, malaise, and right upper quadrant abdominal pain. She has a temperature of 36.7°C (98°F) and a blood pressure reading of 134/78 mm Hg, and her skin and sclera are icteric. Laboratory test results include elevated liver function tests, elevated bilirubin, elevated ammonia, 1+ proteinuria, glucose of 42 mg/dL, and a prothrombin time of 48 seconds.

D **166.** A 31-year-old woman, gravida 3, para 2, presents at 28 weeks of gestation with fever, confusion, nausea, vomiting, and abdominal pain. She has a temperature of 38.5°C (101.3°F) and blood pressure reading of 148/95 mm Hg. Laboratory test results show normal transaminase levels, normal coagulation panel, 3+ proteinuria, creatinine level of 1.4 mg/dL, leukocytes of 28,000/mL, hemoglobin of 7.2 g/dL, and platelets of 15,000/mm^3.

B **167.** A 46-year-old nulligravid woman is admitted to the hospital at 38 weeks of gestation in early labor. She complains of a frontal headache and sees "sparkles" in front of her eyes. She has a temperature of 37°C (98.6°F) and blood pressure reading of 171/113 mm Hg. Laboratory evaluation shows 4+ proteinuria, transaminase levels three times normal, platelets of 80,000/mm^3, and a creatinine level of 1.3 mg/dL.

F **168.** A 23-year-old primigravid woman is seen in triage at 31 weeks of gestation for intense itching that is worse at night. Her temperature is 37.1°C (98.8°F) and blood pressure reading is 102/68 mm Hg. Laboratory test findings reveal trace proteinuria, aspartate aminotransferase of 152 IU/L, alanine aminotransferase of 21 IU/L, total bilirubin of 4.3 mg/dL, prothrombin time of 14 seconds, and elevated serum bile acids.

The differential diagnosis of elevated liver function tests and diseases that affect the liver in the third trimester of pregnancy includes several entities with varying maternal and fetal outcomes. Overlapping clinical presentations often impart a diagnostic challenge. Disorders to be considered are acute fatty liver of pregnancy, HELLP syndrome, acute viral hepatitis, hemolytic-uremic syndrome, thrombotic thrombocytopenic purpura, cholelithiasis, and cholestasis of pregnancy. Clinical and laboratory findings are frequently similar, but management strategies and outcomes may differ (Table 165–168-1).

Patient 165 has classic symptomatology of acute fatty liver of pregnancy, which is a rare condition that is potentially fatal and affects 1 in 7,000 to 1 in 16,000 pregnancies. Acute fatty liver of pregnancy occurs in the third trimester and involves microvesicular fatty infiltration of the liver without inflammation or necrosis. The exact etiology is unknown, but some cases have been linked to the inherited defect in mitochondrial β-oxidation of fatty acids, long-chain 3-hydroxyacyl-coenzyme-A dehydrogenase deficiency. Fetal production of long-chain fatty acids that are not cleared by the mother are toxic to the liver. The maternal mortality rate in women with acute fatty liver of pregnancy is approximately 18%, with a fetal mortality rate of 7-58%. A woman with the condition usually presents in the third trimester with a 1–2-week history of nausea, vomiting, anorexia, malaise, and right upper quadrant pain. The condition is common in women with twin gestations. Elevated transaminases, bilirubin, white blood cell count, and ammonia are often seen. Hypoglycemia and a prolonged prothrombin time are frequent laboratory findings. Decreased fibrinogen and platelets contribute to the coagulopathy. A number of women with acute fatty liver of pregnancy will have features consistent with coexisting preeclampsia, and elevated creatinine and proteinuria may be present. Manage-

TABLE 165–168-1. Differential Diagnosis of Acute Fatty Liver in Pregnancy

	Fatty Liver of Pregnancy	Acute Viral Hepatitis	HELLP Syndrome/Preeclampsia/Eclampsia	Cholestasis of Pregnancy	Hemolytic Uremic Syndrome	Thrombotic Thrombocytopenic Purpura
Onset (I/II/III trimester)	II/III, most greater than 35 weeks, rare reports less than 30 weeks	Any	II/III (after 20 weeks)	III, rare reports II	Any	Any, 60% less than 24 weeks
Clinical findings	Malaise, nausea/emesis, jaundice, mental status changes, abdominal pain, ± hemorrhage, ± preeclampsia	Malaise, nausea/emesis, jaundice, abdominal pain	Malaise, hypertension, proteinuria, nausea, abdominal pain, rare jaundice ± seizures ± oliguria ± coagulopathy	Pruritus (worst in PM, palms and soles) ± jaundice	Hypertension, acute renal failure, nausea/emesis, may have fever and neurologic findings, hallmarks microangiopathic anemia, severe thrombocytopenia	Often neurologic findings, fever and renal dysfunction, hallmarks microangiopathic anemia, severe thrombocytopenia
Laboratory						
Transaminases (units/mL)	↑Usually less than 500 ↑Usually 3–10	↑Commonly greater than 1,000	Normal– ↑50× (more if liver hematoma) ↑occasionally (usually less than 2–3 times)	↑(usually less than 300) Often ↑(usually less than 5)	Usually normal ↑(unconjugated)	Usually normal ↑(unconjugated)
Bilirubin (mg/dL)	↑	±↑	Normal unless DIC/intrauterine fetal distress/abruptio placentae	Usually normal, may be ↑	Usually normal	Usually normal
Prothrombin time	↑	±↑	↑occasionally	↑(up to 4 times normal)	Usually normal	Usually normal
Alkaline phosphatase				↑serum bile acids		
Other	↑Ammonia, very ↓ antithrombin III, ↓platelets, ↓ fibrinogen, ↑WBC, ↑creatinine, proteinuria, ↓glucose	+ hepatitis serology, ↓antithrombin III	Moderately↓ antithrombin III, proteinuria, ↓platelets, ↑creatinine, ↑uric acid		Normal antithrombin III, usually normal fibrinogen, ↑WBC, ↓platelets (often less than 20,000), normal – slightly ↑ creatinine, ± proteinuria	Normal antithrombin III, usually normal fibrinogen, ↑WBC, ↓platelets (often less than 20,000), normal – slightly ↑ creatinine, ± proteinuria
Liver histopathology	Centrilobular microvesicular fat, cholestasis	Marked inflammation and necrosis	Periportal fibrin deposits, hemorrhagic hepatocellular necrosis, inflammation	Centrilobular cholestasis, no inflammation	Unknown	Unknown
Treatment	Immediate delivery, supportive	Supportive	MgSO$_4$ seizure prophylaxis, delivery (delayed in very selected preterm cases), antihypertensive treatment	Ursodeoxycholic acid, corticosteroids, cholestyramine all of reported benefit, vitamin K	Plasma exchange, FFP infusion pending initiation of plasma exchange, corticosteroids/ antiplatelet agents	Plasma exchange, FFP infusion pending initiation of plasma exchange, corticosteroids/ antiplatelet agents

DIC, disseminated intravascular coagulation; FFP, fresh frozen plasma; MgSO$_4$, magnesium sulfate; WBC, white blood cell count.

McNulty J. Acute fatty liver of pregnancy. In: Foley MR, Strong TH, Garite TJ, editors. Obstetric intensive care manual. 2nd ed. New York (NY): McGraw-Hill; 2004. p. 212–3.

ment of the condition includes supportive care and stabilization by treating the coagulopathy, monitoring for hypoglycemia, and providing a transfusion when indicated, followed by prompt delivery.

Thrombotic thrombocytopenic purpura is a rare and life-threatening microangiopathic disorder that may occur in any trimester of pregnancy. The disease process involves aggregation of platelets within arterioles and capillaries that have sustained endothelial cell injury. The small vessel occlusion can produce local ischemia and infarction within the organ system due to platelet thrombi, with resultant thrombocytopenia and mechanical injury to erythrocytes. The classic pentad of thrombotic thrombocytopenic purpura includes microangiopathic hemolytic anemia, thrombocytopenia, neurologic abnormalities, fever, and renal dysfunction (Box 165–168-1). Patient 166 has findings consistent with thrombotic thrombocytopenic purpura. Treatment involves supportive care and plasma transfusions and plasmapheresis, which should be performed daily until the platelet count has normalized and hemolysis resolves. Immediate delivery will not reverse the process.

The HELLP syndrome is encountered frequently in women in the third trimester, as in patient 167. Elevated blood pressure, significant proteinuria, elevated liver function tests, low platelets, frontal headache, and scotomata are characteristic of the disease. The treatment is

seizure prophylaxis with magnesium sulfate, antihypertensive therapy, and delivery.

Patient 168 has normal blood pressure and only trace proteinuria. Her itching, elevated liver function test result and bile acids, and prolonged prothrombin time are indicative of cholestasis of pregnancy. Cholestasis of pregnancy usually presents in the third trimester with intractable pruritus, particularly on the palms and soles, and is worse at night. Some patients develop clinical jaundice. Transaminases, bilirubin, alkaline phosphatase, and serum bile acids are elevated. The prothrombin time in some cases may be prolonged with the resultant risk of postpartum hemorrhage. Treatment includes medications to control maternal itching and vitamin K for the coagulation disorder. Nonstress tests or biophysical profile testing is recommended in women with cholestasis because of the increased risk of nonreassuring fetal heart rate patterns and intrauterine fetal demise. Delivery is recommended at 37–38 weeks of gestation. Cholestasis of pregnancy is self-limited and abates within the first few days after delivery.

Acute viral hepatitis was not represented in the cases described. Hepatitis may occur in any trimester with the clinical presentation of malaise, nausea, vomiting, abdominal pain, and jaundice. Markedly elevated transaminases are found along with elevated bilirubin. Hepatitis serologic testing confirms the diagnosis, and the treatment consists of supportive care.

Cholelithiasis, also not depicted in the cases above, is usually asymptomatic in pregnancy, except when the gallstones obstruct the cystic duct or common bile duct, causing inflammation and pain and, in some cases, acute cholecystitis. Clinical presentation is of intense right upper quadrant, colicky pain, nausea, vomiting, tachycardia, and low-grade fever. Transaminases, amylase, alkaline phosphatase, white blood cell count, and lipase may be elevated. Conservative therapy and stabilization with intravenous fluids, analgesics, and antibiotics may be initiated. Diagnostic modalities such as right upper quadrant ultrasonography, endoscopic retrograde cholangiopancreatography, or magnetic resonance cholangiopancreatography and surgical therapy are options, depending on the trimester of pregnancy and clinical presentation.

BOX 165–168-1

Classic Findings in Thrombotic Thrombocytopenic Purpura*

1. Microangiopathic, hemolytic anemia*[†]
2. Thrombocytopenia*[†]
3. Neurologic abnormalities*[†]
   —Confusion
   —Headache
   —Paresis
   —Visual hallucinations
   —Seizures
4. Fever*
5. Renal dysfunction*

---

*The classic pentad is found in 40% of patients.

[†]This triad is present in 75% of patients.

Foley MR, Strong TH, Garite TJ, editors. Obstetric intensive care manual. 2nd ed. New York (NY): McGraw-Hill; 2004. p. 45.

Fesenmeier MF, Coppage KH, Lambers DS, Barton JR, Sibai BM. Acute fatty liver of pregnancy in 3 tertiary care centers. Am J Obstet Gynecol 2005;192:1416-19.

McNulty J. Acute fatty liver of pregnancy. In: Foley MR, Strong TH, Garite TJ, editors. Obstetric intensive care manual. 2nd ed. New York (NY): McGraw-Hill; 2004. p. 207-15.

Sibai BM. Imitators of severe pre-eclampsia/eclampsia. Clin Perinatol 2004;31:835-52, vii-viii.

169–172

Maternal complications of sickle cell anemia

Match the most likely clinical association (169–172) with the corresponding abnormal hemoglobin (A–D).

(A) Hemoglobin SS
(B) Hemoglobin AS
(C) Hemoglobin SC
(D) Hemoglobin Bart's

A   **169.** Salmonella osteomyelitis

A   **170.** Autosplenectomy

D   **171.** Hydrops fetalis

B   **172.** Asymptomatic bacteriuria

The hemoglobinopathies present a challenge to clinicians at a variety of levels. The genetics of these disorders can be complex and the clinical manifestations quite variable and frequently unique to the specific hemoglobinopathy. Red blood cells first appear at approximately 6 weeks after conception and are accompanied by the production of some unique embryonic hemoglobins until approximately 11 weeks of gestation, when the predominant hemoglobin produced is hemoglobin F, or so-called fetal hemoglobin.

The commencement of synthesis of adult hemoglobin occurs late in the third trimester at approximately 37–38 weeks of gestation. Knowledge of the structures of the embryonic hemoglobins and fetal hemoglobin allows us to conclude that normal α-globin, but not β-globin, is a requirement for normal fetal and early neonatal development.

In hemoglobin Bart's (homozygous α-thalassemia), there is no useful α-globin production. Instead, tetramers of γ-globin are being produced. This abnormal production of γ chains without any production of α chains results in congestive heart failure and hydrops fetalis.

Hemoglobin AS, or so-called sickle cell trait, is the result of heterozygosity that causes the production of both hemoglobin S and hemoglobin A. Clinically, these patients are usually normal but may be at increased risk for painless hematuria and asymptomatic bacteriuria.

Hemoglobin SS is the homozygous state in which only hemoglobin S is produced, resulting from mutation of the β-globin chain and causing the clinical entity of sickle cell anemia. Patients with sickle cell anemia are at risk for a multitude of disorders, including sickle cell crisis, acute chest syndrome, and a variety of more serious vasoocclusive crises that can lead to infarction of multiple organs including the spleen, resulting in autosplenectomy.

Because of the additional immune compromise imposed by autosplenectomy, it is essential that patients with sickle cell disease be watched carefully for signs of infection and that they receive pneumococcus vaccine. Patients with sickle cell anemia also seem to be particularly susceptible to bone infarction and resultant salmonella osteomyelitis. Hemoglobin SC disease is noted for a lesser degree of anemia than that seen in SS disease.

Benz EJ. Hemoglobinopathies. In: Kasper DL, Braunwald E, Fauci AS, Hauser SL, Longo DL, Jameson JH, editors. Harrison's principles of internal medicine. 16th ed. New York (NY): McGraw-Hill; 2005. p. 593–601.

Samuels P. Hematologic complications of pregnancy. In: Gabbe SG, Niebyl JR, Simpson JL, editors. Obstetrics: normal and problem pregnancies. 4th ed. New York (NY): Churchill Livingstone; 2002. p. 1180–4.

173–177
Thrombocytopenia

For each patient (173–177), select the diagnosis (A–H) that best fits her symptoms.

(A) Drug-induced thrombocytopenia
(B) Thrombotic thrombocytopenic purpura
(C) Immune thrombocytopenia
(D) Alloimmune thrombocytopenia
(E) Gestational thrombocytopenia
(F) Systemic lupus erythematosus
(G) Hemolysis, elevated liver enzymes, and low platelet count (HELLP) syndrome
(H) Disseminated intravascular coagulation

E **173.** A 24-year-old woman, gravida 4, para 3, at 32 weeks of gestation has no history of abnormal bleeding, and former pregnancies were normal. Her platelet count is 90,000/mm³.

B **174.** A 21-year-old-woman, gravida 1, at 36 weeks of gestation has a history of seizure, headaches, petechiae, and altered sensorium. She had a fever, nausea, vomiting, and upper abdominal pain about 3 days before coming to the hospital. Her blood pressure is 110/89 mm Hg. Her platelet count is 20,000/mm³.

C **175.** A 27-year-old woman, gravida 1, para 1, at 16 weeks of gestation has a history of easy bruising and heavy menses. Her platelet count is 80,000/mm³.

H **176.** A 21-year-old woman, gravida 2, para 1, at 32 weeks of gestation presented with abruptio placentae. She was delivered of a stillborn and is having postpartum bleeding. Her platelet count is 50,000/mm³.

F **177.** A 28-year-old-woman, gravida 3, para 2, at 36 weeks of gestation presents with fatigue, facial rash, and joint pain. Her platelet count is 60,000/mm³.

Thrombocytopenia is defined as a platelet count less than $150 \times 10^9/L^{-1}$. It is classified as mild with a platelet count of $100–150 \times 10^9/L^{-1}$, moderate at $50–100 \times 10^9/L^{-1}$, and severe with less than $50 \times 10^9/L^{-1}$. It occurs in approximately 10% of pregnant women and is caused by a variety of obstetric and preexisting medical disorders. Thrombocytopenia is caused either by accelerated platelet destruction or decreased production of platelets. A report of a low platelet count also may be an artifact due to platelet clumping. Thus, a first step in the evaluation of a low platelet count should be a manual assessment of platelet number. Box 173–177-1 shows the etiology of thrombocytopenia.

Patient 173 has gestational thrombocytopenia, a condition found in approximately 5–7% of pregnant women. Gestational thrombocytopenia is the most prevalent cause of thrombocytopenia in pregnancy, accounting for approximately 75% of thrombocytopenia in pregnant women. It is defined by a platelet count of no less than $70 \times 10^9/L^{-1}$, chiefly during the third trimester, and the count returns to normal within 12 weeks of delivery. A

BOX 173–177-1

Etiology of Thrombocytopenia

- Pseudothrombocytopenia (platelet clumping)
- Gestational thrombocytopenia
- Immune thrombocytopenic purpura
- Preeclampsia/hemolysis, elevated liver enzymes and low platelet count (HELLP) syndrome
- Disseminated intravascular coagulation
- Microangiopathic hemolytic anemia (thrombotic thrombocytopenic purpura, hemolytic uremic syndrome, acute fatty liver of pregnancy)
- Autoimmune disease (systemic lupus anticoagulant, antiphospholipid antibodies)
- Human immunodeficiency virus (HIV) or other infectious diseases
- Drug-induced thrombocytopenia
- Dilutional
- Myeloproliferative disease/malignancy
- Hereditary/congenital thrombocytopenia

patient with gestational thrombocytopenia will have a normal medical and obstetric history, and the condition usually is diagnosed by exclusion. The etiology is unknown, but is considered to be caused by relative hemodilution in pregnancy, augmented by increased trapping or destruction of platelets. There is no risk of hemorrhage to the mother, fetus, or neonate. Antiplatelet antibodies do not differentiate gestational thrombocytopenia from immune thrombocytopenic purpura.

Patient 174 has thrombotic thrombocytopenic purpura. This condition is characterized by microangiopathic hemolytic anemia, thrombocytopenia, fluctuating neurologic signs, renal impairment, and fever. Neurologic signs are absent in approximately one third of cases, and renal impairment and fever are present in a minority of cases. Approximately 10–25% of cases occur in pregnancy, and pregnancy is considered to be an initiating factor.

Patient 175 has immune thrombocytopenic purpura. This condition is caused by platelet destruction in the reticular endothelial system, due to platelet autoantibodies against several platelet membrane glycoprotein complexes. It is characterized by a moderate to severe decrease in the platelet count. Immune thrombocytopenic purpura constitutes approximately 5% of cases of thrombocytopenia in pregnancy. It is the most important cause of severe thrombocytopenia in the first trimester and is a diagnosis of exclusion. The four consistent features are:

1. Persistent thrombocytopenia

2. Normal or increased number of megakaryocytes by bone marrow aspiration

3. Exclusion of disease or drugs that cause thrombocytopenia

4. Absence of splenomegaly

Most patients with immune thrombocytopenia have a history of easy bruising or bleeding that predates the pregnancy.

Preeclampsia and HELLP syndrome, which none of these patients has, are considered to be the cause of thrombocytopenia in pregnancy in approximately 21% of cases. The maternal platelet count returns to normal within 3–5 days of delivery. The HELLP syndrome is a variant of preeclampsia characterized by hemolytic anemia, elevated liver enzymes, and a low platelet count. It is responsible for maternal deaths and stillbirth, especially as a result of abruptio placentae and preterm delivery. Maternal bleeding may occur because of abruptio placentae and complicating disseminated intravascular coagulation (DIC), as in patient 176.

Abruptio placentae is the most common cause of DIC in pregnancy. A cause of significant mortality and morbidity, DIC can be diagnosed by low fibrinogen level, high fibrin degradation product, low platelet counts, and prolonged prothrombin time. It is important to treat causative factors quickly because delay of treatment worsens DIC. Blood component infusion is a mainstay of management.

In patient 177, the clinical findings are consistent with underlying systemic lupus erythematosus (SLE). Approximately 14–25% of pregnant women with SLE may develop thrombocytopenia caused by antiplatelet antibodies or circulating immune complexes. Maternal autoantibodies also can cross the placenta and cause fetal thrombocytopenia.

Drugs should always be excluded as causes of thrombocytopenia. Heparin-induced thrombocytopenia may increase the risk of thrombosis. Quinidine and sulfonamide are common drugs that cause thrombocytopenia. Viral infections such as human immunodeficiency virus infection also may cause thrombocytopenia and should always be considered.

Alloimmune thrombocytopenia is the platelet equivalent of hemolytic (Rh) disease and affects only the neonate. At least 50% of cases are diagnosed during the first pregnancy. It is associated with fetal hemorrhage, and intracranial hemorrhage occurs in approximately 10–20% of infants. The recurrence risk is very high and may approach 100%. It does not cause maternal thrombocytopenia and the mother is healthy.

American College of Obstetricians and Gynecologists. Thrombocytopenia in pregnancy. ACOG Practice Bulletin 6. Washington, DC: ACOG; 1999.

Castella M, Pujol A, Julia A, Massague I, Bueno J, Ramon Grifols J, et al. Thrombotic thrombocytopenic purpura and pregnancy: a review of ten cases. Vox Sang 2004;87:287–90.

Kam PC, Thompson SA, Liew AC. Thrombocytopenia in the parturient. Anesthesia 2004;59:255–64.

Kobayashi T, Terao T, Maki M, Ikenoue T. Diagnosis and management of acute obstetrical DIC. Semin Thromb Hemost 2001;27:161–7.

Parnas M, Sheiner E, Shoham-Vardi I, Burtsein E, Yermiahu T, Levi I, et al. Moderate to severe thrombocytopenia during pregnancy. Eur J Obstet Gynecol Reprod Biol 2006;128:163–8.

178–181

Management of severe Rh disease

Match each case presentation (178–181) with the most appropriate procedure (A–G).

(A) Analysis of paternal blood for Rh genotype
(B) Amniocentesis to assess fetal RhD-antigen status
(C) Amniocentesis for ΔOD_{450}
(D) Middle cerebral artery peak systolic velocity
(E) Targeted ultrasonography to assess for hydrops fetalis
(F) Maternal exchange transfusion
(G) Fetal blood sampling and fetal intrauterine transfusion

A **178.** A 40-year-old multiparous woman is Rh alloimmune. Her last pregnancy was complicated by Rh alloimmunization, and her neonate required a blood transfusion in the nursery. She is at 18 weeks of gestation and has a new partner. Her anti-D titer is 1:16.

D **179.** A patient who is Rh alloimmune is referred to you with a known affected fetus. She is at 27 weeks of gestation and asks about the most optimal, least invasive test to assess for fetal anemia.

B **180.** A 33-year-old woman, gravida 2, para 1, became alloimmune after failing to receive anti-D immune globulin in her first pregnancy. She is now at 20 weeks of gestation with an anti-D titer of 1:32. Her partner is a known heterozygote for the D-antigen.

G **181.** A 29-year-old woman at 25 weeks of gestation has been followed serially for Rh alloimmunization with a known affected fetus. Ultrasonography performed to assess fetal growth identified gross hydramnios and fetal abdominal ascites.

Maternal alloimmunization is the result of an immune response in the mother to a paternally derived red blood cell (RBC) antigen inherited by the fetus that is foreign to the mother. With Rh-alloimmunization, maternal immunoglobulin G antibodies cross the placenta and bind to the foreign antigens on fetal RBCs, causing hemolysis. Since the introduction of anti-D immune globulin in 1968, cases of Rh alloimmunization are much less frequent. However, despite wide availability of immune prophylaxis, women continue to become alloimmune because of the lack or failure of prophylaxis. Many advances have been made in the detection and management of fetal hemolytic disease, but this entity remains a serious cause of perinatal illness and death.

Most providers are familiar with anti-D alloimmunization, which is the model of RBC alloimmunization. Anti-D is the most common antibody identified, but other antigen groups have emerged with increasing frequency because of the widespread use of anti-D immune globulin (Appendix F). Alloimmunization is first detected with a positive indirect Coombs test. Antibody identification and titer may help assess the degree of alloimmunization. Titer values are reported as the integer of the greatest tube dilution that yields a positive reaction. For example, a titer of 32 is equivalent to a dilution of 1:32. A critical titer is one with a significant risk for fetal hydrops fetalis that requires increased fetal surveillance. The assigned cutoff value for a critical titer may differ among institutions, but the critical value for anti-D usually is defined as between 8 and 32. Next, blood for paternal erythrocyte antigen status is obtained to assess homozygosity versus heterozygosity at the D locus as in scenario one. If a critical maternal titer is reported and the father is heterozygous, an amniocentesis is performed to assess the fetal genotype. Polymerase chain reaction (PCR) on uncultured amniocytes in 2 mL of amniotic fluid is used to determine fetal blood type; PCR is a reliable method to ascertain fetal blood type with a low false-negative rate of 1–3%. In cases involving a heterozygous father, this procedure detects the 50% of RhD-negative fetuses who are not at risk for fetal anemia as in the third scenario.

Several algorithms are available to guide detection of fetal anemia in the alloimmune pregnancy. Ultrasonography is an important modality for detection of anemia and management of affected pregnancies. An initial ultrasonographic examination is performed to confirm fetal gestational age and to evaluate for signs of fetal compromise. Fetal hydrops fetalis is a late sign of severe anemia and is considered end-stage hemolytic disease. Fetal ascites usually precede hydrops fetalis.

Fetal anemia can be detected noninvasively using Doppler ultrasonography to detect an increase in the peak velocity of systolic blood flow in the middle cerebral artery. Blood flow is increased to the brain (autoregulation) with fetal anemia as demonstrated by higher middle cerebral artery values. To obtain a peak systolic middle cerebral artery velocity, an axial section of the fetal brain including the thalami and cavum septum pellucidum is selected. The circle of Willis is identified, and the Doppler gate is placed over the middle cerebral artery just as it bifurcates from the carotid siphon. The middle cerebral artery closest to the maternal skin is evaluated. The angle between the ultrasonographic beam and blood flow should be zero degrees. Middle cerebral artery peak systolic velocities appear to be the most effective noninvasive technique to predict fetal anemia as in patient 179 (Fig. 178–181-1; see color plate). Middle cerebral artery Doppler measurement are obtained serially and graphed based on gestational age. Norms for gestational age have been developed and values above 1.50 multiples of the median (MoM) suggest moderate to severe fetal anemia (Fig. 178–181-2). With values in this range, fetal blood sampling and transfusion for a fetal hematocrit less than 30% are performed. In centers with trained personnel and when the fetus has reached an appropriate gestational age, peak systolic middle cerebral artery velocity is an appropriate noninvasive method to monitor pregnancies affected by red cell alloimmunization.

Amniocentesis is an invasive modality used to detect the presence of fetal anemia by evaluating hemolysis based on elevated bilirubin levels in amniotic fluid. Spectral analysis of amniotic fluid is performed at a wavelength of 450 nm (ΔOD_{450}) to measure the bilirubin level. Originally, Liley curves divided into three zones were used to estimate the degree of fetal anemia. However, more recently a modified curve that uses four zones to monitor fetal disease has been proposed (Fig. 178–181-3). Appendix G shows the atypical antibodies and their relationship to fetal hemolytic disease.

Serial amniocentesis to follow trends can be performed at 10-day to 2-week intervals. If values reach the intrauterine transfusion zone, a fetal blood sampling can evaluate the degree of anemia.

Fetal blood sampling is offered to patients with elevated ΔOD_{450} values, elevated peak systolic middle cerebral artery velocities, or in cases of fetal ascites or hydrops fetalis as in patient 181. Fetal blood sampling is an invasive procedure that is associated with a 1–2% fetal loss rate. Under direct ultrasonographic guidance, a spinal needle is guided into the umbilical vein near the placental insertion. An initial hematocrit is obtained and a paralyzing agent is often administered. When fetal blood sampling is performed, blood should be available for an intravascular transfusion if the fetal hematocrit is less than 30%. The amount of blood transfused is based on the estimated fetal weight, the degree of anemia, and the hematocrit of the donor unit. Final target hematocrit is 40–50%. Fetal blood sampling and transfusion are performed in facilities that are equipped to manage possible complications of severe alloimmunization. A possible approach for overall clinical management of the sensitized gestation is shown in an algorithm in Appendix H. Maternal exchange transfusion is a modality that is sometimes used in women with sickle cell disease or crisis and is not usually employed in cases of alloimmunization.

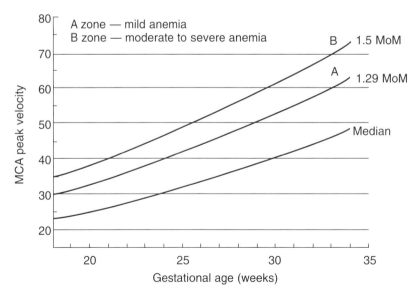

FIG. 178–181-2. Middle cerebral artery Doppler peak velocities based on gestational age. (Moise KJ Jr. Management of rhesus alloimmunization in pregnancy. Obstet Gynecol 2002;100:605.)

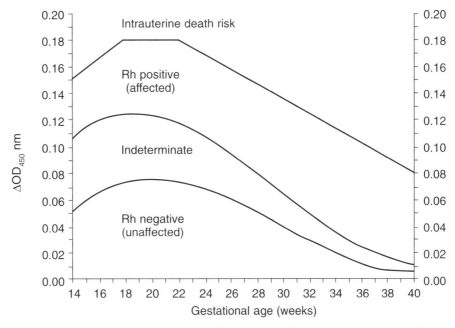

FIG. 178–181-3. Queenan curve for ΔOD_{450} values. Rh, rhesus; OD, optical density. (Moise KJ Jr. Management of rhesus alloimmunization in pregnancy. Obstet Gynecol 2002;100:605.)

Management of alloimmunization during pregnancy. ACOG Practice Bulletin No. 75. American College of Obstetricians and Gynecologists. Obstet Gynecol 2006;108:457–64.

Mari G, for the Collaborative Group for Doppler Assessment of the Blood Velocity of Anemic Fetuses. Noninvasive diagnosis by Doppler ultrasonography of fetal anemia due to maternal red-cell alloimmunization. N Engl J Med 2000;342:9–14.

Moise KJ Jr. Management of rhesus alloimmunization in pregnancy. Obstet Gynecol 2002;100:600–11.

Saade GR. Noninvasive testing for fetal anemia (Editorial). N Engl J Med 2000;342:52–3.

Weiner CP. Fetal hemolytic disease. In: James DK, Steer PJ, Weiner CP, Gonik B, editors. High risk pregnancy management options. 3rd ed. Philadelphia (PA): Elsevier Saunders; 2006. p. 291–312.

Whitecar PW, Moise KJ. Sonographic methods to detect fetal anemia in red blood cell alloimmunization. Obstet Gynecol Surv 2000;55:240–50.

Appendix A

Normal Values for Laboratory Tests*

Analyte	Conventional Units
Alanine aminotransferase, serum	8–35 units/L
Alkaline phosphatase, serum	15–120 units/L
Menopause	
Amniotic fluid index	3–30 mL
Amylase	
60 years or younger	20–300 units/L
Older than 60 years	21–160 units/L
Aspartate aminotransferase, serum	15–30 units/L
Bicarbonate	
Arterial blood	21–27 mEq/L
Venous plasma	23–29 mEq/L
Bilirubin	
Total	0.3–1 mg/dL
Conjugated (direct)	0.1–0.4 mg/dL
Newborn, total	1–10 mg/dL
Blood gases (arterial) and pulmonary function	
Base deficit	Less than 3 mEq/L
Base excess, arterial blood, calculated	–2 to +3 mEq/L
Forced expiratory volume	3.5–5 L
	More than 80% of predicted value
Forced vital capacity	3.5–5 L
Oxygen saturation (So_2)	95% or higher
Pao_2	80 mm Hg or more
Pco_2	35–45 mm Hg
Po_2	80–95 mm Hg
Peak expiratory flow rate	Approximately 450 L/min
pH	7.35–7.45
Pvo_2	30–40 mm Hg
Blood urea nitrogen	
Adult	7–18 mg/dL
Older than 60 years	8–20 mg/dL
CA 125	Less than 34 units/mL
Calcium	
Ionized	4.6–5.3 mg/dL
Serum	8.6–10 mg/dL
Chloride	98–106 mEq/L
Cholesterol	
Total	
Desirable	140–199 mg/dL
Borderline high	200–239 mg/dL
High	240 mg/dL or more
High-density lipoprotein (HDL)	40–85 mg/dL
Low-density lipoprotein	
Desirable	Less than 130 mg/dL
Borderline high	140–159 mg/dL
High	More than 160 mg/dL
Total cholesterol-to-HDL ratio	
Desirable	Less than 3
Borderline high	3–5
High	More than 5

*Values listed are specific for adults or women, if relevant, unless otherwise differentiated.

(continued)

Normal Values for Laboratory Tests *(continued)*

Analyte	Conventional Units
Cholesterol *(continued)*	
Triglycerides	
20 years and older	Less than 150 mg/dL
Less than 20 years	35–135 mg/dL
Cortisol, plasma	
8 AM	5–23 mcg/dL
4 PM	3–15 mcg/dL
10 PM	Less than 50% of 8 AM value
Creatinine, serum	0.6–1.2 mg/dL
Dehydroepiandrosterone sulfate	60–340 mcg/dL
Erythrocyte	
Count	3,800,000–5,100,000/mm^3
Distribution width	10 plus or minus 1.5%
Sedimentation rate	
Wintrobe method	0–15 mm/h
Westergren method	0–20 mm/h
Estradiol-17β	
Follicular phase	30–100 pg/mL
Ovulatory phase	200–400 pg/mL
Luteal phase	50–140 pg/mL
Child	0.8–56 pg/mL
Ferritin, serum	18–160 mcg/L
Fibrinogen	150–400 mg/dL
Follicle-stimulating hormone (FSH)	
Premenopause	2.8–17.2 mIU/mL
Midcycle peak	15–35 mIU/mL
Postmenopause	24–170 mIU/mL
Child	0.1–7 mIU/mL
Glucose	
Fasting	70–105 mg/dL
2-hour postprandial	Less than 120 mg/dL
Random blood	65–110 mg/dL
Hematocrit	36–48%
Hemoglobin	12–16 g/dL
Fetal	Less than 1% of total
Hemoglobin A$_{1C}$ (nondiabetic)	5.5–8.5%
Human chorionic gonadotropin	0–5 mIU/mL
Pregnant	More than 5 mIU/mL
17α-Hydroxyprogesterone	
Adult	50–300 ng/dL
Child	32–63 ng/dL
25-Hydroxyvitamin D	10–55 ng/mL
Iron, serum	65–165 mcg/dL
Binding capacity total	240–450 mcg/dL
Lactate dehydrogenase, serum	313–618 units/L
Leukocytes	
Total	5,000–10,000/mm^3
Differential counts	
Basophils	0–1%
Eosinophils	1–3%
Lymphocytes	25–33%
Monocytes	3–7%
Myelocytes	0%
Band neutrophils	3–5%
Segmented neutrophils	54–62%

Normal Values for Laboratory Tests *(continued)*

Analyte	Conventional Units
Lipase	
60 years or younger	10–140 units/L
Older than 60 years	18–180 units/L
Luteinizing hormone	
Follicular phase	3.6–29.4 mIU/mL
Midcycle peak	58–204 mIU/mL
Postmenopause	35–129 mIU/mL
Child	0.5–10.3 mIU/mL
Magnesium	
Adult	1.6–2.6 mg/dL
Child	1.7–2.1 mg/dL
Newborn	1.5–2.2 mg/dL
Mean corpuscular	
Hemoglobin	27–33 pg
Hemoglobin concentration	33–37 g/dL
Volume	80–100 cubic micrometers
Partial thromboplastin time	30–45 s
Activated	21–35 s
Phosphate, inorganic phosphorus	2.5–4.5 mg/dL
Platelet count	140,000–400,000/mm^3
Potassium	3.5–5.3 mEq/L
Progesterone	
Follicular phase	Less than 3 ng/mL
Luteal phase	2.5–28 ng/mL
On oral contraceptives	0.1–0.3 ng/mL
Secretory phase	5–30 ng/mL
Older than 60 years	0–0.2 ng/mL
1st trimester	9–47 ng/mL
2nd trimester	16.8–146 ng/mL
3rd trimester	55–255 ng/mL
Prolactin	0–17 ng/mL
Pregnant	34–386 ng/mL by 3rd trimester
Prothrombin time	10–13 s
Reticulocyte count	Absolute: 25,000–85,000 mm^3
	0.5–2.5% of erythrocytes
Semen analysis, spermatozoa	
Antisperm antibody	% of sperm binding by immunobead technique; More than 20% = decreased fertility;
Count	20 million/mL or more
Motility	60% or more
Morphology	60% or more normal forms
Sodium	135–145 mEq/L
Testosterone, female	
Total	6–86 ng/dL
Pregnant	3–4 × normal
Postmenopause	½ of normal
Free	
20–29 years old	0.9–3.2 pg/mL
30–39 years old	0.8–3 pg/mL
40–49 years old	0.6–2.5 pg/mL
50–59 years old	0.3–2.7 pg/mL
Older than 60 years	0.2–2.2 pg/mL
Thyroid-stimulating hormone	0.3–3.0 microunits/mL

(continued)

Normal Values for Laboratory Tests *(continued)*

Analyte	Conventional Units
Thyroxine	
Serum free	0.7–2.0 ng/dL
Total	1.5–4.5 micrograms/dL
Triiodothyronine uptake	25–35%
Urea nitrogen, blood	
Adult	7–18 mg/dL
60 years or older	8–20 mg/dL
Uric acid, serum	2.6–6 mg/dL
Urinalysis	
Epithelial cells	0–3/HPF
Erythrocytes	0–3/HPF
Leukocytes	0–4/HPF
Protein (albumin)	
Qualitative	none detected
Quantitative	10–100 mg/24 hours
Specific gravity	
Normal hydration and volume	1.005–1.03
Concentrated	1.025–1.03
Diluted	1.001–1.01

Appendix B

Definitions of Fetal Heart Rate (FHR) Patterns

FHR Pattern	Definition
Baseline FHR	The mean FHR rounded to increments of 5 beats per minute during a 10-minute period. The baseline must be for a minimum of 2 minutes.
	May need to compare the previous 10-minute segment to determine the baseline.
Baseline FHR variability	Fluctuations in the FHR over two cycles per minute or greater.
	Variability is quantitated as the amplitude of peak-to-trough in beats per minute:
	Absent—amplitude range undetectable
	Minimal—amplitude range 5 beats per minute or less
	Moderate (normal)—amplitude range 6–25 beats per minute
	Marked—amplitude range greater than 25 beats per minute
Acceleration	An abrupt (peak within 30 seconds) increase in the FHR from the recently calculated baseline.
	Acme is 15 beats per minute or more above baseline, lasting for 15 seconds or more and less than 2 minutes from the onset to return to baseline.
	Before 32 weeks, acceleration is 10 beats per minute or more above baseline and lasting at least 10 seconds but less than 2 minutes.
	Prolonged acceleration if it lasts beyond 2 minutes but less than 10 minutes.
	If the acceleration is for 10 minutes or longer then it is a baseline change.
Bradycardia	Baseline FHR less than 110 beats per minute.
Early deceleration	In association with a uterine contraction, a visually apparent, gradual (onset to nadir 30 seconds or more) decrease in FHR with return to baseline.
	The nadir of the deceleration occurring at the same time as the peak of the contraction.
Late deceleration	In association with a uterine contraction, a visually apparent, gradual (onset to nadir 30 seconds or more) decrease in FHR with return to baseline FHR.
	The onset, nadir and recovery of the deceleration occur after the beginning, peak, and end of the contraction, respectively.
Tachycardia	Baseline FHR greater than 160 beats per minute.
Variable deceleration	An abrupt (onset to nadir less than 30 seconds) decrease in the FHR below the baseline.
	The decrease in FHR is at least 15 beats per minute, lasting for 15 seconds or more but less than 2 minutes.
Prolonged deceleration	Decrease in FHR from baseline 15 beats per minute or more, lasting 2 minutes or more but less than 10 minutes from onset to return to baseline.
	If the deceleration is for 10 minutes or longer, it is a baseline change.

Appendix C

Prediction of Preterm Birth at Less Than 35 Weeks Gestational Age by Cervical Length Less Than 25 mm by Transvaginal Ultrasonography in Specific Populations of Pregnant Women

Author	N	Preterm Birth (%)	Gestational Age Studied (Weeks)	% Abnormal	Sensitivity	Specificity	Positive Predictive Value	Negative Predictive Value	Relative Risk
Asymptomatic									
Singleton low-risk (cross-sectional) Iams, 1996*	2,915	4.3	22–25	10	37	92	18	97	6.2
Singleton: Prior preterm birth Owen, 2001[†]	183	26	16–24	—	69	80	55	88	4.5
Twins									
Goldenberg, 1996[‡]	147	32	22–24	18	30	88	54	74	3.2
Symptomatic									
Singletons with preterm labor Murakawa, 1993[§]	32	34	25–35	31	64	86	70	82	3.9

*Iams JD, Goldenberg RL, Meis PJ, Mercer BM, Moawad A, Das A, et al. The length of the cervix and the risk of spontaneous premature delivery. N Engl J Med 1996;334:567–72.

[†]Owen J, Yost N, Berghella V, Thom E, Swain M, Dildy GA, et al. Mid-trimester endovaginal sonography in women at high risk for spontaneous preterm birth. JAMA 2001;286:1340–8.

[‡]Goldenberg RL, Iams J, Miodovnik M, Van Dorsten PJ, Thurnau G, Bottoms S, et al. The preterm prediction study: risk factors in twin gestation. Am J Obstet Gynecol 1996;175:1047–53.

[§]Murakawa H, Utumi T, Hasegawa I, Tanaka K, Fuzimori R. Evaluation of threatened preterm delivery by transvaginal ultrasonographic measurement of cervical length. Obstet Gynecol 1993;82:829–32.

Appendix D

Antiviral Treatment for Herpes Simplex Virus

Indication	Valacyclovir	Acyclovir	Famciclovir
First clinical episode	1,000 mg twice a day for 7–14 days	200 mg five times a day or 400 mg three times a day for 7–14 days	250 mg three times a day for 7–14 days
Recurrent episodes	500 mg twice a day for 5 days	200 mg five times a day or 400 mg three times a day for 5 days	125 mg twice a day for 5 days
Daily suppressive therapy	500 mg once a day (10 recurrences or more per year) or 1,000 mg once a day or 250 mg twice a day (less than 9 recurrences per year)	400 mg twice a day	250 mg twice a day

American College of Obstetricians and Gynecologists. Management of herpes in pregnancy. ACOG Practice Bulletin 8. Washington, DC: ACOG; 1999.

Appendix E

Risk Factors for Preterm Birth

History

- Obstetric–gynecologic history: prior spontaneous preterm birth (spontaneous preterm birth of twins is not a significant risk factor when the next pregnancy is a singleton pregnancy); prior second trimester loss; two or more prior dilation and evacuations; prior cone biopsy; uterine anomalies; diethylstilbestrol exposure; myomata; extremes of interpregnancy interval; assisted reproductive technology
- Maternal lifestyle (smoking, drug abuse, sexually transmitted infections)
- Maternal prepregnancy weight less than 50 kg (120 lb) or low body mass index (weight in kilograms divided by height in meters squared [kg/m^2] less than 18.5); poor nutritional status
- Maternal age (younger than 19 years; 35 years or older)
- Race (especially African American)
- Education (less than 12th grade)
- Certain medical conditions (eg, diabetes mellitus, hypertension)
- Low socioeconomic status
- Limited prenatal care
- Family history of spontaneous preterm birth (poorly studied)
- Vaginal bleeding (especially during second trimester)
- Stress (mostly related to above risks)

Identifiable by screening

- Anemia
- Periodontal disease
- Cervical length less than 25 mm on transvaginal ultrasonography (especially before 30 weeks of gestation)
- Positive fetal fibronectin test result (greater than 50 ng/mL between 22 and 34 weeks of gestation)

Usually symptomatic

- Uterine contractions

Indicated preterm birth

- Abruptio placentae
- Fetal demise/major anomaly/compromise/hydramnios
- Placenta previa
- Major maternal disease (eg, hypertensive complications, diabetes mellitus)

Appendix F

Antigens That Cause Fetal Hemolytic Disease

Common
    Rhesus family: D, C, E, c, e
    Kell
Uncommon
    JK^a (Kidd)
    Fy^a (Duffy)
    Kp$^{a\ or\ b}$
    k
    S

Modified from Weiner CP. Fetal hemolytic disease. In: James DK, Steer PJ, Weiner CP, Gonik B, editors. High risk pregnancy management options. 3rd ed. Philadelphia (PA): Elsevier Saunders; 2006. p. 292. Copyright Elsevier 2006.

Appendix G

Atypical Antibodies and Their Relationship to Fetal Hemolytic Disease

Blood Group System	Antigens Related to Hemolytic Disease	Hemolytic Disease Severity	Proposed Management
Lewis	*		
I	*		
Kell	K	Mild to severe[†]	Fetal assessment
	k	Mild	Routine obstetric care
	Ko	Mild	Routine obstetric care
	Kp^a	Mild	Routine obstetric care
	Kp^b	Mild	Routine obstetric care
	Js^a	Mild	Routine obstetric care
	Js^b	Mild	Routine obstetric care
Rh (non-D)	E	Mild to severe[†]	Fetal assessment
	C	Mild to severe[†]	Fetal assessment
	c	Mild to severe[†]	Fetal assessment
Duffy	Fy^a	Mild to severe[†]	Fetal assessment
	Fy^b	[‡]	Routine obstetric care
	By^3	Mild	Routine obstetric care
Kidd	Jk^a	Mild to severe	Fetal assessment
	Jk^b	Mild	Routine obstetric care
	Jk^3	Mild	Routine obstetric care
MNSs	M	Mild to severe	Fetal assessment
	N	Mild	Routine obstetric care
	S	Mild to severe	Fetal assessment
	s	Mild to severe	Fetal assessment
	U	Mild to severe	Fetal assessment
	Mi^a	Moderate	Fetal assessment
MSSs	Mt^a	Moderate	Fetal assessment
	Vw	Mild	Routine obstetric care
	Mur	Mild	Routine obstetric care
	Hil	Mild	Routine obstetric care
	Hut	Mild	Routine obstetric care
Lutheran	Lu^a	Mild	Routine obstetric care
	Lu^b	Mild	Routine obstetric care
Diego	D1^a	Mild to severe	Fetal assessment
	Di^b	Mild to severe	Fetal assessment
Xg	Xg^a	Mild	Routine obstetric care
P	PP$_{1pk}$ (Tj^a)	Mild to severe	Fetal assessment
Public antigens	Yt^a	Moderate to severe	Fetal assessment
	Yt^b	Mild	Routine obstetric care
	Lan	Mild	Routine obstetric care
	En^a	Moderate	Fetal assessment
	Ge	Mild	Routine obstetric care
	Jr^a	Mild	Routine obstetric care
	Co^a	Severe	Fetal assessment
	Co^{1-b-}	Mild	Routine obstetric care
Private antigens	Batty	Mild	Routine obstetric care
	Becker	Mild	Routine obstetric care
	Berrens	Mild	Routine obstetric care
	Biles	Moderate	Fetal assessment
	Evans	Mild	Routine obstetric care
	Gonzales	Mild	Routine obstetric care
	Good	Severe	Fetal assessment
	Heibel	Moderate	Fetal assessment

(continued)

Atypical Antibodies and Their Relationship to Fetal Hemolytic Disease *(continued)*

Blood Group System	Antigens Related to Hemolytic Disease	Hemolytic Disease Severity	Proposed Management
Private antigens *(continued)*	Hunt	Mild	Routine obstetric care
	Jobbins	Mild	Routine obstetric care
	Radin	Moderate	Fetal assessment
	Rm	Mild	Routine obstetric care
	Ven	Mild	Routine obstetric care
	Wright[a]	Severe	Fetal assessment
	Wright[b]	Mild	Routine obstetric care
	Zd	Moderate	Fetal assessment

*Not a proven cause of hemolytic disease of the newborn

[†]With hydrops fetalis

[‡]Not a cause of hemolytic disease of the newborn

Adapted from Weinstein L. Irregular antibodies causing hemolytic disease of the newborn: a continuing problem. Clin Obstet Gynecol 1982;25:321.

Appendix H

Algorithm for Overall Clinical Management of the Sensitized Gestation

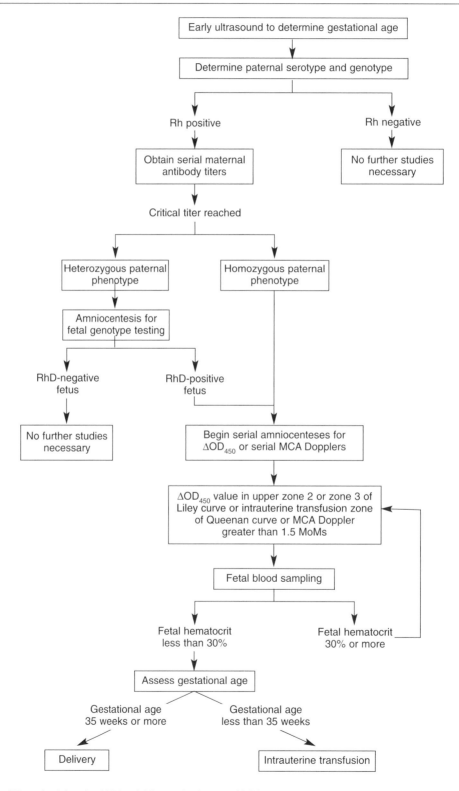

Rh, rhesus; OD, optical density; MCA, middle cerebral artery; MoM, multiples of the median. (Modified with permission from: Moise KJ Jr. Diagnosis, management, and prevention of Rhesus (Rh) alloimmunization. In: Rose BD, editor. UpToDate. Wellesley [MA]: UpToDate Inc.; 2007. Copyright © 2007 UpToDate Inc. For more information visit www.uptodate.com)

Appendix I

Revised Classification Criteria for the Antiphospholipid Syndrome

Antiphospholipid antibody syndrome is present if at least one of the clinical criteria and one of the laboratory criteria that follow are met.*

1. Vascular thrombosis[†]

One or more clinical episodes[‡] of arterial, venous, or small vessel thrombosis[§], in any tissue or organ. Thrombosis must be confirmed by objective validated criteria (ie, unequivocal findings of appropriate imaging studies or histopathology). For histopathologic confirmation, thrombosis should be present without significant evidence of inflammation of the vessel wall.

2. Pregnancy morbidity

   a. One or more unexplained deaths of a morphologically normal fetus at or beyond 10 weeks of gestation, with normal morphology documented by ultrasonography or by direct examination of the fetus, *or*

   b. One or more premature births of a morphologically normal neonate before 34 weeks of gestation because of: 1) eclampsia or severe preeclampsia defined according to standard definitions, or 2) recognized features of placental insufficiency[‖], *or*

   c. Three or more unexplained consecutive spontaneous abortions before 10 weeks of gestation, with maternal anatomic or hormonal abnormalities and paternal and maternal chromosomal causes excluded.

In studies of populations of patients who have more than one type of pregnancy morbidity, investigators are strongly encouraged to stratify groups of subjects according to a, b, or c above.

Laboratory Criteria[¶]

1. Lupus anticoagulant (LA) present in plasma, on two or more occasions at least 12 weeks apart, detected according to the guidelines of the International Society on Thrombosis and Haemostasis.

2. Anticardiolipin (aCL) antibody of immunoglobulin G (IgG) isotype with or without immunoglobin M (IgM) isotype in serum or plasma, present in medium or high titer (ie, greater than 40 G phospholipid (GPL) or M phospholipid (MPL) or greater than the 99th percentile), present on two or more occasions, at least 12 weeks apart, measured by a standardized enzyme-linked absorbent assay (ELISA).

3. Anti-β_2 glycoprotein-1 antibody of IgG isotype with or without IgM isotype in serum or plasma (in titer, greater than the 99th percentile), present on two or more occasions, at least 12 weeks apart, measured by a standardized ELISA.

---

*Classification of antiphospholipid antibody syndrome should be avoided if less than 12 weeks or more than 5 years separate the positive aPL test and the clinical manifestation.

†Coexisting inherited or acquired factors for thrombosis are not reasons for excluding patients from antiphospholipid antibody syndrome trials. However, two subgroups of antiphospholipid antibody syndrome patients should be recognized, according to a) the presence, and b) the absence of additional risk factors for thrombosis. Indicative (but not exhaustive) such cases include age (men, older than 55 years; women, older than 65 years) and presence of any of the established risk factors for cardiovascular disease (ie, hypertension, diabetes mellitus, elevated low-density lipoprotein cholesterol or high-density lipoprotein cholesterol, cigarette smoking, family history of premature cardiovascular disease, body mass index [weight in kilograms divided by height in meters squared (kg/m^2)] of 30 or greater, microalbuminuria, estimated glomerular filtration rate less than 60 mL/min^{-1}), inherited thrombophilias, oral contraceptives, nephritic syndrome, malignancy, immobilization, and surgery. Thus, patients who fill criteria should be stratified according to contributing causes of thrombosis.

‡A thrombotic episode in the past could be considered a clinical criterion, provided that thrombosis is proved by appropriate diagnostic means and that no alternative diagnosis or cause of thrombosis is found.

§Superficial venous thrombosis is not included in the clinical criteria.

‖Generally accepted features of placental insufficiency include: 1) abnormal or nonreassuring fetal surveillance test(s), eg, a nonreactive nonstress test, suggestive of fetal hypoxemia; 2) abnormal Doppler flow velocimetry waveform analysis suggestive of fetal hypoxemia, eg, absent end-diastolic flow in the umbilical artery; 3) oligohydramnios, eg, an amniotic fluid index of 5 cm or less; or 4) a postnatal birth weight less than the 10th percentile for the gestational age.

¶Investigators are strongly advised to classify antiphospholipid antibody syndrome patients in studies into one of the following categories: I, more than one laboratory criteria present (any combination); IIa, LA present alone; IIb, aCL antibody present alone; IIc, anti-β_2 glycoprotein-I antibody present alone.

Modified from Miyakis S, Lockshin MD, Atsumi T, Branch DW, Brey RL, Cervera R, et al. International consensus statement on an update of the classification criteria for definite antiphospholipid syndrome (APS). J Thromb Haemost 2006;4:297.

Appendix J

Bilateral Uterine Artery Ligation

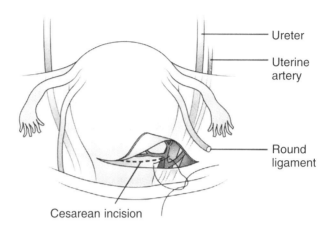

Operative technique for uterine artery ligation. The vesicouterine fold of peritoneum has been incised transversely and the bladder mobilized inferiorly. A number 1 chromic catgut suture on a large smooth needle has been placed through the avascular space of the broad ligament and through the uterus. The suture includes the uterine vessels and several centimeters of myometrium. (Rogers MS, Chang AM. Postpartum hemorrhage and other problems of the third stage. In: James DK, Steer PJ, Weiner CP, Gonik B, eds. High risk pregnancy. 3rd ed. Saunders Elsevier; 2005. p. 1569. Copyright 2005 by Elsevier.)

Index

NOTE: Numbers refer to questions, not pages.

NOTE: Numbers refer to questions, not pages.

NOTE: Numbers refer to questions, not pages.

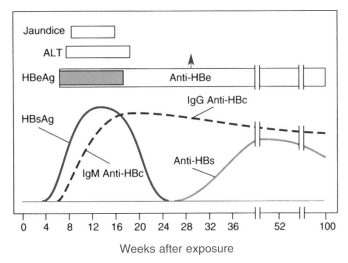

FIG. 2-1. Typical clinical and laboratory features of acute viral hepatitis B. ALT, alanine transaminase; HBeAg, hepatitis B e antigen; HBsAg, hepatitis B surface antigen; HBc, hepatitis B core; IgG, immunoglobulin G; IgM, immunoglobulin M. (Dienstag JL, Isselbacher KJ. Disorders of the gastrointestinal system. In: Kasper DL, Braunwald E, Fauci AS, Hauser SL, Longo DL, Jameson JH, editors. Harrison's principles of internal medicine. 16th ed. New York: McGraw-Hill; 2005. p. 1825.

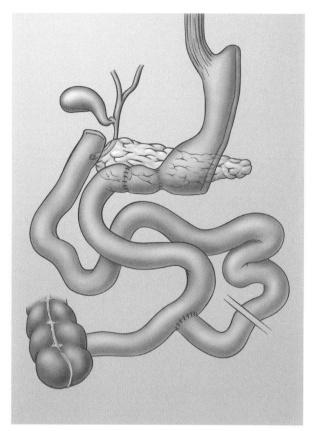

A

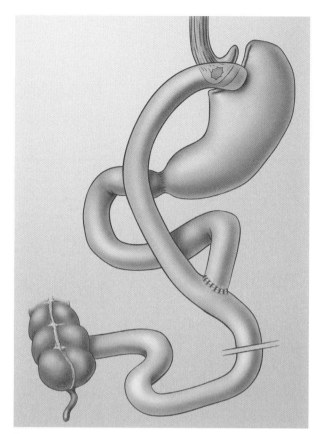

B

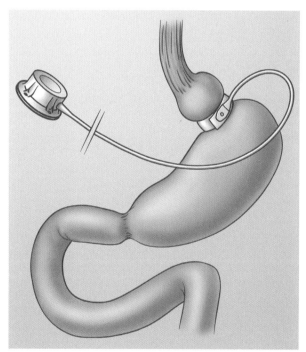

C

FIG. 27-1. An illustrated guide to common weight-loss procedures. **A.** Biliopancreatic diversion with duodenal switch. The biliopancreatic diversion with duodenal switch procedure includes a partial gastrectomy, which reduces the stomach along the greater curvature, restricting capacity while maintaining normal function. The procedure also keeps the pyloric valve intact, eliminating the possibility of the dumping syndrome. The most serious potential complication is protein malnutrition. **B.** Roux-en-Y gastric bypass. In the Roux-en-Y gastric bypass, the cardia is partitioned off or completely separated from the remainder of the stomach. Gastric bypass prevents the ingestion of a large amount of food at one time. This procedure is associated with the dumping syndrome if a patient ingests a high-fat, calorie-dense liquid such as a milkshake; the liquid is dumped directly into the Roux-en-Y limb of the gastric bypass, causing unpleasant symptoms. **C.** Adjustable gastric banding. In this procedure, a band is wrapped around the stomach to create a small opening from the upper pouch to the lower stomach, which controls the rate of emptying. The band can be tightened or loosened over time to change the size of the opening by inserting saline into a balloon that lines the interior of a flexible band through an access port under the skin. © Sharon & Joel Harris / illustrationOnLine.com

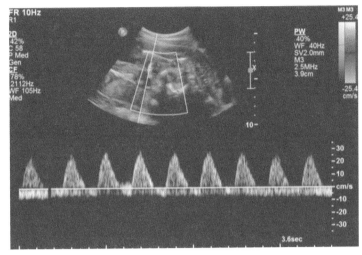

FIG. 56-1. Umbilical artery with absent end-diastolic flow.

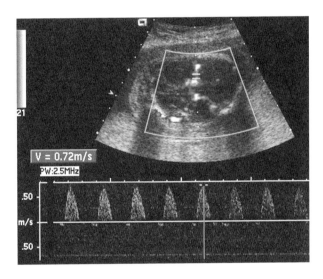

FIG. 178–181-1. Middle cerebral artery Doppler ultrasonogram.

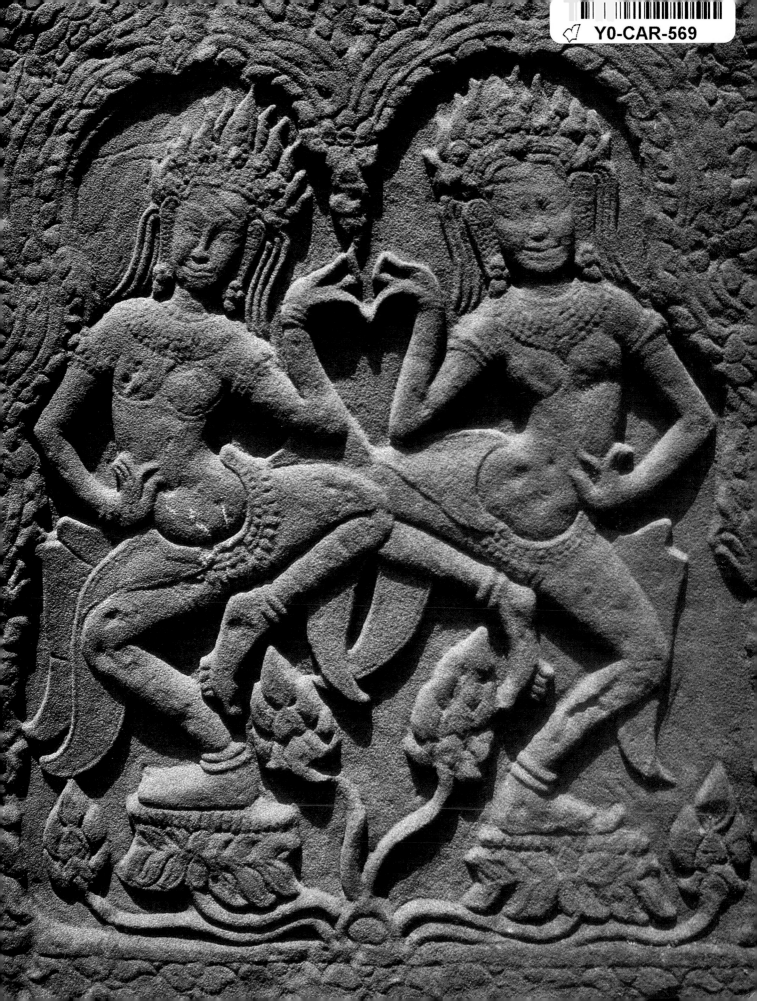

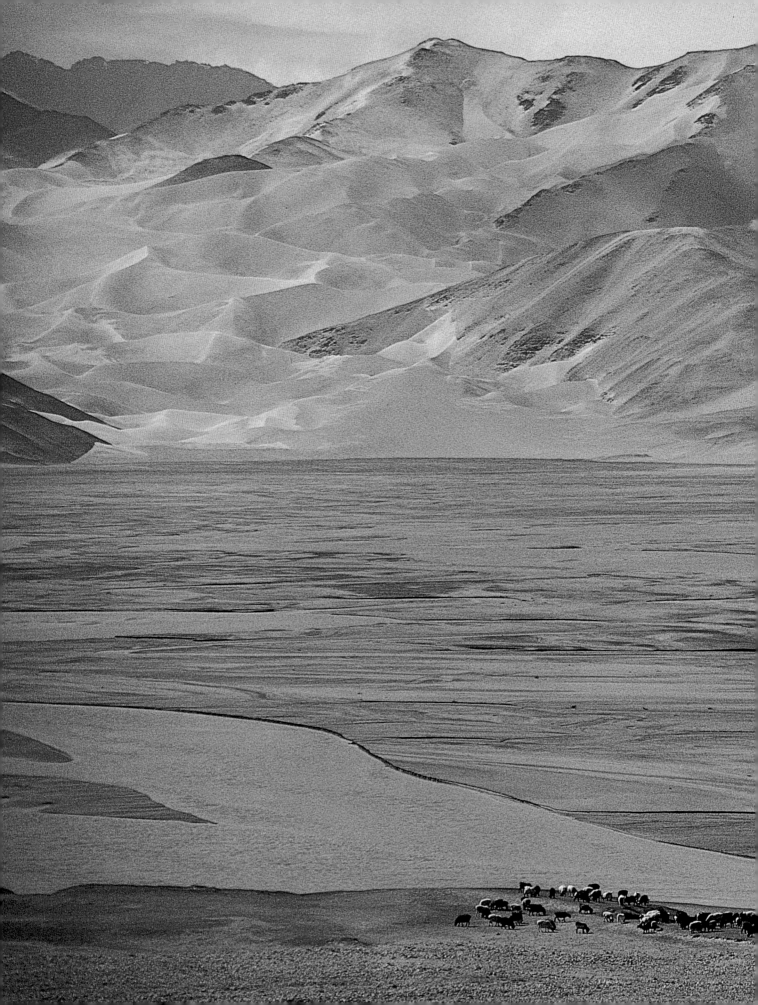

ADVENTURE TRAVEL PHOTOGRAPHY

NEVADA WIER

WATSON-GUPTILL PUBLICATIONS/NEW YORK

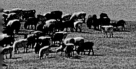

Nevada Wier is a professional photographer who specializes in remote-travel photography, particularly in Asia. Her photographs have been published in such magazines as *Audubon, Discovery, Geo, Natural History, Popular Photography, Sierra,* and *Smithsonian.*

Editorial concept by Robin Simmen
Edited by Liz Harvey
Designed by Areta Buk
Graphic production by Ellen Greene

Copyright © 1992 by Nevada Wier
First published 1992 in New York by AMPHOTO,
an imprint of Watson-Guptill Publications,
a division of BPI Communications, Inc.,
1515 Broadway, New York, NY 10036

Library of Congress Cataloging-in-Publication Data
Wier, Nevada.
    Adventure travel photography: how to shoot great pictures off the
beaten track / by Nevada Wier.
    Includes index.
    ISBN 0-8174-3275-2   ISBN 0-8174-3276-0 (pbk.)
    1. Travel photography.   I. Title.
TR790.W54   1992
778.9'991—dc20   92-13989
                                                  CIP

Manufactured in Singapore

1 2 3 4 5 6 7 8 9 / 99 98 97 96 95 94 93 92

I OWE A BIG THANKS TO EVERYONE WHO SUPPORTED ME DURING THE
COMPLETION OF THIS BOOK, ESPECIALLY LISL AND LANDT DENNIS,
SHELLY O'CONNELL, AND, MOST OF ALL, SALLY BUTLER.
I ALSO OWE THANKS TO ALL THE PEOPLE WHO'VE TRAVELED WITH
ME OVER THE YEARS IN THE WILD CORNERS OF THE EARTH.

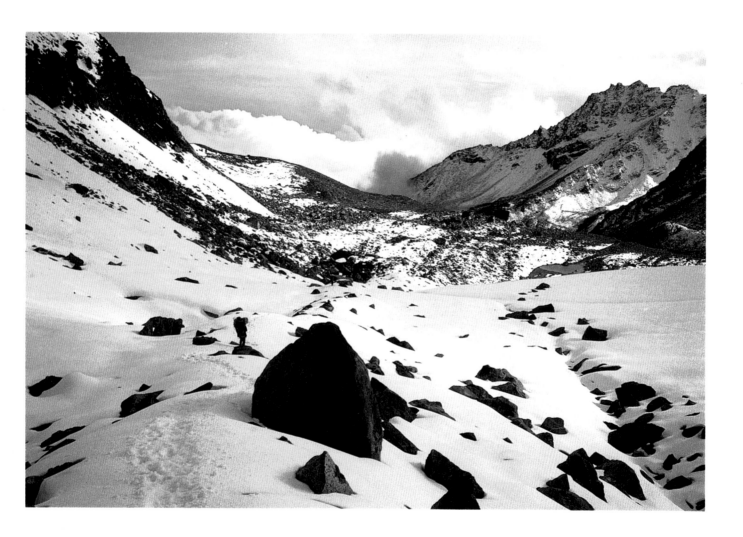

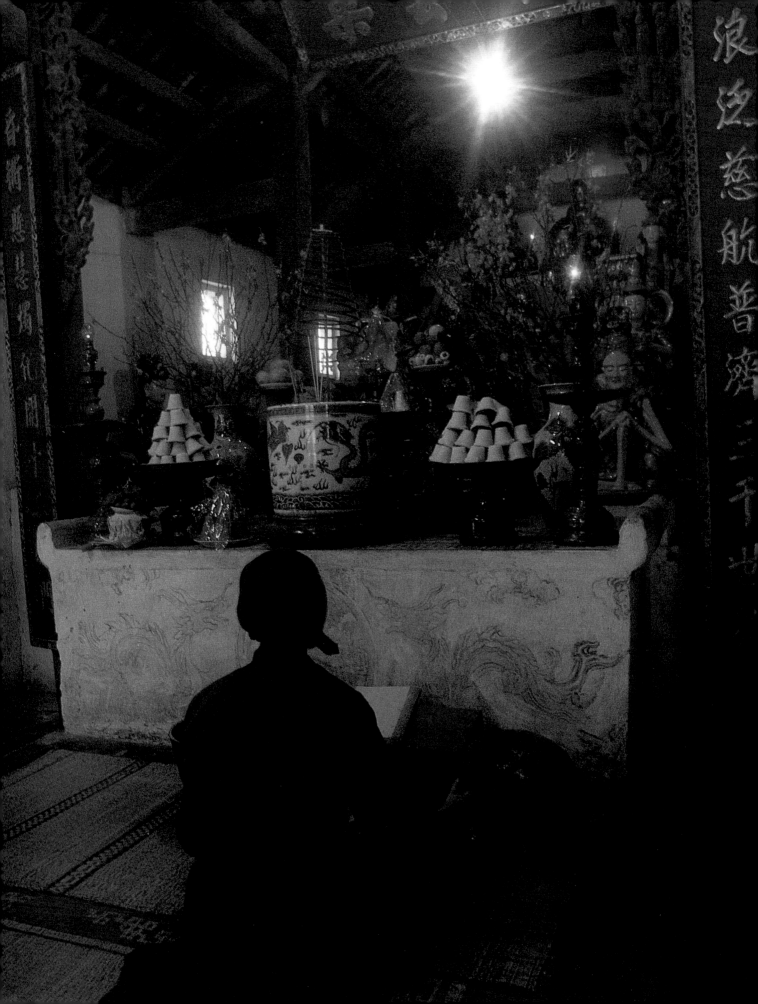

CONTENTS

PART ONE

THE DESIRE TO WANDER

Hearing the names Kathmandu, Rangoon, La Paz, Samarkand, and Nairobi evokes hazy images of unabashedly romantic and seemingly unreachable destinations. People sometimes assume that these are places where only missionaries, scientists, mountaineers, wealthy individuals, and *National Geographic* photographers travel. Today, however, distances in time and space have shrunken; it doesn't require months of sailing, riding camels, or trudging across deserts to reach these remote outposts. Within two days you can be sipping tea in the most fabled cities on the globe. But for the truly adventurous, the journey is just beginning. Turning your back on the cities, you can head into the surrounding terrain: mountains, deserts, vast plains, jungles, and seas. In these windswept, sunshine-drenched worlds you visit the land of your dreams and people of the past—places where you truly understand the meaning of the word "remote."

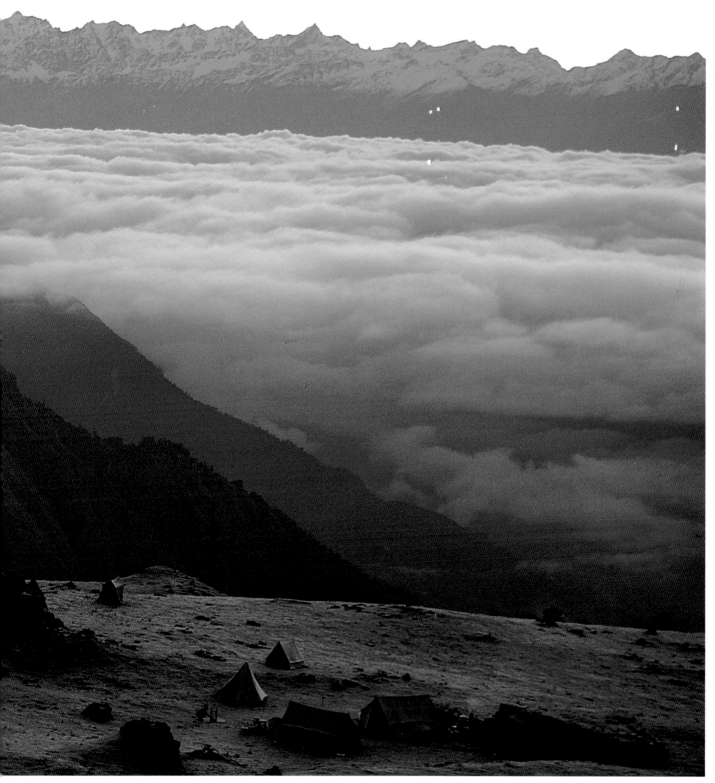

I photographed this tranquil morning scene on the Tiradanda Ridge in Nepal, below Singla La with my Nikon F3 and a 50mm lens. The exposure was 1/60 sec. at f/4 on Kodachrome 64.

HOW I GOT STARTED

Twenty years ago I began exploring the canyons, mountains, deserts, and rivers of the American Southwest. As I learned the skills to feel comfortable and confident in various challenging outdoor situations, I was inspired to venture farther. Sometimes with friends, sometimes alone, I explored deeper canyons, wilder rivers, and more remote mountains.

In 1972 while hiking in Escalante Canyon, Utah, I turned a bend and confronted an immense sandstone wall. It was late afternoon, and the canyon resonated with an intense orange glow that seemed to radiate from within its massive walls. I wanted to keep that image with me forever. I owned a book by Eliot Porter called *Glen Canyon—A Place No One Knew*, and the beauty of his photographs echoed my immediate feeling. However, those were his images. I wanted to record my own viewpoint. I remember thinking, "If Eliot Porter can photograph these walls, so can I!" I was naive to assume that I could be Porter's rival, but that flash of inspiration and intent changed my life forever. From that moment on, I aspired to incorporate photography into my philosophy of travel and life. The camera became a tool for investigation and my photographs expressions of a quest to explore my personal vision and relationship to the world in its largest sense.

My travels began to take me farther afield, from the shores of Lake Titicaca, Bolivia, to Xinjiang Province, China. I'd found my niche and calling in combining my outdoor skills with an intense desire to explore remote destinations and interact with people of other cultures. At that point I didn't realize I was joining the ranks of a long line of photographers who set out on voyages to record foreign places and cultures.

I supported myself by guiding adventure tours in Nepal and China initially, until I began to develop enough professional contacts to absorb the cost of film and travel. Travel photography isn't an easy field in which to make a living, and adventure-travel photography is even more difficult. Amassing assignments requires a prodigious dose of perseverance and what I call the "tenacity quotient." I sometimes feel that amateur photographers are in an enviable position; they don't have to worry about hustling a story, meeting deadlines, or having heart palpitations if their camera breaks down. They can enjoy their travels unencumbered by imposed photographic restraints or time schedules and can dive 100 percent into discovering artistic thresholds.

Whether you're traveling alone or with an organized tour, in the Appalachian Mountains of Tennessee or in the Himalayas of Nepal, the key is to take advantage of a chance to travel beyond familiar places and comfortable facilities. Whenever I venture into "terra incognito," which is anyplace outside my normal frame of reference, and encounter new cultures and traditions, I experience a revitalization of my physical, sensory, and perceptual self.

Adventure and photography are natural partners. If your instincts are sharp and your eyes are open wide, you can translate your experience into an evocative, revealing, informative, or dazzling photograph—however you define your purpose. Unfortunately all too often, photographs are taken with an acquisitive intent and become a substitute for the real experience. As Susan Sontag remarks in *On Photography*, "Most tourists feel compelled to put the camera between themselves and whatever is remarkable that they encounter. Unsure of other responses, they take a picture. This gives shape to experience: stop, take a photograph, and move on."

Photographers have been accused of hiding behind cameras and viewing the world as a small rectangle. But I find that photographing doesn't divorce me from a situation; it motivates me to become more involved. I find myself searching out light, colors, emotions, and patterns more intensely and relating to people I might otherwise feel too shy or reluctant to greet. Photographing forces me to interact with other people, and it demands that I concentrate and be open and genuine. I find that the source of the real joy in photographing is the relationship between my subject and me, which becomes much more important than the actual image I take home.

To raise a photograph above the average, traveling photographers must be willing to develop sufficient intellectual and aesthetic capabilities in order to interpret a situation and translate it into a personal photograph. Just as you search for meaning and value in your travel experiences, you need to look beyond the obvious in your photographic investigations. There is a tendency to romanticize and perpetuate myths about foreign destinations and cultures. People tend to photograph only blue skies, gleaming mountains, and smiling natives— what I call the "waist-level-up-viewpoint." And by continually recording these images, traveling photographers are ignoring their own vision, unfairly glamorizing the world, and losing credibility as responsible communicators.

When I first conceived the idea of this book, I had some reservations. Environments and cultures are fragile, and certain species are becoming extinct. You have to delve into the densest jungles to find a culture untouched by the modern world. Each passing year and each passing traveler bring changes to the farthest reaches of the globe. I was concerned that writing a book encouraging travel to remote areas would

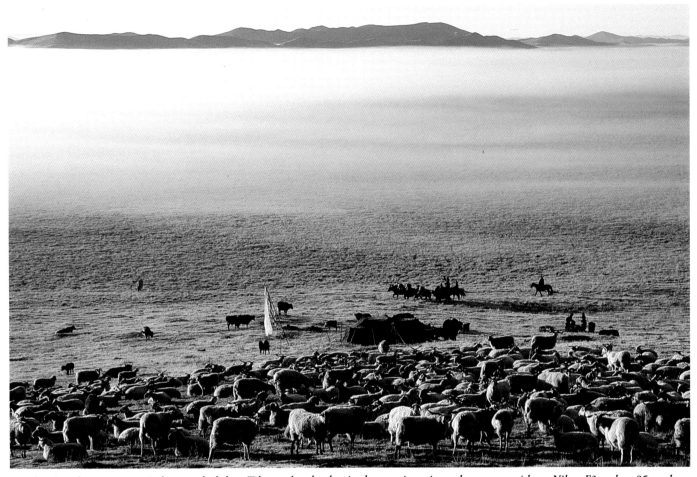

In China's Sichuan Province I photographed these Tibetan sheepherders in the morning mist as the sun rose with my Nikon F3 and an 85mm lens, and exposed Kodachrome 64 for 1/60 sec. at f/5.6.

contribute to cultural annihilation and the spread of America's pop-cultural dogma.

On the other hand, this has never been a static world and never will be. Civilizations have risen and fallen and cultures and languages have mixed and flourished since the beginning of humanity. Ironically some individuals in the Western world, the purveyor of change, lament cultural evolution for developing countries. Change is inevitable, but unfortunately there is a tendency now toward cultural homogeneity instead of diversity. I believe that it is important to venture beyond your own culture in order to cultivate global awareness as well as an appreciation of foreign mores and customs, rather than to smugly stay at home with a false sense of cultural superiority. As you travel you need to be sensitive to your impact, as well as to abandon your self-absorption and become more responsible for relating to the world and yourself as a continuum.

Images are usually your first encounter with the myriad of cultures and environments outside your own. Movies, television, and photography books and magazines bombard you with information. The camera has done more to enlarge your awareness of the world than any other invention of modern society. Ours has become a culture addicted to cameras and their resulting images. A camera is the one item people rarely leave at home, and the one they rarely take full responsibility for.

Travel and photography have become my profession and my lifestyle. This isn't a lifestyle that I encourage you to emulate in its entirety: it is certainly less romantic than it sounds. Hauling around between 25 and 50 pounds of photographic gear isn't fun. Sometimes I yearn for an Instamatic and a daypack. Just as important as your physical stamina is your mental stamina. You have to cultivate a willingness to endure delays, hardships, infuriating bureaucrats, inclement weather,

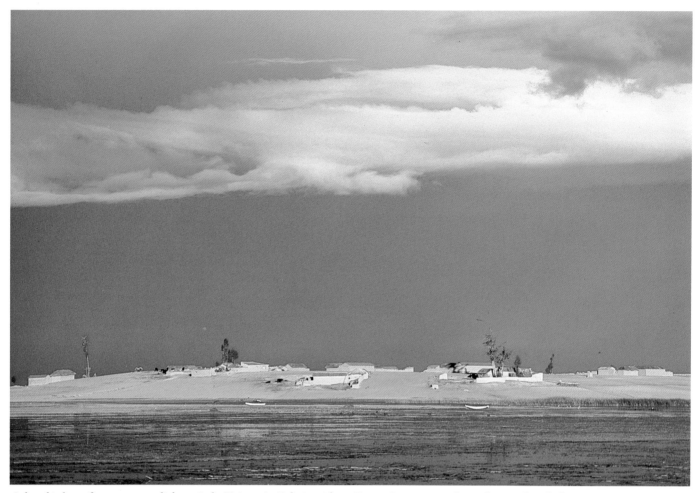

I shot this late-afternoon storm light on Lake Titicaca in Bolivia with my Pentax Spotmatic, a 40mm lens, and Kodachrome 64.

fouled-up air schedules, and unforeseeable and uncontrollable events that are impossible to resolve quickly. But once I am out in the field becoming acquainted with a new place and people, experiencing new food, and saturating myself with sensory stimuli, I realize that the struggle is worth it.

I can't tell you in this book how or what to photograph in foreign situations. I can only give you a kind of map to start you on your own photographic journey. Curiosity and circumstance are your best personal tour guides. Of course, you don't have to go to China or Africa to make a great photograph. "Remote travel" is really only a term that signifies your allowing the exploration of your interior world to reflect your image of the exterior world. Remote travel often involves using primitive modes of transportation, such as walking, riding animals, and traveling in dugout canoes, thereby offering the ultimate luxury in this fast-paced, frenetic world: time. You have time to think, to observe, to explore all your

senses, and to investigate all photographic possibilities. By taking time and being deliberate, you can pursue encounters and experiment with compositions that can lead you to your singular vision.

When you do decide to explore new terrain, I hope that this book encourages you to venture off the beaten track; helps you deal with the nuts and bolts of logistics, equipment, and technical and cultural situations; and propels you toward a greater personal photographic vision.

The source of my desire to wander is still a mystery to me. I didn't grow up in a family of explorers, athletes, or even armchair travelers. I didn't pore over *National Geographic* magazines as a youth and fantasize about riding camels across blowing dunes. I was a city girl, seemingly destined for an urban academic existence. However, through a series of fateful events, I was propelled in a very different direction, and the fire of a latent wanderlust was ignited. My journey to Lake

Titicaca, Bolivia, was my first impromptu foreign adventure, and I was just beginning my photographic career.

On my previous outdoor trips in America, I often set out on one path only to end up on another. In fact without any forethought or predictions of the outcome on my part, many of my travels have taken a 90-degree turn into an unexpected adventure. Such was the case in Bolivia. It was like sliding down a dark chute and not knowing where I was going to land.

SAILING A REED BOAT ON LAKE TITICACA IN SOUTH AMERICA

In 1978 I went to South America originally intending to go climbing with my friend Jeff for two months. I didn't have a photographic assignment when I left home. But I ended up staying in Bolivia for over half a year and went on one of the most remarkable journeys of my life, a seven-week voyage circumnavigating Lake Titicaca in a tortora reed boat (tortora is an indigenous reed that grows prolifically in the lake).

Jeff and I'd hoped to set out immediately to climb in the Cordillera Real of the Bolivian Andes. However, my climbing gear was held up in customs, so we looked in the direction of the altiplano, a high plateau, for a different type of adventure. Jeff had seen Lake Titicaca on his earlier wanderings around Bolivia and mused about the possibility of kayaking or sailing around it. Lake Titicaca, pressed between earth and clouds at 13,000 feet, is the highest navigable lake in the world. Spanning 3,200 square miles in Bolivia and Peru, it has the temperament of a miniature ocean: moody, capricious, and often dangerous. Winds sweep down from the Andes, instantly transforming the placid lake into a raging sea with surfing

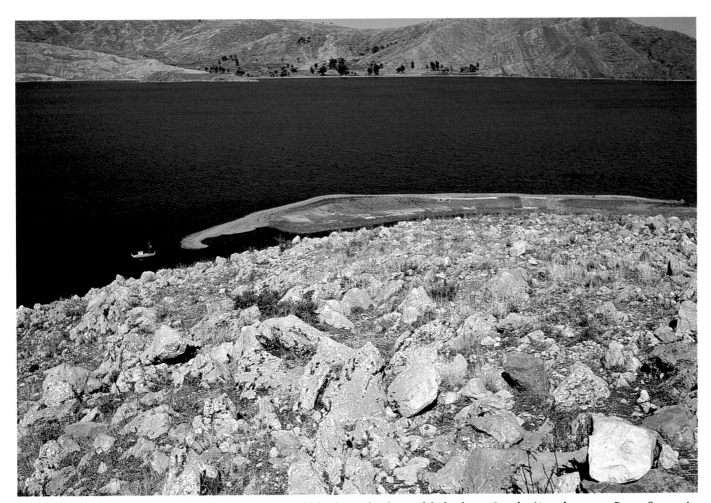

I climbed above the boat to get a high-angle view and was struck by the graphic design of the landscape. I used a 40mm lens on my Pentax Spotmatic to include a wide expanse of foreground, so the composition accentuates the insignificance of the boat in comparison to the spacious landscape.

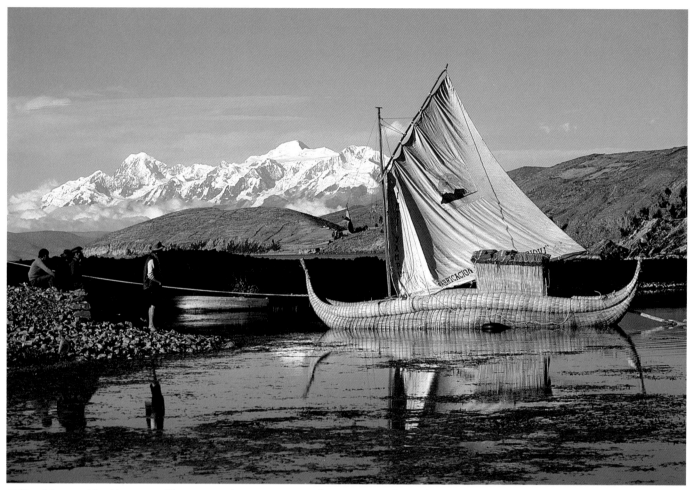

Jeff and I stopped in this protected lagoon to make some repairs to the ropes on our boat. Shooting with my Pentax Spotmatic and a 100mm lens, I stood back to photograph our Bolivian friends and the inti yampu with the Andes Mountains in the background.

waves. Along the shore the population is predominantly Aymara, a people whose ancestry dates back to the mysterious pre-Inca civilization of Tiawanaku.

Intrigued by the lake, Jeff and I abandoned our climbing plans in an impulsive moment of naiveté and commissioned the island men of Suriqui to design and build a 23-foot-long, 6-foot-wide, and 6-foot-high tortora reed boat. Most tortora boats are small and made for riding around placid lagoons, but not ours. The inti yampu, which is the Aymaran term for sun raft, took five weeks to build. It was an elegant bundle of reeds, fitted with a eucalyptus mast, a handsewn sail, an anchor made by the Bolivian Navy, a massive handcarved oar in the back that served as a rudder, and two oars 6 feet apart that required both of us to row simultaneously.

Neither Jeff nor I had ever sailed before. On the first day, we began drifting sideways across the lake, out of control and

away from the safety of the shore. We knew there was a terrible flaw in the boat design. There wasn't a keel or sideboard to help keep us on course. We were at the mercy of the wind. We couldn't sail against it because we'd be swept in the middle of the turbulent lake, and we couldn't row into it. Jeff and I realized that we could sail only when the wind was directly behind us, or row during a lull in the wind. We also found out that circumnavigating the lake was a bigger undertaking than we'd originally expected.

As we struggled our way northwest, we proudly told the curious Bolivians that we were heading to Peru and around the lake. "It would be faster in a car," one Aymaran woman remarked. "Yes, I'm sure it would," I replied, "but I would miss out on the adventure." They stared at us and at the reed boat. Shaking their heads matter-of-factly, they said, "If you get to Peru, you're going to die there. Very cold in lake. The waves

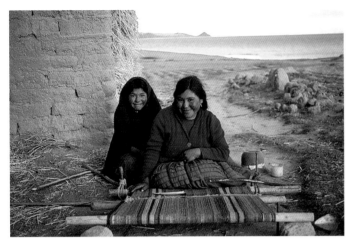

As I was returning to the boat after visiting an Aymaran family, I was attracted by the soft light on the daughters' round faces and knelt down to take their portrait. I used my Pentax Spotmatic, a 40mm lens, and Kodachrome 64.

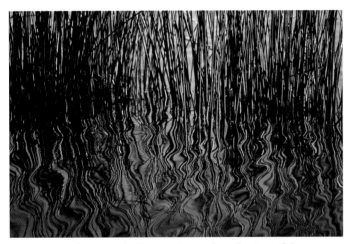

I spent many hours on the boat staring at the reflections of the tortora reeds in the water. Finally recognizing their photographic appeal, I captured them on Kodachrome 64 with my Pentax Spotmatic and a 40mm lens.

hit rocks. Boom. Boom. Boom. You will be smashed." Living daily in a rough, difficult world, it was impossible for them to understand why anyone would intentionally want to inflict hardship on themselves. A couple of months later, I began to have a profound insight into their point of view.

After two months passed and Jeff and I were only halfway around the lake (we originally estimated five weeks for completion), we were discouraged and tired. We'd weathered storms, fierce winds, and incredible waves, as well as a glut of boring days sitting on the boat waiting for the winds to change in our favor. However, we were still determined and kept

plodding onward from the tortora patch to the sheltered harbor praying our boat would hold together. Finally on Thanksgiving Day, 11 weeks after we began, we sailed our battered, soggy, 2-ton boat into our home port of Huatajata to the astonishment and relief of everyone.

I've traveled for longer periods of time, and I've been on numerous outdoor trips from four to six weeks. But this was the longest outdoor trip using one mode of transportation in one region that I'd ever gone on. I'd never choose to repeat this particular voyage, but I expect to go on more extended journeys. Jeff and I had no idea when we started how long the trip was going to take. We had no set agenda on this trip, except to complete it. And if I knew then what I know now, I might not have gone. Still, despite the boredom, hardships, cold, and worry, it was a grand adventure. There is definitely something very special about traveling with no plan or schedule whether you're walking, sailing, or riding horseback. You connect intimately with the country, the people, and yourself.

This was my initiation into photographing outside Western countries and using color-transparency film. Before this, I'd used only black-and-white film, a large-format camera for landscapes and portraits, and a 35mm camera for sports photography. I decided that I didn't want to cart a large-format camera around the world; a 35mm camera seemed better suited to traveling. I took two camera bodies, a Pentax MX and a Pentax Spotmatic, and three lenses, a 40mm, a 100mm macro, and a 135mm. I kept my cameras in individual leather cases in a ratty old daypack. I also brought some lens paper, a few filters, and a small screwdriver. It was a very simple and lightweight arrangement. For this trip I decided to shoot color transparencies. I took with me only about 25 rolls of Plus-X and 25 rolls of Kodachrome 64, which at the time seemed very excessive. I shot the black-and-white film with one camera, the color with the other.

At that time I took only one or two photographs of a scene. Now, looking back over my photographs, I see some gaps and lost opportunities but not as many as I could expect. This reinforces the idea that you don't need a motor drive and a large assortment of lenses to create excellent images. When you're just beginning to shoot, it is important not to overwhelm yourself with too much technical information. Remember, photographs primarily come from within yourself, not the camera. Since I had a minimum of equipment, I learned everything about the limitations and advantages of my lenses.

I also learned many lessons on that trip: watch out for pickpockets, eat only peeled fruits, drink only boiled water, and, second to my life, save and protect my cameras at all

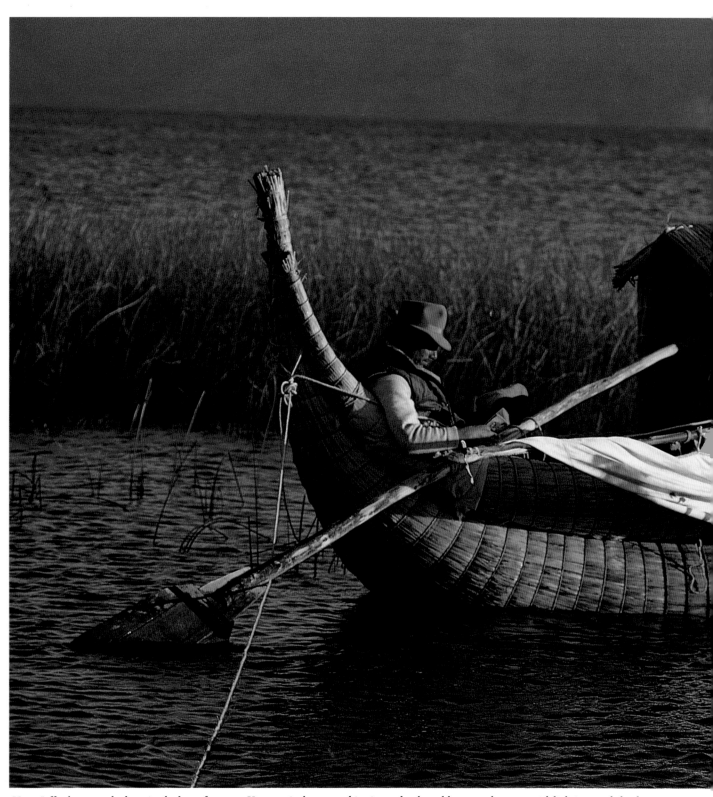

Here, Jeff relaxes on the boat in the late afternoon. Your eye is drawn to this picture by the golden sun, the strong sidelighting, and the deep shadows on the tortora boat. Shooting Kodachrome 64, I used my Pentax Spotmatic and a 135mm lens.

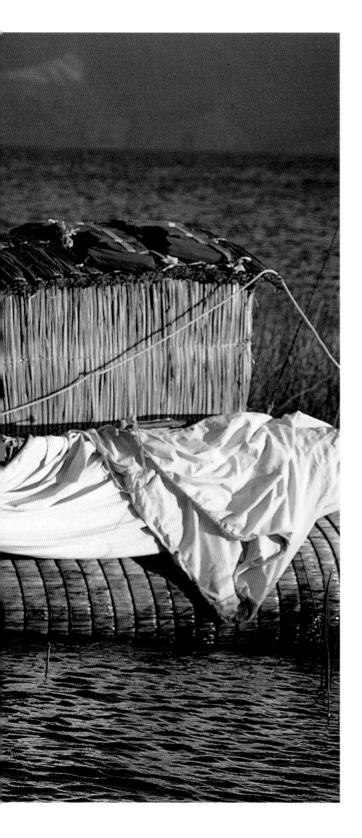

costs. In my journals I wrote more than once, "We almost lost the boat, but I saved my cameras." However, about halfway around the lake, my Pentax Spotmatic camera with the 100mm macro lens on it fell into 5 feet of water. I jumped into the frigid water, fished out the camera, shook out the water, and laid the camera in the sun to dry. Amazingly the camera dried out and worked fine, but the lens never recovered. (For more information on dealing with water, see page 28.)

One of the most difficult tasks on a long journey is maintaining photographic momentum. It is easy to roll over in the morning mumbling, "I'll take a sunrise photograph tomorrow." Inevitably you'll miss the quintessential sunrise, and the next day it'll rain. Only you know the difference between a well-deserved rest and laziness.

Sometimes when I go on longer trips I give myself an assignment. I try to narrow the theme to an object, color, or expression and portray it in as many different ways I can. For example, in Vietnam I photographed conical straw hats. And in Nepal I've focused on the color red and temple details, while in the Chinese Pamir Mountains I photographed the buttons on young girls' coats and in their hair. On Lake Titicaca I shot the tortora reeds. Giving yourself an assignment on a long trip can help keep your photographic momentum alive. Also, don't forget self-portraits on the trip, and be creative.

Keep good notes and records of the photographs you take. Over a long period of time your memory can fade, and you might not remember the Aymaran name of the weaver, the town she was in, or what she was weaving. Write down precise notes of names, dates, events, and photographic exposures in a notebook. Finally, on long trips you have time to be experimental, not just three days to photograph everything. Experiment with night shots, low-light indoor shots, and slow exposures.

Not only was my sailing trip around Lake Titicaca a great journey, but also, in retrospect, a pivotal event: the prelude to a new thrust to the rest of my life. I cultivated flexibility, stamina, and a sense of humor. And I learned not to rush but to take time and listen to people, and to keep my eyes open and genuinely "see" what was around me. I began to understand what it means to see with a camera. Photography and travel became indispensable partners.

PART 2

THE THRILL OF ACTION

Some of my travels have turned into unexpected adventures that require a flexible mindset and time frame. My trip to Lake Titicaca, Bolivia, falls into this category. These are exceptional experiences. However, I also like succinct, well-planned (and usually shorter) kinds of journeys, when I know where I'm going beforehand and basically what I'll be doing once I get there.

Each type of trip has its own travel and photographic appeal. The more time you spend in a region, the greater the possibility of capturing intimate images. However, it is easy to lose your photographic momentum over a long period of time. On a short trip the impetus is strong, but sometimes it feels as if you're just beginning to detect the essence of the place or the people when you have to leave. How much time you spend on a journey is subject to personal needs and limitations. There is something to be gained from every trip, whether you head out for one year or one day.

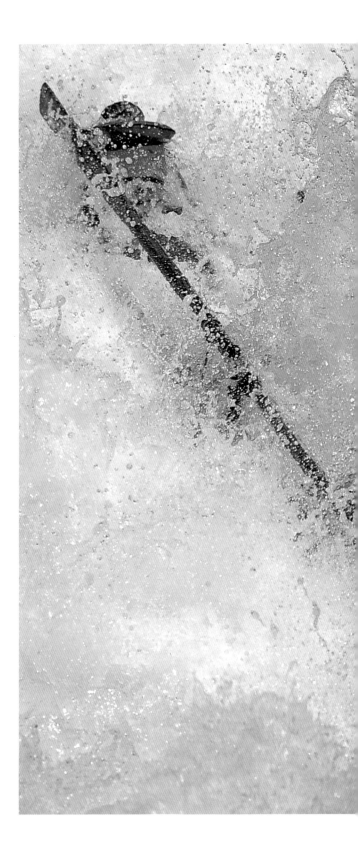

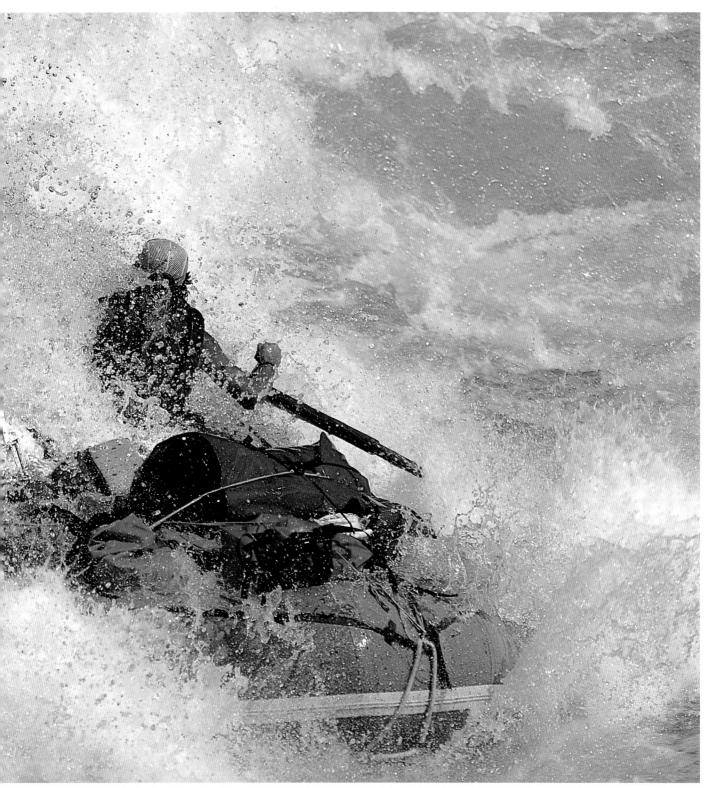

After we stopped on the bank to photograph the other two rafts running the eighteenth rapid on Africa's Zambezi River, I positioned myself above a huge "hole" of recirculating water and photographed the raft as it attempted to punch through the water. Shooting with my Nikon N8008, an 80-200mm lens, and Fuji Velvia, I exposed for 1/500 sec. at f/4.

DOG SLEDDING IN THE BROOKS RANGE IN ALASKA

Since very few people are able to take 11 weeks off in order to go on an international, outdoor photography trip, I say, "Take it while and when you can." On a 5-to-10 day trip you can journey to a remote place and have an unforgettable adventure. Time seems to expand when you aren't at home or at work. I've marveled many times at what I've experienced and seen in only a week.

Recently I went on an eight-day dog-sledding trip in Alaska. It had been 13 years since I'd gone sailing on Lake Titicaca. I have more experience and gray hair, but I still feel the same excitement about being in an unfrequented, pristine environment.

The Gates of the Arctic National Park reaches from Alaska's central Brooks Range into the far-north Arctic region. Southerly foothills sweep into waves of mountains that have limestone and granite peaks over 7,000 feet in elevation. The Brooks Range is wild, immense, and inspiring.

I flew by skiplane with three other people into the Gates of the Arctic near Tinyaguk Cabin, a rustic and very primitive log cabin on the edge of the Koyukuk River. We were 67 degrees north of the Arctic Circle. At the end of March the sun rose around 6 A.M. and set at 9 P.M. Because of the northern latitude, we were gaining eight minutes of sunlight per day. Yet the angle of the sun was low, maintaining a warm glow during midday and languidly setting in the evening for a protracted sunset. Even though it was the beginning of spring and we had 16 hours of sunlight, the temperature rarely rose above 20°F during the day. And after the sun set, the temperature was in the minus range. Luckily, we were blessed with windless, sunny days.

I carried two packs of equipment. One was a fannypack I attached to the top of the dog sled, so that I could open it while I was moving. In it I kept a Nikon F3 with a motor drive, a 20mm lens, a 24mm lens, and an SB-24 flash. I had an 80-200mm autofocus (AF) lens in a separate hard case also clipped and tied to the sled in a handy position. Around my neck I wore a Nikon N8008 with a 35-105mm AF lens tucked inside my jacket. I often use chest straps or a torso harness, but in this instance my jacket kept the camera from bouncing around. I cinched a belt high around my torso for the camera to rest on and to keep its weight from pulling on my neck.

Inside the sled on top of all my gear, I put a Tamrac camera bag with another F3 body, a spare motor drive, and several lenses, a 35mm $f/1.5$, a 50mm macro, an 80mm, and a 180mm. This camera bag wasn't accessible while I was moving on the sled, so I used these lenses while I was in camp, when we stopped for lunch, or if I stopped for a special shot. The next time I go dog sledding, I'll put my cameras in waterproof cases; this way, in case there is a storm or I encounter unexpected overflow, or water melting on top of the ice in a river, they'll be completely protected.

There is nothing like dog sledding. It is breathtaking and exhilarating to be on a sled with your own team of dogs barking and lunging forward enthusiastically at the release of the break. Since I'd never mushed a dog sled before, for the first few hours I traveled without my cameras around my neck to get used to being on a sled and controlling the dogs. Once I hit a bump while I was shooting and found myself practically hanging off the sled on my belly and being dragged along an icy river. I managed to grab onto the sled with one hand, tuck my camera into my jacket, and pull myself back into position. If I hadn't, my dogs would've gleefully raced on without me for miles, glad to be rid of the extra weight.

We headed north toward the Gates of the Arctic on the north fork of the Koyukuk River; Boreal Mountain was on the right, and the Frigid Crags on the left. We broke trail into the Gates of the Arctic along frozen rivers, snowbanks, and pure white valleys. White was the theme. There were snowy hills, white furry dogs, icy rivers, and blinding sun.

There is very little incentive to be up and on your sled early in extremely cold weather. Between warming up, cooking, packing the sleds, and harnessing 50 dogs, we often didn't get moving until early afternoon. There wasn't much stopping once we mounted the sleds. I found that my camera's motor drive and autofocus capabilities were indispensable; I hung onto the sled with one hand and leaned over or out to the side and shot.

When shooting from the sled, I tended to use either the 35-70mm AF lens or the 20mm lens. The greater the angle of a lens, the greater its depth of field. With ultrawide-angle lenses, depth of field extends from a few feet in front of the camera to infinity. When I used either lens, the front part of my sled was in focus and the background was crisp. Because my Nikon cameras don't have a built-in autobracket, I had to be exact in my light readings. If you have an autobracket you might consider using it: snow needs to be exposed precisely in order for you to capture its luminous quality. Although the physical conditions can be difficult to deal with, snow offers a welcome change from the usual tonal arrangement of land and sky. By coating the land, it tends to simplify images.

On this trip I used Kodachrome 64 for its sharpness, saturation, and neutral color cast. However, keep in mind that Fujichrome is superb in overcast lighting conditions where its inherent contrast brings out the best in subdued tones, particularly in the green areas. I shot about five rolls of film a day.

Because of the cold weather, I had to pay close attention to keeping my batteries warm. At night I took the batteries out and placed them in my sleeping bag. During the day I had AA batteries in practically every inside pocket of my clothing to warm them with my body heat. When I wore my camera on the outside of my chest, thereby exposing it to the cold and wind, I usually had to switch my batteries at least once. I had only one battery pack for my Nikon N8008 so when the temperatures dropped, I took the battery pack out of the motor drive and kept it next to my stomach or under my arm. Then when I needed to use the camera, I slipped the battery pack back into the camera.

When I went inside a heated tent or cabin, I put one set of cameras inside the camera bag (after taking out the batteries) and left them in a moderately cold place, such as under the cots or next to the door; the cameras remained cool and ready to be used outdoors. I put the second set of cameras in heavy-duty plastic bags, squeezed out as much air as possible, and sealed up the bags before entering a warm room. When

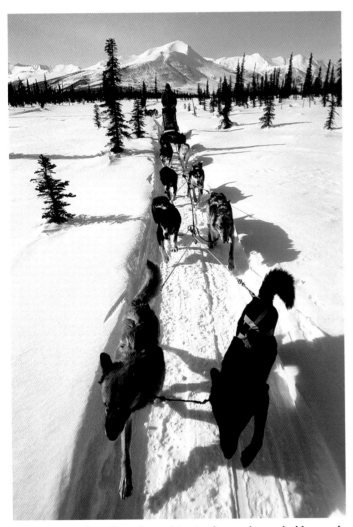

As we were mushing down the trail I twisted around, crouched low, and held onto my moving sled with one hand to photograph the sled behind me with a 20mm lens. Tightly holding onto my Nikon N8008, I exposed for 1/1000 sec. at f/5.6 on Kodachrome 64. The drama of the event is enhanced by the converging lines of the sled, which direct the eye to the top of my friend's head and the mountain in the background.

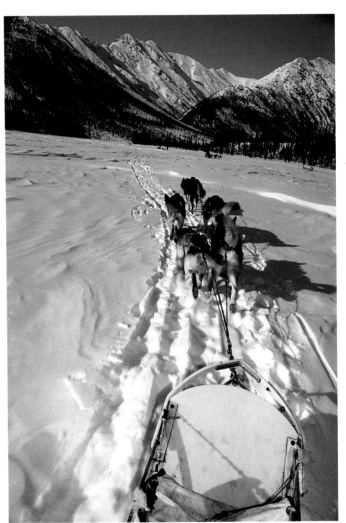

Once we were on our sleds we rarely stopped until we reached our destination. So I did much of my photographing from the moving sled. For this photograph, made with my Nikon F3 and a 20mm wide-angle lens, I leaned forward and low over the sled with in order to photograph the dogs and to include a portion of my sled and the landscape. The exposure was 1/500 sec. at f/5.6 on Kodachrome 64.

the warm inside air hit the cold bag, condensation formed on the bag, not the camera.

I remember the first day I went out to photograph the sunset. It was after 8 P. M., and the sun was very low on the horizon. I panicked and raced around trying to find the perfect shot. Then I remembered that I was in the northern latitudes, the land of the slow sunset. So I calmed down and strolled around for more than an hour, photographing the sun's sweet, pale glow. I was ready to move to the Arctic Circle.

After reaching the actual Gates of the Arctic, we turned back down the Koyukuk River and headed over a series of passes, vast snow meadows, pine forests, and wide ice rivers toward Wiseman, a small town on the Alaskan highway. At this point I reflected on the trip. I'd learned a new outdoor skill, experienced the call of the unbridled landscape, and augmented my repertoire of winter photography in a completely different venue. I could've kept going for weeks, but eight days was all I had. I felt very satisfied and elated. Besides, it is good to leave a place a little hungry for more.

TECHNIQUES FOR SHOOTING IN THE COLD

The hardest winter picture to shoot is a perfectly exposed snow landscape in the middle of a sunny day that holds detail without underexposing its whites. Photographing white as white is a challenge. The margin of error is slim. Because snow is white, the in-camera meter reads that white as 18-percent gray and exposes accordingly. Unless you override the meter reading, the picture is probably doomed; the usual result is a dense image with muddy whites and darker colors often in the hue of blue. So for the best results, use an incident meter or make your own personal adjustments to your in-camera meter reading.

Meter off something that approximates 18-percent gray, such as the sky, your hand, a piece of neutral-colored clothing, or a neutral-gray card. I normally gauge the exposure by metering directly off the back of my hand because I am familiar with its skin tone. When it is tan, I use the exact reading or maybe open up half a stop; if it is pale, I open up 1 to 1 1/2 stops. You can also take a reading off a blue sky, which approximates a gray card, if you point your meter away from the sun. I also carry a gray card in my camera bag that I can use instead of my hand if I'm wearing gloves.

Another option when shooting a snow scene under the midday sun is to increase the in-camera exposure reading by one to two stops depending upon the direction of the light: one stop for light over the shoulder, and two stops for strong light in the face (see page 88). Don't be fooled, though. The whites that you're looking at often aren't really white. As an

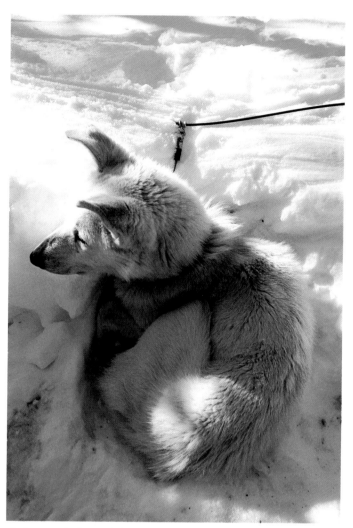

I photographed one of the sled dogs as we hitched them to their sleds. This was a particularly difficult exposure because of the monochromatic scene, although the shadows in the snow helped to separate the whites. Using my Nikon N8008 and a 35-70mm zoom lens, I metered off my hand to get the correct exposure and bracketed my shots. Here, I exposed for 1/60 sec. at f/8 on Kodachrome 64.

efficient reflector snow picks up the color of its surroundings, particularly the blue of a clear sky. Shadows in snow on a bright, sunny day are inevitably blue, so by exposing for the whites you lose the blue. If you want "white whites," open up to override the 18-percent-gray syndrome of reflected-light meters. The creative decision is yours.

When you're looking at a snowfield, examine the light. Check its direction, color, and shadows, and become aware of the shapes and the texture. Texture in snow is a function of the angle, direction, and intensity of light. The stronger and more parallel the light rays are to a surface, the better the light reveals the texture and shapes of that surface. If you make the exposure only for the white snow and not the shadows, you lose that magic.

I never turn down the opportunity to photograph in a snowstorm. It is easier to predict exposure on an overcast day when the light is constant. I use the camera's reflected meter because it wants to expose everything to make it appear neutral gray, turning the snow darker than normal and blacks lighter than normal. I'll back myself up by bracketing $^1/_3$ to $^1/_2$ stops. Err in the direction of a half-stop underexposure to make the storm scene appear dark and dangerous. Blues and purples dominate long exposures in overcast or snowy weather, creating even more dramatic results.

The middle of a cold, sunny day is my least favorite time to photograph. To increase color saturation when the sun provides a uniformly boring light, you should underexpose by $^1/_4$ to $^1/_3$ stop. When you photograph right before or after sunset, you can usually be within half a stop of the meter readings. I'll usually bracket for the subtleties of color. Long exposures give an exaggerated color cast to certain parts of the photograph, which actually enhances the scene.

With the exception of a polarizing filter and a Nikon A2 warming filter, I rarely use filters when shooting snow and ice. Occasionally I use the A2 warming filter on overcast days to offset the cool color of the light by warming up skin tones and colors. I use a polarizer to reduce glare and reflections, to sharpen the contrast between the snow and the blue sky, and to enhance the prismatic spectral colors of frost crystals. Be careful when you use a polarizer. Sometimes the sky turns an unnatural navy blue, especially at high altitudes.

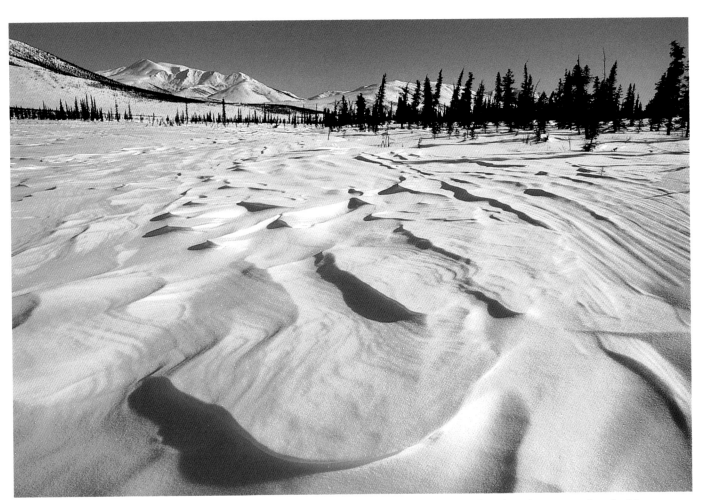

I went snowshoeing one morning to explore the area around our camp and came upon a pristine valley of windswept snow. I used a 20mm zoom lens on my Nikon N8008 to accentuate the textured patterns delineated by thin shadows, and a polarizer to deepen the blue of the sky. With Kodachrome 64, this exposure was 1/60 sec. at f/11.

To photograph glowing tents—your protection from the cold and the elements when you aren't shooting—first you need to add a small amount of ambient light to the scene so you can see the details. Set up the shot with someone inside the tent, and have the individual use a flashlight or lantern to paint the inside with light. Expose for the natural light outdoors if the tents are just one element of your composition. Expose for the light inside the tent if it dominates the frame. Use an exposure time of at least 4 sec. because the longer the exposure, the better the glow.

To get closer shots of people in action in the cold, such as mushing, skiing, dog sledding, or skating, in front or in back of me, I use an 80-200mm zoom lens. By using an autofocus (AF) lens you can shoot a follow-focus series of sledding shots, keeping the focus at the head while capturing a succession of images. To freeze action you need a shutter speed that is fast enough to stop the movement of the subject as well as camera motion. A good rule of thumb is to double the focal length of your lens and use that number as the minimum handheld shutter speed.

While dog sledding in Alaska, I usually shot for 1/1000 sec. since the subject and I were both moving and I was worried about camera shake. I had to hold on to the sled with one hand and shoot with the other, so I had to preset a focal length and shoot or wait for a smooth section of the trail, take my hands off the sled, and shoot with both hands, a potentially hazardous maneuver. I always used my motor drive in order to take a number of shots to ensure that my subject was in optimum focus, and I made at least one shot with a level horizon.

When using a manual-focusing lens you have to concentrate. During this trip I used one basic focusing technique when working with a manual lens. A few times I set up shots where I knew the person would be coming to a prearranged point. I focused on that particular spot and fired the camera at the moment the subject arrived. Since cameras often have a microsecond delay after you fire the shutter, you should press the shutter a microsecond early. You can also use a high-speed motor drive and blast away (although you may miss the decisive shot when the subject leapfrogs away from the point of focus). You can practice this technique while sitting on a road; using a telephoto lens, try to keep the oncoming cars in focus. It takes some time but soon you'll be able to follow the focus from infinity until the car fills the frame.

The longer the focal length of a lens, the less depth of field it provides at any focusing distance except infinity. For example, using a 200mm lens instead of a 400mm lens enables more space around your subject to be in sharp focus. As a result you are less likely to cut off part of it, and it is easier to compose. Longer lenses allow for a larger image on the film, but a larger image isn't an advantage unless it is as sharp as the image taken with one of the shorter lenses. So for me the 80-200mm zoom lens and the 300mm lens are ideal.

A long lens also comes in handy when you want to capture the action in falling snow. It compresses the scene and enhances

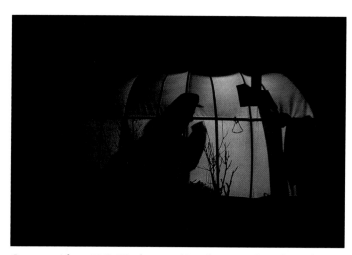

I was outside at 11 P. M. photographing the aurora borealis with my Nikon F3 and a 50mm lens and turned my head to see the exaggerated shadow of one of my friends drinking tea inside the group tent. I abandoned my intended shot, set up my tripod outside the tent, and asked my friend to hold his pose so that I could take a slow exposure. I took a light reading of the tent and bracketed my shots. This exposure was 1/2 sec. at f/2.8 on Kodachrome 64.

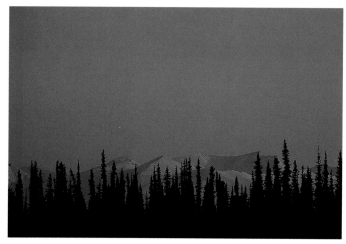

I was entranced by the prolonged sunsets of the northern latitudes. The first evening I strolled down the valley photographing the pink glow of dusk. This silhouette of a line of trees against the luminescent sky was one of my last shots. Shooting Kodachrome 64 with my Nikon N8008 and an 80-200mm zoom lens, I exposed for 1/60 sec. at f/5.6.

the snow in motion. A shutter speed of at least 1/125 sec. stops the flakes, while a slower shutter speed blurs the snow. Make sure that you step back from your subject. You need to put a good amount of snow between you and the action.

Follow-focus shooting is hardest when you're working with a longer lens because you have to be exact about depth of field. A sled running parallel to you is an easy subject to photograph because it's running on approximately the same plane you are. So the focus remains the same, but you need a faster shutter speed. It is more difficult to focus on a sled running at a 45-degree angle to you because the angle masks the speed of the sled. And it is even more difficult to focus on a sled running directly toward you because it's either coming toward or going away from you quickly. Actually, between these two shooting situations, it is easier to focus on a sled heading directly away from you because as it's running, you're approaching the infinity setting on your lens. You can stop the action with a shutter speed as slow as 1/125 sec. if you have a steady hand. If, however, the sled's running directly toward you, focus in front of it and trip the shutter when it appears sharp in the viewfinder.

Be careful if you're using a wide-angle lens: the subject goes in and out of the framing so quickly that you barely have time to shoot, let alone focus. In order to successfully use a wide-angle lens, you must be extremely close to the action. But this shooting position can be dangerous since you may suddenly realize that the dog sled in your lens is also right on top of you.

COLD AND YOUR EQUIPMENT

There are different levels of severity of coldness. From 32°F down to 0°F you need to follow common-sense precautions of keeping your equipment as dry and warm as possible. Below 0°F, however, some of the materials' characteristics are altered. Some lubricants thicken, which causes moving parts to slow down or jam. Film becomes brittle and less sensitive. To avoid tearing or breaking, advance the film lever very slowly. If you use a motor drive or load or wind the film too quickly, you might get small flash marks from static discharge on the film. Of course, the amount of time you spend out in the cold will help to determine how severe the negative effects are. In very cold weather be careful when using ultrafast speeds, such as 1/1000 sec. and 1/5000 sec. The shutter curtain can drag, leaving a dark, unexposed portion at the side of each frame.

Some photographers talk about winterizing cameras, but hardly anyone does this anymore. The process involves replacing normal lubricants that might congeal at very cold temperatures with others based on silicon, molybdenum, or Teflon. This is an extreme and costly process. Furthermore once this is done, you need to "de-winterize" your camera in order to use it again in more temperate climates. With the new lubricants and compatible metals used in modern cameras, winterizing is unnecessary for all but a few makes.

Some people swear by taking only manual cameras in cold climates. I don't have any problems with my automatic cameras and motor drives as long as I keep the batteries warm. Battery failure is the most common technical problem photographers encounter in winter; no batteries like cold weather. As the temperature drops, so does their efficiency. At 32°F, the freezing temperature of water, fresh batteries operate at about a third of their rated capacity. Specifications for most batteries indicate that they can be used to –4°F, but temperatures can fall much lower than that in Alaska and other mountain terrain. Always bring plenty of spare batteries for your camera. The newer rechargeable nicads have a greater capacity in cold conditions. However, it usually isn't possible to recharge batteries on an extended, outdoor winter trip.

Several camera makers have remote battery holders. One end screws into the battery compartment on the bottom of their manual cameras. A long cord connects to the other end, which holds two AA batteries. The battery holder can be slipped into a shirt or coat pocket, so you can protect the batteries from the cold. You can also use a chemical hand warmer to keep your camera or battery pack warm. When shooting with my Nikon F3 with a motor drive, I usually have several battery cartridges readily accessible in my jacket or pants pockets, close to my body. When I start to shoot, I slide one cartridge in and then rotate the cartridges as they cool in the camera.

Expose your equipment to the cold only when shooting. The rest of the time you should keep your equipment insulated in a padded, waterproof bag or under as many layers of clothing as possible. In Alaska I hung my camera around my neck and snuggled it inside my outer jacket, but I had to be careful when I removed it because of the condensation that formed on the lens and body. If you find condensation on your camera, wait a few seconds for it to stabilize and then wipe it off carefully with some lens tissue. Never blow the snow off your lenses. Your breath is warm and wet, and trying to blow moisture or snowflakes off the lens element in freezing weather produces a coating of fog or ice. I use a camel-hair brush for the lens and a soft chamois cloth for a foggy eyepiece.

Finally, don't put your cameras next to a fire to warm them up. Accidents can happen. Furthermore, this is a radical approach. Using body heat and letting your equipment slowly come to room temperature are best.

STAYING WARM

Pay close attention to your field equipment, particularly your clothing. You want to make sure that you're protected adequately from all the elements. The most efficient cold-weather clothing is available through mountaineering shops or catalogs. Some of the equipment is expensive, but it can last a lifetime. Another key to staying warm is maintaining a high caloric intake, up to 5,000 calories a day.

Keeping your hands warm is essential. It isn't a good idea for bare skin to touch metal parts in freezing weather. To protect my fingers, I put three or four layers of black gaffer tape over all the areas of my "winter" cameras, lenses, and tripod that I touch or hold. You can also purchase commercial leg covers for your tripod. These "Tri-Pads" are made from standard foam pipe insulation, covered with a durable cloth material, and secured with Velcro. Wrapping a cushioned bicycle handlebar around the tripod legs also works.

I wear a pair of lightweight, capilene glove liners. I can feel the camera controls through them, and they protect my hands against the numbing cold. Over the liners I wear protective outer mittens. When I want to shoot, I take off the outer shells and stuff them into a pocket. You can also use a safety pin to attach an "idiot cord" from your mittens to your sleeve, so you can drop them at any critical moment without losing them. But be careful not to include the ends of the mittens or the cuffs of your jacket in your shots.

WHITEWATER RAFTING ON THE ZAMBEZI RIVER IN AFRICA

Rafting on the Zambezi River is one of the world's greatest whitewater adventures. From the base of Musi-O-Tunga, the local name for Victoria Falls that means "the smoke that thunders," the Zambezi River careens down a narrow corridor of black volcanic rock between Zambia and Zimbabwe. I joined a commercial trip down the Zambezi. We put into the river in three rafts at the Boiling Pot directly beneath Victoria Falls (the spot where Dr. David Livingstone abandoned his exploration in 1885). We had 60 miles of challenging whitewater before we hit the flat water of Lake Kariba. The Zambezi has 38 named or numbered rapids, and boasts 10 of the world's biggest rapids. I sat in the back of the middle raft because this was the best vantage point for photographing the front of the boat when it hit the rapids and was flung sharply upward. I was also positioned to shoot the raft in front of or behind mine.

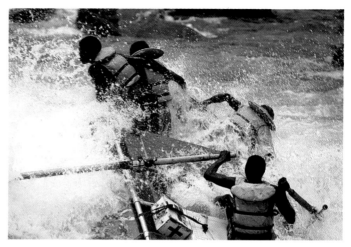

I made this shot of the first boat as it plunged into the Ghost Rider rapid with my Nikon N8008, an 80-200mm zoom lens, and Kodachrome 64. Standing on a platform at the back of the second boat, I exposed at f/4 for 1/500 sec.

For photographing in the whitewater, I had a Nikonos V with a 35mm lens mounted on it around my neck, across my chest, and under my arm with a neoprene strap. The rest of my camera gear was in a Tundra #613 waterproof case, which measures $13\frac{1}{2} \times 9$ inches, and was attached to the raft but accessible. The case held a Nikon N8008 camera, an 80-200mm AF $f/2.8$ zoom lens, a 50mm macro lens, a 24mm $f/2.8$ lens, a 20mm $f/2.8$ lens, and an SB-24 flash. I opted to travel compactly. I was able to untie the case quickly whenever I left the boat. It was light and small enough to clip with a carabiner, a piece of rock-climbing gear that acts like a large safety pin, to a strap on my life jacket. This was awkward, but left my hands free at critical moments. My tripod, extra film, and backup equipment was in a waterproof rubber bag made expressly for river rafting. But this gear was available only when we unloaded the boats at the end of the day.

On the first day we had a nonstop series of huge rapids to run. As we approached the first rapid, I grabbed onto the boat line with my left hand and clutched my Nikonos in my right, eye to the viewfinder. We plunged into the current, and a wall of water blasted the raft. The raft pitched to the left and right as we were battered again by curtains of water. Dazed, swamped, but intact, we slid into the calm water. I'd been able to shoot a few frames during the turbulence, but it was harder than I thought to keep a firm stance and secure grip. Pools of calm water separated the dizzying succession of rapids, but the current was swift and we barely had time to bail out the boats before we were attacked by another set of rapids. I didn't even have time to open up my camera case and shoot the other rafts with my regular camera and long lens, so I concentrated on capturing the commotion in my raft.

As we entered the seventh rapid I was able to see the lip of a massive wave directly in front of us. I had my camera cocked and was as steady as a two-legged, one-armed tripod could be. Just as I was making the shot, I felt myself submerged in a cascade of water. I was ripped from my handhold and as I lurched for another grip, I knew I was being catapulted out of the boat. I was immediately sucked down into the frothy, turbulent water. I tried to get a shot on one of my brief excursions to the surface, but it was too tumultuous. Finally I was spat out, and a boatman threw me a line and dragged me into his boat. I didn't lose my camera, but from that moment I clipped the strap to my life jacket with a carabiner.

SHIFTING POSITIONS

The next day we continued our adventure through impressive rapids. I changed my position in the raft so that I'd be able to photograph from the bow of the boat and concentrate my attention on the expressions of our boatman, Vinnie. I wedged myself down low, bracing against the tubes and the other rafters, and shot up toward Vinnie. Then we plunged into the rapids, and the river jumped over my head into Vinnie's face.

Shooting from a raft gives you the chance to capture an intimate and dramatic photograph. However, you're shooting under volatile conditions, so you risk being washed overboard if you don't have a firm stance. Inevitably since you're pitched unpredictably and unexpectedly around the raft, you often miss the decisive moment. Shooting a rapid from the banks of the river, on the other hand, means that you can previsualize

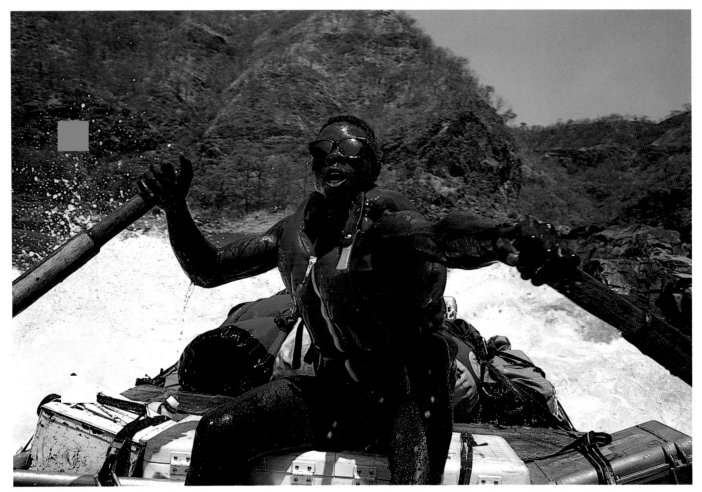

I often knelt in the bow of the raft and shot up toward the oarsman as we negotiated the rapids. Here, I captured him in action through the "Let's Make a Deal" rapid with my Nikonos V and a 35mm lens. The exposure was 1/250 sec. at f/5.6 on Kodachrome 64.

the shot. And by not being limited to a waterproof camera, you also have a bigger selection of lenses to choose from as well as the ability to use a motor drive to catch quick movement. Each perspective has advantages and disadvantages; try both.

Since I was with an amenable crew, I spent some time hanging off the back end of my raft and photographing the raft following very close behind. If the Zambezi River didn't have hippopotamuses and crocodiles, I also would've jumped into the river to photograph for a water-level viewpoint. I experimented with various positions within the boat trying to find intriguing camera angles, such as sitting directly behind the oarsman and shooting with a 20mm or 24mm lens to capture a portion of his movements with the crew and the rapids in the background.

By the last day the river was wide, cutting through the flat, arid countryside, as it does above Victoria Falls. We languidly, and cautiously, floated around the hippos and crocodiles until we reached the exit point at the near-still waters of Lake Kariba.

EXPOSING FOR ACTION

Exposure is the Achilles heel of sport photography. The subject moves fast and is usually in the frame for only a microsecond. You may have time for only one shot and no time to bracket. And you can never be absolutely sure if the meter's electronic circuitry will be fast enough to see the subject. In addition if the subject is wearing white or black, your meter reading will be way off.

The feeling and rendition of whitewater movement vary greatly with the exposure interval. For example, a shutter speed of 1/500 sec. freezes a breaking wave so that you can clearly see what's happening but you are more likely to sense the dynamics of water against rock when you shoot the same wave with a shutter speed of 1/2 sec. And there are times when a 6-sec. exposure may best express the movement of water.

Sometimes the exposure is simple and straightforward, and other times it can be extremely complex. Your eyes and brain have the uncanny ability to adjust to almost all lighting variations. You don't look at the world as if it's underexposed or overexposed; you can handle a 15-to-20-stop range perfectly, from snow white to coal black, while your camera can handle only a 5-stop range.

Like snow, the highly reflective quality of water or bright sand can cause your in-camera meter to give you an underexposed reading. To correct this, use an incident-light meter or take a reading off a middle-tone subject, such as your hand or gray camera case. If you're metering off the water, open up one to two stops. You can also apply the "sunny 16 rule" to the film you're using (see page 105).

CHOOSING WATERPROOF EQUIPMENT

Nikonos cameras have been the choice of professionals specializing in underwater photography for years. One of the most recent incarnations, the rugged Nikonos V, is especially practical. It has through-the-lens (TTL) metering for both ambient light and high-power strobes. You can select from six lenses, ranging from 15mm to 80mm. Each lens requires a matched optical or open-framed sportsfinder. The extension tube offers magnification up to life-size, thereby allowing photographers to focus on even the smallest marine life or micro images. The Nikonos V also has aperture-priority automation, which comes in handy when there is no time for fully manual exposure control. You might also want to take a look at Nikon's newest model, the Nikonos RS camera. It offers reflex viewing without the need for bulky housings, as well as autofocus capabilities, TTL flash, and matrix metering. The Nikonos RS can be used to depths of 300 feet and is the first camera to have a 20-35mm $f/2.8$ zoom lens. Another choice is the Sea and Sea Motor Marine II. This camera provides TTL flash control, automatic film advance, power rewind, and a wide variety of accessories, and has the added advantage of enabling photographers to change lenses underwater.

A less-expensive option is to buy a flexible housing from Ewa Marine. These high-strength bags are available for virtually any lens-and-camera combination, from 35mm compact and SLR cameras to medium-format cameras and camcorders. The housings are tested to 100 feet, feature optical glass ports for lenses, and allow for unrestricted autofocus operation. Some are designed with built-in gloves, making it easy to manipulate camera controls. An adapter is available to accommodate most lens types and sizes.

These are only a few of the numerous options available. Many manufacturers are beginning to produce smaller waterproof and water-resistant cameras. (For up-to-date information, contact your local camera store.)

Don't panic if a few unexpected drops of spray or flying sand hit your non-waterproof camera; the chance of this causing serious damage is practically nonexistent. But be sure to dry off your camera as soon as possible. If you don't immediately attend to your camera equipment, it could get ruined. And if there is any chance that water has entered the interior of the camera body, remove the batteries at once, dry them, and clean them with a pencil eraser. Rubbing the contacts lightly with an eraser or cotton removes corrosion. Once you are in a sheltered area, remove the lens and the film and thoroughly check for water. Dab away any you find, and pack the camera in a plastic bag with a few packets of fresh desiccant overnight. If salt water has entered the camera or strobe, flush it with fresh water to remove any salt or battery acid.

Trying to air-dry or blow-dry a camera is controversial because it can help internal rust and corrosion begin. However, in situations where keeping a camera sealed or frozen isn't practical or possible or getting to a repair shop isn't an option (such as on Lake Titicaca), this technique can be quite effective. If you need to use a blow-dryer, select a medium or low setting and thoroughly dry the camera or strobe. A high-heat setting can damage rubber or plastic parts. Then open the equipment and allow the warm, dry air from the dryer to get inside. You can make a simple drying oven by placing the camera or strobe inside a plastic bag. Tape the nozzle of the blow-dryer to the inside of the bag, and make a small hole at the other end of the bag so that the air can escape. By following these steps after a camera or

strobe is flooded, you'll probably be able to use it until you can take it to a repair shop.

When a non-waterproof camera gets a good soaking, it usually stops working immediately. But even in this dire situation there is still hope. Take out the battery and film, seal the camera in a plastic bag to prevent evaporation, and take or send the sealed camera to a competent repairperson immediately. If you can't get to a camera repair shop soon, freeze the camera to retard rust formation. Sometimes the cost of repairing the camera is more than the cost of the camera itself, but if it is a valuable camera it is usually worth fixing.

Sand can do nearly as much damage as water; it just takes a little longer. Use a soft brush to gently remove sand from the camera and lens exteriors, and a blower brush to carefully clean the camera interior. Take great care when cleaning lens surfaces. Begin by removing any dust or grit with a few puffs

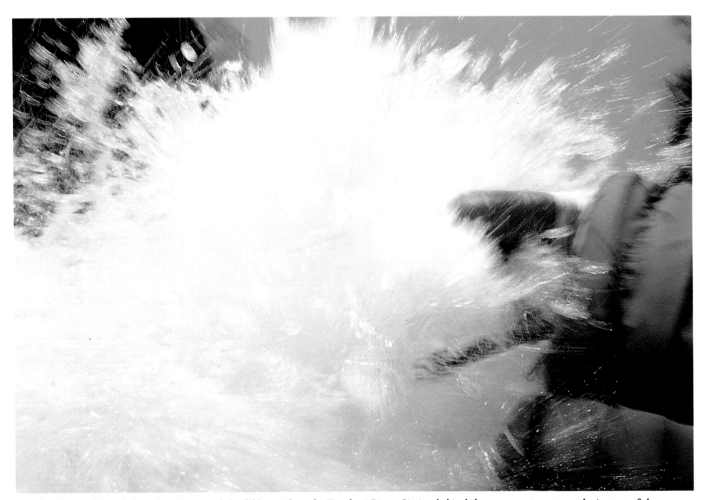

A colossal wave blasted the raft as it entered the fifth rapid on the Zambezi River. Sitting behind the oarsman to capture the impact of the mammoth hydraulic, I used my Nikonos V, a 35mm lens, and Kodachrome 64; I exposed for 1/30 sec. at f/11.

At Moemba Falls we carried all our gear and the rafts around a large waterfall, and then lowered them from a rock cliff into calm water. I climbed around the cliffs to a pinnacle across from the cliff and photographed the scene with my Nikon N8008 and a 35-70mm zoom lens. The exposure was 1/125 sec. at f/5.6 on Kodachrome 64.

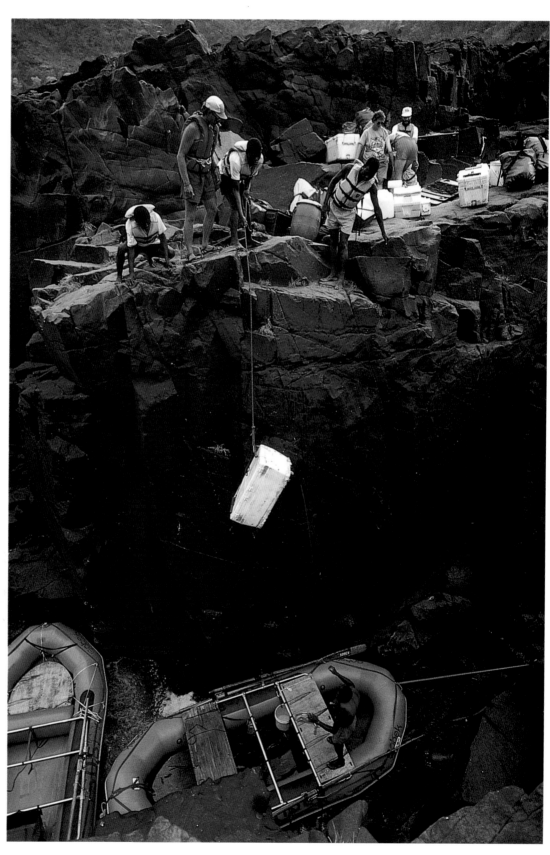

from a second blower brush, then brush the lens surface gently to remove any remaining material. If necessary clean any smudges with a lens tissue lightly wetted with a commercial lens-cleaning solution or blow gently on your lens to create a moisture film, then delicately wipe it with lens tissue.

Two of the best waterproof camera cases for whitewater rafting are made by Pelican and Tundra SeaKing, and are available in a number of sizes. Both cases are made of a lightweight, noncorrosive material; high-impact ABS polycarbonate resin; and injection-molded construction; both have an O-ring seal. They are waterproof, airtight, dustproof, dentproof, and shockproof. Some models are even equipped with a pressure purge valve that compensates for changes in temperature and altitude.

The Tundra SeaKing offers the option of replacing the top foam padding with the SeaKing Palette. This lid insert is actually a nylon-mesh storage device with loops and see-through pockets that hold film, lens-cleaning supplies, filters, batteries, lens hoods, and other sundry items.

Because the difference in interior temperature between a dark and a light case is significant, always purchase a reflective gray color instead of black. Despite this precaution, when the temperature soars on a river trip, I stow all my cases beneath a white towel that I've drenched in water. I bring along several towels specifically for this purpose.

An alternative means of transporting photography equipment is a large ice chest. An 80-quart cooler holds a lot of camera equipment, but be aware that it doesn't offer the same watertight security commercial waterproof cases do. This is only an alternative for a mild float trip with no possibility of the boat flipping over. Another option is to buy an Army-surplus metal ammo can and customize it with foam inserts. These were the standard before the Tundra and Pelican cases were available. In fact boatmen still use these cans for carrying various necessary items during the day. They can be rigged to the raft so that you have only to flip a latch to open them; however, they are heavier and have sharper edges than the newer cases.

You can also carry your cameras on a river trip in a padded camera bag or a convertible bag that doubles as a backpack. Wrap the backpack in a plastic bag, and clip it with a carabiner to the tied-down gear on board. On a mild river I cover my camera with zip-lock bags and keep it around my neck. Then when I see a potential photograph, I take off the bags, stuff them in my pocket, and shoot.

When you are on a river trip, make sure that you secure your camera at night. Dew can collect on a camera if it's left unprotected overnight. Use your camera bag or water-resistant case; either can combat most moisture problems. You can also wrap your camera bag in a plastic bag. Use a desiccant to absorb potentially dangerous moisture in all your equipment bags.

In addition I always bring a tripod with me. Shooting doesn't end after the whitewater run of the day is over. You'll make some of your best shots—of camp, the river, sandstone walls, or campfire scenes—during the magic hours of twilight and dusk. But sometimes you'll find that it is tough to keep your tripod steady in the sand. Even when you've cranked it down into the sand until it seems steady, it often isn't. To help solve this problem, you can either weigh the tripod down with a bag of sand hanging from the middle of it or make "tripod sandshoes" from pieces of cardboard, plastic lids, or books. These keep the tripod afloat and steady.

It is important to guard your film, as well as your cameras, against heat. Keep your film in a small waterproof case inside a cooler to protect it from dampness. If this isn't possible, do what I often do: I stuff my film into a stuff sack and place it inside the center of my sleeping bag. Every evening I remove exposed film from my daytime camera case and replace it with fresh film for the next day.

In addition to the regular tool kit you should carry the following on a river trip: a dry towel, plastic bags, an O-ring removal tool (a bobbypin works well), silicone grease (to lubricate O-rings), and spare O-rings.

SEA KAYAKING ON THE BAY OF ISLANDS IN NEW ZEALAND

A friend, Shelly, and I unloaded our kayaks at Whangaroa Harbor, north of the Bay of Islands, New Zealand, during a downpour and gale-force winds. We couldn't help glancing at each other and wondering, "What are we doing?!" The waves were smashing furiously on the basalt cliffs of the sheltered bay, and I dreaded to think about what was happening on the open seas. Nevertheless we stuffed our kayaks with sausage-shaped bags of clothes, food, sleeping gear, tents, diving gear, stoves, fuel, and other essential items. Next I tied my waterproof camera boxes tightly on top of the front and rear decks of the kayak. A Nikonos V hung around my neck, tucked into the pocket of the kayak's spray skirt.

We shrugged and shoved our boats into the mayhem, committing ourselves to a 10-day excursion south along the coast. As my muscles struggled with the paddle against the wind and waves, I noticed that I never remember to work out enough before a trip. After a grueling two-hour paddle Shelly and I arrived at a Park Service hut. Malcolm, a calm, competent fellow and our local guide for the trip, underscored that July brings the worst weather to the Bay of Islands. For most of the year the seas are tranquil, with clear waters and good diving possibilities. The Bay of Islands is reputed to have some of the most superb sea kayaking in the world, from its mangrove swamps to rocky islands, calm bays, and river estuaries, to open water and coastal surf beaches. However, it was difficult to picture halcyon days as the waves crashed and frothed at the rock cliffs outside our door. Unfortunately, I happened to arrive right in the middle of an uncommon series of severe storms. But that didn't matter. I was committed and willing to confront whatever came my way.

The rain abated in the morning, and Shelly and I set out for a day foray in the kayaks. The wind was having the party of its life, blowing up to 50 knots and creating 10-foot-high swells. It was impossible to kayak and shoot at the same time. I didn't want to take my hands off the paddle, fearing it would immediately blow away or flail out and knock me off balance. I also had to keep a forward momentum against the wind, so that I wouldn't be blown backward. We inched our way around the cove, straining against the wind. I was very concerned that the wind was going to torment us for the next eight days. Despondent, I visualized returning to America having shot just one roll of film. Fortunately the next couple of days were a bit calmer: the swells were only 3 to 8 feet high. I was becoming stronger and more confident; nevertheless, it was still a challenge to photograph while maintaining my equilibrium in the surges and swells.

On the front of the boat, tied to the deck, was a small Tundra case rigged so that I could open the box easily. Inside I kept a Nikon N8008 with several lenses, a 20mm, a 24mm, a 35-70mm, and a 180mm. I had a Nikonos V with a 35mm lens around my neck. Tied to the back of the kayak was a larger Pelican case with a Nikon F3 and motor drive, an SB-24 flash, a 50mm macro lens, an 85mm $f/1.4$ lens, a 300mm $f/4$ lens, and assorted filters. Inside a waterproof bag stuffed in the boat I had a tripod, a repair kit, more filters, spare items, and the bulk of my film. I also had a small waterproof diving box with film that I kept available during the day. Coupled with all the camping gear, this equipment made my kayak weighty but fairly stable.

The breaking waves made it difficult to undo the front box, and I was afraid of water flooding it. So I often had to ask Shelly or Malcolm to stabilize my boat in order to change film

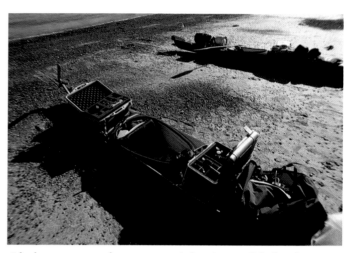

I had two waterproof camera cases tied to the top of the kayak. The front one was accessible while I paddled, so I kept gear that I used while on land in the back one. I made this shot with my Nikon N8008, a 20mm lens, and Kodachrome 64, and exposed for 1/60 sec. at f/8.

or shoot with both hands. Primarily I used my Nikonos V. I felt as if I were shooting from a bucking bronco, hanging on to the paddle with one hand and the camera with the other. Still I had better balance and more nerve than I did on my first day of kayaking, and I was desperate to get some photographs. I prayed that a wave wouldn't knock me over; a rescue in that water would've been a nightmare. I draped a towel from my visor so that I could easily wipe the spray off the lens.

The hardest part wasn't taking pictures, but advancing the film. I had to press the camera against my chest, maneuver my fingers to rewind the film, check my distance dial, and then prepare to shoot. The weather was partly cloudy, which made it impossible to have a consistent light reading. Since I didn't always have time to take a light reading with every shot, occasionally I changed the setting to automatic (something I rarely do) to give me an aperture-priority setting. Because I had to preset the focusing distance on my Nikonos, I used Kodachrome 200 film to obtain as much depth of field as possible with a shutter speed of 1/500 sec. Later when I edited the film, I was amazed to see that most of my horizons were straight and my exposures acceptable.

The Nikonos is really best for conditions when you can use both hands to manipulate the controls. One-handed photography was quite difficult. It was virtually impossible to change film and lenses in the conditions I faced. I wish that I'd brought two Nikonos cameras with me, so I could've had one with a wide-angle lens and the other with an 80mm lens.

On our last day Shelly, Malcolm, and I kayaked back from Deep Water Cove to Waipiro Bay. The waves were savagely flogging the rock walls as we paddled our way across the open, unprotected waters. The troughs were irregular and ugly, often breaking on top of the kayak and spitting into my face. My camera cases made the boat top-heavy and a better target for the battering waves. Sometimes I'd look over and see my companions 5 feet or more above or below me on a large gray swell. I had to concentrate on keeping my balance and staying relaxed. We had to keep moving; the wind was against us, and the current was coaxing us out to sea. It was a grueling, tense paddle, and yet an exhilarating experience in terms of all the great personal challenges we faced. The three of us paddled into the harbor exhausted and relieved. This trip was splendid—and worth every aching muscle.

ACTING LIKE A HUMAN GYROSCOPE

Working from a kayak, or any other boat, requires that you, the photographer–kayaker, act like a gyroscope in order to absorb the movements inherent to kayaking. The trick is to isolate the camera and lens from the boat. One technique is to use a "tele-stock" to hold the telephoto lens and maintain the position as the boat shifts around you. Most of the time you'll find yourself trying to keep your upper body steady while your hips and legs absorb the motion of the kayak. When shooting from the kayak in shallow areas, I run the boat up onto the sand and rest my elbows on the stabilized edge of the boat. Using an Ewa Marina bag while kayaking is difficult. It is hard to move your hands in and out of the waterproof bag to operate the camera. However, this is more manageable when you use a motor drive and an AF lens.

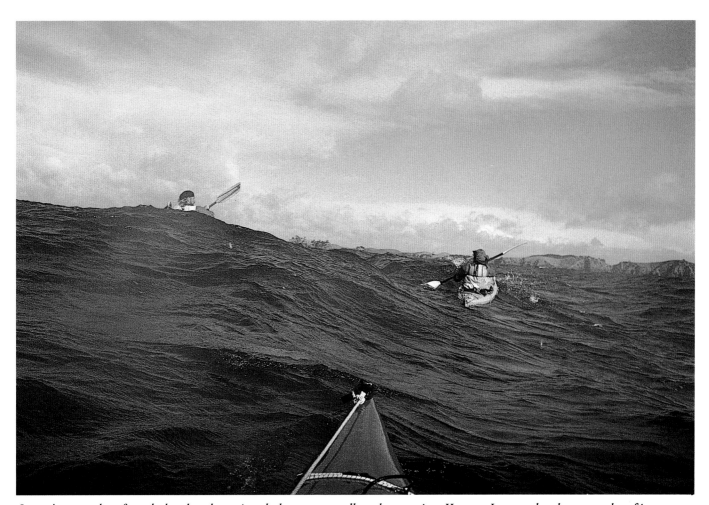

It wasn't easy to shoot from the kayak and negotiate the large ocean swells at the same time. However, I managed to shoot a number of images as we crossed a particularly turbulent stretch. Working with my Nikonos V and a 35mm lens, I exposed at f/5.6 for 1/250 sec. on Kodachrome 200.

SHOOTING FROM THE HIP

Perspectives change quickly when you're continually moving. In some situations you have very little time to previsualize images, and you have to shoot literally from the hip. This is when I switch the camera to autofocus and shoot. I also take a lot of "insurance shots" when working this way. For an unusual perspective, try taking a swim with your camera among the kayakers. Be careful not to get speared by the bow of a kayak if you're using a wide-angle lens. And make sure that you wear a diving mask and a snorkel so you can breathe.

There was only one evening during the sea-kayaking trip that the winds and seas abated. I was able to stop during a magnificent sunset and choreograph my kayakers. Sea kayaks don't turn as fast as river kayaks, so it takes more time to get into a good shooting position. Carefully observe what you want to include in the shot and get into position. Direct the kayakers clearly. Look through the viewfinder with both eyes, so you can track them as they come into the frame. You don't, of course, want to miss the perfect moment.

Don't forget to focus on the activities outside of kayaking. Take advantage of photographing from different vantage points, such as hills, promontories, and ledges. One benefit of bad weather is the quality of light. I had fabulous sunsets, sunrises, and rainbows to shoot on every day of this trip.

PROTECTING YOUR EQUIPMENT AT SEA

Always use a skylight filter, a lens hood, and an eyecup when shooting out on open water. The lens hood cuts the flare, and the filter slightly warms the cold light of stormy scenes. The eyecup reduces ambient light in the viewfinder, thereby giving you a better view and ensuring an exposure that isn't confused by stray light. Eyecups also help protect your camera by blocking drips, spray, and blowing sand. I have neoprene straps on all my cameras. They are durable, absorb the camera weight, and are perfect for humid and wet environments.

A common problem I face regularly when photographing on salt water is spray on my camera and lenses, which can be almost as bad as dropping the camera into the ocean. Salt, moisture, and salty air can create rust or oxidation, which in turn causes photo equipment to age rapidly. You can prevent this after your shooting is completed by taking a soft cloth with a small amount of WD-40 oil sprayed on it and gently wiping the camera and lens barrel. Make sure, however, not to get any of the WD-40 on the glass lens or eyepiece. This process leaves a protective film on the camera. Then wipe the camera with a soft, dry cloth to remove any excess WD-40 and any salt loosened during the process.

If I'm going out for an extended period of time, I always take extra 0-rings for the waterproof cases with me. I take special care to keep the case closures clean. When I get home I wash out all the cases in clean water, dry them well, check them in the bathtub to see if there are any leaks, and dry them again. When a case isn't in use, I remove its O-rings and let them swell back to their original size.

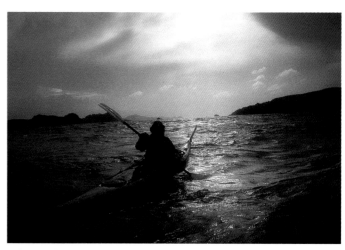

The weather was very stormy during our kayaking expedition. Not only was I contending with maneuvering the kayak, but also with shooting in unsettled conditions. While I made this photograph, we were in a bay sheltered from the waves, but the winds were gusting up to 50 knots. In between the powerful gusts, I managed to photograph Shelly with my Nikonos V and a 35mm lens, exposing Kodachrome 200 for 1/250 sec. at f/5.6.

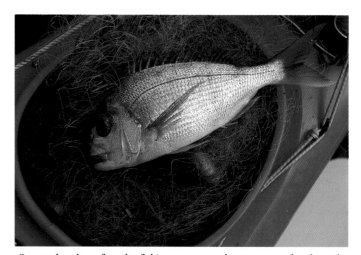

On one beach we found a fishing net snagged on a group of rocks and pulled it loose. Then we stuffed the net into a hatch of a kayak, and I arranged this red snapper on top for this closeup. Shooting with my Nikon N8008 and a 50mm macro lens, I exposed Kodachrome 64 for 1/125 sec. at f/8.

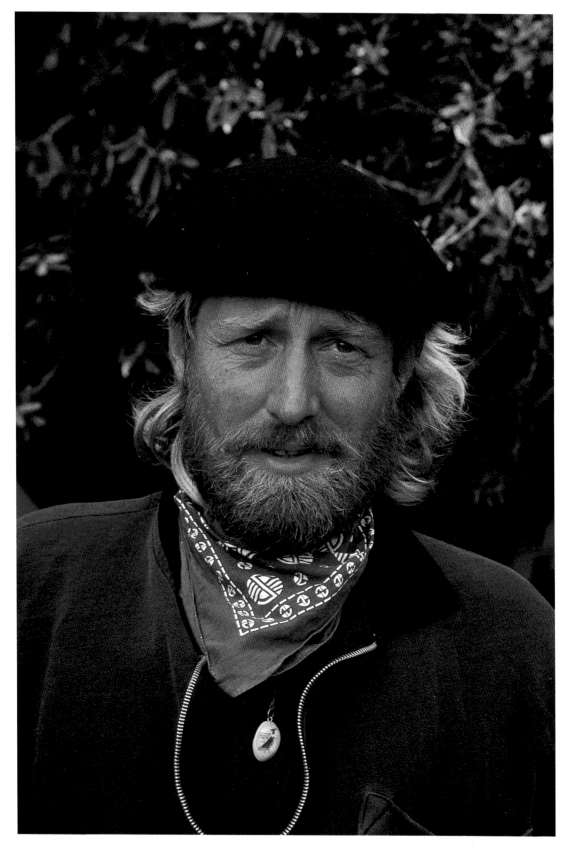

In New Zealand I had the good fortune to travel with an interesting and knowledgeable native. He had a wonderful face, but was very shy and reluctant to have his photograph taken. It was only after we'd spent a number of days together and established a rapport that he felt comfortable enough to look directly into the camera. I exposed for 1/60 sec. at f/11 and used my Nikon N8008, a 35-105mm zoom lens, and Kodachrome 64.

PART 3

WHILE YOU TRAVEL

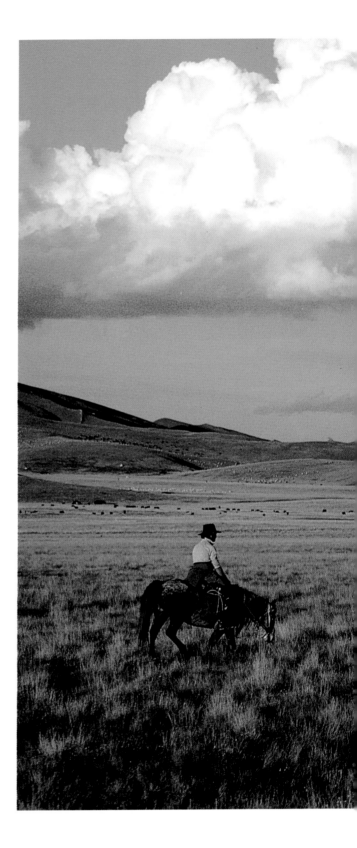

Today you can travel in many ways. Part of the adventure in remote travel is using a mode of transportation that the locals themselves use or is appropriate to the terrain, such as trekking in Nepal, horseback riding in Mongolia, and bicycling in China.

In order to find out about local methods of transportation, you need to thoroughly research the area you're thinking about going to. Read historic and recent travel accounts, look at guidebooks, talk to people who've been in that region—anything that will give you a feel for the area, its people, and its ways. If you've never been to the country before, don't expect to be able to waltz in and make local arrangements in a day or two without backup from a government liaison office or travel company unless, like Nepal, Kenya, or Thailand, the country is accustomed to tourists. Even then, if you want to travel in unfrequented regions, it takes time and experience to navigate the local bureaucracies and regulations. If this kind of travel is new to you, go with a reputable adventure-travel outfitter.

This isn't a definitive guide to all of the different modes of adventure-travel transportation, which might mean skiing or riding pony carts or motorcycles. However, with a little imagination you can apply my traveling suggestions to almost any method of travel.

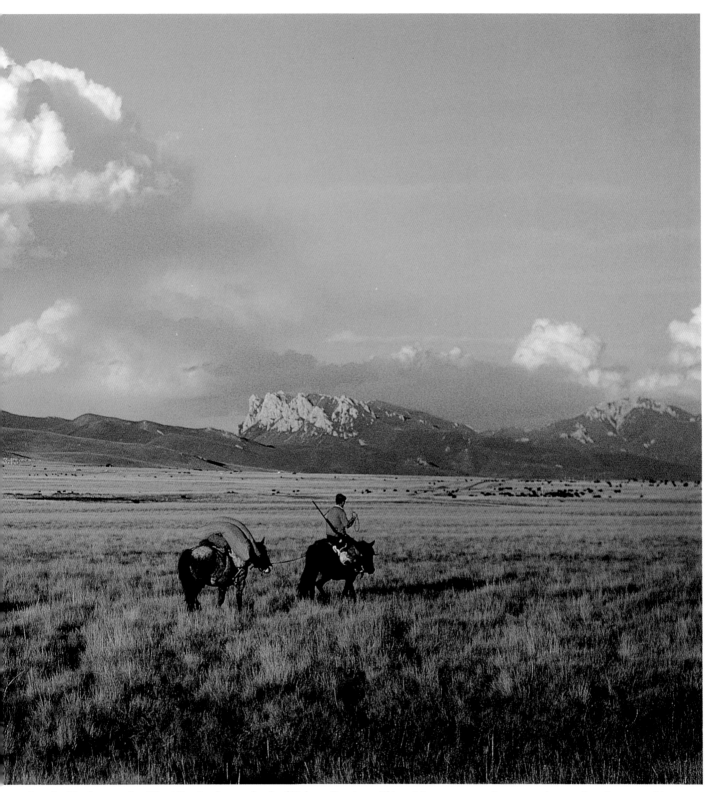

I made this photograph while riding in the grasslands of Sichuan Province, China. My camera was slung around my neck and supported by a Velcro strap around my waist. I prefocused my Nikon F3 and waited until my companions were ahead of me and under the white cloud. Then I quickly took this shot using an 85mm lens and Kodachrome 64, and exposing for 1/250 sec. at f/5.6.

USING PACK ANIMALS

When you're planning an extended journey, it is difficult if not impossible to carry all your gear and food on your back. If you're bringing a large quantity of camera equipment, it certainly helps to have the assistance of an animal or two. I've been on legions of trips with pack animals in China, Tajikistan, and Nepal. Animals add a different dimension and flavor to your trip. They can also restrict where you can travel. For example, horses, mules, yaks, and camels are impressively sure-footed, but they can't go over ice falls or rocky cliffs. And you have to worry about not only your own welfare and meals, but also those of your animals and handlers.

On one trip to the Pamir Mountain range of western China, four companions and I used a medley of horses, mules, and camels to carry our packs and duffels. The Kirghiz look scornfully upon you if you travel on foot and carry your gear on your back. We journeyed from one Kirghiz village to another, negotiating for animals for the next day's journey in each settlement.

The Kirghiz who live in the Pamirs may be far removed from cities, but they are extremely savvy bargainers and traders. My friends and I were continually renegotiating the rental cost of our pack animals. The locals had the advantage—they had the animals and we were strangers—and they knew it. We bargained fiercely, sometimes for hours. We'd come to a friendly agreement, pay for seven mules and two men for two days, or whatever, and then the next day they'd show up with only five mules. "Well, you may have paid for seven mules, but if five can carry the load, so what?" they'd shrug. Their logic was hard to

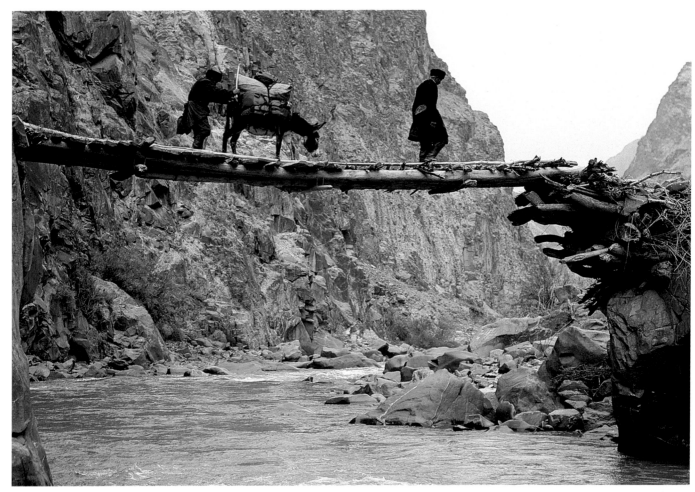

While traveling through one of the canyons, we had several bridges to cross. The mules were far from enthusiastic and had to be prodded and cajoled across the shaky wooden trestles. I positioned myself upstream and below the bridge in order to combine the mules with a sense of place. With my Nikon F3 and a 35mm lens, I exposed at f/5.6 for 1/250 sec. on Kodachrome 64.

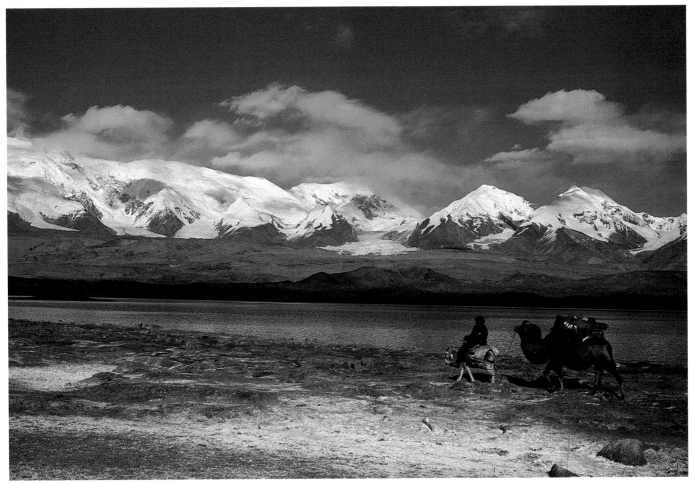

On the first leg of our journey in the Pamir Mountains in China, we hired a Kirghiz guide and a camel to carry our gear. I walked to the side so I could photograph our entourage with the mountains as a backdrop. I used my Nikon F3, a 35mm lens, a polarizer, and Kodachrome 64, and exposed for 1/125 sec. at f/5.6.

disagree with, especially when you don't know the language and you're using gestures, drawings in the sand, and a smattering of badly accented Kirghiz and Chinese words to communicate.

Loading the animals was a time-consuming morning ritual, taking at least one hour. We had put all our gear in soft backpacks and duffels. All of the bags had shoulder straps in case there was a rock fall or a river crossing where we'd have to haul the gear ourselves. We brought webbing and straps with us to tie up the loads and purchased extra cord in the Kashgar market.

I wore a camera vest laden with lenses and accessories and carried extra equipment in my daypack. I securely tied my tripod and my camera bag that held my spare camera bodies and miscellaneous items onto the most sure-footed pack animal in a place where they wouldn't be banged or get wet. Still I was taking a risk because an animal can decide instantly to sit down or roll over and flatten your camera bag.

This was a memorable month in the Pamirs. My friends and I negotiated narrow trails in steep canyons, river crossings, and mountain passes while traveling from village to village. Then winter began to set in, and we prodded our irascible mules back toward Kashgar.

TRAVELING ON HORSEBACK

Horseback riding across the vast Mongolian plains and with the Tibetan cowboys on the Songpan Grasslands are five-star memories. In Inner Mongolia I rode across the vast, pastoral plains past mud villages and yurts, which are Mongolian tents made of heavy felt wrapped around a collapsible wooden frame, with windmills powering the radios and television sets. Mongolians ride as if they were born on horses, standing

At a rest stop in Inner Mongolia, I noticed a young girl peering shyly at me from a doorway. I backed up, composed so the doorway was underneath a wooden frame, and made this shot. I especially like the saddle and the bucket on either side of the image. Here, I used my Nikon F3, a 35mm lens, and Kodachrome 64; I exposed for 1/60 sec. at f/8.

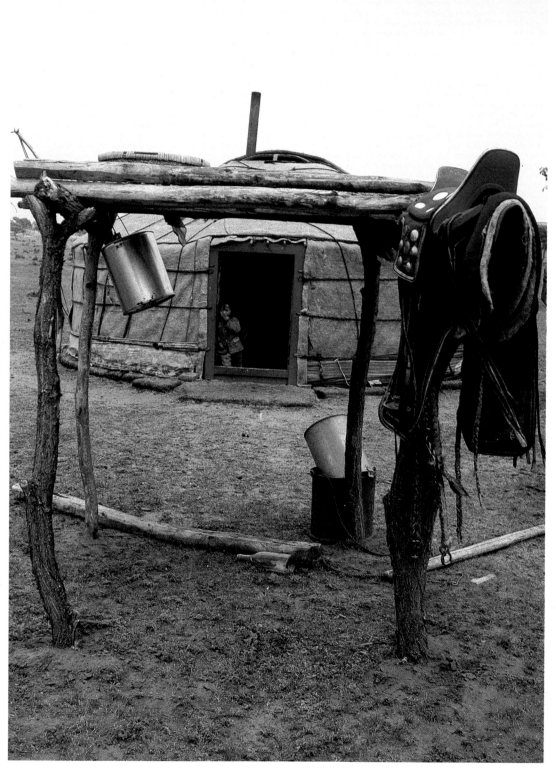

straight up in the stirrups, proud and laughing, with the wind battering their faces as they gallop ahead. Tibetans are more restrained, but are equally brilliant horsemen. There are very few vehicles on the eastern edge of the Tibetan plateau; horses, however, are everywhere. People gather around pool tables set outside on the dusty streets, and swarthy Tibetans in thick yak coats trimmed with fake leopard fur send pool balls slamming wildly across the old, warped tables. Their horses stand placidly beside them, reins tucked securely into the players' leather belts.

Photographing from a horse is a completely different experience than photographing on the ground. Not only do you have the obvious technical problems, such as camera motion and dealing with your camera's controls, but you also have to manage the spirit and will of your horse. An autofocus camera with a motor drive is indispensable for shooting from a horse. Unless you are an expert rider on a docile horse, it isn't wise to take your hands from the reins to focus and to advance the film. And since it is even more difficult to be continually changing lenses, zoom lenses are your best bet.

How to wear your camera so that it is accessible, protected, and comfortable is a dilemma. Having a camera hanging around your neck while riding is a miserable experience; for the duration of your ride, one hand has to grip the camera while the other holds the reins. For more comfort and security use either a Quick Shot, a nylon pouch with a quick release, or a CamJacket, a chest bag for one camera and mounted lens

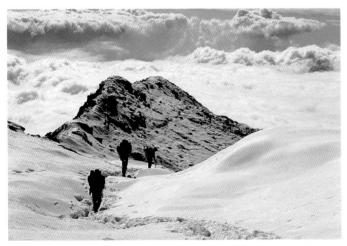

We experienced a series of bad storms in eastern Nepal on one trip to Makalu Peak. The snow was very deep on the trail. While crossing a high pass, I photographed three porters as they reached the crest of the ridge ahead of me. The three figures in the middle of a triangular hill and the monochromatic nature of the scene are what make this composition so strong. Shooting Kodachrome 64 with my Nikon F3 and a 180mm lens, I exposed for 1/250 sec. at f/4.

that is secured with a chest strap. You can also wrap your camera around the horn of your saddle when your horse is at a walk. I wear a photography vest for keeping film and filters available and strap my camera bag tightly onto the back of my horse, making sure any lenses inside are wrapped in chamois cloth or well padded and secure in the bag. Some photographers who frequently ride customize their saddlebags with padded pockets and pouches.

TREKKING WITH PORTERS

I've been going to Nepal every fall since 1978. The Himalayas have some of the most spectacular scenery found on earth, as well as some of the oldest living cultures. I've worked as a guide for various adventure-travel companies, and now I guide my own custom treks in the more remote regions of this remarkable kingdom.

Most of the trails in Nepal are too steep, narrow, and rugged for pack animals. For a great many people, trekking with porters who carry gear and cook is the best way to walk in the Himalayas. On nearly every trek, whether I am with a group or alone, I hire porters to carry the loads. These usually weigh around 65 pounds and are transported by means of a tumpline; this is a band that goes around the load and around the forehead. You only need to put the load in a duffel bag or a doko, which is a conical basket.

Much like having pack animals, having a porter to help you shoulder your load frees you to enjoy the Himalayas, which is the reason you came. You can take your time along the trail, photographing, talking, or pursuing whatever interests you. Traveling with local people also means that you have companions to photograph as you travel along the trail, and they introduce you to much that might otherwise pass by unnoticed.

Being a porter is a well-respected job in Nepal. Every time you hire a local, you're supplying him with much-needed income. If you have a guide, he'll take care of all the porter arrangements. If you're traveling with only porters, you are responsible for arranging everything yourself. Be sure to treat your porters well: check to see that they have the proper equipment and sufficient food for the undertaking.

When traveling in the Himalayas, I wear a photo vest on the trail, keep bulky lenses in my daypack, and put my extra gear in my duffel. I make sure that my gear is well protected with padding. By using a vest I make my lenses immediately available; I don't have to stop, take off a daypack, and dig inside for my lens of choice. I try to travel as light as possible since

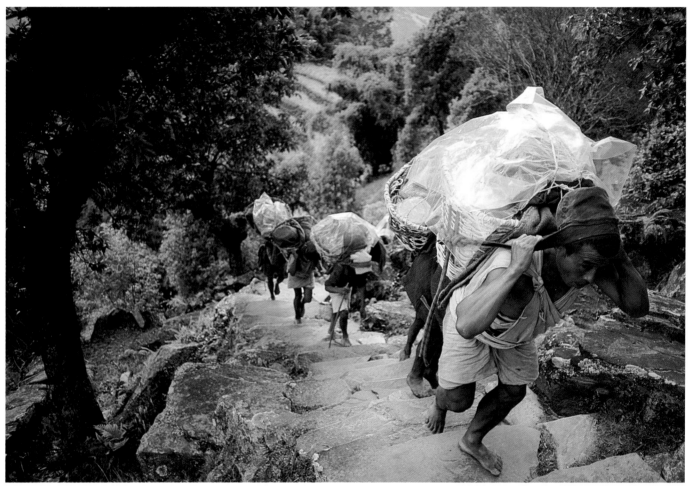

On a trail in the Annapurna region of Nepal, I stepped to the side, knelt down, and photographed the porters as they walked past me with their loads. For this shot, I used my Nikon F3 and a 24mm lens and exposed for 1/125 sec. at f/5.6 on Kodachrome 64. *over exposed*

I'm also carrying a heavy daypack. I bring zoom and wide-angle lenses with me; the longest lens I carry in my vest is an 80-200mm zoom lens. Usually I carry a small tripod with me in my daypack and a larger one in my duffel bag. If you're going to be seriously photographing, you can hire a porter to carry your photographic gear and stay close to you as you trek.

TRAVELING IN CANOES

Canoes come in different forms, including African mokoras and Malaysian dug-out canoes, and are found all over the world. Canoeing is fun and relatively easy to learn, and you can carry more gear in a canoe than in a kayak. I had my first experience on the lower section of the Zambezi River, a wide and easygoing river with an impressive parade of wildlife and birdlife.

Canoes are great to photograph from, especially if you have an amenable partner. My canoeing partner gingerly paddled me astride the carmine bee-eater nests and grazing buffaloes and elephants while I endlessly photographed. Needless to say, as you maneuver through the pockets of hippopotamuses and crocodiles, you need an experienced guide with you.

Because my waterproof case hadn't made it to Africa, I had to bring my regular camera bag on the trip. Inside I had two Nikon F3s, a Nikon N8008, and various lenses: a 300mm, an 80-200mm zoom, a 35-105mm zoom, a 24mm, and a 20mm. I selected the most experienced canoeist as my partner and prayed that we wouldn't capsize. I kept the camera bag in front of me on the canoe floor, on top of an upside-down cooking pot. A strong wind was lapping waves and tossing spray into the canoe and, unfortunately, my camera bag. So I put it into two garbage bags with the opening toward me in order to protect it. I was still able to reach in and remove my camera easily. I had my tripod, extra filters, accessories, and film in a waterproof bag tied into the canoe. After the wind subsided the next day, I dispensed with the garbage bags but kept the camera bag on top of the pot in order to keep it out of any stray water on the canoe floor.

I took a tremendous risk with my gear, one that I hope never to repeat. But the point is that you often don't have the perfect gear for each trip. Be creative, make do with what is available, and try to minimize the hazards you expose your equipment to.

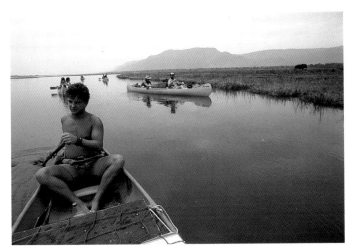

On the lower Zambezi River in Zimbabwe, I made this shot from the front of the canoe with a 20mm wide-angle lens on my Nikon F3. I wanted to include my boat, the other boats, and the elephant on the shore. The exposure was 1/125 sec. at f/8 on Kodachrome 64.

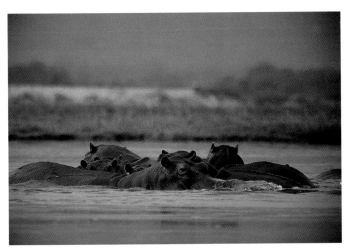

I always had my cameras ready while we were canoeing. At one point a group of hippopotamuses emerged next to us. I grabbed my Nikon N8008 already fitted with a 300mm telephoto lens and quickly made this shot. Here, I exposed for 1/500 sec. at f/2.8 on Fuji Velvia.

CARRYING YOUR OWN GEAR

Being completely independent by carrying your gear yourself in a backpack has positive and negative points. On the positive side you aren't restricted by the limitations of an animal, other people, or a vehicle. You can traverse difficult terrain, climb high-altitude peaks, and rappel down canyons. On the negative side you have to carry the backpack.

During one trip in the Pamirs the camel driver belatedly informed the group that the upcoming pass was too treacherous for the camels. So we unloaded them; gave away our extra flour and sugar; and pushed the tents, stoves, food, and too many other things into our packs. I strapped my 20-pound camera bag on top of my 50-pound pack and trudged up the trail, leaning like the Tower of Pisa. It wasn't any fun crossing an 18,000-foot glaciated pass with that load of gear. I cursed my heavy cameras and my stupidity for not anticipating such a situation. Luckily, on the other side of the pass we descended into a village and were able to continue on with mules.

Whenever you travel it is important to carry the minimal amount of equipment possible. Pare down to the essential items. Leave your heavy cameras at home, and bring the simplest and lightest one you own. I always wear my photo vest and keep any extra gear in a small fannypack that I put on top of my expedition backpack. I usually carry one camera body, a few essential lenses, film, flash, and a small tripod. You'll also probably want to get a chest strap; it prevents your camera from swinging when you climb trails and from bouncing against your chest on descents. I also recommend the Quick Shot, CamJacket, or Galen Rowell's new system from Photoflex. Another option is to place your camera inside your camera vest and cinch up the belt to your backpack, so it holds your camera firmly in place.

RIDING BICYCLES

Bicycles are the primary vehicles in China, and riding them is a grand way to tour the villages. On my first trip I brought my mountain bike over from the United States and joined a tour into the back roads of Sichuan Province. It isn't easy to bring a bicycle into China, but if you are persistent you can wind your way through the bureaucracy. On my second trip to the area, I led a guided tour and used the company's bikes.

I felt very cavalier and free, peddling down the roads, stopping when the mood struck me or when I saw potential photographs. The local people found my mountain bike

Paddling through Mana Pools National Park in Zimbabwe, we came upon spectacular wildlife. As we drifted past this elephant, I quickly framed its body and reflection and made this shot before we moved out of range. Shooting with my Nikon F3 and an 80-200mm zoom lens, I exposed for 1/500 sec. at f/4 on Fuji Velvia.

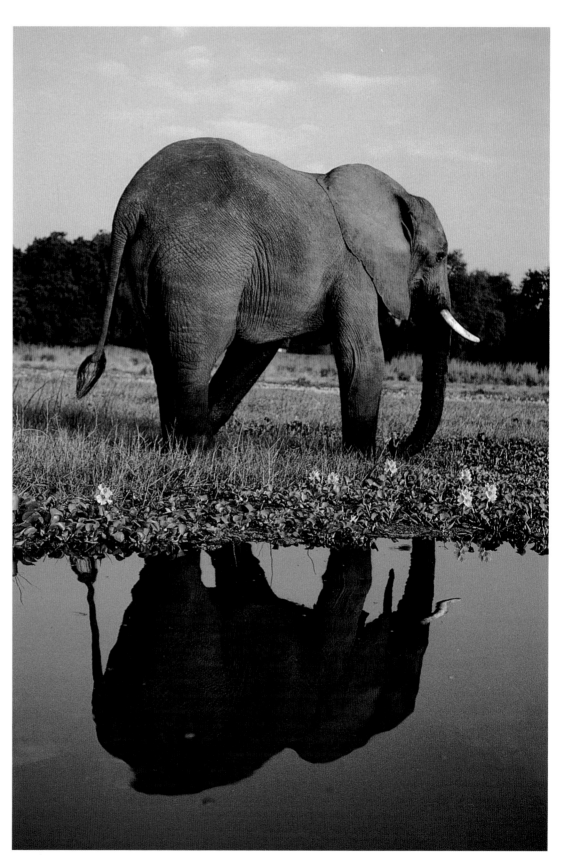

fascinating. It was much lighter, had more gears, and was brighter than their basic black models. Support vehicles accompanied me on the trip, which meant that I was able to bring extra equipment and plenty of film. If, however, you have to carry all your gear on your bike, you have to travel light.

I wore my indispensable photo vest and slung my camera over my head and around my shoulder. Some days I brought a fannypack and tied it into the basket on the front of my bicycle. You might want to consider custom-made paniers; these are small, rigid packs made of padded foam and nylon that attach to the front handlebars of your bicycle. Some bicycle companies make paniers that are designed specifically for photographers. But you have to be careful not to overload them or you'll have a difficult time steering your bicycle.

SHOOTING FROM THE AIR

If you want to photograph from the air in third-world countries, you must plan ahead. Getting the necessary government permission to do aerial photography can be a nightmare. It can sometimes take six months or longer to receive clearance to shoot aerials in a small country. And once you've got the papers there isn't any guarantee that you still won't be arrested on a technicality. Always expect the worst.

Around takeoff and landing you can shoot satisfactory aerial landscapes from a commercial passenger aircraft, provided that you avoid the vibration of the fuselage and reflections from the window. A rubber lens hood near or pressed up against the glass helps to eliminate both problems. You can also avoid vibration by not resting your arm or the camera on the aircraft body as well as by using a high shutter speed, 1/250 sec. or faster. Small planes are a better option, especially if the door is off or open. Don't—under any circumstances—lean out of the aircraft without a harness on. And be sure to attach the camera well to your body because the airflow may tear the camera from your hands.

If you shoot from a helicopter, you can usually open the windows to shoot. But pay attention when you compose so that you don't get the helicopter rotary blades in your wide-angle shots. One advantage to shooting from a helicopter is its ability to fly lower than an airplane and to land places where planes can't.

Because exposure meters often give misleading readings in aerial photography, you need to take a reading on the ground before takeoff and a second one in-flight. Split the difference to find the ideal setting. Depth of field isn't a problem because the whole scene is distant; just be sure to set the fastest shutter speed you can. And since the principal enemy of aerial photography is haze, shooting on a clear day is best. Take pictures as soon after dawn as possible; when you shoot later in the day, heat blurs the view. Photographs taken in the early morning have the additional advantage of long shadows that help delineate indistinct landscape features. Finally, be careful when you photograph animals that you don't fly so low that they become upset.

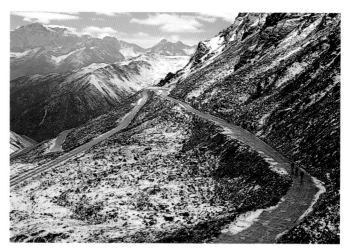

On one trip we rode down 5,000 feet from the top of Balan San Pass, which is 15,000 feet high. I waited at the top of the pass and photographed my companions peddling around the curves before I jumped on my bike to catch up. I exposed at f/5.6 for 1/250 sec. on Kodachrome 64 and used my Nikon F3 and an 85mm lens.

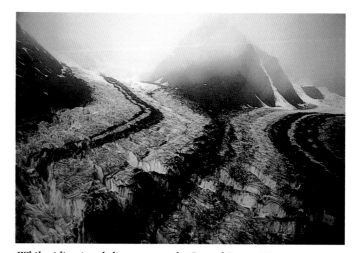

While riding in a helicopter over the Central Pamir Mountains in Tajikistan, I opened a window and shot with a 24mm wide-angle lens on my Nikon F4. I like this image because of the repeating curves of the glacier and the ominous weather. The exposure was 1/500 sec. at f/2.8 on Kodachrome 64.

PART 4

VISUAL INTUITION

During my travels I've observed photographers who arrive somewhere and expect "the-picture-taking-place" to be right in front of them. They have one preset image in their minds and believe that there is one and only one right spot to stand. It is better to search instead for whatever is meaningful to you and the image that expresses it. When your mind becomes set on one thing or one way of doing things and is relentlessly determined to pursue this course, you inhibit your intuition and miss much of the wonder of the world around you. Traveling fosters my intuitive response to the world. When I place myself outside of my normal context, I'm forced to become more aware of my surroundings and pay more attention to the sensory and visceral undercurrents.

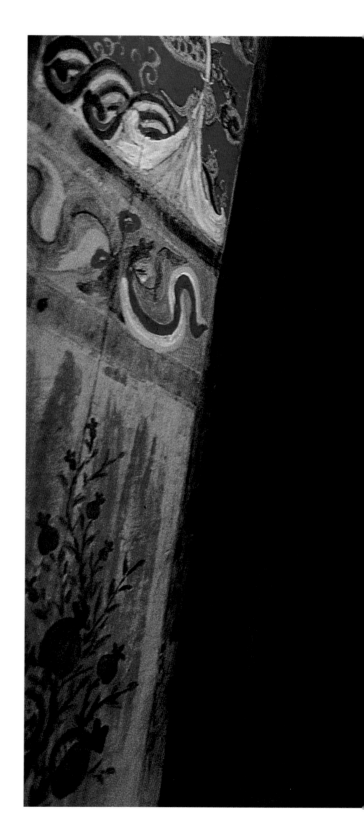

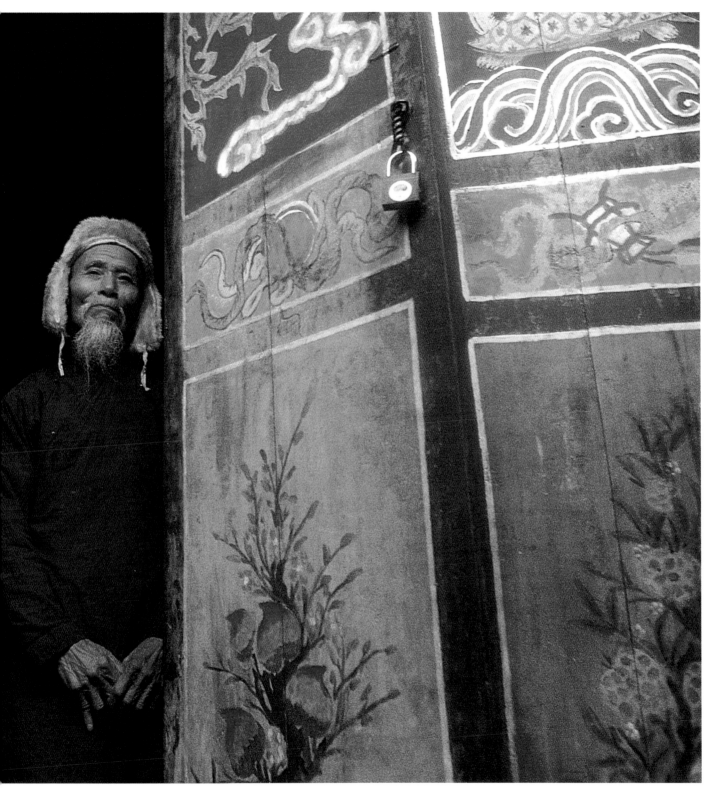

Along the Yen River outside Hanoi, Vietnam, I visited a small pagoda. After photographing one of the icons, I saw the pagoda keeper leaning against the door. I immediately knew that this was the image I was looking for. So I pulled out my Nikon F3 and a 20mm lens, knelt down, and gestured for him to lean farther into the doorway and to clasp his hands. I exposed for 1/30 sec. at f/5.6 on Kodachrome 64.

The word "intuition" means various things to different philosophers, psychologists, and artists, but the basic sense of the word is captured in the dictionary definition: "the act or faculty of knowing directly without the use of rational processes." You know something but don't know how you know it. You can no more force intuition than you can force

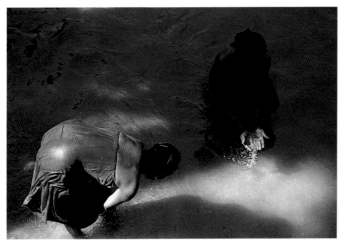

While standing on a bridge over the Bagmati River in Kathmandu, Nepal, during the Magh Purnima festival, I noticed that the river was crowded with people taking a ritual bath. Because there was quite a tangle of activity, I waited until I sensed a perfect combination of light, composition, and action before shooting this scene with my Nikon F3, an 85mm lens, and Kodachrome 64.

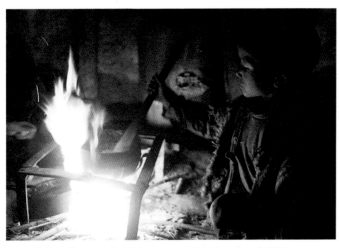

I made this photograph while visiting a Nepalese family I'd become very close with over the years. While sitting at the family hearth waiting for dinner, I was struck by the glowing firelight illuminating the young son's face. I replaced the Kodachrome 64 in my camera with Fuji P1600 and pushed it to ISO 800. The grainy aspect of the film precisely reflects the moodiness of the atmosphere. With my Nikon F3 and a 24mm lens, I exposed for 1/15 sec. at f/5.6.

someone to fall in love with you. You can prepare yourself for your intuition to manifest itself, invite it, and create attractive conditions to coax it, but you can't say, "Now I'll have intuition." Intuition can defy your expectations by suddenly veering off in a new direction, rearranging the material you've been working with, or bringing in something that seems entirely out of place.

If you work too hard at seeing, you never will. If you over-intellectualize a photograph and try to make images filled with information instead of emotion, you aren't getting to the soul of your vision. Intuition can't be ordered, commanded, implored, or contrived. You simply have to be ready for it.

Taking real photographs—photographs that mean something to you—doesn't come easily. This takes a tremendous amount of effort and even suffering when you feel that your effort hasn't given you what you wanted. You can't will yourself to be intuitive, but you can will yourself to be open to what comes your way.

INTEGRATING INTUITION AND TECHNIQUE

Photographing is a fine-tuned combination of thinking and feeling, and of intellect and intuition. The more technical information you have to integrate into your picture-taking, the more complex your decisions about photography become. At the same time the more technically competent you become, the easier it is to photograph with greater awareness. Of course, you need to know the technical aspects of photography in order to operate your camera and lens. But when it comes down making the actual photograph, that comes from your gut.

Sometimes expertise can actually work against intuition because it can make you overly dependent on a particular frame of reference or on a stylized, orthodox approach. You can try to "wow" yourself and others with tricks, filters, and unusual effects, relying completely on your knowledge of technique and equipment. But by doing this you lose your heart and soul, as well as inhibit the free working of your heart. Follow your inner voice; it is far more central to your photographs than technique is.

You can't leave yourself open only to luck and chance and the hope that you'll miraculously find a photograph. Shooting in a wild, crazy way without any discipline doesn't mean that you're being intuitive. If you don't have inner discipline and technical discipline, you might not be able to decipher what pleases you. Choice encourages you to define your own vision.

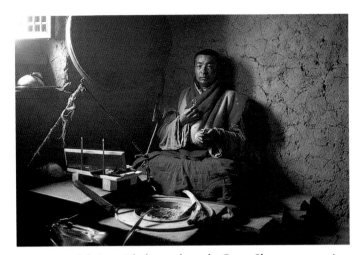

I spent a week living with the monks at the Gonga Shan monastery in Sichuan Province, China. While I was there a visiting Tibetan lama, Tu Den Shi Long Lama, beckoned me to come into the room where he was praying with the other monks. Although I didn't want to intrude, I sat down to listen to the chanting. Toward the end of the ceremony, he paused and looked at me; I knew then that taking his portrait was fine. For this shot, I used my Nikon F3, a 24mm lens, and Kodachrome 64, and exposed for 1/15 sec. at f/5.6.

If someone tells you what you should be photographing, you might make a photograph that looks pretty but it won't reflect you. However, if you go into a shooting situation where you have a choice, and no one dictates or inhibits your expression, you may find a new inspiration and a startling image.

LETTING YOUR INTUITION EMERGE

The most important thing anyone can do to develop intuition is to cultivate a higher state of awareness. Some photographers meditate or practice yoga to keep the mind fresh and open. I like long solo walks in the outdoors. Inner silence and heightened clarity are the hallmarks of a consciousness conducive to quality intuition and vision. Most artists and athletes spend a few moments preparing themselves before they perform. The orchestra tunes up, the tennis pro hits a few balls, and the painter fiddles with the paints. I usually take a few insignificant photographs. This ritual puts me in a clear and fresh frame of mind and disperses erratic and undisciplined energy.

People often work against intuition by taking themselves, their work, their dilemmas, and their problems too seriously. A certain playfulness and an appreciation of whimsy and absurdity seem to favor intuition. The most creative and innovative people are those who revel in unsolved problems and play with their imaginations the way children play with toys. Curiosity is a lightening rod for intuition.

All photographers have experienced a run of mediocre photographs, and then, suddenly, "the one" appears. It is possible that you might not even recognize that you'd seen something profoundly moving until you edit your photographs and say, "Of course! How could I have not seen it?!" But eventually, you come to recognize "the one" when it emerges. It may not even be anything you can intellectualize; you just "know."

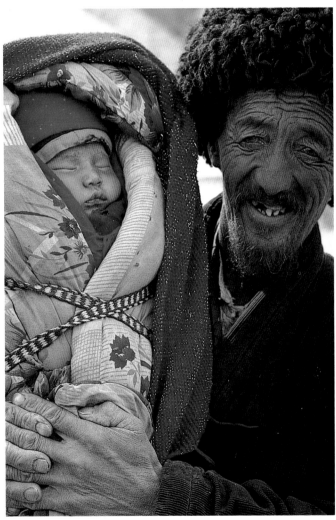

As I was walking through a Kirghiz village in the Pamir Mountains of northwestern China, I passed an old man holding his newborn grandchild. He stopped me and raised the baby, hoping that I'd take a picture. I knew this was a wonderfully poignant expression of young and old, so I quickly captured it on Kodachrome 64 using my Nikon F3 with a 50mm lens.

It is fine to have some preconceived ideas about what you're going to photograph, but don't let your plans blind you to other photographic possibilities. Never be afraid to reformulate or drop your original intentions. Keep your eyes and your mind open. Those who can free themselves of old mindsets, open themselves up to new information and surprise, play with perspective and context, and focus on process rather than outcome are likely to become the most creative and expressive photographers.

THE ESSENTIALS OF COMPOSITION

Most photographers are better at making sweeping statements in their photographs than paring down to the essentials of an image. This is usually because even when they focus on one particular object, design, or color, their eyes also see the environment surrounding it. For example, if you focus on an orange cup on a table, your mind concentrates on the cup while your eyes also see the desk it's sitting on, the room, and any objects surrounding the cup. So often when you take a picture, you include all that your eyes see even though your intent is to show only a detail of the whole; this clutters the photograph with unnecessary information and objects. Simplicity in design is critical to a strong photograph. What you omit from an image is as important as what you include in it.

Photographing a detail of an object or place can provide a sense of the bigger picture and can elicit subliminal responses to the subject's shape, form, or pattern. Colors also evoke latent emotional responses. While you travel it is important to key into essential details and color, to enhance not only the quality of your journey but also that of your photographs. You need to carefully observe and be aware of the wondrous designs, details, and colors found in the larger perspective of people and the landscape.

USING COLOR AND DETAIL EFFECTIVELY

Some photographers have a penchant for light, others for action, and a rare few for the quality of color. I try to have a balance of all three. However, color often becomes the motive and justification for a photograph. Everyone varies considerably when it comes to perceiving color. People filter out a scene and truly "see" only certain portions of it unless

they concentrate. The ability to see the quality of color and its different relationships is an art, as well as a skill that must honed through continual exercise.

Color relationships can make or break a great photograph. Placing warm colors next to cool colors or vice versa can make a dull subject come alive. Warm colors usually prevail over cold colors that are next to them in the same picture. Shades from yellow to red are associated with fire, the sun, and tanned skin, and brilliant scarlet subjects sometimes seem to leap from a picture. On the other hand, blue shades communicate cold, isolation, and silence; they are the colors of ice, cloudy skies, and night. Cold tones—blues and greens—also intensify the

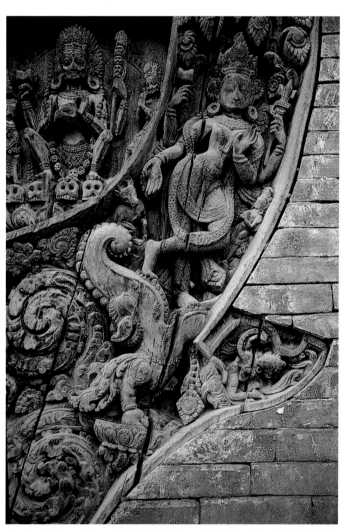

At the Gorkanath temple in the Kathmandu Valley, Nepal, I admired the intricacy and craftsmanship of this ancient wood carving. I came in close with my Nikon F3 and a 180mm lens to isolate one piece as well as to emphasize the repetitive curves. The exposure was 1/250 sec. at f/5.6 on Kodachrome 64.

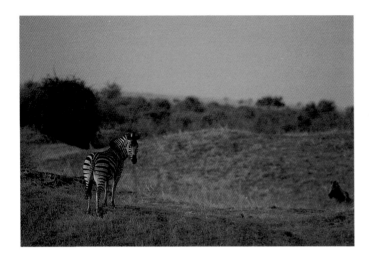

As we were heading back to camp in Botswana, Africa, I spied a zebra set aglow by the last remnant of light from the setting sun. I yelled to the driver to stop, quickly steadied my camera on a sandbag on top of the roof, and shot a number of frames, aware that the red would be enhanced by a slow shutter speed and Kodachrome 200. With my Nikon F3 and a 300mm lens, I exposed for 1/15 sec. at f/2.8. One of my companions was surprised that I was able to photograph in the late twilight and was doubtful that the images would be sharp, but I knew that because the sandbag was as sturdy as a tripod, the images would be fine.

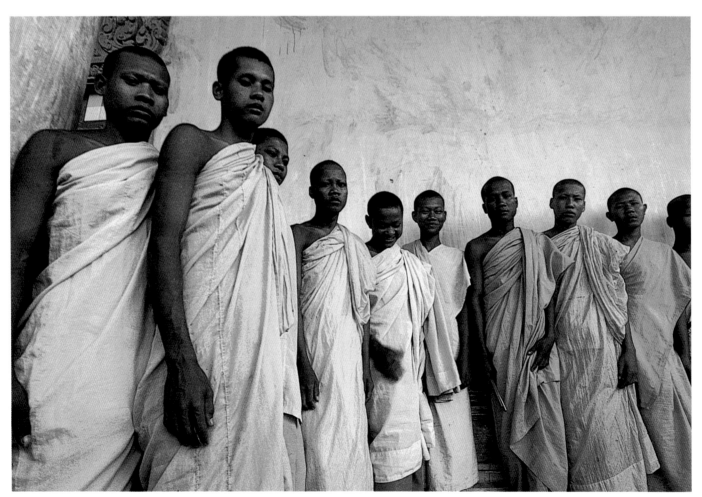

At the Soc Soai pagoda in Vietnam's Kien Giang Province, I was struck by the bold robes the young Buddhist monks wore. To emphasize the yellow robes, I placed the monks against a cool-blue wall, came in close with a 20mm wide-angle lens, and shot with my Nikon F4 from a low position. The exposure was 1/60 sec. at f/8 on Kodachrome 64.

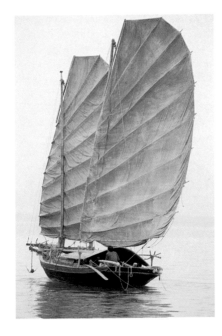

On the only day I was at Hailong Bay in Vietnam the weather was miserable and rainy, and the light was even worse. I knew that all the photographs I was taking were terrible, as shown on the right. So as a last resort I decided to use Cokin colored filters to alter the light. I combined a sepia and an orange filter to mimic late-afternoon light for the shot below. Working with my Nikon F4 and a 35-70mm zoom lens, I exposed for 1/125 sec. at f/4.

mystery and suspense of a scene, and cool-colored subjects appear to recede. When you want to suggest depth, you can use this effect to your advantage by composing pictures with warm hues in the foreground and cooler colors behind them. Including black in your images intensifies and isolates a color.

A hue is the tint of a color. Color saturation is a fairly relative, subjective quality that refers to how vivid a color is. Some films, such as Ektachrome, favor hues over saturation, but no film delivers color exactly as you see it. I achieve intense color largely either by underexposing transparency film to saturate the colors in the scene or by using a polarizing filter, also called a polarizer, that cuts glare in a landscape shot, thereby making colors richer and darker. I routinely rate Kodachrome 64 film at ISO 80 and process it normally; this automatically underexposes the film a bit. With Fujichrome and Fuji Velvia I don't change the film-speed rating, but I always bracket with a bias toward underexposure to saturate the colors in my photographs.

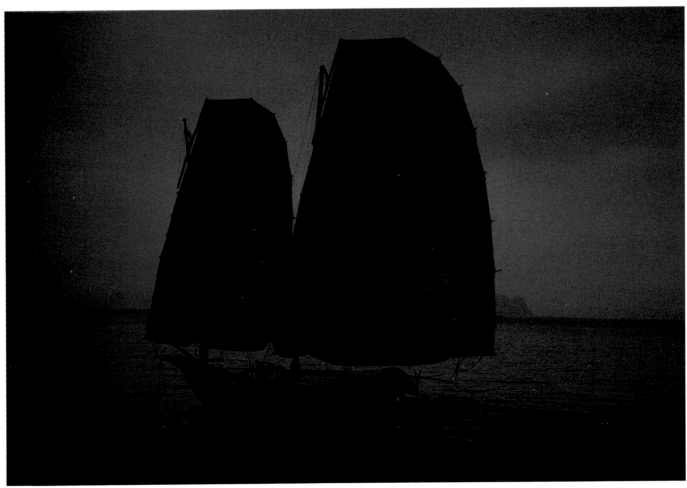

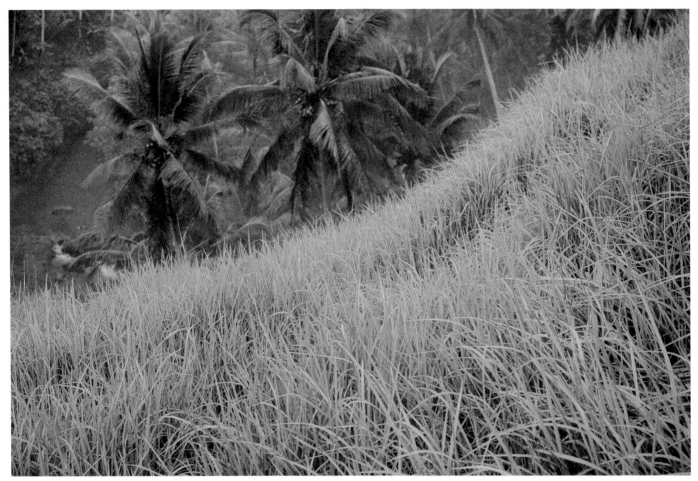

During an afternoon walk through the rice fields in Pejeng, Bali, a light rain was falling, diffusing the light and saturating the green of the surrounding fields. I found the deep color and the sinuous double curve of the hill enchanting. I photographed this scene with my Nikon F3 with a 35mm lens; the exposure was 1/60 sec. at f/8 on Kodachrome 64.

Manipulating exposure to produce saturated or pastel colors can bring a spirited mood to your images. You can also create a mood via the use of monochromatic color or even the absence of color. Capturing the colorful mood of landscapes means observing and understanding the cycles of nature, as well as the direction and color of the light. There is a great temptation to go looking only for images that incorporate nature's brightest colors yet subtle colors can weave as powerful a spell. Overcast weather provides subtle, more delicate colors than sunlight does, and some of the most beautiful hues appear just after the sun slips down below the horizon. By restricting the field of view, a telephoto lens makes it easier to crop out brightly colored details.

Scenes of a single color are also pleasing to the eye. Remote third-world villages tend to be monochromatic. Here, light combines with mud adobe buildings and the desert sand to make everything seem one color. I frequently photograph in countries where mud and stone are the predominant materials for houses, walls, and streets. The real challenge is to separate objects and enhance their color. I look for long shadows to create definitions and to put contrast into monochromatic situations. Like black-and-white images, monochromatic-color photographs express more about tone and texture than color ones do. Haze and mist restrict color and act like a pale-blue filter over a scene.

Some countries are meccas for photographers who prefer shooting color. The people of India, Nepal, Burma, and Africa, to name just a few, have a color style uncommon to that of Western countries. They boast color, parading every shade in the spectrum. Male birds may flaunt the colors in the aviary, but in the human realm rural women are inevitably the most brilliant. In regions where men now wear drab Western

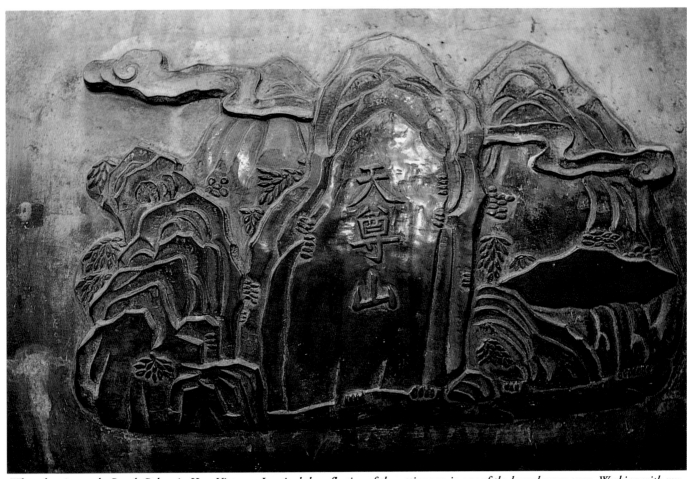

When shooting at the Purple Palace in Hue, Vietnam, I noticed the reflection of the setting sun in one of the large bronze urns. Working with my Nikon F3 and a 50mm macro lens, I came in close to concentrate on the light and design and exposed for 1/125 sec. at f/8 on Kodachrome 64.

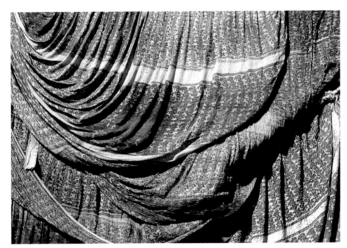

This is one of the hundreds of prayer flags surrounding a Buddhist shrine in Tibet. With a 50mm macro lens on my Nikon F3, I tightly framed to accentuate the patterns formed by the thin gauze and hand-stamped prayers. The exposure was 1/125 sec. at f/8 on Kodachrome 64.

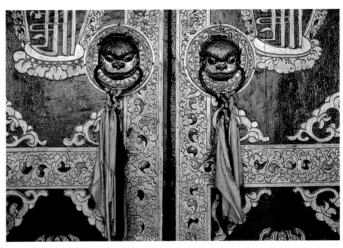

While photographing a monk at a Buddhist temple in Damiao, Inner Mongolia, China, I became fascinated by this door. Using my Nikon F3 and a 35mm lens, I zeroed in on its ornate handles and symmetrical design. The exposure was 1/125 sec. at f/5.6 on Kodachrome 64.

trousers, women still don their traditional colorful attire. And each minority group has its own personal dress, colors, and design sense. Red seems to be the color of choice, but all the primary colors are on display. They're embroidered in skirts and jackets, stitched into hats and boots, and printed on cottons and silks.

Although I rarely use colored filters, they've saved me on a couple of occasions. For example, I've found that a sepia-colored filter or a blue filter improves dull-gray rainstorms. I've also used a weak-orange warming filter to enhance sunsets and a yellow filter for early-morning scenes.

While it is important and natural to photograph both large vistas and human events, it is just as important to look beyond the big scene at the details that are an integral part of it. Vast expanses, such as the Tibetan Plateau, are as interesting in detailed closeups as they are in wide-angle shots. By shooting details you can make your own personal statement.

Some of my favorite travel photographs are graphic-detail shots in which I drench the frame with as much color as possible. If I am in a market and see a woman wearing a red scarf next to a group of bright yellow flowers, I move in close and fill the frame from edge to edge with an explosion of color.

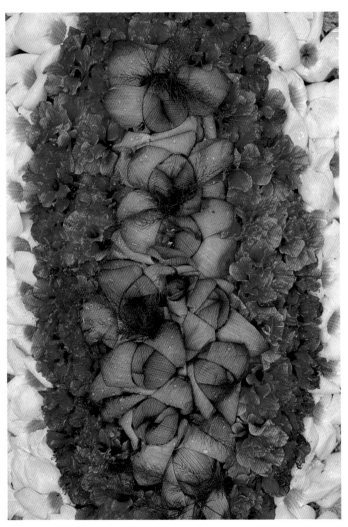

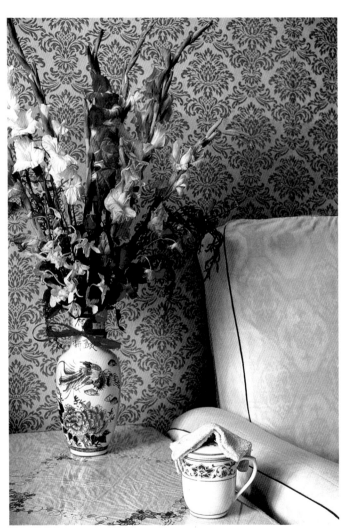

I was walking down a street in Hanoi, Vietnam, when my eyes were filled by the brilliant yellow and red of a display of funeral wreaths. I decided to come in close with my Nikon N8008 and a 50mm macro lens to fill the frame with only color and form. Here, I exposed Kodachrome 64 at f/8 for 1/125 sec.

The subjects of travel photographs shouldn't be limited to people and landscapes. I like to shoot interesting vignettes, such as elements of my hotel rooms. In Datong, China, I composed a photograph of the objects common to most of the hotel rooms in the area: a teacup, elaborate wallpaper, covered chairs, and fresh flowers. Here, I used my Nikon F3 with a 35mm lens and exposed for 1/15 sec. at f/8 on Kodachrome 64.

At Wat Phra Maha That in Ayuthaya, Thailand, I found this ancient stone carving of Buddha embedded in the roots of a Banyan tree. With my Nikon F4 and a 50mm macro lens, I focused tightly on the head and the tangled roots. The exposure was f/8 for 1/60 sec. on Kodachrome 64.

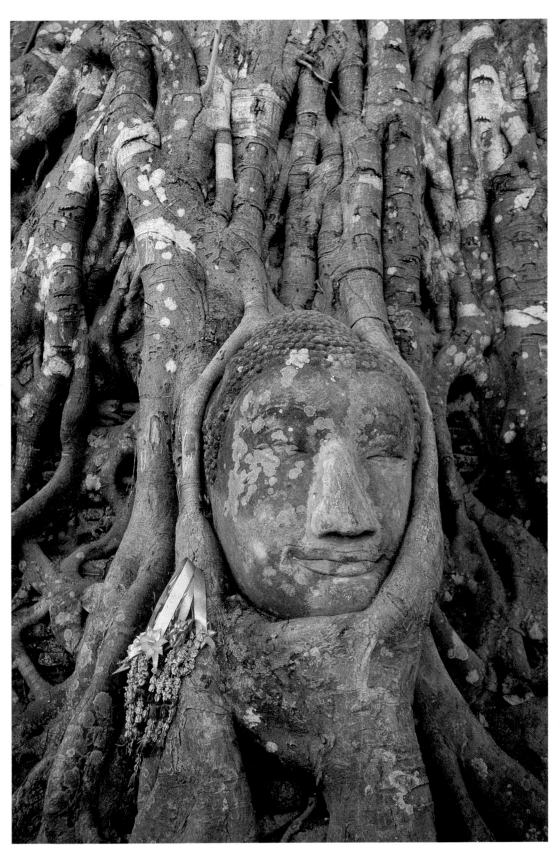

I've found that most people are reluctant to come in close with their cameras. However, sometimes the closer you move in, the easier it is to reduce an object to its intrinsic essence or form. You can even make it appear abstract. For example, if you're photographing a sunset and you include the shore and the sun, the resulting image is a beautiful rendition of a recognizable sunset. But if you use a telephoto lens and capture only the reflective colors on the water, you can transform the scene into a symbolic image of color and light. Mystery can be created by showing only a small fragment of a familiar subject. Less can often mean more.

When you begin creating abstract or symbolic images when you photograph other people or objects, you'll find that the act of seeing becomes more complex and interesting. Being able to see detail or abstract patterns in the subjects you're considering shooting broadens your approach to photography and expands your vision, and at the same time narrows your focus. Once you begin to recognize what holds your interest in a potential image, whether it is the necklace a woman is wearing, a rhythmic repetition in nature, or someone else's hands, then you'll begin to photograph not only what you see but also what you sense.

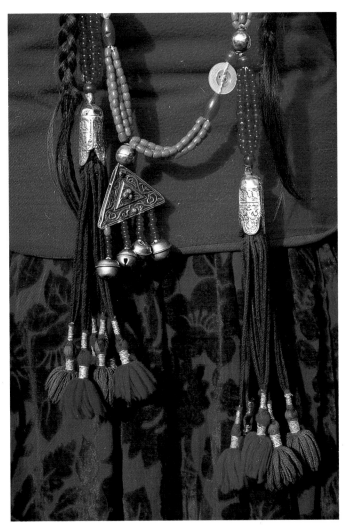

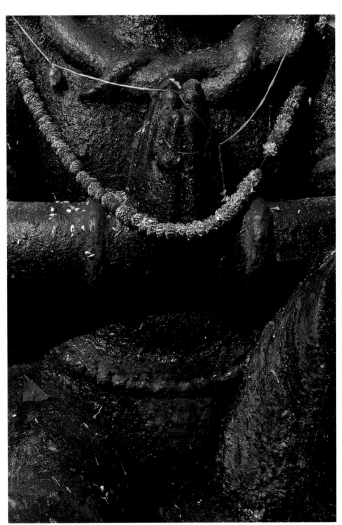

I was fascinated by the hair braids of the young Kirghiz girls in the Pamir Mountains in China. The braids were adorned with buttons, ribbon, silver, and beads. I asked one of the girls to turn around so I could photograph the braids up close. I particularly like how the hair seems to be moving in this photograph. I used my Nikon F3 and a 50mm macro lens, and exposed for 1/125 sec. at f/8 on Kodachrome 64.

While shooting a statue of Garuda in Kathmandu, Nepal, I moved in close on the meditative pose of the hands. I felt that an intimate photograph would be more compelling than one of the entire body. I especially liked the three repetitive curves around the neck, under the hands, and around the belly. Working with my Nikon F3 and a 50mm macro lens, I exposed at f/8 for 1/125 sec. on Kodachrome 64.

PHOTOGRAPHING PEOPLE IN THEIR ENVIRONMENT

Whenever you point your camera at someone, you have a precise reason for doing so whether it is conscious or unconscious. The crux is to understand this reason and translate it into your photograph. In order to do this, you must have a clear idea about what you want to say and to whom. You also need to decide on the appropriate technique and logical approach to produce the image.

There are many important elements in composing a good photograph of a person, such as the light source, composition, color details, and expressions. (Take a look at some of the excellent books that are dedicated entirely to photographing people.) But when photographing people in a travel situation, I find it critical to express the essence of an individual in his or her own natural and home environment.

I'm interested not only in unspoiled nature but also how humans can find intimacy within it. Most of my travel photography focuses on people, what I call "ethnographic photography." I am curious about how people relate to each other and their environment. Population density isn't as great in rural areas as it is in urban areas. And rural people are more aware of their natural surroundings and spend more time outdoors working and playing.

People add interest and intrigue to a photograph. The human figure is the most potent of all introduced objects. It draws the eye and can easily dominate the scene, so that even

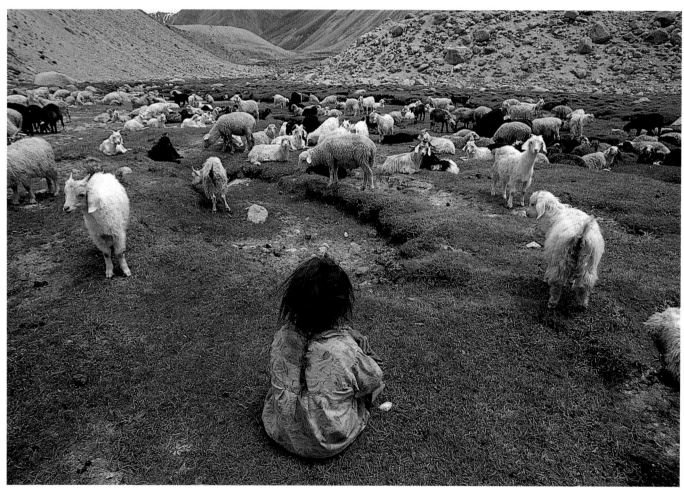

In the mountains of Tajikistan I happened on a little girl tending a flock of sheep and goats. Overwhelmed by a feeling of aloneness and contentment, I stood behind her and shot from above with a 20mm wide-angle lens on my Nikon F3 in order to position her prominently in the image with the animals in the background. Because I kept her back to the camera, I was able to maintain the sense of isolation. The exposure was 1/60 sec. at f/8 on Kodachrome 64.

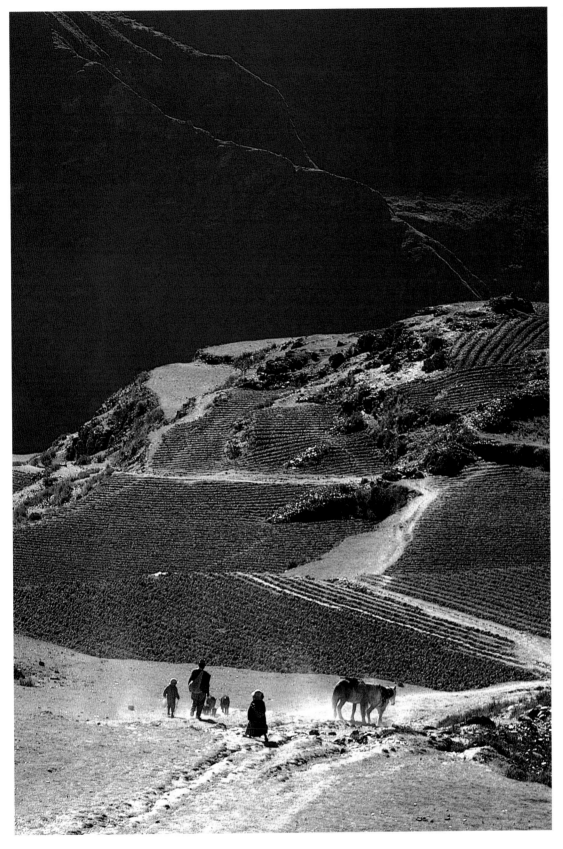

As I was exploring the terrain around Caata at the foothills of the Cordillera Apollobama in Bolivia, I spied this family ahead of me on the trail. The frontlit fields and the shadows on the hills were wonderful, but without the people to add a human touch and perspective the image wouldn't work. Here, I used my Pentax Spotmatic, a 135mm lens, and Kodachrome 64.

a tiny figure on the horizon is a counterpoint to a towering landscape. A human form in a large landscape provides scale and perspective. In an unfamiliar environment, the eye seeks out familiar objects as points of reference. Because the human figure is instantly recognizable and relatively constant in size, it is a valuable yardstick for measuring distance in landscape pictures. Trees, animals, and familiar structures can also form a focal point and suggest depth, but they don't catch the eye quite so readily.

When put in perspective against the landscape, the human figure also defines the situation. Often the environment is the key to a portrait. It sets the atmosphere and the tone. If the sun is about to break through the clouds and you see someone heading toward the rays of light, don't be afraid to quickly get into position in order to capture the special moment. Although the people may be the essential element, the background answers unspoken questions about the subjects, their life, and their work. You can make many landscape photographs more interesting—and more publishable—by adding people. Some photography magazines demand that you get the whole picture. They're interested in photographs that set the stage for the action and give readers more information.

Wide-angle lenses can create a sense of closeness and involvement between subjects and their environment. You can position a figure in a photograph in relation to a vast landscape in two ways. The figure can dominate the landscape, or the landscape can be the main subject and a small figure can be included to add perspective and the human element. This is a personal choice and

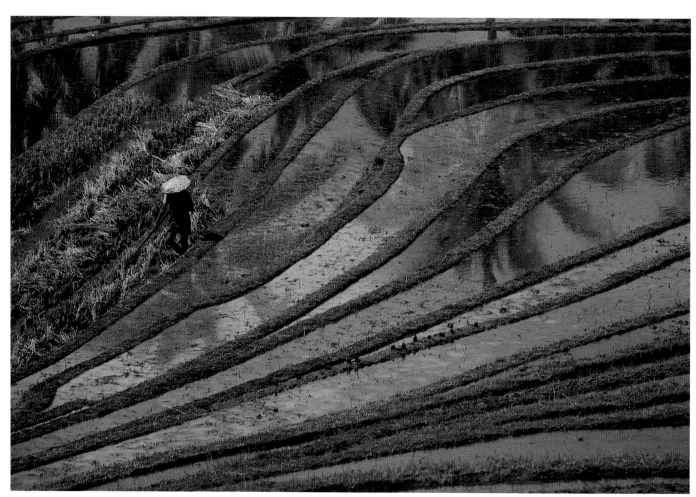

While riding a motorcycle around Bali, I noticed a worker harvesting the rice field below me. I leapt off the bike and grabbed my camera out of the camera bag, which I'd secured between my knees. I framed the figure off to the left to balance the weight of the field and to keep the water reflections in the frame. Working with my Nikon F3 and a 180mm lens, I exposed for 1/250 sec. at f/4 on Kodachrome 64.

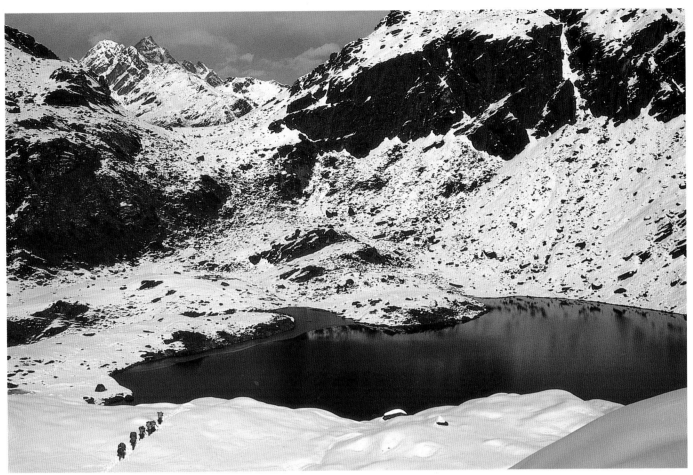

En route to the Makalu Basecamp in Nepal, my traveling companions and I crossed three high passes. From the top of the second pass I photographed the porters walking toward the third pass. The small figures add perspective and dimension to the landscape. Here, I used my Nikon F3 and a 35mm lens; the exposure was 1/125 sec. at f/8 on Kodachrome 64.

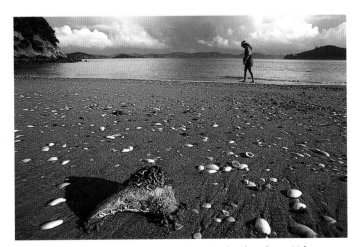

Lying on my stomach on a beach in New Zealand with my Nikon N8008 and a 20mm lens, I shot at eye-level to the shell so it would dominate. The exposure was 1/60 sec. at f/11 on Kodachrome 64.

depends on what you decide you want the predominant focus of the image to be.

Take advantage of using the people you're traveling with as subjects for your photographs. They may not seem as interesting or colorful as the local people, but they may be more accessible and willing to be in your photographs. In addition they are the obvious choice of subjects when it comes to showing your activities and undertakings against a landscape backdrop. You can also capture any spontaneous interaction between your traveling companions and the locals.

So whether you're just traveling through a region or spending time in one place, you should be aware of the human relationship to the natural world. It is something photographers in the Western Hemisphere often ignore, and it's quickly slipping away in all parts of the globe.

PART 5

THE CHALLENGE OF PHOTOGRAPHING PEOPLE

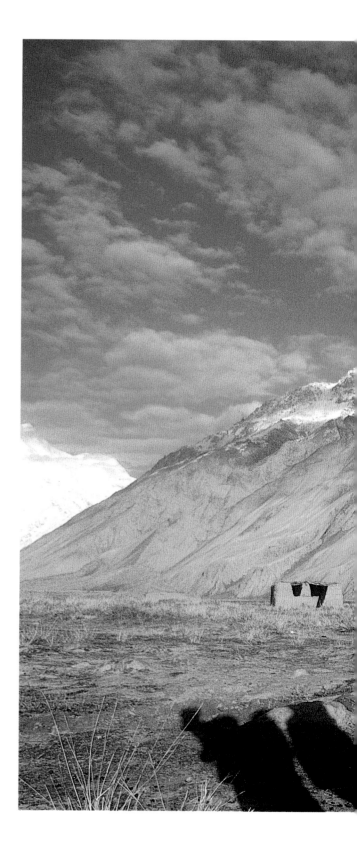

My raisons d'être for photography are interaction, exploration, and knowledge. Although I take many different types of photographs, such as shots of landscapes, details, and sports, it is people photography that I connect with most deeply. It isn't the image I'm searching for; it is an expression of interaction. Taking a photograph is the pathway to learning about someone else and ultimately about myself. I often see people and details better with a camera in my hand, and I pay more attention to peoples' gestures, expressions, and movements. My camera becomes my tool for exploration and helps pave the way for a personal exploration of life and people.

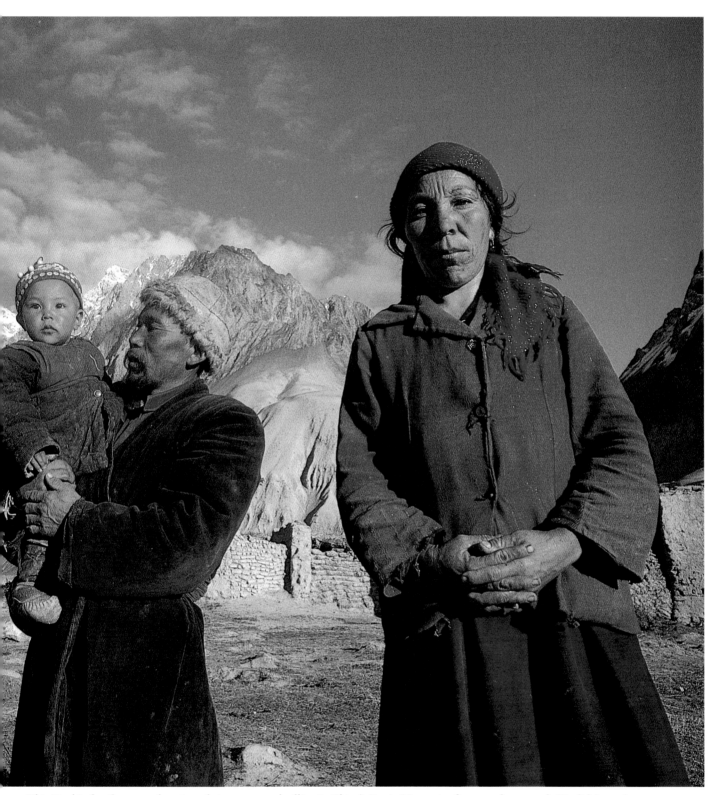

This Kirghiz family accepted me into their one-room dwelling in China's Pamir Mountains for more than a week. We didn't speak a common language, but we communicated fairly well with gestures, expressions, and even drawings. I photographed the family outside their house; I like the asymmetrical quality and different eye contacts. With my Nikon F3 and a 24mm lens, I exposed for 1/125 sec. at f/8 on Kodachrome 64.

Photography has opened the doors to many memorable experiences for me. I've been asked to shoot weddings, ceremonies, and sacred rituals. The photographs were good; the experiences were even better. This is important to remember: you are there first for the traveling experience, and second for the photograph. Of course, if I am on an assignment or have a time limitation, the pressures are greater. However, if I don't have a genuine interest in my subject, even if I express it with only a smile and a thank-you, then I shouldn't be there. As a photojournalist once said, "My job is to parachute into people's lives and establish intimacy in two days."

For most people communication isn't one of their greatest abilities. When they travel outside their comfortable sphere of customs and habits, they're confronted with situations and attitudes that can be confusing, frustrating, and often irritating. The keys to transcending these moments are patience, open-mindedness, and curiosity.

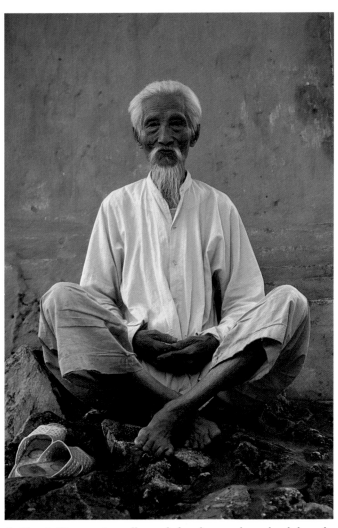

In Hanoi, Vietnam, I usually rose before dawn and wandered through the narrow, old streets. One morning as I was photographing people doing their morning exercises around Hoan Kiem Lake, I came across this gentleman on a pile of rocks, meditatively basking in the faint sunlight. I approached him and nodded a greeting. When he acknowledged me with his eyes, I raised my camera and he kept his pose. I shot nearly a roll of Kodachrome 64. Using my Nikon N8008 with a 35-105mm zoom lens, I exposed for 1/60 sec. at f/5.6.

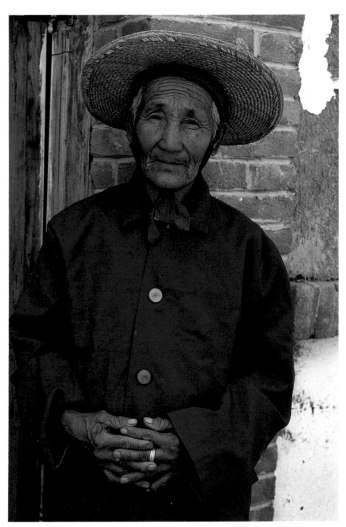

I am attracted to weathered faces; they can tell a story on their own. In Inner Mongolia, China, a woman saw me photographing, came out of her house, and called to me. When I looked over, I saw her calm face and profound eyes. The serenity of this woman is expressed in her solemn, simple pose. The two buttons complete the image. For this shot, I used my Nikon F3 and a 35mm lens, and exposed Kodachrome 64 for 1/125 sec. at f/5.6.

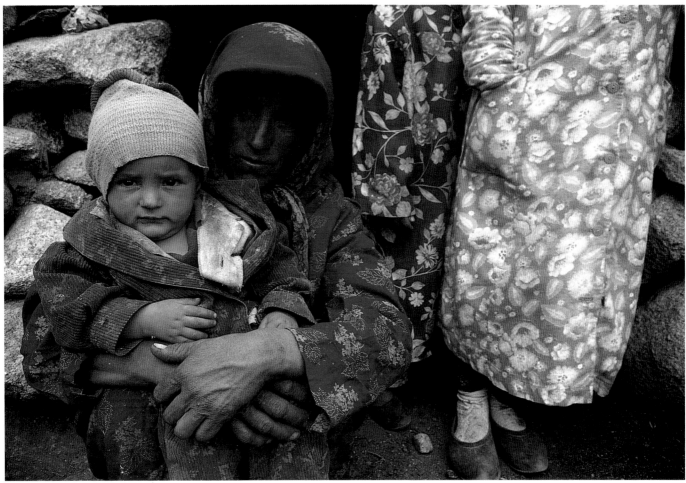

While on a trek through the Central Pamir Mountains of Tajikistan, I passed by numerous stone sheepherder huts. Hospitality is an unwritten law in this part of the world. The women in this home invited me in for a simple meal of yogurt and bread. As I left the hut I was struck by the color combinations in their dress fabrics. I leaned down and with my Nikon F3 and a 20mm lens, I photographed a mother with her son, making sure to include the skirts of her two daughters. The exposure was 1/60 sec. at f/8 on Kodachrome 64.

TAKING TIME

The longer you stay in one place and establish an intimacy with the locals, the better chance you have of experiencing special and unexpected moments. Ideally it would be wonderful to have unlimited time with no government restrictions or family obligations—and an endless bank account. I am in awe of Alexandra David-Neel, a Frenchwoman who traveled intrepidly through Tibet to Lhasa in 1924 disguised as a beggar and wrote about this remarkable journey. Fortunately her husband continually sent her funds for her travel and scholarly work, even though she was gone for periods of time as long as 14 years. Sadly I usually don't have that luxury of time or that kind of financial support. Often the

accelerated pace of modern publishing, not to mention individual time and money constraints, dictate the limitations of a photographer's schedule.

If, however, you're going to be in an area for an extended period of time, it is helpful to have personal introductions and letters of reference. Then once you arrive take the time to build relationships and break down shyness or suspicion. Share in the locals' work, and play with their children. Don't isolate yourself; become part of the daily world. I know one photographer who spends months in a village or community before he even takes out his camera.

That isn't my style. But when I arrive in a village, I don't take my camera out immediately and start shooting. I spend the first day walking around, becoming familiar with the area, noticing people and their habits, and checking out places I may want to photograph eventually. (I may take a few unobtrusive shots. I usually get some good ones during this time, when my mind is fresh and open and I don't take anything for granted.) I try not to become obsessed with the time limitation on my shooting. I make time to socialize without my cameras.

APPROACHING POTENTIAL SUBJECTS

Sometimes I wonder if cameras shouldn't be licensed. I can always tell where hordes of cameras have come before me. I'll put my camera to my eye and people immediately cringe,

duck, or flee. This is a completely opposite reaction to the friendly curiosity I notice in places where few foreign cameras travel. Of course, having one person in six months come along and photograph you is very different from 16 people approaching you in one day.

Newcomers to travel photography are led to believe that only a combination of stealth and long lenses can guarantee the travel trophies they want. My guess is that most people feel guilty taking photographs of other people; they feel that they're being obtrusive and invasive, so they use a long lens to shield themselves. Still, even with a 200mm lens you need to be as close as 15 feet to your subject for a portrait from the waist up.

All photographers develop their own distinctive manner and style with other people. Some are pushy, some are silent, and some are flamboyant and loud. All kinds of approaches work.

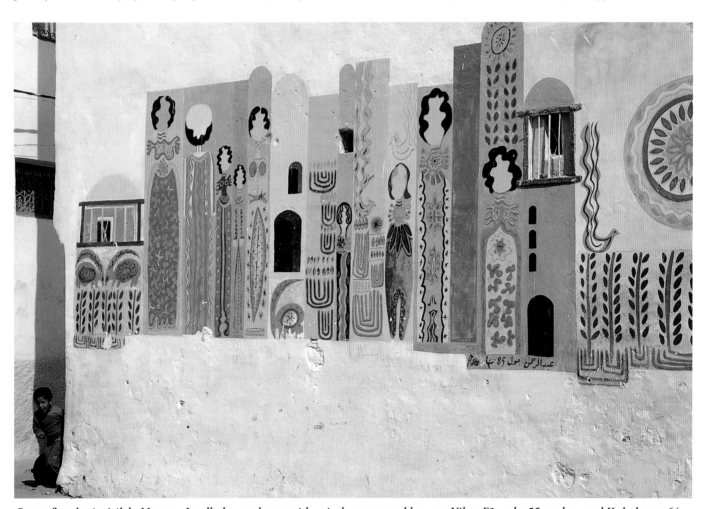

On my first day in Asilah, Morocco, I walked around town with a single camera and lens, my Nikon F3 and a 55mm lens, and Kodachrome 64. I was getting to know the area and scouting places for future shots. As I rounded a corner I was struck by this large, colorful mural and photographed this young boy as he turned the corner.

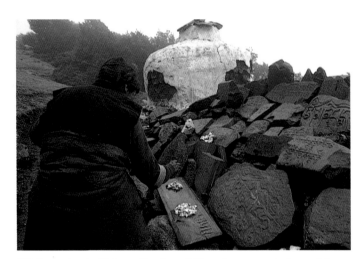

While staying in Sichuan Province, China, I accompanied two old Tibetan women on their early-morning walks to the sacred shrines around the Gonga Shan monastery. As we walked I photographed them, as well as participated in the different prayers and prostrations to Buddha. Since I was an active participant, they were comfortable with my presence; this enabled me to capture spontaneous moments. For this photograph, I used my Nikon F3, a 24mm lens, and exposed Kodachrome 64 for 1/125 sec. at f/4.

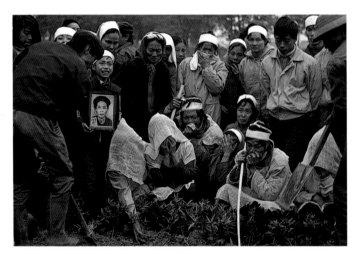

At times you have to distance yourself from an emotional situation while remaining empathetic, which isn't always easy. In Vietnam I waited at the Hanoi National Cemetery for a funeral; I wanted to photograph the mosquito-net clothing worn by the family. Even though I knew I was there specifically to photograph a funeral, I was unprepared for how intensely their grief affected me. When a group of mourners arrived at a burial site, at first I stayed back. But I soon realized that I wasn't capturing the impact of the occasion, so I asked my interpreter if I could go closer. When he said yes, I moved to the front of the grave and photographed until I felt that my presence was becoming intrusive. With my Nikon N8008 and a 35-70mm zoom lens, I exposed for 1/125 sec. at f/8 on Kodachrome 200.

I've seen some wonderful shots made by photographers who fit in every one of these categories. I have a simple approach. I rarely use a telephoto lens; I prefer direct photographic contact with people. Since I enjoy a personal exchange, I go right up to someone and engage in a conversation or make some kind of contact.

Success in photographing people is the result of the manner of your approach. Suppose you are in a village market, and you see an intriguing woman selling beautiful red tomatoes. The light is perfect. You know the best shot is a candid shot, so you quickly hold up your camera and you snap the picture. Suddenly, she senses you and looks up. If you meet her gaze with a guilty look and scurry around the corner, you're sending a message that you've done something wrong or you've violated something. I've seen this happen far too many times.

Don't slink furtively away. Instead, put down your camera, smile, and wave. Go over and shake the person's hand in gratitude. You might even buy a tomato from her. After you establish good, friendly terms, take out your camera, put on a wide-angle or macro lens, and continue shooting. I find that people love this approach, and that the person in the next market stall may also be willing to pose for you. By then you have the market on your side and have shown that being photographed can be fun. Be open and flexible. What you first envisioned might evolve into something better. For example, the woman's twin sisters might come out in pink checkered dresses and stand on either side of the tomatoes.

Sometimes, though, you'll find that a person notices you, becomes annoyed, and waves you away. With experience you learn to tell the difference between people who are sincere in their wish to be left alone and people who say, "No, no, no!" but mean "Yes, yes, yes!" Often these individuals wave you away, saying, "Oh, I'm not dressed in my best clothes" or "I'm not pretty enough." I laugh and dismiss that assertion, which is usually exactly what they want me to do. Most often they agree to have their picture taken. I never patronize people or talk down to them, but I do reassure them and try to put them at ease. However, if people give me an obvious abrupt "No!" in response to my request or ignore my pleasantries, I smile, thank them, and walk away. I never sneak a photograph. It is their choice whether they want their picture taken or not. There is always another photographic opportunity. No picture is worth irritating someone over.

Don't spend too much time photographing one person in front of their family or friends; it begins to embarrass them. Often I'll intensely photograph one person, then leave or turn to his or her neighbor. Later I'll return and continue photographing the person who initially interested me.

Photographing people isn't for the shy at heart. You need a certain amount of impudence to overcome natural reserve. You have to be friendly and forthright and have a lot of panache in order to approach people. Confidence and friendliness open the gates to communication. People are as curious about you as you are about them, and often all that is necessary to unlock this curiosity is a friendly word or two. And it doesn't matter if you don't speak the same language. I have the longest conversations with individuals who don't speak English. I talk in my language and they talk in theirs. None of us, of course, can understand anything that's being said, but we have a wonderful time.

Sometimes it helps to have a local with you, whether the person is a paid guide or someone who befriends you on the street. I've worked with guides from the Foreign Press Center in Vietnam and local agencies in China, as well as with guides assigned to me in Africa and even little boys who tugged on my shirt in the temples of Nepal. Frequently you find people who are happy to walk with you because they want to practice their English. In Vietnam a teenager who wanted to speak English approached me so we walked together around the streets. As we visited his friends in local cafés, he set up photographs for me, pointed out shots, and dragged me over to likely subjects. I had a wonderful time, and the locals saw me with a neighborhood kid who was also having fun. He broke the ice and paved the way for others to relax with me. The teenager certainly wasn't shy, and he felt very proud that he was showing a foreigner around his town. But you should be wary. Sometimes people want more than friendship.

I always wear jewelry that I think might interest the local women. For example, if I'm around Tibetans, I wear some turquoise rings or necklaces. The women and I inevitably end up admiring and comparing each other's jewelry. Then when the time feels right, I ask if I can photograph them. When dealing with a shy woman, I might ask to take a photograph of her earrings or necklace; this minimizes the emphasis on her face. You may have to do some conventional overall shots and tactfully see if you can work your way in closer. It is rude to immediately zoom in on a subject's chest. And be sensitive when using a flash. Remember how blinding it is to have a flash go off directly in your eyes.

Make your camera a bridge rather than a barricade. If your subjects are unfamiliar with a camera, you might let them look through the viewfinder. Sometimes I even have them take a photograph of me (make sure you put the motor drive on single-frame exposure). You might get an interesting portrait of yourself.

Many photographers prefer not to use a motor drive when photographing people. I can certainly understand the sentiment. Motor drives can be noisy, obtrusive, and confusing. However, they are invaluable for catching fleeting expressions and a sequence of action. After I've reeled off a series of motor-driven shots, I usually drop the camera from my face, laugh at its antics, and then begin photographing again if necessary. It helps to have a quiet camera. The Nikon F3 with a motor drive is one of the worst in terms of noise: it sounds like a submachine gun. A Leica is a great stealth camera because it is one of the quietest on the market.

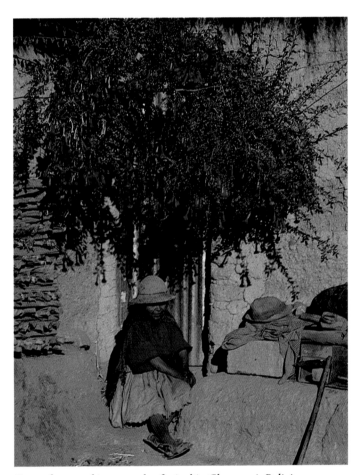

I was photographing a market festival in Charazani, Bolivia, when I noticed a young girl sitting under a flower bush with her mother. I approached and asked the mother if I could take her daughter's photograph. Because the young girl was pleased but embarrassed, I photographed her as quickly as possible, thanked the two of them, and moved on. Here, I used my Pentax Spotmatic, a 40mm lens, and Kodachrome 64.

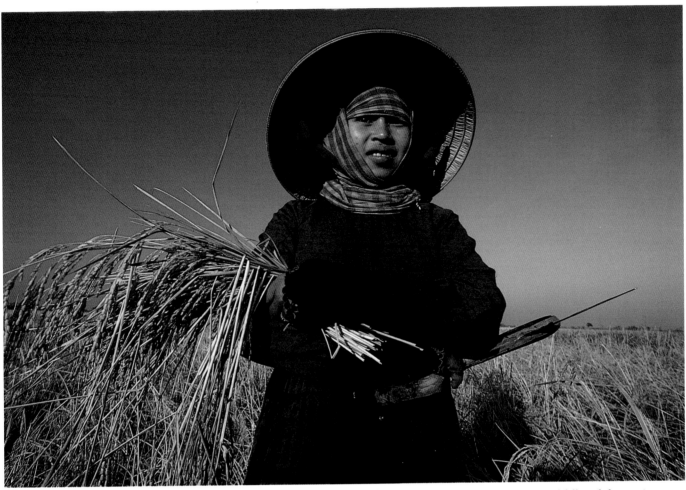

Driving down Highway 1 in Vietnam, I saw an ox cart heading down a narrow dirt road. I jumped out of the van and followed the cart into a field where a few women and girls were harvesting rice. Smiling, I walked right up to them and clasped their hands in mine. Since I was being friendly and effusive, they gleefully posed for me; this girl willingly moved into direct light for me, and I adjusted her position. I used my Nikon N8008 and a 20mm lens, and exposed for 1/125 sec. at f/11 on Fuji 100.

If you're shooting with other photographers, whether they are your friends or people on a photo tour, you need to remember an important rule of etiquette. If you see a person talking with someone and establishing a rapport, don't sashay over and shoot over his or her shoulder. Not only is this action annoying for the person who has set up the shot—as well as rude—but it is surprising for the person who's being photographed.

The key word is sincerity. If people feel that you're trying to use them, they won't communicate with you. If potential subjects find you amusing, go ahead and laugh with them. Laugh at yourself, your clumsiness, and your inept language skills. If you be yourself and are open and honest, in one afternoon you can find yourself taking photographs that

sometimes can only be made after you are in one place for a long period of time.

Even though you want to be sensitive to other country's mores, don't be shy. And don't be afraid to explore the back alleys and tracks not mentioned in the guidebooks. Stretch yourself beyond your own cultural boundaries and inclinations. I find the people of most cultures to be very tolerant; they expect foreigners to make mistakes. As I walk through small towns in foreign countries, I'm not afraid to peer into doorways or go into stores and talk with people. These acts are usually construed as friendly gestures, not intrusions. You'll get the message if you've overstepped boundaries. Seek out the unexpected; if you expect the predictable, that is what your photographs will be.

I gravitate to old women; they have an ease and an acceptance of life that I admire. This Yi woman in China was sitting on her step having a morning smoke as I passed by. From the moment I saw this woman, I felt a rapport with her. I sat down next to her for awhile, silently taking in the scenery. As I got up to leave, she nodded at me and gave me a pat on the hand; then I took this photograph using my Nikon F3 with a 35mm lens. The exposure was 1/60 sec. at f/8 on Kodachrome 64.

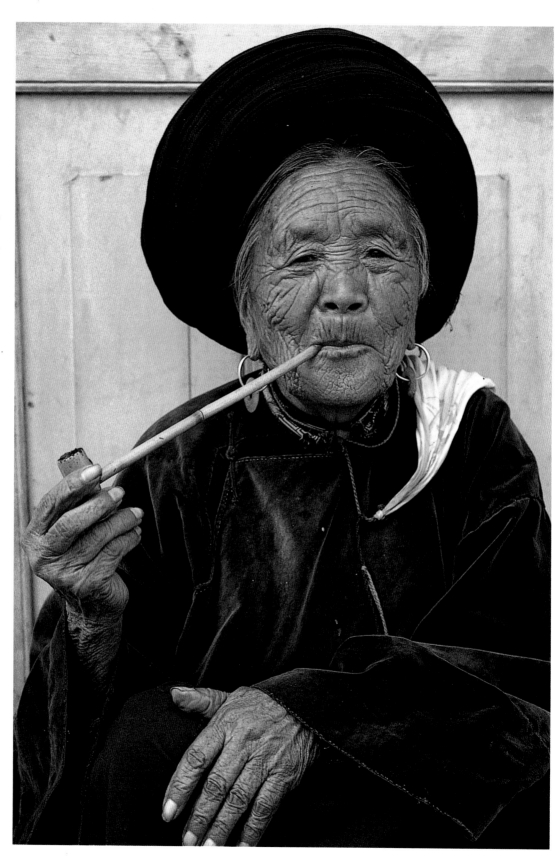

COMMUNICATING ACROSS CULTURES

Try to learn a little of the language. You can easily learn important words and simple phrases, such as "hello," "goodbye," "thank you," and "please," as well as numbers. Your goal isn't to be able to discuss quantum physics, but to extend a thread of contact. Some languages are easier to pick up than others. I find tonal languages nearly impossible. Even if you mangle a language, most people are pleased and honored that you've taken the time to try to learn to speak some of their language.

Lonely Planet Press publishes excellent compact phrase books for some of the more obscure languages. For non-Roman script languages it is helpful to have a phrase book that provides phonetic pronunciation and writes out the phrase in the local script. So if you can't pronounce the words, you can at least point to them in order to have someone read them for you.

I've passed phrase books back and forth in restaurants, trains, and buses, carrying on lively and humorous "conversations."

Phrase books have their limitations, as well as an abundance of useless comments, such as "Excuse me, where can I find a pencil box?" And questions and requests that photographers might need certainly aren't included. I have a list of frequently used expressions that I take with me on each trip; these include "Please, may I photograph your child?" and "Please move over here so I can take your photograph." I usually can find an accommodating hotel-staff member or a friendly person willing to translate them for me. When you liberally mix such remarks with gestures, imagination, good humor, and an outgoing nature, it is impressive how quickly and effectively you can communicate in a short period of time.

Nonverbal communication is an easy art to learn. All it takes is practice and confidence. It involves using your whole body:

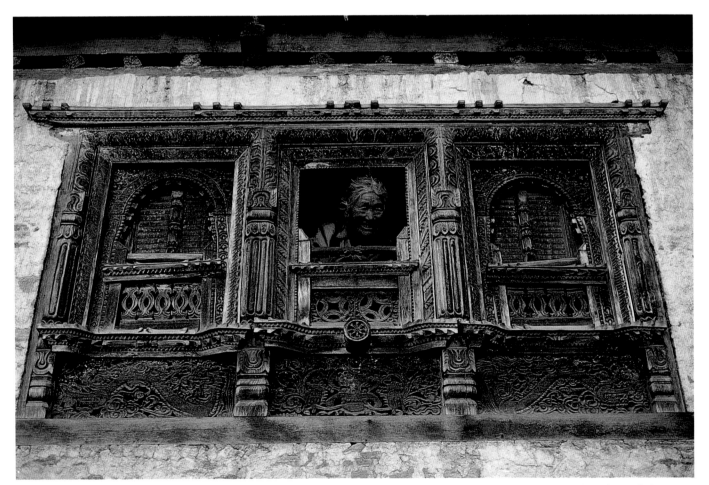

I saw an old woman peering out of an elaborately carved window in a Tamang village in central Nepal. When she ducked inside, I called out to her in Nepali, asking her to come back and talk to me. She returned, laughed that I could speak her language, and readily agreed to be photographed. For this shot, I used my Nikon N8008 with an 80-200mm zoom lens and exposed at f/4 for 1/250 sec. on Kodachrome 64.

your face, hands, and head and torso movements. If your first attempt fails, try a different approach or another set of gestures. While photographing people I've found nonverbal communication to be as successful as verbal communication. Be aware, however, that cultural gestures vary from country to country. For example, in India when a man moves his head languidly from side to side, it looks as if he is indifferent and bored. But he's actually saying, "Yes!"

Asking permission to take a photograph isn't always the best choice. In some cultures women are very reluctant to verbally agree to be photographed, and certainly not in the presence of men. Instead, I might ask with my eyes and body language, and expect a similar response, such as a nod, a smile, or simply continued eye contact as I raise my camera. However, if I'm not sure about how the person feels, I always ask.

One of the most exhausting parts of travel is perpetually maintaining a good mood. If you aren't in a good mood your body language expresses this, and people are instinctively repelled from you and your camera. It takes more energy to relate nonverbally than verbally. The best travel photographers are open and indefatigably friendly. Of course, everyone inevitably has down days. That is the time to put down your camera and go do something else.

BEING SENSITIVE, DIPLOMATIC, AND UNOBTRUSIVE

When you travel you may feel as if you're representing only yourself, but to the eyes of the world you're also representing your country. You are a foreign ambassador, for better or for worse. I can't count the number of times that I've been referred to as the "American woman." I've learned not to bristle at this attack on my individuality but to accept it gracefully.

The richest opportunities to photograph people arise when the tourist bus stops and the road ends. You may be the one making the rules for the photographers to come. Learn the local customs and traditions before you go, or ask about them along the way. Being familiar with them will make it easier to interact with the people. For example, before I leave on a trip, I do some research into what the local dress is. This is usually a more important issue for women than men, but not always. I don't believe in wearing only native clothes when I travel. I wear simple, neat, unostentatious clothes to blend into the crowd as much as possible. If I see the local women wearing long skirts and long-sleeve blouses, I mimic their level of modesty in my Western style. Men also need to pay attention

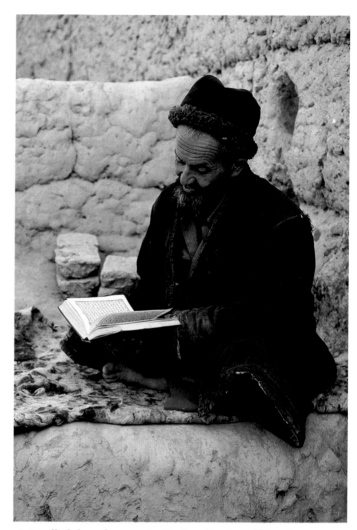

As I walked through a town in Xinjiang Province, China, I saw this Kirghiz man reading the Koran. I didn't want to disturb him, so I slowly walked into his courtyard and stood respectfully to the side with my camera lowered. He looked up, saw me, and went back to his studies. Since he didn't object to my presence and was aware of my camera, I felt comfortable photographing from a discreet distance. Shooting with my Nikon F3 and an 85mm lens, I exposed for 1/125 sec. at f/5.6 on Kodachrome 64.

to whether or not it is appropriate to wear shorts. In some cultures they're viewed with disdain or worn only by men of the lowest social rank.

It is always a good idea to meet the leader of the community when you arrive at your destination. Make sure that you take the individual's photograph, explain why you are there, and present any letters of introduction you might have. Your reputation will be judged by the company you keep. Tactfully inquire as to the standing of the family you're being housed with.

Talk to the people about what you're doing, so that they understand. Keep your communication open and honest. The more people know, the more they'll help you. Explain how your photographs will be used, such as for personal use, in a magazine, in a slide show, or in schools. One Moroccan woman refused to have her picture taken saying, "You will take my picture. It will be in a magazine and someone will use it as toilet paper." I tried to explain, but to no avail. If you're going to be in one city or village for a few days or more, begin making "shop friends." Eat at the same local restaurant, and buy from the same shopkeeper. Soon you'll become familiar to the local people, and they'll relax in your presence. Then you'll have the opportunity to shoot unobtrusively. I usually carry photographs of my family, friends, and house with me in a small book. They are big hits.

As you travel, keep in mind that food is the confluence of a people and their environment. If you have special dietary needs, you might experience trouble when you travel. I rarely refuse hospitality even though I might want to. People usually go to a huge effort to honor me with a meal, so I don't ask what I'm eating; as long as the food is well cooked, I accept it graciously. Since I often travel alone, I'm faced with being the sole ambassador and thus lone imbiber of food and spirits. I've spent many a hazy evening drinking toasts to friendship and goodwill. If you are lucky enough to be traveling with a partner or a group, you can usually share the ambassadorial duties.

Be aware that your hosts might want to find out what you're made of. They might ask you to do menial chores, such as fetching water or making noodles. It helps if you can laugh at yourself and whatever situation arises.

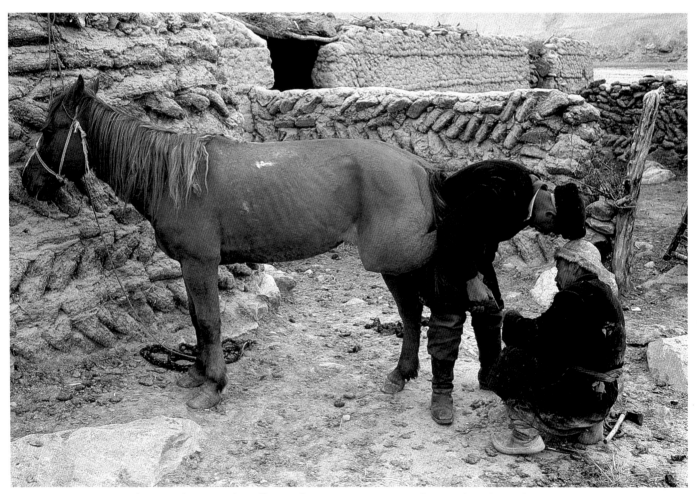

On one trek I spent more than a week in a Kirghiz village in the Pamir Mountains in China. At first the people were self-conscious around my camera, but after a few days they forgot about me and went about their daily tasks as if I weren't there. I used my Nikon F3, a 24mm lens, and Kodachrome 200 to photograph these two men shoeing a horse.

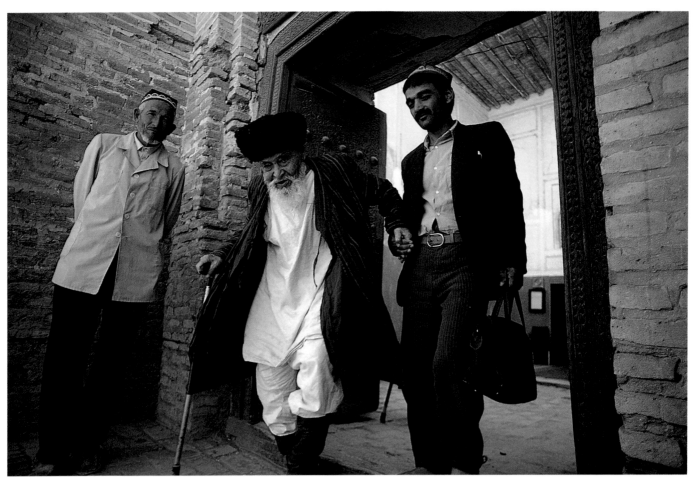

I was wandering the streets of Bukhara, Uzbekistan, when I chanced upon a small mosque; I asked what time the evening service was held. Later on I returned at the end of service, crouched outside the door, and photographed the men as they left. Working with my Nikon F3 and a 20mm lens, I exposed Kodachrome 64 for 1/125 sec. at f/5.6.

WORKING QUICKLY

Photographing people requires you to think and act fast. Before I lift the camera, I get my light reading, think about my composition, and decide which lens to use. Then I swiftly raise my camera, focus, and shoot as many pictures as I want or as many as my subject is comfortable with. Because expressions change quickly, a motor drive helps you catch all the ephemeral reactions. Don't be afraid to change your position or your angle.

It is essential to know your equipment so well that the camera is simply an extension of your hand and eye. Dexterity with your equipment comes from long hours of shooting and familiarity with your gear. Without quick reflexes and an automatic knowledge of your equipment, those instantaneous, decisive moments will pass unrecorded on your film.

Sometimes it is possible to compose your picture without raising the camera to your eyes; doing that reveals your intentions immediately. If you can frame a scene this way, you are more likely to go unnoticed, even from pretty close range. This technique of instinctive shooting is quite easy with wide-angle lenses. You must, however, allow for a margin of safety and leave space around the subject because you can't be sure of the results. Finally, avoid noisy cameras. The classic "click" is a giveaway every time. Take advantage of a sudden sound to cover the noise the shutter makes.

As with wildlife photography, it is helpful to know the habits and customs of the people you're photographing. If you want to photograph people streaming out of the door of a particular temple, you have to find out what time the services are, return before they begin, and find the right photographic angle. It takes practice and effort to time your shooting to coincide with an event so you can catch that spontaneous moment.

Spending time in one area certainly helps you capture spontaneous moments. I once stayed in a Tibetan monastery in the mountains of Sichuan Province, China, for a couple of weeks. When the people became accustomed to me and my camera, I wasn't a novelty any longer and I was able to catch spontaneous and remarkable moments of their everyday lives.

Most third-world cultures have a different orientation to the camera than Americans do. Having a portrait taken isn't a time to be spontaneous and open for these people; it is a serious, special event. They're expected to pose straight-backed and stare somberly into the camera. In Vietnam I once photographed an older Black Thai woman. I really wanted her to smile and show her black enameled teeth (until recently in Vietnam, Black Thai women traditionally enameled their teeth black as a sign of beauty), but her natural reaction was to assume the usual rigid pose. After I shot a few photographs so that I wouldn't seem rude, I tried to change the mood. I talked to her and the crowd, hoping to dispel the somber atmosphere. I mimicked a smile and made everyone laugh, including the woman. Fortunately I succeeded. But this was only because when she laughed, I was ready and shot fast. My camera's motor drive proved indispensable in capturing the fleeting moment.

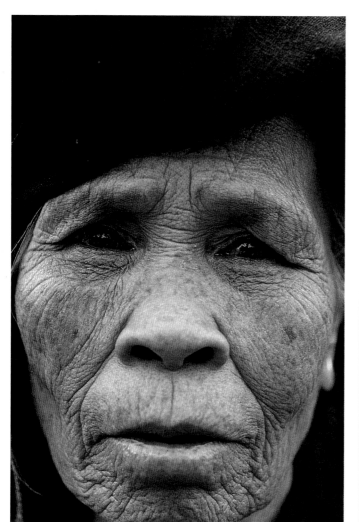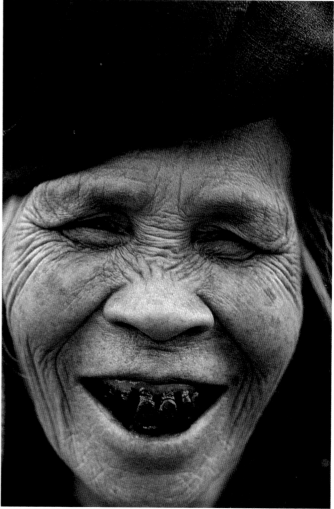

During one of my trips to Vietnam, I photographed an older Black Thai woman in at the Chieng Pac village market in Son La Province. Although the woman's natural reaction was to assume the usual rigid pose shown on the left, I made her smile and show her black-enameled teeth. I made these two portraits with a Nikon N8008, a 55mm lens, and exposed for 1/125 sec. at f/5.6 on Kodachrome 64.

DIRECTING THE PHOTOGRAPH

After you've made a connection with people who are amenable to being photographed, don't be shy about repositioning them if, for example, you don't like where they're standing or if the light is bad. Ask them to move a few inches, sit down, or even follow you to a better place. They'll get the message that you're trying to portray them in a flattering fashion.

When I want subjects to rearrange themselves but we don't speak a common language, I mimic the posture or action I'd like to see and imply that they follow my lead. I put my hands together and give them an "Okay, how about you?" look. Usually they immediately understand. If not, I go over and politely move them to where I'd like them to sit or reposition their hands myself.

POLAROIDS AND TIPPING

The subject of deciding whether or not to bring a Polaroid camera on a trip elicits a variety of disparate opinions. Some people swear by their usefulness, claiming that they unlock doors. Others say that they may briefly unlock a door, but that they close doors for the next person who might not have a Polaroid. I tend to agree with the "anti-Polaroid" faction. I don't believe in fostering a type of instant gratification. Polaroids breed more Polaroids, and eventually people will refuse to have their photograph taken unless they can immediately have an image. Then the sole purpose of a camera becomes an instrument for a quick snapshot of the person and the entire village.

You also have to be aware of the "Polaroid syndrome." You pull out a Polaroid camera, and suddenly the entire town is at your tent door demanding a print. If someone traveling with me has a Polaroid camera, I ask the person to keep it inside a suitcase. Of course, there are times when these cameras are definitely useful, such as when you want to photograph government officials or to give pictures to families you've spent a long time with. But to casually meet someone on the trail and hand out a Polaroid is inappropriate and very expensive.

Sometimes people come up to me and ask to have their picture taken, expecting that it'll come out instantaneously. I have a stock gesture in such situations. I hold up my camera and make my right palm flat as if it is a photograph coming from the camera and say, "No instant," in whatever is the closest approximation of their language. Usually they understand and leave. I prefer sending photographs to people later. I have the subjects write down their addresses, in their native language and script, in a book I keep for this specific purpose. Then when I'm ready to send the photograph, I photocopy the address and tape it to an envelope.

I try to avoid paying for a photograph. As I mentioned before, my main reason for shooting is primarily for the interaction and the experience. I don't pay someone to say hello to me, so I don't pay to photograph. It is my responsibility to convey that in my approach and manner. If you act frenzied and pushy, you can expect the person to feel like an object and to want to be paid.

In a small town in Mongolia I noticed a woman with a beautiful yellow turban standing in the warm afternoon sunlight. I motioned that I'd like to take her photograph. She agreed, but as she turned toward me, she moved out of the sunlight into the shade, as shown on the left. Although I photographed her with my Nikon F3, exposing Kodachrome 64 for 1/60 sec. at f/4, I knew that I'd lost the drama. So I asked her to move back into the red light of the setting sun where the shadows flatteringly framed her face, as shown on the right. After changing the aperture to f/5.6, I quickly took a series of shots because the sun was hurting her eyes, and then thanked her for cooperating.

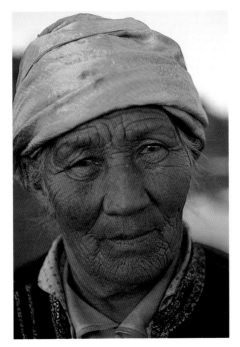
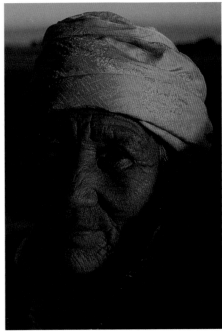

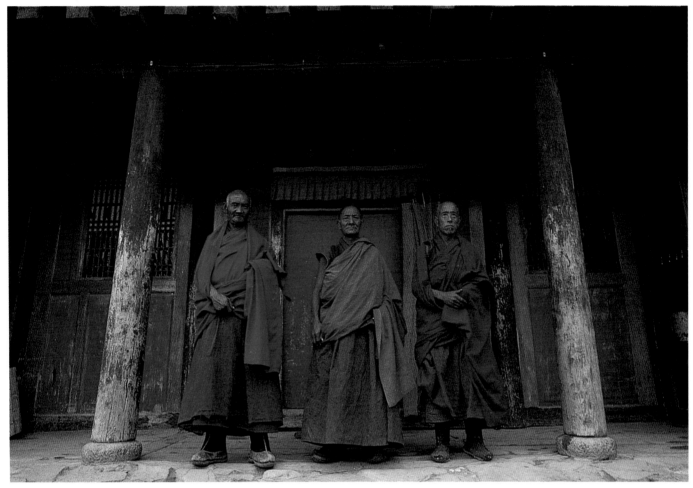

I coaxed these three lamas out of their monastery in China's Sichuan Province and onto the front steps for a group portrait. I was intrigued by the redness of the scene. To emphasize the grandeur and magnitude, I shot from below with a 24mm wide-angle lens on my Nikon F3. The exposure was 1/60 sec. at f/8 on Kodachrome 200. When I finished shooting, I placed a donation on the altar.

If you're shooting in a country or region where a million cameras have come before you, such as the Everest trail in Nepal or the villages in Kenya, you can expect to be greeted by outstretched palms. I never cavalierly saunter into an area and distribute money for photographs. I won't demean people by viewing them as only a photograph and a business deal.

Be aware that there are opportunistic people who'll try to squeeze whatever pennies you have in your pockets into theirs. Trust your intuition about someone, be direct, and don't let yourself be intimidated. I've encountered one scam numerous times. Lively young boys approach me and say or gesture, "Take my picture!" If I agree, their palms come out and they ask for 1 ruppee, 100 bhat, or 10 dollars. I never hand out money on these occasions. I simply smile, wave graciously, and continue on my way.

However, there are a few situations in which I'll pay money or present a small gift in exchange for photographs. For example, I give subjects a token gift when I ask them to take time out from their work or from their home duties to pose for me. And when I photograph a religious beggar or an educational, religious, or art institution, I'll make an appropriate contribution. Keep your gifts modest and personal in nature, such as food or something else that the subject will find useful. Extravagant gifts and excessive amounts of money increase the schism between people and immediately set you apart from the local people. You may even become an object of disdain, since people will think that you don't know the value of money. Before you throw your money around freely and foolishly, think carefully about how the power of money and greed can transform a culture.

DEALING WITH OFFICIALS

If you spend your time traveling in remote third-world countries, inevitably you'll be spending more time than you like dealing with officials and a lumbering bureaucracy. Waiting is an essential part of traveling in remote areas. Always carry a book or magazine in your camera bag.

Even if you judicially do your homework before you go and know what is permissible legally and culturally, there always comes a time when you are a captive of red tape. It is best to be flexible and maintain a sense of humor because everything that can go wrong probably will. If you do get stopped in mid-shutter on the street by an official, don't become rattled or angry. It is probably only a minor hassle. Diplomacy always

works best. Smile or feign innocence if necessary. If it becomes clear that there truly is a problem, put away your cameras and move on. If you happen into one of those unfortunate situations when you're asked to speak to the official's superior, relax. The request is rarely serious and is usually just a case of flexing muscles.

I've never had any serious trouble with authorities during my travels. I take special care not to bend too many rules if possible, but sometimes that is unavoidable. I've spent a few occasions nervously waiting in stuffy offices, but usually after I apologized and professed ignorance I was sent on my way with a brief reprimand. I don't like bribery or extortion, and I always feign confusion if that seems to be the official's intent. Occasionally I've been forced to pay small "fines." Ask for a receipt.

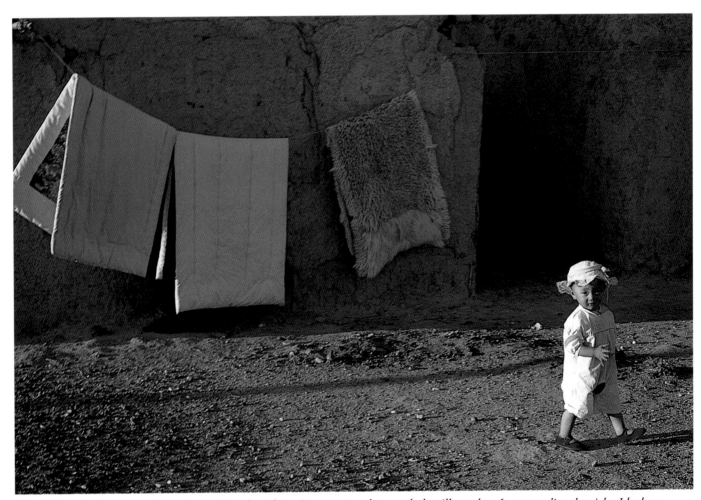

After a long day horseback riding in Inner Mongolia, China, I went out to photograph the village where I was spending the night. I had one camera in my hand and my camera bag slung over my shoulder. As this little girl sauntered by, I quickly photographed her as she passed the mattresses on the clothesline. I like the way the red in the mattress mirrors the red in her shoes. Here, I used my Nikon F3, a 35mm lens, and Kodachrome 64, exposing for 1/125 sec. at f/5.6.

RECORDING SPONTANEOUS MOMENTS

Photographing a spontaneous action requires a combination of intellect, intuition, anticipation, and luck that brings you to the right place at the right time and enables you to "pre-sense" what's about to happen. At times I come into a new situation ready and watching, and grab the decisive moments as they occur. Other times I pick a spot where something unusual or interesting might happen, such as a market street corner or a charming wall or doorway, study the composition, decide what I need, and wait for someone to come along and complete the photograph.

I don't like to have a multitude of cameras around my neck, so I keep my cameras in my bag until I'm ready to use them. When you have cameras and lenses dripping all over you, everyone notices you. Suddenly you are the object of stares and curiosity. And you're inviting thieves. I try to use my equipment as discreetly as possible. Often I see what I want to photograph, go over to a quiet corner, and arrange my cameras. Then I return and pull out the cameras as quickly and inconspicuously as possible.

However, sometimes I find that it is a good idea to have one camera in my hand ready at all times, with either a 24-50mm AF lens or a 35-70mm AF lens with a motor drive or automatic advance. Then if I see something interesting happening or about to happen, I can begin shooting immediately.

Don't look directly at your subjects; follow them out of the corner of your eye. It is easy to become conscious of someone staring at you. Furthermore, eye contact both reveals your intentions and prejudices your chances of success. You should combine this ability to look as if nothing is on your mind with a capacity for acting out roles suitable for the place and time you are in.

MANIPULATING YOUR SUBJECT

Some photographers never move a leaf or a twig for a photograph. Eliot Porter's images, for example, are expressions of found objects. Other photographers, especially commercial photographers, always create photographs from scratch. Both require control and paying attention to the intent of the photograph. I fall into the middle. I like the process of both taking and making a photograph. I'm willing to move an object in order to form a more pleasing composition or color arrangement. For example, I move objects on a table or a

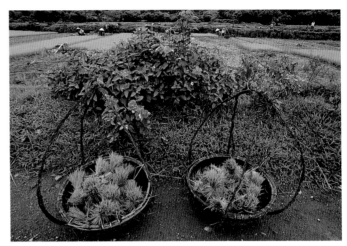

While shooting in Vietnam's Nghia Binh Province, I was struck by a beautiful bush in front of some people planting rice. Still, something seemed to be lacking to complete the picture. Then I noticed two baskets of small rice plants off to the side. So I placed them in front of the bush and made this shot using my Nikon N8008 and a 20mm lens. The exposure was 1/60 sec. at f/11 on Kodachrome 64.

windowsill a fraction of an inch for a more harmonious design. I rearrange objects in a person's house into an interesting pattern or put them in a better light source, such as under a window. I also rearrange the folds in a skirt or the position of a hat, and I brush back stray wisps of hair. I direct poses and hand placements. And if someone's tie is crooked or shirt is unbuttoned, I ask the person to fix the problem.

I don't believe that I'm being dishonest. Everyone is guilty at one time or another of composing a roadside scene with signs, buildings, and power lines until it looks like a pristine wilderness. Changing a hand position or moving a vase isn't much different from changing your shooting angle or the focal length of your lens. Yet to be successful the images mustn't look conspicuously artificial or labored.

Since I rarely travel with more than one flash, I'm forced to be very creative with available light. I often move subjects in direct sunlight into open shade outdoors, near a wall or under a portal, to get a soft, even light.

I'm obviously not shy, but I don't march into a situation and brazenly begin moving objects and people around. I always ask permission when necessary and involve the subjects in the process as much as is appropriate. I find that people aren't put off then; in fact they appreciate the effort and time I spend on the image or their appearance.

Still you don't always have the time or the fortune to wait for serendipity to lead you to a good shot. Sometimes you have to rely on your wits and ingenuity, experience, and

I arrived at this floating market in Hau Giang Province, Vietnam, at dawn. I mounted my Nikon N8008 and an 80-200mm zoom lens on a tripod and photographed from a bridge in order to look down on the activities. I was attracted to the composition formed by the hats and the vegetables, and exposed at f/5.6 for 1/125 sec. on Kodachrome 64.

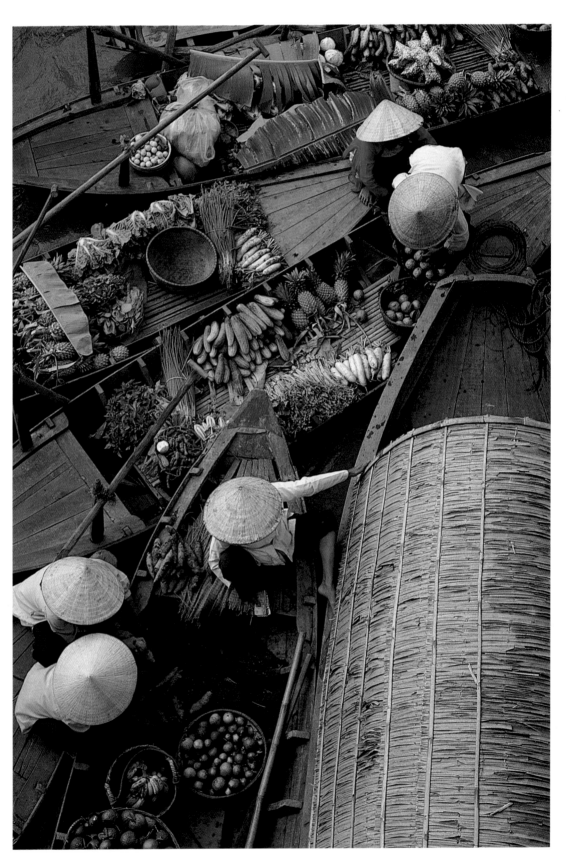

imagination to turn a good opportunity into a great photograph. You don't take great pictures; you make them.

FESTIVALS AND MARKETS

One of the most stimulating moments of any journey comes when you discover a weekly bazaar or market. Rural villagers don't have the convenience of buying food at a local supermarket. They plan their shopping around a weekly market that lasts for only a day or two. Festivals are usually annual events, but can also occur on a 12-year cycle. They can go on for days, even weeks. If you happen onto or get the chance to go to a local festival, do it; it could be the experience of a lifetime. Markets and festivals are grand events. People are animated and active, and the colors, smells, and sounds are sublime.

Exploring a market and photographing one are two entirely different experiences. I find shooting these festive occasions to be extremely challenging. They are usually crowded, chaotic, and overwhelming. You can easily return home with great stories and disappointing photographs. When a place is teeming with activity, it is difficult to separate out details and situations. You have to pay strict attention to your framing and edges. You have to be aware of people walking in front of the camera, your subject moving, and elbows and legs sticking in from the side of the frame. Photographing festivals and markets is exciting but exhausting work.

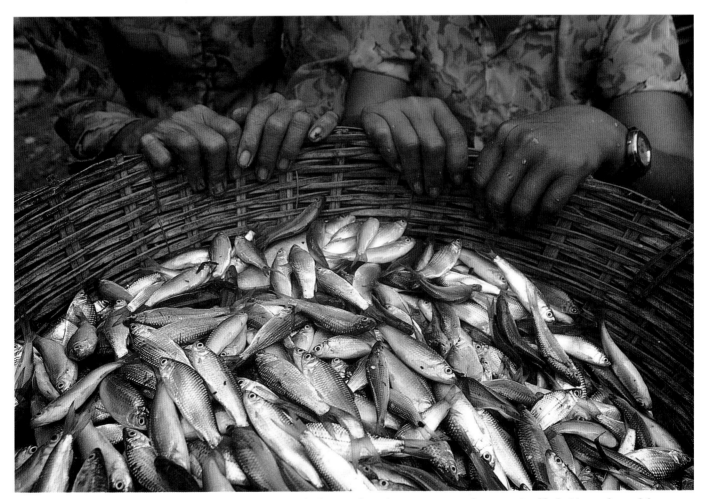

Driving along Highway 1 in Vietnam, my companions and I had to stop for a short time at a road-construction block. I jumped out of the van and walked around a small market while we waited. I saw two women with blue shirts sitting behind a basket of fish. One woman had her hands on the basket, so I knelt down and moved the other woman's hands next to her friend's hands. I made this shot with my Nikon N8008 and a 20mm lens; I exposed for 1/30 sec. at f/8 on Kodachrome 64.

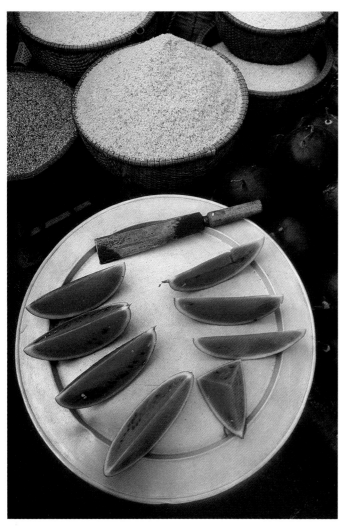

At a small local market in Hau Giang Province in southern Vietnam, I was drawn to the design and color of a plate of watermelon and some baskets of rice. Using my Nikon N8008 with a 20mm lens, I shot from above at a slight angle. The exposure was 1/60 sec. at f/8 on Kodachrome 64.

WHEN AND WHERE TO SHOOT

If you're heading to a big market or festival, get up at first light and venture out as the stalls are just beginning to be set up. Use fill flash or fast film in order to capture the early-morning commotion. Then stay late or at least return at the end of the day. Usually there are fewer people in the early morning and late afternoon, so it is easier to move around and get uncluttered photographs. In addition the light is softer, and the shadows are less harsh at these two times of day. Also, I find that people are more relaxed at the end of a successful business day, as well as more willing to pose in front of a camera.

When the activity starts to pick up, a few hints will help you combat the bedlam. Don't try to include too much in a shot unless you specifically want to shoot an overall scene. Narrow in on one person, area, or activity while looking for details, colors, light, and interesting moments. In a crowd of people it is difficult to see or get a perspective on anything. For an overall shot, get above the masses by standing on a roof or climbing up a pole. Frame your shot tightly or expansively depending on the effect you want.

Back on the ground, either shoot with a telephoto lens to frame situations tightly or come in close with a wide-angle lens. I usually carry three camera bodies, one with a 20mm lens, an 80-200mm lens on the second, and a 35-70mm or a 55mm macro on the third. If a lot's happening and I need to shoot quickly in a short period of time, I wear all three cameras. If I have more time for shooting, then I wear just one and keep the rest accessible in my camera bag.

What is so great about festivals and markets is that with so much going on, people tend not to notice you or be bothered by you. And, of course, it is easier to get candid shots in a crowd. You can stand in one place, waiting for the perfect shot without disturbing anyone or making people feel uncomfortable. Zero in on important details and activities that capture the essence of a situation. For example, you might want to concentrate on the exchange of money and goods in a market, the lighting of candles and the beating of gongs in a monastery, or the reactions of the crowd to the festival or dance. Often a very simple image says more than a jammed overall shot. Try shooting a series of shots, isolating the important moments of an event or activity, in order to tell a story.

Don't stand timidly in the back of the crowd. Get in close, especially if you're shooting with a wide-angle lens; otherwise you'll end up with distracting elements at the edges of the frame. When shooting closeups in a market, you have to wait for a lull in shopping activity or work fast so that you don't disturb the commercial transactions. Have your exposures and framing in mind before you step in for an intimate photograph.

I continually move around the area, visiting the same place dozens of times because light changes and there is always something new to see. It is boring when all of your shots of someone show the person only directly facing the camera. Shoot low, high, and from the sides; explore creative angles. Wide-angle lenses are my favorite choices for photographing markets. I can stand above people and shoot down onto their wares, or shoot directly into the vegetables to create a spray of color with a portrait in the back.

If, on the other hand, you want or need to photograph from a conspicuous position or one where your presence might annoy participants or onlookers, you have to honestly judge the appropriateness of your intentions and actions. If you decide that your shooting position won't be an intrusion, go in and out discreetly and quickly. However, I often have to let go of great shots when I think my presence would be rude or disturbing. This is a hard call to make because there is a very fine line between being shy and being restrained.

HOW TO FIND LOCAL FESTIVALS AND MARKETS

I try to arrange my travel plans to coincide with as many local markets and festivals as possible. Sometimes it is very difficult to find out where and when they take place, particularly in the more obscure regions. Such remote areas don't have tourist boards, and information can be quite localized. The dates of some festivals are commonly based on a lunar cycle, which makes it difficult to calculate the date from one year to another.

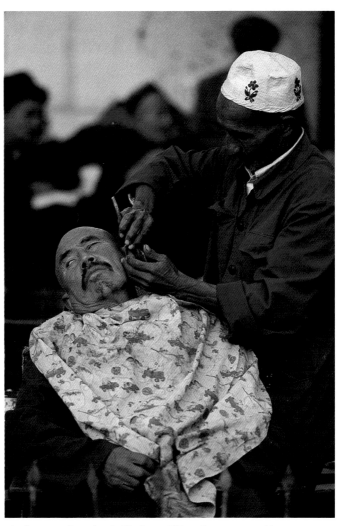

The Sunday market in Kashgar, China, is one of the world's greatest bazaars. There are hundreds of stalls, with thousands of buyers and sellers from the region. As I was walking around the lumberyard at the end of a very long day, I noticed this Uighur man leaning against a cart filled with logs. The light was soft and muted. After I approached him, he held his stance while I took his portrait using my Nikon F3 and a 24mm lens. I exposed for 1/60 sec. at f/8 on Kodachrome 64.

At the central market in Kashgar, China, I came upon this man getting a shave. So I moved back and waited until I got a clear view of him through the crowd. When that happened, I shot a number of photographs quickly and unobtrusively using my Nikon F3, a 180mm lens, and Kodachrome 64. The exposure was 1/250 sec. at f/4.

They're also often planned according to auspicious signs, the deliberations of a shaman, or the impulsive decision of the village headman, making it even harder to pin down a date.

For the best information, consult travelers who've visited the regions before, guidebooks, and government bureaus. Keep your ears open, and continually ask about local festivals as you travel. Make sure that you get a few similar answers before you trust this information, or you might find yourself traveling for days in a crowded bus to a remote town only to find an empty field littered with festival debris. Sometimes you are lucky, but often you aren't. On a trip in Vietnam, every place I visited I heard the refrain, "If only you had come yesterday (or last week, or last month)." Of course, there are also the fortunate times when you arrive at a fabulous festival you had no idea about.

Some festivals are carefully guarded and restricted to foreigners. Be sure that you have the proper permits to be there. Also, be very careful of your camera gear. Markets and festivals invite pickpockets and thieves. Carry your camera bag diagonally over your shoulder to prevent it from being grabbed off your body. Although this has never happened to me, I've heard of camera straps being cut. So if you have a bag with a waist belt, use it. If you're carrying a thin-canvas camera bag, line it with a towel. This way if the bag is slit, the contents won't fall out. Never leave your bag open or unzipped. In a crowd you'll never feel slippery fingers creeping inside your camera bag and stealing your favorite lens. Don't put your camera bag down unattended. It is helpful to go with a friend who can watch your bag. If you do have to put it down, keep your foot or knee on it with your strap around your leg.

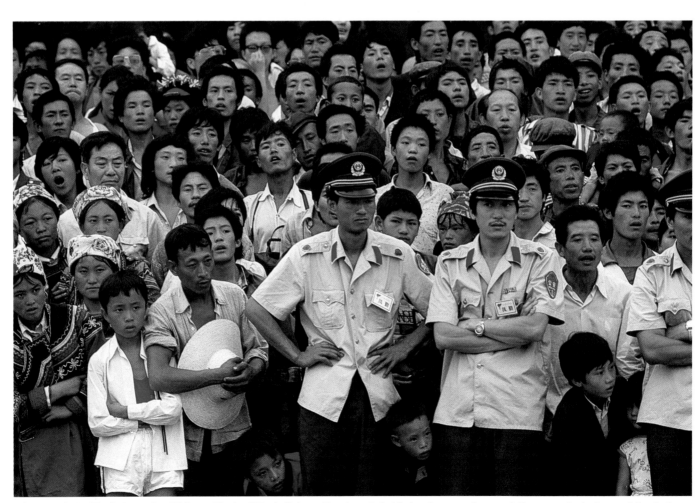

Shooting the Yi Torch Festival in Xichang City in China's Sichuan Province, I decided to focus on the crowd. I was particularly struck by the boy peering out from in between some onlookers' legs. For this shot I used my Nikon F3 with a 180mm lens, and exposed for 1/250 sec. at f/4 on Kodachrome 64.

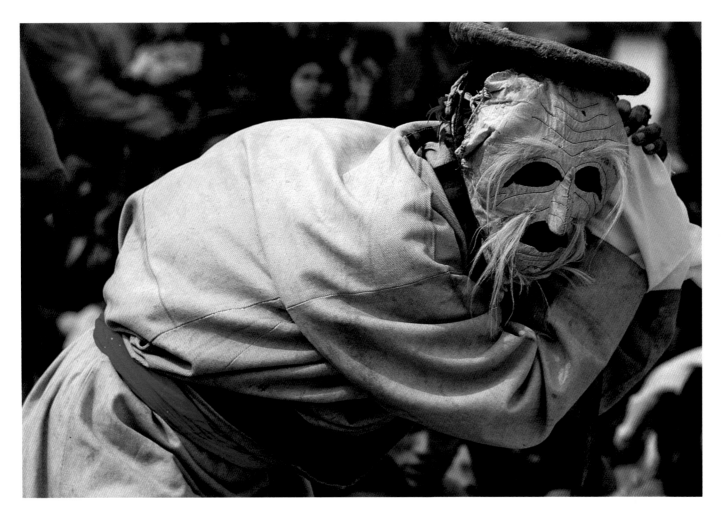

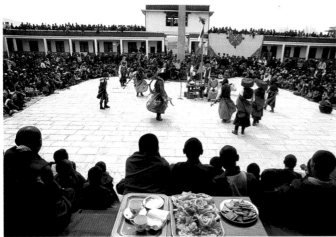

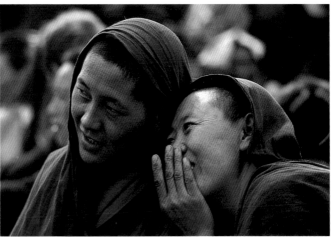

During the Tibetan New Year celebration in Kathmandu, Nepal, I concentrated on the details of the dance and the crowd. I was careful to be unobtrusive, but I still managed to wedge into spaces to get an unusual angle, such as the area filled with food behind the monks, shown above. Shooting the scene with my Nikon F3 and a 24mm lens,

I exposed Kodachrome 64 for 1/125 sec. at f/8. Then when I sat in the crowd, I focused on individuals, such as these two Buddhist nuns enjoying the dance. The masked dancer particularly interested me. I used my Nikon F3, a 180mm lens, and Kodachrome 64 to photograph these two scenes; the exposure was 1/250 sec. at f/5.6.

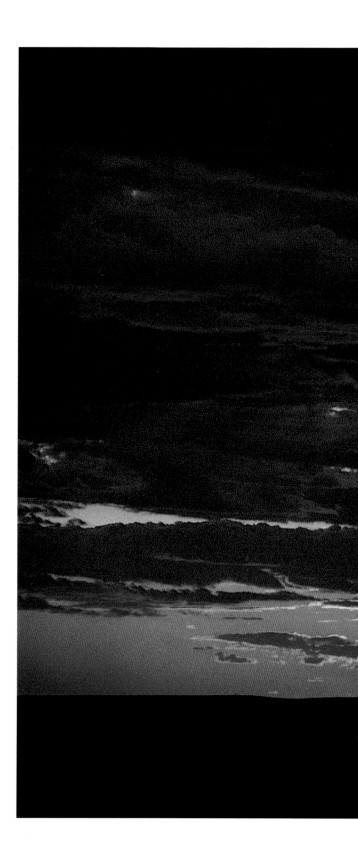

PART 6

THE LIGHT IN THE WILD

The aim of photography is to parent shape, tone, texture, and color into a personal expression. Light is the substance that makes this miracle possible. It can transform and exalt the most commonplace subjects. I can't emphasize strongly enough that light is the most important element in photography. Use it inappropriately, and all of your technical skill is wasted; use it successfully, and many of your technical flaws will go unnoticed.

Every photograph is a manifestation of light. I am a rapt admirer of its forms and epiphanies. I marvel at rainbows, thin rays of light streaming through a window in a dark room, shadows, and reflections. For me, light is the ultimate wonder of the world. While I travel through remote landscapes and wilderness, whether I'm photographing people or elephants, I am aware that their very existence is a kind of magic performed by light.

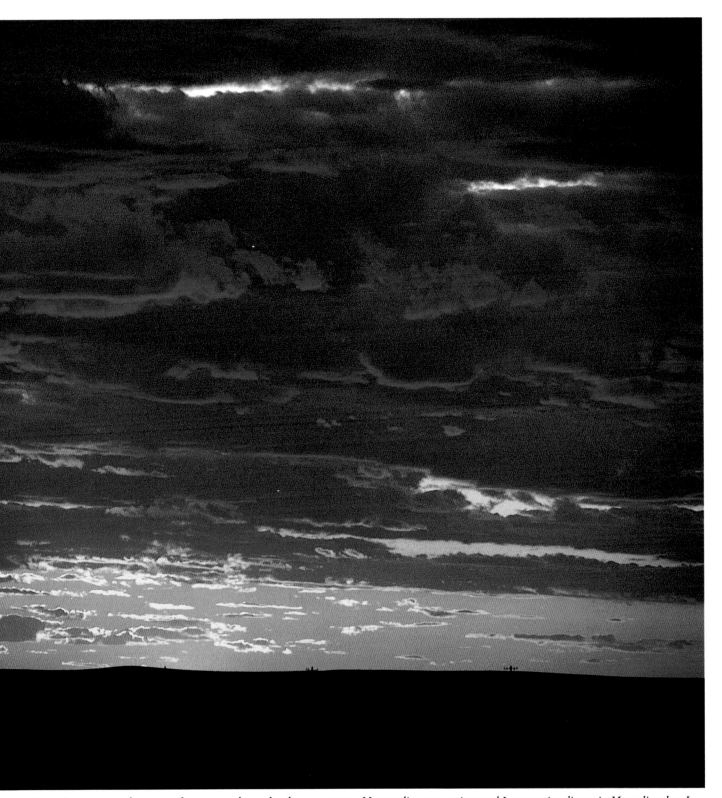

You can't create a perfect sunset, but you can be ready when one occurs. My traveling companions and I were eating dinner in Mongolia when I happened to look out the window and saw a symphony of crimson in the sky. I grabbed my camera and tripod, ran outside, found a good vantage point, and shot until the light disappeared. Working with my Nikon F3 and a 35mm lens, I exposed for 1/30 sec. at f/8 on Kodachrome 64.

THE PERFECT LIGHT

Photographers are always in search of the "perfect light." But "perfect" is a very subjective word. What is inspirational illumination to me may seem disastrous to someone else. Some photographers love the rain, while others thrive in late-afternoon, low-angle light. I am partial to fog and mist; I like the romance and monochromatic qualities.

Luck plays a part in the search for your perfect light. You can plan all you want, but whether you get rainbows or simply rain to shoot ultimately has more to do with chance than skill. When you're traveling, you rarely have time to return to the same spot over and over in order to capture a rainbow or a full moon. So how you respond to an opportunity is often as important as the opportunity itself.

Be aware and anticipate; make your photograph happen. When something lucky happens, quickly assess the situation. Perhaps you can improve on the image by running 100 yards down the trail. Of course, although it doesn't always pay off, sometimes it is necessary to be an active participant when making your photograph rather than a passive one waiting for the world to create your photograph.

SIDELIGHTING

Light coming in at right angles to the subject provides wonderful texture, emphasizing the subject and creating an illusion of depth. Because of the resulting shadows, the sculpted surface of the earth or the individual hairs and other parts of a person's body stand out in bold relief. Sidelighting also produces a partial rim lighting, which accentuates human

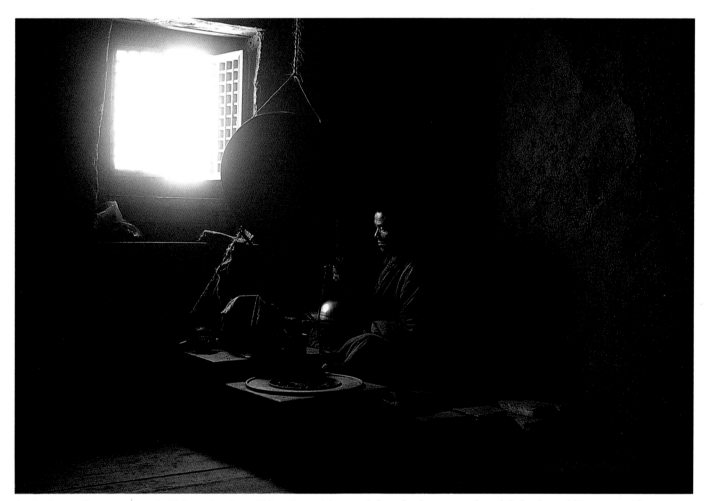

At the Gonga Shan monastery in Sichuan Province, China, I sat with a monk for a few hours everyday while he chanted his prayers. After a couple of days, he agreed to let me photograph him. The light coming in from the side window illuminated his profile. I used a 24mm wide-angle lens on my Nikon F3 to minimize his figure in the image and exposed for 1/8 sec. at f/5.6 on Kodachrome 64.

you can otherwise reduce your flash to ⅛th or ¹⁄₁₆th power if you want to keep some detail in the shadowed side.

BACKLIGHTING

Some of the most dramatic outdoor photographs feature backlit subjects, particularly people, animals, and small plants. When the sun is directly behind a subject, a halo of light separates it from the background, emphasizing the subject's form and texture. Subjects that the light can shine through look soft and translucent.

The correct exposure for a backlit photograph depends on the background and how tightly you frame the subject. A backlit head-and-shoulders shot should contain a background that is also backlit or in the shade; if it doesn't, it'll look overexposed. Take a reading by pointing your meter at the shaded side of a gray card, a neutral background, or your hand in the same light falling on the subject. The background will then be perfectly exposed in the photograph, and the closer side of your subject will be slightly darker than normal but still acceptable. A full-length backlit shot will be one stop less exposed, or darker, than the head-and-shoulders shot. Here you can see the sunlit ground the person is standing on, so it is obvious that you're looking at the shaded side of the subject. You expect to see the subject a little darker than usual. Sometimes to balance the photograph, you may need to add some fill flash (see page 95).

Always use a lens hood on your lens to prevent flare; this is caused by stray light hitting your lens. If the sun shines into your lens, you or a friend need to shade the lens with a hand or a piece of cardboard while you shoot or to tape a piece of cardboard or commercial black foil around your lens.

Extreme backlighting causes a silhouette. In these shooting situations detail is blanked out to give an unusual, often mysterious feel to the image. This is particularly effective for subjects that have graphic, recognizable forms, such as people, buildings, animals, and trees. To create a silhouette, simply meter the light area near the sun. The resulting exposure will be three to four stops overexposed, making your subject appear black and dramatic.

SUNRISES AND SUNSETS

An intense and rewarding time to photograph is just before and after sunrise and sunset. These are the times when the light is magical (the weather gods permitting, of course), when the world is full of brilliant, efflorescent colors. For an hour before dawn and following sunset, a cool-blue light casts an air of mystery across the landscape. During the 5 to 10 minutes

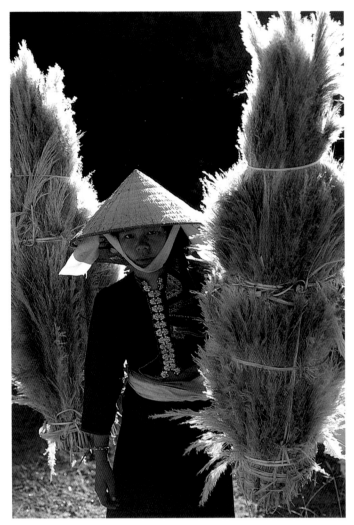

One day while I was photographing the ethnic hill tribes in Son La Province in northwestern Vietnam, a young Black Thai girl walked by carrying two bundles of Lau flowers used for stuffing mattresses. The sun was shining from behind, dramatically backlighting her and her load. I motioned to the girl to stop, metered off my hand, and shot a series of photographs. For this image, I used my Nikon F4 and a 24mm lens. The exposure was 1/60 sec. at f/5.6 on Kodachrome 64.

hair and animal ears, horns, or antlers. Because sidelighting effectively reduces the strength of the sun by at least 1 full stop, you'll have to open the aperture or reduce your shutter speed by 1 to 1½ stops.

One of the most flattering types of indoor illumination is window light; it bestows on the subject an attractive sidelighting. But when light falls on the subject from the side, sometimes the contrast between the illuminated and shaded areas is very high. This causes the subject to appear to be cut in half. You might need to fill in the darker side of the face with a reflector;

right before sunrise and after sunset, the air is imbued with a golden glow emanating from the sun, and frontlit subjects are bathed in this spectacular illumination.

You have to work quickly and decisively to catch this mystical time. In the temperate latitudes in summer, the sun touches the horizon for less than two minutes after it first appears in the morning and before setting at night. In the northern latitudes the sun moves much more slowly, but as you get closer to the equator the sun drops like a lead ball at sunset.

I prize sunsets in dusty or humid places. These atmospheric conditions filter out the blue light, leaving only the red to produce splendid sunsets. Humidity and haze screen the sun so that it appears to be a crimson sphere when it drops below the horizon.

The most reliable way to determine exposure at sunset and sunrise when you want to include the sun in the picture is to meter an area of sky just to one side of the sun, excluding it from the frame. Then lock in the exposure indicated, and swing the camera back to compose the view as you want. I always bracket copiously in these situations, so that I have a range of color saturations to choose from later. Check your exposure often because light levels change by the minute. If you are a serious photographer, you might want to consider investing in an incident-light meter, which measures the light that falls on the subject. This will ultimately save you a lot of trial and error, especially when you photograph people at sunset.

If you want to correctly expose for the foreground subject without losing the color saturation of the sunset or sunrise sky, use a one- or two-stop split neutral-density (ND) filter. Don't use an aperture smaller than $f/8$ with a wide-angle or standard lens or $f/11$ with a telephoto lens because the filter's gray line of density will sharpen up on the film and cause a noticeable line in your composition.

The sun always seems bigger when it is low in the sky, but you need a surprisingly powerful telephoto lens to magnify it significantly on film. For a rough guide, dividing a lens' focal length by 100 gives the sun's size on the negative in millimeters. For example, with a 200mm lens, a setting sun fills just $1/12$th of the picture width. You'll find that using a teleconverter to increase the sun's size is worthwhile, and needle-sharpness isn't usually crucial in sunset and sunrise pictures.

On the other hand, knowing exactly when and where the sun rises and sets is obviously critical to help you anticipate and set up a shot. Local newspapers usually publish these

times but often you are far away from such conveniences or they're printed in a language you don't understand. I always have a compass in my camera bag in order to orient myself to the sun. However, the positions of the rising and setting sun can vary as much as 60 degrees in the middle latitudes over the course of the year. The least-complicated method of

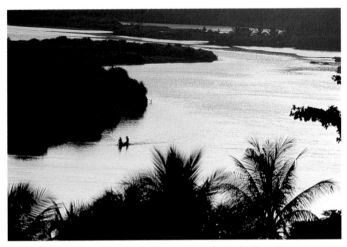

I set up my tripod on a stone outcropping above the Cay River in Nhatrang, Vietnam, and waited for the sunset. As the river began to turn golden, a small boat happened to paddle down it. I metered off my hand in the sun and bracketed while I shot. Here, I used my Nikon N8008 with a 35-70mm zoom lens and exposed for 1/60 sec. at f/8 on Kodachrome 64.

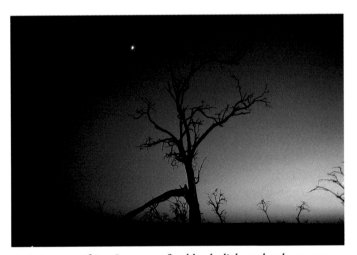

In Botswana, Africa, I was transfixed by the light and woke up every morning before dawn to photograph in the sweet light just before the sun rose. One afternoon in Savuti National Park, I noticed a group of magnificent dead trees; checking my compass, I realized that the sun rose directly behind them. So I returned the next morning with my Nikon F3 and a 20mm lens to capture this scene. The exposure was 1/15 sec. at f/5.6 on Kodachrome 64.

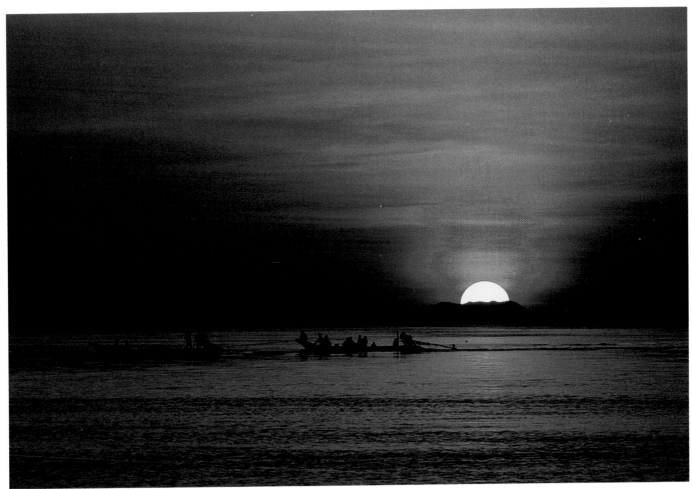

I was photographing the sunset off the coast of Cambodia in Kien Giang Province when, fortuitously, a long boat appeared just as the sun began to drop below the horizon. I metered to the left of the setting sun and quickly bracketed a series of photographs, using the motor drive on my Nikon N8008. Working with a 35-70mm zoom lens, I exposed for 1/125 sec. at f/8 on Kodachrome 64.

accurately forecasting sunrises and sunsets is being in the same place two days in a row and simply making observations.

You can also use the *Nautical Almanac,* which is published by the United States Naval Observatory and is available in any United States government bookstore. To use this almanac you need a map that depicts latitude and longitude and a good compass. Calculating the sun's rising and setting times is a little complicated, but it comes quickly and easily with practice.

Computer enthusiasts have another option: choosing from the dozens of software programs at a good computer-software store that tell you everything about what's going on in the sky. Visual Departures makes a software program for pocket computers called "Focal Ware." It determines the sun's angle at any time of day at any inputted longitude and latitude, and gives sunrise and sunset times.

TWILIGHT

At twilight the land is painted with the colors of sunset, but without the glare of the sun itself. So the colors are subtle across the whole frame, not just the sky. There is no direct sunlight illuminating the hard edges of the landscape, but there is still enough light in the sky to photograph.

Most photographers put their cameras away too soon. As it gets dark out you may lose the ability to detect color, but photographic film doesn't lose its sensitivity in the same manner; it can still record the fading colors. Twilight is an especially good time to shoot city lights and traffic. City lights give a cityscape a certain ambience, and if you shoot traffic at twilight with a long exposure, you'll get dramatic long trails of light from both the headlights and taillights of the vehicles. The longer the exposure, the longer the trails. At twilight the lights of the city and the light of the sky are basically equal in their exposure values. Meter off the dusky twilight sky, not the city lights, and use the longest possible exposure to emphasize the flow of the traffic. For accurate exposures, use a handheld meter. I've also had excellent results with my in-camera meter, but I bracket extensively. Handholding your camera in this low light is impossible. Mounting your camera on a tripod is ideal, but you can also prop your camera on a wall or a chair.

Film speed drops in dim conditions. Allow $1/2$ stop extra when the shutter is open for more than 1 sec., 1 stop for shutter speeds longer than 10 sec., and 2 stops for those longer than 60 sec. If your camera doesn't have these long shutter speeds, set the shutter-speed dial to "B," hold the shutter open with a cable release, and time the exposure with your watch or count the seconds. To compensate for reciprocity failure, which is a radical shift of color noticeable at shutter speeds longer than 1 sec., allow more exposure than the meter indicates, usually $1/2$ to 1 stop. Personally I like the odd color shifts, but I always bracket long exposures since it is difficult to predict all the variables.

SHOOTING THE MOON

The moon adds drama and romance to a landscape photograph and is relatively easy to capture on film when you know a few of the basic rules. I try to shoot the "full" moonrise the day before it is actually full. At that time the moon rises in conjunction with sunset, casting a gentle glow onto the landscape and enabling you to photograph detail in both the foreground and middleground. If you wait until the next day for the true full moon, you'll find that the moon will rise approximately an hour later. By then the foreground will be too dark, and the moon will appear as a white hole in your photograph. If you do shoot on the eve of the full moon, be aware that there is a three- to four-stop exposure difference between the land and the sky. You can compensate for this with a split ND filter.

To get a good-size moon on film, use a 135mm or longer telephoto lens. Telephoto lenses that are 400mm and longer in length produce the most dramatic results. However, there are no rules. I've seen some stunning moonrise photographs that were made with wide-angle lenses. Whatever size lens you choose, mount the lens on a sturdy tripod, set it at wide open, and use the fastest shutter speed possible to minimize any image blur that can result from the shaking of the camera lens and tripod.

To retain detail, try to photograph the moon when it is just a little paler than the sky. The moon reflects direct sunlight at a reflectivity of only 7 percent, so it demands a near daylight exposure. The trick, therefore, is to have enough ambient light in the scene to hold detail in both the moon and the sky. A landscape with a moonrise should be metered no differently than a landscape without one. At sunset on the day

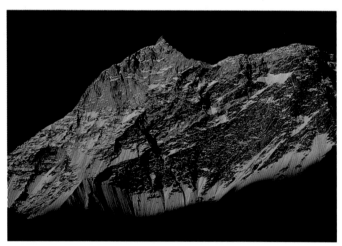

At the Makalu Basecamp, at an altitude of 16,000 feet, I mounted my Nikon F3 and a 180mm lens on a tripod and then made this image of the top of Makalu Peak, the fifth-highest mountain in the world. Shooting right before sunset, I exposed for 1/125 sec. at f/8 on Kodachrome 64.

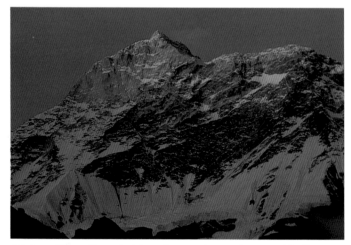

I left my Nikon F3 and 180mm lens in place and returned half an hour later to capture the last scarlet remnants of light on Makalu Peak. For this shot, I exposed for 1/60 sec. at f/4 on Kodachrome 64.

before the actual full moon, the sky and landscape are equally bathed in the final remnants of light from the western sky; their exposures are as close to identical as you can get. Be sure to meter off the sky just above the horizon, not off dark shadows. If there is a one- or two-stop difference between the land and sky, you'll find it best to split the exposure with a bit of emphasis on the sky and to bracket.

The moon ascends in the sky roughly one diameter every two minutes. So to prevent blur and to keep the moon round, you need to expose for no longer than 10 sec. with a standard lens and a shorter duration with a telephoto lens. To photograph the moon one hour after dark and even later, set the fastest shutter speed possible with the lens wide open. For example, if you're using ISO 64 film, shoot at $f/5.6$ for 1/250 sec.

The time of the moonrise can vary greatly from day to day, a result of the angle of the moon's orbit around the earth. If possible scout the location beforehand, so you can see where the moon comes up in relation to the surrounding landscape. Plan your composition; you don't want to be running around at the moment you should be taking your photograph. Once again, you can use the *Nautical Almanac* or a computer program for times of the moonrise and moonset.

Just as you do with the full moon, you want to photograph the crescent moon immediately before or after the sunset in order to try balancing the brightness of the moon with the ambient light. The best time is just before the sky has lost its color or light. When shooting Kodachrome 64, you should photograph a half moon at $f/5.6$ for 1/60 sec. and a crescent moon at $f/5.6$ for 1/8 sec. Be sure to bracket your exposures $1/2$ to 1 full stop on either side of the indicated exposure; this will guarantee your getting a successful shot.

For unusual coloration and time effects, take a long time exposure solely by the light of the moon. Photographing by moonlight is a fairly straightforward but time-consuming process. Trial and error is essential here because so much depends on your lens and film. As a beginning point, Kodak recommends a 15-sec. exposure at $f/2.8$ with ISO 400 film. Add at least one stop for reciprocity failure, and two or even three stops for some films. With Fujichrome 400 I find that two-, four-, and six-minute exposures at $f/4$ gives me interesting results. Since you'll want to bracket exposures, it is clear that one successful image can take at least 30 minutes to produce.

Ideally your camera should feature manual exposure control, a tripod socket, a cable-release socket, and a mirror lockup button. Use a sturdy tripod, and bring a penlight to help you determine exposures in the dark. Since color film exposes moonlight quite vividly, be sure to include star trails or distant artificial lights, such as car lights or building lights, in your framing. Otherwise the photograph might appear as if it were taken during the day.

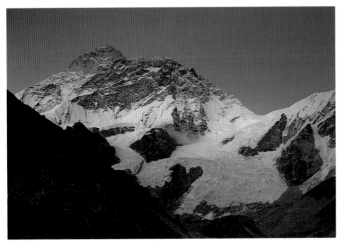

Later that night, after a virtually full moonrise, I ventured outside my tent to shoot Makalu Peak. Because I was at a high altitude, the light was especially brilliant and pure, almost like daylight. I used the automatic meter on my Nikon F3, which had a 50mm lens on it, for the basic reading and then bracketed. Here, I exposed at f/5.6 for 5 sec. on Kodachrome 64.

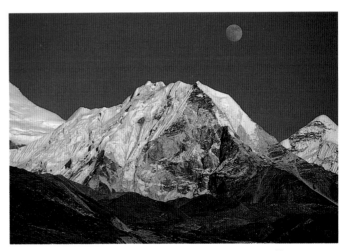

In Chukung Valley, Nepal, I steadied my camera on a wall to photograph the full moonrise over Island Peak. Since I was shooting the day before the actual full moon, I was able to take a light reading from the sky and still maintain detail in the mountain. Here, I used my Nikon F3 with an 80-200mm zoom lens and exposed for 1/125 sec. at f/5.6 on Kodachrome 64.

Including the moon as an integral part of a daytime photograph isn't always easy. Unless the sky is exceptionally clear, a moon of any kind during the day might simply be too faint to record well. One exception is a half moon at 90 degrees from the sun; it can often be made to "pop out" by using a polarizer.

RAINBOWS

Stormy weather and intermittent sunlight should alert you to be prepared for rainbow possibilities. To find a rainbow, stand with your back to the sun. If one is present, it'll be visible in the sky directly in front of you. Even faint rainbows are easy to spot in the sky because they move across a static background when you move.

The sun must be low on the horizon in order to form one of those enormous, spectacular rainbows that seem to form an arc from the ground to the zenith of the sky. This often conveniently occurs just before sunset as the sun bursts from the storm clouds before sinking into local cloud cover.

On film, rainbows often appear fainter than you remember because the colors aren't always bright enough to make a good picture. The key is the background: a rainbow photographs best against a dark backdrop. I usually meter and expose for the sky and the rainbow. If the sky is dark, I'll close down one or two stops to retain the drama and keep the rainbow colors saturated. Since the double-refracted light of a rainbow is polarized, you can brighten a faint rainbow or completely erase it by using a polarizer.

I am also always on the lookout for unconventional light reflections and refractions. Rainbow streamers are produced when sunlight is refracted through humidity or light mist and, as their name suggests, manifest themselves as streamers of light. They can be found when it is humid and misty out, but only if you use a polarizer.

IMPERFECT LIGHT

When you travel you have to accept whatever comes your way, opening yourself to the vagaries of the unknown. This applies not only to experiential encounters, but also to photographic endeavors. Often you'll end up somewhere during less-than-ideal light conditions. Your goal is to turn imperfection to perfection. Sometimes the "imperfect light" is an illusion or a curtain in front of a great photograph. If you walk away with a rigid preconception, thinking, "I can't shoot—it's the middle of the day, it's raining, and it's too dark," you might miss out on a photographic gem.

HIGH NOON

Sometimes it seems as if everything and everybody are conspiring against your photographic efforts. For instance, on one trip to Africa my companions and I always seemed to arrive at the game parks right in the middle of the day when the light was flat and the landscape was washed out. A scenario like this is frustrating, but there are ways to

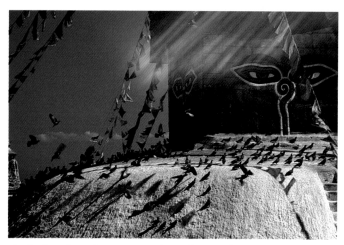

At the Syambunath stupa in Kathmandu, Nepal, I was photographing with a polarizer on my 80-200mm zoom lens to darken the sky after a light rainfall. I noticed a series of rainbow streamers and framed them next to the famous Buddha eyes on top of the stupa. Shooting with my Nikon F3, I exposed for 1/250 sec. at f/4 on Kodachrome 64.

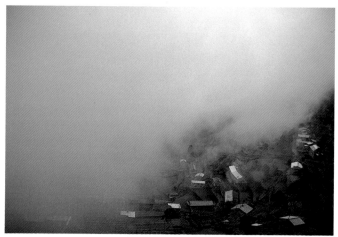

I was trekking in the Everest region through a thick fog. As I crested a ridge, the fog lifted slightly so I was able to get a brief glimpse of Namche Bazaar. It was dark, but I steadied my Nikon F3 and 85mm lens and shot this mystical image. The exposure was 1/15 sec. at f/2.8 on Kodachrome 64.

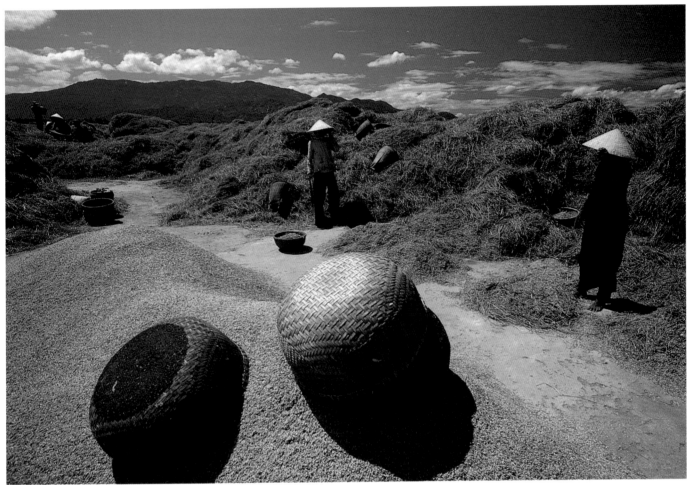

I usually avoid shooting at high noon, but one midday in Vietnam I was driving toward Nhatrang and passed some people winnowing rice. Struck by the deep shadows and the color of the rice, I got out of the car and talked to the locals while checking out the photographic possibilities. I used a 20mm wide-angle lens on my Nikon F3 to come in close on a couple of baskets that were resting on a pile of rice for a strong foreground and to include the activity in the background at the same time. I used a polarizer to help saturate the colors and exposed at f/8 for 1/60 sec. on Kodachrome 64.

salvage the situation. One option is to use a polarizer to cut the glare and squeeze some color out of a less-than-optimal shooting situation.

At midday people tend to linger in alleyways and doorways as well as inside buildings, mosques, and churches to escape the sun and heat. So these places are great opportunities for photography. Shadows saturate color. By waiting for the right person to complement a wall or a door, you can explode a dull scene with a vivid splash of color. Midday is also an excellent time to scout for potential photographic sites; this simple but often underutilized practice enables you to know exactly where the best photo opportunities are.

USING FILL FLASH

When you shoot at midday, another option is to use a bit of fill flash. This is a relatively easy procedure. Basically, you're adding light to the shadows to bring them closer in value to the highlights. In a sense, you're filling in the shadows—hence the term "fill flash"—although a more accurate term would be "balanced fill." If some fill light is impractical, you either have to live with the shadows or make them a graphic element of your photograph. Come in close to isolate an image, and make color or a detail, not light, the main event.

If you can use fill flash, the world of high-noon photography opens up to you. When the sun is at its zenith, it casts harsh, deep shadows (under the eyes or from hats) that normally ruin portraits. A touch of fill flash opens the shadows and adds direction to the light. With the addition of as little as $^1/_{16}$th to $^1/_2$ the flash power of your strobe light, you can transform a contrasty setting into a stunning image.

Using fill flash has always been a common technique among professionals, but it has been incorporated only recently into the mechanisms of modern cameras, even point-and-shoot cameras, to make it easier for the amateur photographer. The older, direct full flash erased all shadows and texture of the subject, caused "red eye," or reflected light back into the camera from glasses or shiny surfaces. Now fill flash in combination with sunlight is becoming increasingly common

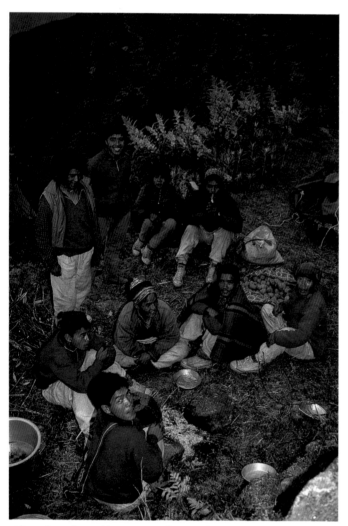

After a long day trekking in Nepal I passed by some of the porters preparing their evening meal as I arrived at camp. I put an SB-24 flash on my Nikon N8008, set it to matrix fill flash with a -2 EV, and shot a couple of photographs. I used a 35-70mm zoom lens and Kodachrome 64.

in outdoor photography. Balanced fill minimizes shadows across your portrait subject and blends your subject naturally with the background.

If your flash unit offers variable-power levels, you can experiment with fractional power to achieve just the right intensity of fill in the shadow areas of your shot. When I use a Nikon N8008 or F4 in conjunction with a Nikon SB-24 flash unit, all the fill-flash calculations are made for me. Combining TTL flash exposure with the camera's matrix-metering system produces accurate overall results. The strobe fills to the ratio of your choice between the main light and the fill flash (1:+1 EV, which stands for "exposure value," to 1:–3 EV) and continues to automatically maintain that ratio as you move from subject to subject.

If you set the strobe on the fully automatic mode, it'll fill somewhere between equal balance and –1 EV under the main light source. I feel that this is usually too much fill. In most situations I like to keep the SB-24 flash set on –2 EV to achieve a natural ratio between highlights and shadows; this is just enough to soften shadows or to add catchlights to the subjects' eyes to give portraits a professional look.

You don't have to be concerned about midday exposures because most of the newer cameras sync at 1/250 sec. In a bright sunlit situation requiring an exposure of $f/11$ for 1/125 sec., a sync speed of only 1/60 sec. calls for an $f/16$ aperture to maintain proper background exposure. Depending on the flash-to-subject distance, however, this aperture might be too small to produce adequate fill-flash exposure in the shadows. High sync speeds also help minimize the possibility of ghost images, which are additional existing-light images caused by subject movement.

Some professional photographers have made a career out of shooting strobe-filled photographs at sunset. With the recent advancements in modern cameras, amateurs can make the same type of shots without having to do elaborate calculations. Some photographers let the backgrounds and perimeters of their subjects blur with slow shutter speeds, and then freeze the subject with a blast from an on-camera strobe. The resulting images are called "fades."

If you can't adjust your strobe, you do have another choice. You can vary the ratio of the strobe to the main light by changing the film-speed rating or the exposure compensation of the camera. (Don't forget to reset your camera when you remove the strobe.) The critical element in your camera's exposure system is the aperture. You can also substitute a strobe with a reflector card or a Flexfill. This is a circular reflector made of silver, white, or gold cloth bound by a

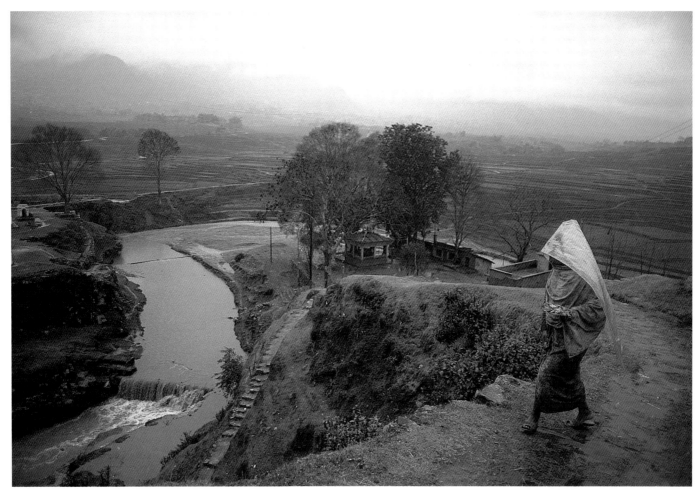

In the Kathmandu Valley in Nepal during a monsoon, it was raining heavily as I was heading to a friend's house to participate in a local festival. Behind me I saw a young girl coming up the trail with a religious offering. I moved to a spot above her, sheltered my Nikon F3 and 35mm lens with an umbrella, and shot unnoticed as she approached me. The exposure was 1/60 sec. at f/5.6 on Kodachrome 64.

flexible metal ring; it can be twisted to smaller than half its size, so it is portable. Both the reflector card and the Flexfill reflect sunlight back onto the subject from a different angle. One advantage to using a reflector is that you actually see the effect of the reflector on your subject: the light produced is much softer than the harsh, direct light of a flash. The disadvantage is that you need someone to hold the reflector.

If you're shooting a portrait with the background in the sun, you should calculate the exposure using the sun as the light source; otherwise the background will look overexposed. Since your subject is backlit, you need a fill light, one or two stops less than the full sun exposure (depending on your personal preference), from a reflector or a flash in order to avoid underexposing your subject. You usually want to keep the light soft, even, and natural looking, but not too flat.

OVERCAST SKIES AND RAIN

Many photographers head for the hotel or the tent when the clouds roll in and the sun disappears. This is unfortunate because gray, overcast skies are perfect for shooting portraits, markets, and subjects with intricate details or saturated colors, such as leaves, plants, and flowers. There are no harsh shadows; the light is diffused and evens out abrupt contrasts between sun and shade. The shadows have full detail, and there are soft, gradual transitions to the parts illuminated by the main light. You can shoot almost anything that doesn't require a blue sky or shadows to delineate land contours.

Sometimes inclement weather is as much a part of a place as sunshine is in the Sahara desert. The Brazilian rain forest, for example, looks terrible in the sun. If you get to the rain forest on a rainy day, be thankful—that is the way it's supposed to be. Rain saturates and evens out colors, and evokes a special mood. Raindrops flash past so fast and their translucent quality makes them so indistinct that they often disappear in the picture. To prevent this, include an area of water, such as a puddle, in the foreground. You can also take advantage of strong backlighting from the sun to distinctly reveal the raindrops. You can even use a flash to capture the droplets of rain.

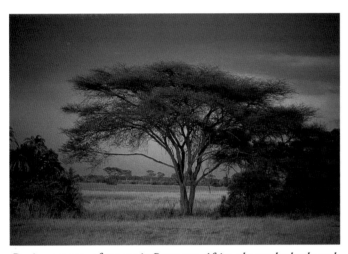

During a stormy afternoon in Botswana, Africa, the sun broke through the clouds for a few minutes to dramatically illuminate an acacia tree at the edge of the Moremi Reserve. I yelled for the driver to stop and reeled off a few exposures. Seconds later, the sun disappeared and the scene looked uninteresting again. With my Nikon N8008 and a 35-70mm zoom lens, I exposed for 1/60 sec. at f/5.6 on Kodachrome 64.

Storms often create unexpected and sensational lighting, with the foreground brilliantly illuminated against a navy sky. Catching these moments requires being instantly ready. Your camera meter usually responds to the extreme highlights of storm light and produces underexposed pictures. Bracket the exposure one stop over and one stop under.

HAZE, MIST, AND FOG

These conditions can spawn very romantic images. Haze creates a sense of distance and depth in a picture. It makes distant parts of the scene look bluer and lighter than the foreground, such as a series of ridges one after another that fade into the distance. If you want the clearest possible pictures, use a polarizer. This often darkens and improves the contrast of distant parts of the scene.

Light mist adds atmosphere to any scene, but you need to be out very early. Once the sun appears above the horizon, it is only a matter of minutes before thermal air currents lift the mist from the ground. Select subjects that have inherently strong outlines, such as buildings, boats on a lake, fences, and rock outcroppings. Subjects that rely on texture or form for their impact are weakened in such soft light. The prevailing white tones easily confuse the camera's exposure meter, so the resulting photographs tend to look too gray and dull. Open up 1 to 1 1/2 stops.

Thick mist and fog isolate and soften the forms of buildings and intrusive objects, creating a dreamy scene that might

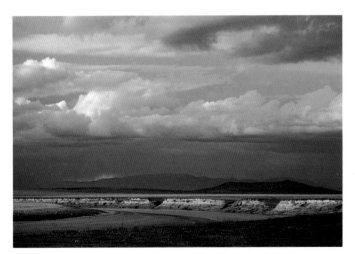

While I was riding across the Songpan Grasslands in the Tibetan Plateau in China, the sun unexpectedly broke through the clouds right before sunset to inject a thin line of yellow light across the landscape. Here, I used my Nikon F3 and a 35mm lens, and exposed for 1/125 sec. at f/4 on Kodachrome 64.

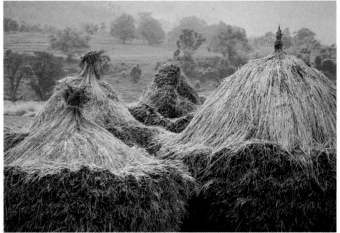

On an overcast, rainy day in the Modi Khola Valley in Nepal, I photographed a group of freshly stacked hay. I was attracted by the saturated colors and textures, which were emphasized by the diffused, misty light. Shooting with my Nikon F3 and a 35mm lens, I exposed at f/4 for 1/60 sec. on Kodachrome 64.

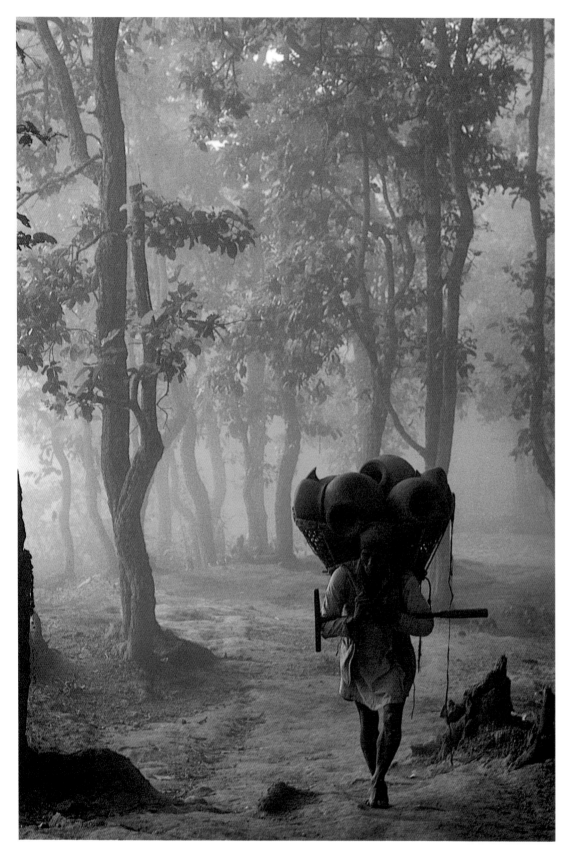

At the low elevations in Nepal, a fog often blankets the ground in the early morning. I photographed one of our porters carrying his wares to the weekly market in Khandbari Village through a light, hazy mist. With my Nikon F3 and an 85mm lens, I exposed at f/5.6 for 1/125 sec. on Kodachrome 64.

not be interesting in sunlight. If you want to retain the moody atmosphere of a dark-gray, misty morning, use the exposure indicated by your in-camera meter. The pastel tones of the fog will be amplified, and the objects in the image will loom mysteriously.

HIGH CONTRAST

Unlike the human eye, film has trouble coping with the broad contrast range between highlights and shadows that is prevalent in outdoor scenes. Most color-transparency films have a total exposure range of only four to five stops, and often the exposure range of a potential photograph is much

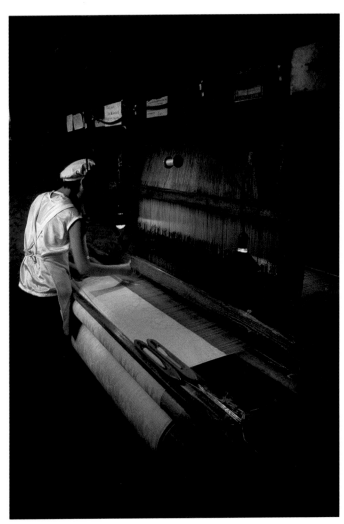

The light was extremely dim in this brocade factory in Chengdu in China's Sichuan Province. So I loaded my camera with a special push film, Fuji P1600, and rated it at ISO 800. Leaning against the wall to steady my Nikon F3 and 35mm lens, I made a number of shots using the motor drive.

greater. Your choice is either to expose for the highlights and let the shadows go dark, or to expose for detail in the shadow areas and wash out the highlights.

This is when a split-field ND filter, also called a graduated filter, becomes essential. It increases the latitude of your film, enabling it to record a much wider range of light values. It helps balance, for example, bright skies and glaring snowcaps with dark rocks and shaded foregrounds. This type of filter is dense at one edge, and the density tapers so the other edge is clear. There are many variations of these filters. They can be rectangular or round. Screw-on filters come in glass, plastic, and different tones and colors. Select a system that allows you to move the filter up and down in the frame and to rotate it 360 degrees.

Graduated filters work best when there is a sharp edge, or a horizon line, between the elements of differing brightness in a photograph. When you place the filter in front of the lens, the part covered by the neutral-density half of the filter is reduced in brightness, while the rest of the photograph remains unaffected.

I've begun to find more and more uses for graduated filters, such as sunsets with dark foregrounds, canyon shots in which one wall is in shade and the other is in bright sunlight, and backlit skies. I use a graduated filter whenever I feel there is a disparity of more than three or four stops between two essential elements of an image. These filters aren't the solution for all situations, but if used properly they allow you to make a successful image out of a potential loss.

I primarily use two Cokin Graduated Gray density filters: a G120, which results in a one-stop loss of light, and a G121, which results in a two-stop loss of light. I can also combine these filters for a three-stop change in light loss. It is important to note that Cokin filters aren't true graduated ND filters, but rather filters that range from clear to gray in color. They're made from an optical-resin compound and conform to the standards of neutral density.

Because Cokin filters are plastic, they hinder image sharpness more than glass filters do. They also tend to harbor static electricity, attract a lot of dust, scratch easily, and aren't always as neutral or evenly colored as I'd like. However, they are inexpensive enough to replace frequently if they become scratched, and light enough to carry in your pocket.

If your wallet allows, I recommend buying either the more expensive, sharper Tiffen glass-square filters that fit the Cokin P series holder, or the Heliopan optical-resin or optical-glass rectangular filters that come with their own rotating filter holder.

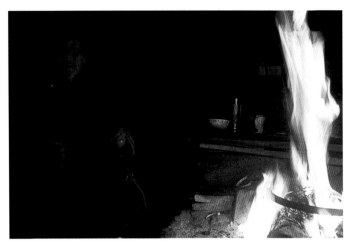

I photographed a Tibetan woman sitting by a fire spinning her prayer wheel. Because there was no natural light in the house, I set up my Nikon F3 and a 35mm lens on a tripod and took a light reading off her face and the fire. I used a slow shutter speed, 1/8 sec., to accentuate the flames and exposed Kodachrome 64 at f/5.6.

LOW-LIGHT SHOOTING

Modern photographic technology has effectively made it possible to photograph virtually anything that can be seen with the naked eye. This is important for photographers who travel to parts of the world with dark temples and small-windowed houses. Often some of the best photographic opportunities are in light that is too low for Kodachrome 64 or Fujichrome 50, and when your tripod is at home, fill flash isn't appropriate, or your lens is too slow. I love the grainy texture and ruddy color of Kodachrome 200, especially for indoor candlelight, firelight, and lamplight portraits. Films faster than ISO 200 are grainier and have slightly washed-out colors but work beautifully in low-light situations, especially in fog or by firelight.

When you photograph people in dark settings, such as inside a dim hut, using a slow shutter speed, wait for a relatively quiet moment or a pause in the action to avoid a blurred subject. Mount your camera on a tripod if possible, or brace your camera firmly so you can shoot with a very slow shutter speed. I can handhold my camera down to 1/4 sec. with a wide-angle lens and a motor drive. I press the camera against my forehead, pull my elbows into my body, and try to lean against a wall, a tree, or a friend to steady myself even more. Then I take a breath and exhale before pressing the motor drive, shooting between four and eight photographs. At least one image is always sharp; more usually are. The longer the focal length of the lens you use with this technique, the worse your odds at preventing camera shake are.

You can also consider pushing your film. For outdoor scenes, I've found that Fujichrome 100 can be pushed acceptably to ISO 200. I've talked to a number of photographers who actually prefer Fujichrome 100 pushed to ISO 200 over Kodachrome 200. When you push most slide or print film, you suffer increased grain, higher contrast, and an attendant loss of both shadow detail and color saturation. If you push film too far, usually more than about $2^{1}/_{2}$ stops, reciprocity failure will occur. Some slide films are specifically designed for push processing, such as Fujichrome P1600 and Ektachrome P800/1600 Pro films. Experiment with them to satisfy your own chromatic taste. I never push Fuji Velvia or Kodachrome 64; the color tones shift off scale. I've also found that Velvia is particularly bad for Caucasian complexions—they become very ruddy—and there is too much contrast.

Pushing film is a simple technique of resetting the film-speed dial to the desired film speed. Then when it comes time to process the roll, simply inform your E-6 lab that you shot it at a different ISO rating and want it push-processed accordingly. To ensure there are no mistakes, I write, for example, "push to ISO 200" with a marking pen directly on the canister or on a piece of masking tape on the canister. (Kodak sells ESP-1 prepaid mailers for one-stop push processing. Each mailer costs $2, and the price covers the additional expense for push-processing when used in conjunction with the standard PK36 mailer for Ektachrome and Kodachrome.)

In low-light situations selective focusing is extremely important. Since depth of field is probably limited, it is critical to focus directly on the person or object of interest. As long as the subject's eyes are in focus, it usually isn't disturbing if the rest of the photograph isn't. You can also use a bit of fill flash, $^{1}/_{2}$ to $^{1}/_{4}$ the power of the strobe. To match light given off by a fire, I tape an 85B acetate filter over my flash.

The problem with most automatic cameras with built-in automatic flash is that the camera often sets itself at 1/60 sec. or 1/250 sec., whatever is the camera's maximum sync speed. In low-ambient-light situations, this speed won't keep the shutter open long enough to give you a good background exposure. Backgrounds become black voids, and foreground subjects seem to be standing in a spotlight.

The Nikon SB-24 flash and other advanced strobes permit you to work with slow shutter speeds for low-light backgrounds by either setting the rear-curtain sync (when the strobe fires at the end of the shutter curtain opening), or setting the camera on shutter priority. The matrix meter reads the background perfectly while the SB-24 flash provides a balanced main light in the foreground.

ELUSIVE LANDSCAPES

A good landscape photograph is more than a mere record of where you were. It reflects your basic understanding of yourself in nature at that moment and is an important element of your traveling experience. There is no such thing as an objective landscape photograph. All photographers make subjective decisions at every stage of picture-taking, right from the moment they stop to view a scene and evaluate it. Often what they choose to leave out is more important than what they include. And packing in too much tends to confuse and ultimately weaken the image. Simplicity in design is the key.

CONTEMPLATING THE LANDSCAPE

Approach your landscapes with the same open mind with which you approach people, having no fixed ideas or preconceptions. I often try to steer a course between spontaneity and control. On one hand, I want to give the impression that I am in full control of technique; however, I don't want to rob a picture of its vitality. Sometimes I'll sit and look at a particular landscape for a long time before it becomes clear to me what I'm trying to express. At other times, what I want to say hits me right away. Great landscape photographs are usually the result of intuition, anticipation, thinking, and planning—and a bit of luck.

VARYING YOUR VIEWPOINT

Mobility is a more valuable photographic tool than owning a vast number of lenses is. By moving around your subject, you can totally change the composition of a picture, aligning different foreground and background elements or cropping out unwanted details close to the camera.

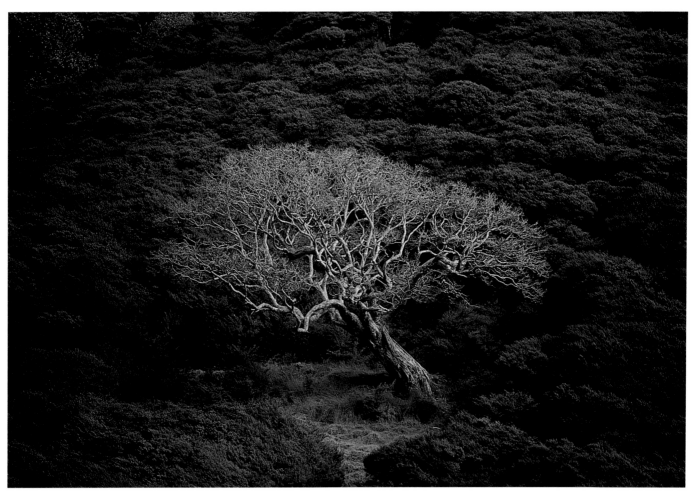

In New Zealand I was intrigued by the contrast of the gray, dead limbs of a Putukawa tree against the live green foliage. Shooting with my Nikon N8008 and a 180mm lens, I framed the image tightly. I exposed for 1/250 sec. at f/4 on Kodachrome 64.

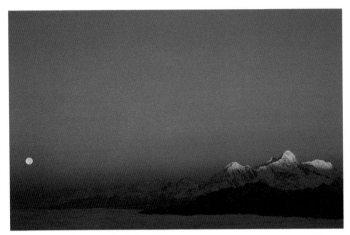

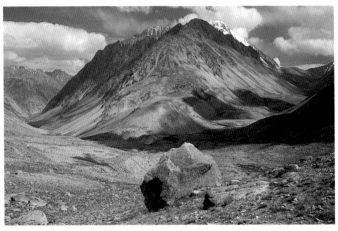

In Nepal, I photographed the full moon and the Annapurna massif using a 24mm wide-angle lens on my Nikon F3. I wanted the sky to dominate the frame, and the mountains and the moon to anchor the image. The exposure was 1/60 sec. at f/5.6 on Kodachrome 64.

In the Central Pamir Mountains of Tajikistan, I watched the shadow patterns flit across the landscape. I framed the large boulder in the foreground to echo the large hill in the background. With my Nikon F3 and a 24mm lens, I exposed for 1/60 sec. at f/11 on Kodachrome 64.

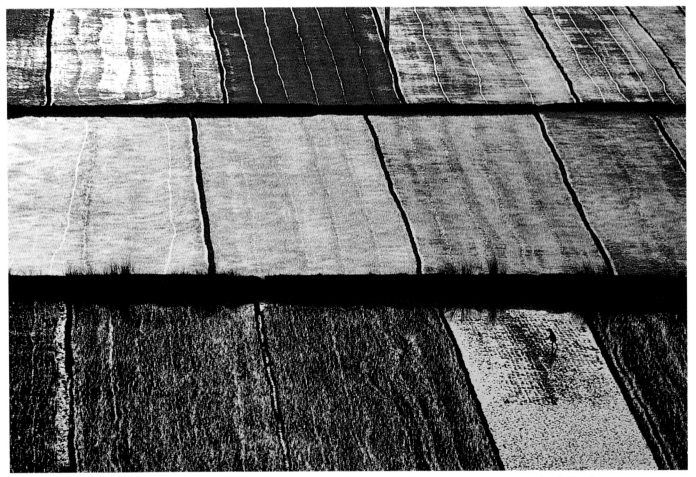

I was photographing the glare of the setting sun in some rice paddies in Vietnam's Nghia Binh Province when I realized that the composition would be improved by a higher perspective. So I ran up a hill and took this shot just before the sun disappeared. The small figure in the fields adds needed perspective. With my Nikon F3 and a 180mm lens, I exposed at f/8 for 1/125 sec. on Kodachrome 64.

USING WIDE-ANGLE LENSES

It is easy to be seduced into collecting lenses by the expectation that they'll help you make better photographs. They won't, and they don't make you a better photographer either, although they do extend your range and give you a wider choice of viewpoints. Each photographer has a preferred lens for landscape photography. I tend to favor wide-angle lenses even though I've heard that 18mm to 28mm wide-angle lenses are the hardest to learn to use properly. This may be true, but once you master the techniques, you'll find wide-angle lenses to be perfect for landscape photography.

Wide-angle lenses enable you to provide an interesting foreground while including background information for viewers. They give a perspective to the entire image. These lenses simply increase the area that can be included in a photograph beyond what is possible with standard lenses.

Wide-angle lenses also help you in tight places, such as narrow canyons, creating a sensation of dynamic space that strongly involves viewers. Using a longer-focal-length lens in such places won't give you the feeling of the space you're trying to photograph.

Changing your viewpoint has the most dramatic effect when you use wide-angle lenses. Because they include more of the subject close to the camera, moving just a yard or two to the left or right brings a completely different foreground into view. A high camera position is very effective on flat terrain where the horizon is relatively distant. Extend the tripod fully, and point your camera down to show just a sliver of the sky; this emphasizes the immensity and vastness of the open space.

A low camera angle is one of my favorite shooting positions. It is most effective when an object or large subject is relatively close to the camera, and the terrain isn't the most

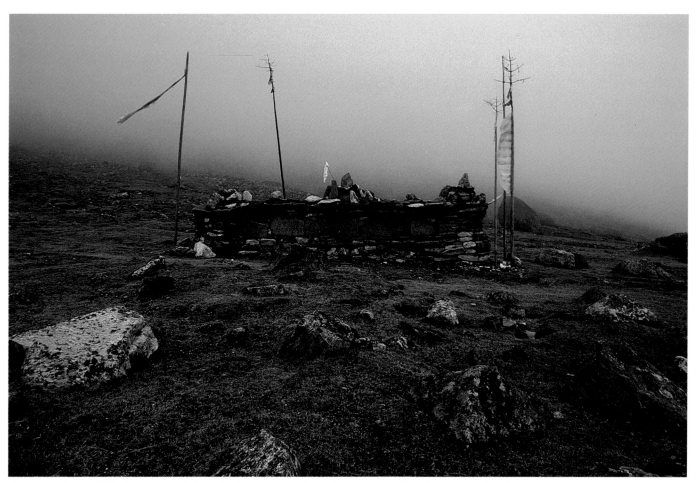

In Nepal's Barun Valley I accentuated the rocky field in front of a Buddhist mani wall, a bench stacked with stones carved with a prayer, to draw the viewer's eye toward the wall. Shooting with a Nikon F3 and a 24mm lens, I exposed for 1/30 sec. at f/8 on Kodachrome 64.

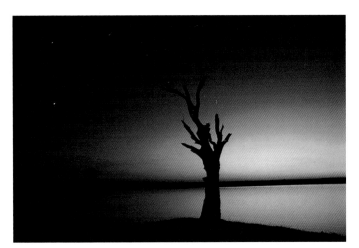

At sunrise along the Chobe River in Botswana, Africa, I set up my Nikon N8008 and a 20mm lens on a tripod low to the ground and shot up toward brightening sky from under the tree. The exposure was 1/15 sec. at f/8 on Kodachrome 64.

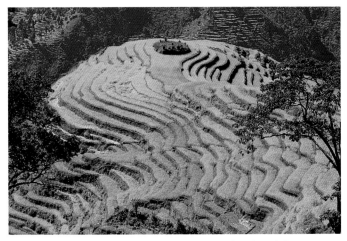

I was fascinated by the sinuous design and bright color of these rice fields in Nepal. I waited for the sun to illuminate the pattern. Then, for impact, I cropped the image close. With my Nikon F3 and a 180mm lens, I exposed for 1/250 sec. at f/5.6 on Kodachrome 64.

important element in the composition. It also works well for waterfalls and swiftly moving streams where the water appears to be flowing directly into your camera.

I often try to get close to my subject when I work with wide-angle lenses. Sometimes I'll be directly on top of a subject. For example, when I photograph flowers with a waterfall in the background, I am just inches from the flowers. As a result, the flowers dominate the larger scene.

I also try to use the smallest aperture I can to ensure all elements are sharp. And the best way to visually minimize

the effects of distortion is to compose so that there is no pronounced horizontal line. When you use a lens wider than 18mm, the distortion becomes harder to compensate for. In fact, it becomes so difficult to capture a true perspective of the scene that it is best to include the distortion as part of the image.

Trusting your camera's exposure meter is asking for trouble when you shoot with wide-angle lenses. An averaging meter opens up for the larger shadow areas, thereby overexposing the image. Aim a spot meter or center-weighted meter directly at whatever part of the scene is the most important to you.

When you use wide-angle lenses, your images are more susceptible to lens flare. If you use a lens shade or a polarizer, be careful that it fits the lens properly. Otherwise vignetting will occur. Pay attention to the edge of your frame. Unwanted objects somehow creep inside the frame if you aren't careful.

LENS SHARPNESS

Most lenses aren't at their sharpest at either end of their aperture scale. The best aperture for sharpness is two to three stops up or down from the limits of this scale. For example, if your 300mm telephoto lens has an $f/5.6$ minimum aperture, $f/11$ or $f/16$ will be the sharpest setting. Today's lenses are far better optically than those manufactured just a few years ago. The better telephoto lenses, such as the Nikon ED IF lenses made with low-dispersion glass, provide close-to-optimal sharpness even at the widest apertures. However, you pay significantly in cost and weight for this feature.

DETERMINING EXPOSURE

When shooting on a bright sunny day between midmorning and midafternoon, you can obtain correct exposure by using the sunny 16 rule. This calls for using an aperture of $f/16$ and the shutter speed that most closely approximates the film speed. For example, according to the sunny 16 rule, ISO 64 film calls for a shutter speed of 1/60 sec. at $f/16$, and ISO 100 film calls for a shutter speed of 1/125 sec. at $f/16$.

At most photography stores you can buy a Kodak Gray Card, which is invaluable when it comes to determining exposure. The card has an 18-percent reflectance, which is called middle gray. All light meters are calibrated to meter objects equal to a gray-card reflectance. I always keep one (or half of one) in my camera bag. In most low elevations at midday in the northern hemisphere, a cloudless sky is close to middle gray. At higher elevations, above 6,000 feet, the light reflected is darker than 18-percent gray. Pointing your camera away from the sun, meter off the middle-blue of the sky. You can also meter off green grass during the summer because it is also close to middle gray in tonal value.

In order to accurately determine exposure, keep in mind that for most Caucasians, the skin tone on the back of the hand is approximately 1 to 1 1/2 stops brighter than middle gray. If you are tan or have a red, yellow, brown, or black skin tone, experiment and adjust accordingly.

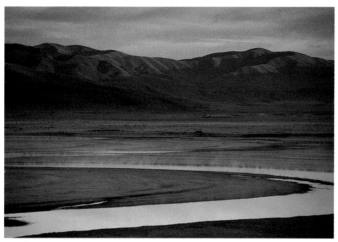

I took this photograph right before sunrise as the mist was lifting off the water. The curve of the river suggested motion as it wound its way across the landscape. Here, I used my Nikon F3 and a 50mm lens and exposed for 1/30 sec. at f/5.6 on Kodachrome 64.

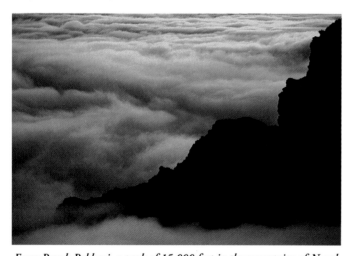

From Panch Pokhari, a peak of 15,000 feet in the mountains of Nepal, the clouds stretched below me like a giant sea. At sunset I photographed the changing colors, keeping a portion of a ridge in the frame to anchor the image. I exposed for the clouds, continually checking the meter reading as the light faded. With my Nikon N8008 and an 80-200mm zoom lens, I exposed Kodachrome 64 for 1/15 sec. at f/4.

ON SAFARI

There is more to adventure travel than an adrenaline rush, and there is more to adventure-travel photography than people, action, and landscapes. I'm not a wildlife photographer, but I knew that I had to go to Africa to see and photograph the animals in a vast, unbridled environment.

I was late coming to Africa. I always assumed that it was ruined—wrecked by decades of tourism. But a good friend kept encouraging me to go to Botswana, saying, "You won't be disappointed." So I went, and he was right. There is a majesty and mystery to Africa. The country has piqued the fantasies of writers and explorers for centuries. For me, Botswana evoked a visceral feeling that exposed a new viewpoint of the world. It was all those huge animals. I've spent many years in the outdoors, hanging from cliffs and being roughed up by raging waters, but all of those experiences seemed very tame and insignificant when I heard a lion roar outside my tent.

I didn't have the time, money, or experience to travel solo in the African bush. So I joined an organized safari. I was with seven other people who weren't photographers and who had their own agendas. Not only did I have to adapt my journalistic style to wildlife photography, but also to group demands. I had to make compromises to the group while remaining resolute to my photographic goals. This balancing act required diplomacy, stubbornness, good humor, and the ability to let go of photographs that weren't critical.

The same phenomenon that I've witnessed in foreign countries involving people photography is true for wildlife photography, too. Photographers become so excited about seeing something new that they immediately begin clicking shots without really looking to see what is around them. It isn't enough to just see the right animal; you have to consider the light source, the angle, the composition, the background, and the animal's behavior. All of these elements rarely come together at the same time, and hardly ever when you are ready to shoot.

Wildlife photography is demanding and rightly deserves its own special place in photography. Wildlife photographers don't just cavalierly saunter off in a jeep for a few hours and return loaded with rolls of brilliant photographs. Recording special wildlife images on film requires infinite patience, an insatiable curiosity, and a reservoir of behavioral knowledge.

It is inevitable that you'll miss a lot of shots. Capturing the emotion and behavior of animals is excruciatingly difficult. Those are the elusive, great moments. It seems like every time you get a chance, the sun is in front of you or you have the wrong lens on the camera. Sometimes you are lucky and get a great shot immediately. Usually, however, you have to sit, wait, and relax. The longer you linger near an animal, the more relaxed it'll become, and the better photographs you'll get. If you are serious about photographing wildlife, encourage your guide and safari group to stay awhile with a troupe of animals.

While on safari, I saw people driving their vehicles up to animals, taking a few shots, and then zooming on to the next attraction. Often people feel that after only a couple of pictures or even a couple of rolls of film, they've expended enough time, money, and energy on a particular animal and they just want to see something else.

No matter what you're shooting, you have to anticipate the best image and, if possible, move into position to get it. Often the most interesting picture isn't, for example, of an animal's head and horns, but of an environmental portrait. I approach many of my wildlife shots as if I'm photographing a landscape, incorporating the animals into the image.

Since I'm not an amateur zoologist, I didn't know what to anticipate in an animal's behavior. I often wasted film before I captured the relaxed or dynamic behavior. An animal's positions and expressions change continually, so you always have to be ready, with your camera to your eye. At the moment I intuitively know that I have a great shot, I don't hesitate to shoot a lot of film, sometimes even a whole roll or two. I bracket as I shoot, so that there are different exposures to choose from. I like heavily saturated images, but magazines often like ones that are less dense. Also, it is cheaper and easier to duplicate in the camera, and these bracketed exposures are insurance against loss or damage.

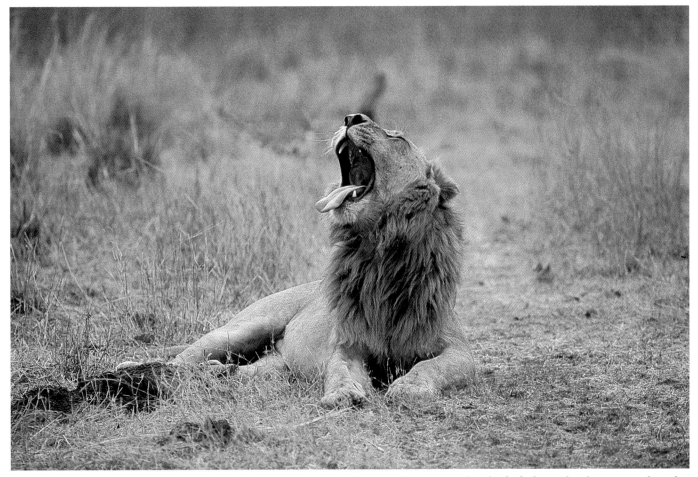

What safari would be complete without a lion? In Botswana, Africa, the lions usually laze around in the shade, languid and unconcerned. At the edge of the Moremi Reserve, my traveling companions and I parked our safari van next to a lion and lioness and watched them while they sunned themselves. Suddenly the lion raised its head and let out a loud roar. Since I had my Nikon N8008 and an 80-200mm zoom lens poised at my eye, I was able to catch this fleeting expression. The exposure was 1/250 sec. at f/4 on Kodachrome 64.

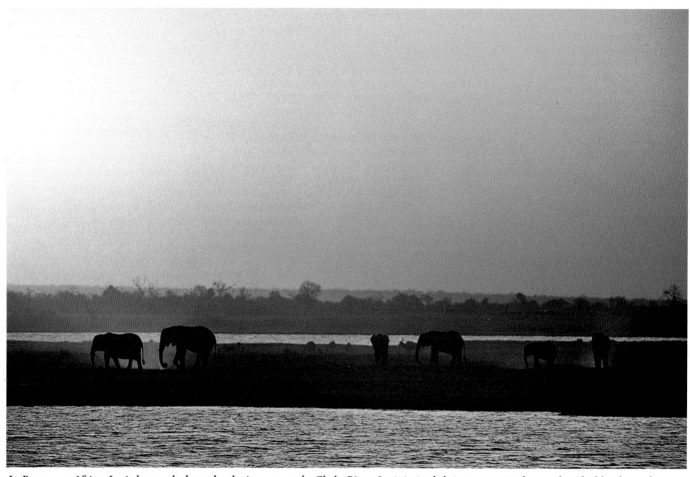

In Botswana, Africa, I spied some elephants lumbering over to the Chobe River. I minimized their presence in the sun-drenched landscape by including a lot of sky. Here, I used my Nikon N8008 and an 80-200mm zoom lens, and exposed for 1/250 sec. at f/5.6 on Kodachrome 64.

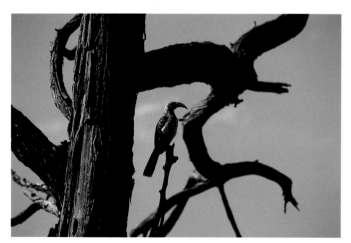

I find bird photography especially demanding. One day, however, I was fortunate enough to see a yellow hornbill perched on the limb of a dead tree. Its curved bill mimicked the curved branches so well that he seemed to become part of the tree. Shooting with my Nikon N8008 and a 300mm lens, I exposed for 1/500 sec. at f/4 on Kodachrome 64.

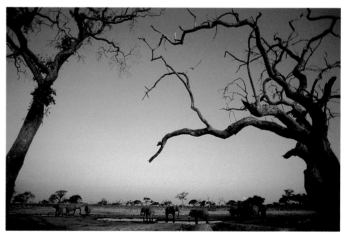

After photographing the elephants drinking water from every conceivable conventional angle at the famous watering hole at the Savuti swamp in Botswana, Africa, I decided to use a 20mm wide-angle lens on my Nikon N8008; I wanted to incorporate the limbs for an unusual image. The exposure was 1/60 sec. at f/8 on Kodachrome 64.

LOOKING BEYOND THE ANIMALS

The light in Botswana is fabulous. I had a very accommodating guide who uncomplainingly woke up at 4:30 A.M. and drove with me at dawn to the spot I'd selected the day before. Sometimes animals were present, but often they weren't. I focused on dead trees, termite mounds, branches, and the vast, interminable landscape.

It is easy to become myopic in a traveling situation, especially when there is a definite focus of attention, such as the wildlife in Africa. Occasionally it is important to take your attention off the parading wart hogs and shoot some of the other peripheral events around you, such as your safari mates and guides and

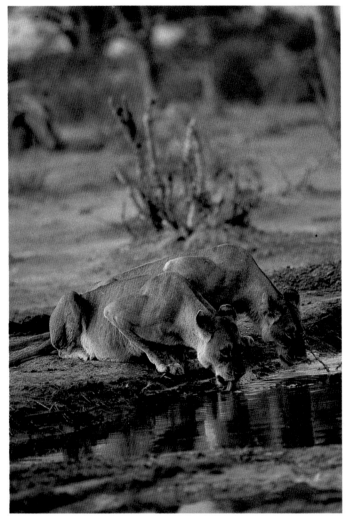

Just as my companions and I were leaving the waterhole at the Savuti swamp in Botswana, Africa, a pride of lionesses ambled over. The light was very low, but I placed my Nikon N8008 and a 300mm lens securely on a sandbag and shot a series of photographs using the motor drive. For this image, I exposed for 1/15 sec. at f/4 on Kodachrome 200.

camp scenes, particularly if you plan on putting together a slide presentation or album when you get home. Be alert to any details and lifestyle images that convey an element of the trip, such as coffee mugs on the table, the inside of your tent, or the campfire. Make a still life with found objects, baskets, feathers, and bones. Not only will this enhance your presentation, but also lead you toward an awareness of the entire journey.

WHAT TO BRING

While on safari in Africa I used two Nikon F3s with motor drives and a Nikon F4 with an array of lenses. These ranged from a 300mm f/2.8 lens with a 1.4X tele-extender to a 20mm wide-angle lens. I'd mounted different lenses on the three camera bodies and loaded two with Kodachrome 64 and one with Kodachrome 200. I shot a lot of Kodachrome 200 on this trip; I needed the speed for handholding long lenses and shooting in low light. I had one camera around my neck, and I kept the other two in my camera bag at my feet or beside me wrapped in a towel on the seat of the jeep, ready to be used in an instant. If you do wear more than one camera, adjust the camera straps so that they are at different lengths to prevent them banging into each other.

I carried this large arsenal of photographic gear in a Tamrac Super Pro camera bag that measured 18 inches wide, 10 inches deep, and 9 inches high. It was a formidable bag, big and heavy. Actually I brought too much equipment with me; there were a number of lenses I never even used.

The next time I go on safari, I plan to bring: two or three camera bodies, a 400mm lens (with 2X and 1.4X tele-extenders), a 300mm f/2.8 or f/4.5 lens, an 80-200mm f/2.8 lens, a 35-70mm f/2.8 lens, a 24mm f/2.8 lens, and a 20mm f/2.8 lens. If I want to travel really light, I'll bring only: two camera bodies, a 400mm lens (with 2X and 1.4X tele-extenders), a 100-300mm f/4.5-5.6 lens, a 35-70mm f/2.8 lens, and a 20mm f/2.8 lens.

A 400mm lens is a great choice, but it is expensive and requires a tripod. A 300mm f/2.8 lens is also expensive, heavy, and difficult to hold steady without a monopod or tripod. Using a 300mm f/4.5 lens means losing 1 1/3 stops of light, but it can be handheld. One stop can often mean the difference between being able to shoot a fine-grain film, such as Fujichrome 50 or Kodachrome 64, rather than a grainier ISO 200 film. Bear in mind that depth of field at 25 feet with a wide-open 300mm f/2.8 lens is a mere 2 inches. An autofocus lens can be indispensable for a range that small.

You can also use a 300mm lens with two tele-extenders (2X and 1.4X) to achieve the equivalent of three large lenses—a 300mm, 420mm, and 600mm—but with the weight of only the 300mm lens and two small tele-extenders. You lose some quality when you attach a tele-extender to a lens. If, however, you use a lens of good optical quality, the loss won't be significant. But if you use a marginal-quality lens, the loss will be perceivable. You lose one stop of light with a 1.4X tele-extender and two stops with a 2X tele-extender.

Bring a camera bag that is large enough so that all of your equipment is readily accessible and your lenses don't pound against each other as the jeep bounces along on the rough dirt roads. Be sure to bring a flash, too. You can use it for fill at any time of the day, and it adds a sense of mystery to and enhances the mood of dusk shots. Keep your camera on the quietest mode possible.

Tripods can be an awkward item to have in a safari jeep. Monopods are better, and you can find tripod clamps specially made for attaching to windows or jeep bars. I brought an empty pillowcase with me, filled it with Kalahari sand the first day of the trip, and kept it on the roof of the jeep for the remainder of the safari. It supported both the camera body and lens, and I was confident that my photographs were free of camera motion at the lower f-stops. However, I did have a tripod with me for shooting outside the jeep.

To protect your cameras and lenses from the all-pervasive dust, wrap them in cotton scarves or a small towel. You can also use Domke Protective Wraps, which are padded cloths with Velcro corners. Keep skylight filters on all your lenses.

A pocket minicassette recorder makes it easy to quickly make a log of photo notes, animal and bird names, and your guide's anecdotes. A tan lightweight vest is indispensable for holding your small lenses, binoculars, tape recorder, and

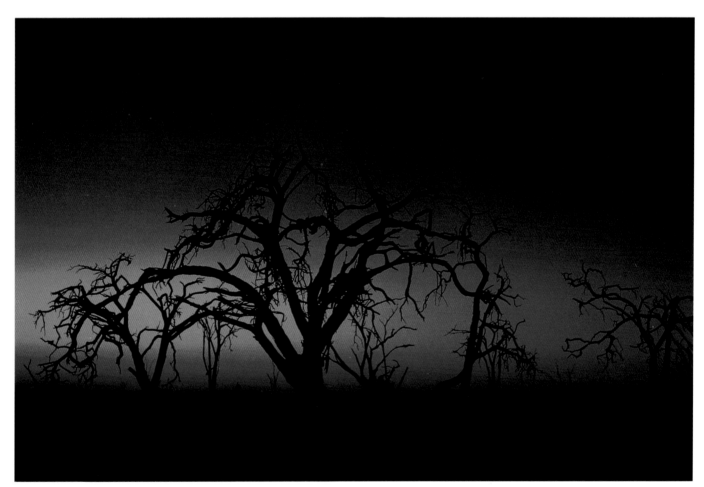

I was captivated by the light in Botswana, Africa, as well as by the whimsical shapes of the dead trees. One evening I pleaded with my guide to drive me to a particular spot at 4:30 A. M. the next morning so that I could photograph the trees silhouetted against the red sky at dawn. Luckily he agreed, and I was able to get this dramatic shot. Working with my Nikon N8008 and a 20mm wide-angle lens, I exposed at f/8 for 1/15 sec. on Kodachrome 64.

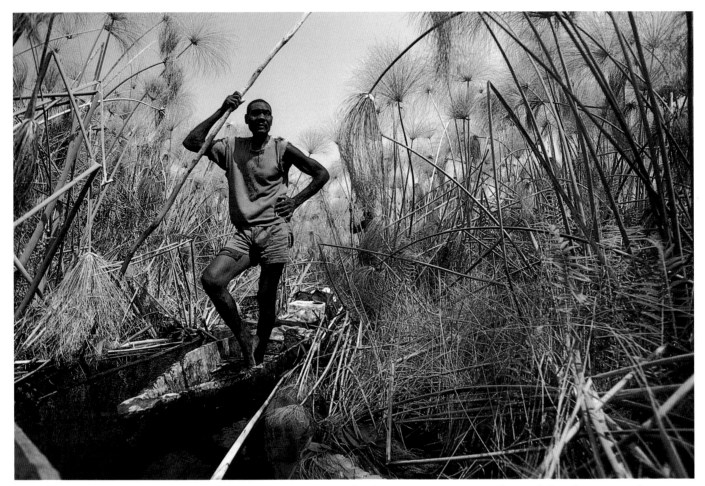

I traveled through the Okavango Delta on a wooden makoro boat for a few days. As my companions and I passed through papyrus reeds on channels created by hippopotamuses, I turned around and photographed the guide as he paused for a rest. I used a 20mm wide-angle lens on my Nikon N8008 in order to include him and the encroaching reeds. The opposing triangles formed by the guide's arms and right leg draw the viewer's eye. The exposure was 1/125 sec. at f/8 on Kodachrome 64.

sundry items when you take short walks outside the jeep. Always wear cool, lightweight-cotton clothes to combat the heat. Khaki is the best color for not showing dust or disturbing the animals. Don't forget a travel alarm clock for early-morning wake-up calls, sunscreen, and a hat or visor.

TRAVELING ON A SAFARI TOUR

On a photo tour you have the advantage of being among like-minded people who wake up before dawn and are out until dark photographing. You're also jockeying for space and position, with elbows, tripods, and long lenses perpetually in your way. I enjoyed being with people with diverse interests. The avid game- and birdwatchers sat up on the roof of the jeep keeping an eye for movement and any breach in their prey's camouflage, while I stalked the light and promising compositions.

There is a fine line between being courteous to your jeep-mates and getting the shot you want. Be intent on taking the photographs you want, when you want, for as long as you want. Simply be as patient with your colleagues when they want to stop and gaze at a yellow hornbill.

I was on a "luxury-tented safari." The luxury was certainly nice, but the invaluable part was not having to sacrifice any of my photography time worrying about logistics. A less-expensive alternative is a participatory safari, where you set up the tents and help with the meals. These trips are great fun, but not always appropriate for photographers who want to be in the field at first light, rather than cooking breakfast. A small group is best, certainly no bigger than eight. Finally, traveling with guides who are knowledgeable, patient, and sympathetic to, or at least tolerant of, your photographic needs is critical.

PART 7

PREPARING FOR YOUR TRIP

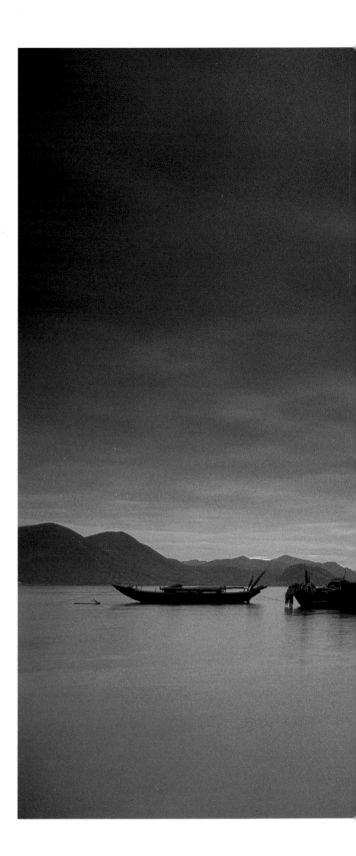

When planning your adventure, you must first decide what kind of adventure suits you. If you are an experienced traveler and have outdoor skills, you can penetrate deep into remote regions on your own or with a harmonious group of friends. If you've never been on a wilderness trip or traveled outside the United States, you should join an organized adventure-travel trip with a reputable company. There are many varieties of adventures, from jeep safaris in Africa to rugged mountaineering trips in the Himalayas. Pick one that suits your skills, fitness level, and dreams. And while you travel, remain flexible and maintain a sense of humor because everything that can go wrong probably will.

Don't expect that you can suddenly go from a sedentary lifestyle into a wild "Indiana Jones" adventure. Whatever type of journey you decide to take, you should be in excellent physical health. I recommend getting a thorough physical examination before you set off on any rugged journey. In fact, most adventure-travel companies require one.

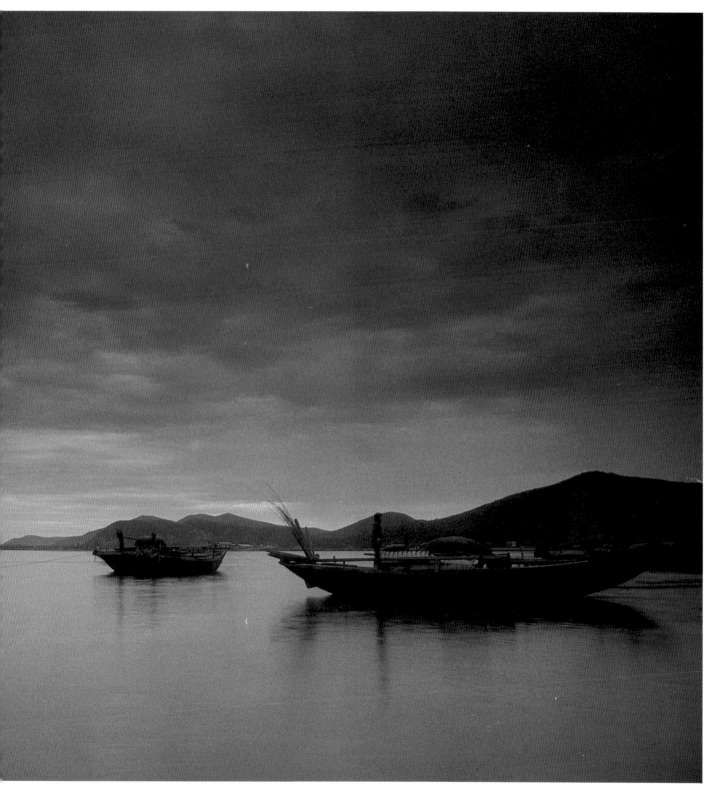

One morning in Vietnam's Nghe Tinh Province, I drove down to the beach at Cua Lo to shoot the fishing boats against the red sunrise. But when the darkness began to lift, I saw a deep blue sky; a storm was approaching. I mounted my Nikon F4 on a tripod and put a split ND filter on my 85mm lens to darken the sky. The overall cold blue tone enhances the mystery of this scene. I exposed for 1/8 sec. at f/5.6 on Kodachrome 64.

Just as important as your physical stamina is your mental stamina. Cultural shock is considerable in the so-called "undeveloped" countries. Customs, religions, and government regulations differ, and laws can be confusing and convoluted. Other problems are matters of comfort and convenience. Tap water isn't always suitable for drinking. And inclement weather, fouled-up air schedules, and other unforeseeable and uncontrollable events may cause delays or other situations that are impossible to resolve quickly. If you can't accept these kinds of problems graciously or if rude surprises cause you to blow your stack, you should think twice before undertaking a journey that is too far off the beaten track.

HOW TO GET THERE

In the modern world of transportation buying an airline ticket and finding yourself on the other side of the globe the next day are relatively effortless processes. Since the deregulation of the airlines, there are numerous ticket options and prices available. Finding the best offer just takes a little research. If you can travel Monday through Thursday and are willing to buy a "nontransferable, nonrefundable, restrictions-apply" ticket at least three weeks ahead of time, you can save a substantial amount of money. Consider an "around-the-world" excursion fare if you'll be traveling to different continents. To find these bargains, look in the Sunday travel sections of the *New York Times* or the *Los Angeles Times* for advertisements for inexpensive ticket fares. If you need a ticket that is open-ended, refundable, and changeable, you'll have to pay a higher price.

There are also more exotic modes of overseas transportation, such as traveling on steamer ships or hitching rides on sailing cruises. Although more romantic in concept, they are also more expensive and require a greater time commitment. Some tramp steamers, which are cargo-carrying freighter ships, are licensed to carry passengers in conjunction with their standard freight. Tramp steamers can take you virtually anywhere in the world, from Sri Lanka to Melbourne, or from Rotterdam to Mombasa; they embark from a number of East Coast, West Coast, Gulf, and Canadian ports. Depending on the freighter company and the itinerary, you can travel anywhere from two weeks to six months. The accommodations can be quite plush and the atmosphere convivial. The cost is less than that of a luxury cruise, but still more expensive than that of an airplane ticket. Also, you sometimes have to make your plans a year or more in advance. It is essential to remember that the major function of freighters is transporting cargo, so schedules and ports of call are solely determined by the shipping needs of the companies whose products the freighters are carrying. As a result, the ports of call may change at any time. Consult a local travel agent for names of freighter lines.

Hitching a ride on a small yacht is a good idea if you are a seasoned sailor, but captains often look for cooks or inexperienced deckhands. This kind of travel requires time and a commitment to hanging around yacht clubs and marinas in order to find out about potential openings on cruise ships.

Once you arrive at a foreign destination your options multiply: you can ride trains, buses, and trucks (in some places truck travel replaces local-bus travel). You can also hitch, but this isn't one of your safer options in most parts of the world. It is best to consult with other travelers about the various local-transportation options. Always hedge on the side of safety; pay attention to your instincts. The naive often end up with their luggage being stolen, or worse, by trusting the wrong people.

TRAVELING ALONE

Sometimes I have a yen to travel somewhere at a particular time, and no one is able to join me. So I go alone. This isn't as impressive as it sounds, but it is rewarding. The truth is that when you are by yourself, you meet more people than when you travel with a companion. You also experience a country and its people in a way that is impossible when you are with another person or a group. Being solely responsible for transporting your gear and arranging all the logistics is tiring and time-consuming, but you're compensated by a very real freedom to come and go exactly as you please.

It is easier for me to travel alone when my primary purpose is photography. I can go at my own pace and not feel guilty for holding anyone up. I can stand on a street corner or on the top of a Himalayan ridge for hours and wait patiently for my perfect moment without having to account to anyone. Traveling alone isn't for everyone, but if you are an avid traveler, I definitely recommend going on a solo trip once in your life.

Some places off the main traveling arteries aren't suitable for women alone; other areas can even be dangerous, such as some Moslem countries, southern Pakistan, and the hills of Morocco. Although I've never had any trouble traveling alone, I am aware that as a woman I need to be more cautious and alert in places where a man wouldn't think twice. This is unfortunate, but it is a reality. When I feel uncomfortable in places or situations, I'll often team up with a group of people that I met along the way.

TRAVELING IN A GROUP

Traveling in a remote area with friends over an extended period of time can mean experiencing camaraderie at its finest. However, it takes a good deal of cooperation to plan the details and the route and to coordinate all the different aspects of a long trip. Mountaineering and other expedition leaders very carefully consider not only the skill level of their potential members, but also the compatibility. The dynamics of the group often can make or break the success of an expedition's outcome.

Some of my best trips have been with friends. Nevertheless, I'd be very wary about going to a remote, rugged mountain range with people who had very limited experience traveling outdoors. Choose an expedition that matches the experience and expertise of the group, and vice versa. On all the remote-travel trips I've gone on, I've been with companions who have extensive experience in the outdoors and traveling experience in foreign countries.

Unless your companions are photographers as well, chances are that they won't be too enthusiastic about stopping every two minutes for you to shoot pictures, or about your dashing out in the middle of dinner to chase the sunset. The key in situations like this is to make deals, such as "If I don't have to cook dinner, I'll clean the dishes," and stick to them. This will not only mollify your companions, but will also help you to relax and enjoy your trip.

There are often many bewildering and perplexing moments when you travel, especially in places like China and India. It is helpful to be with someone in order to support each other through the difficult moments, such as missing a train or finding a good place to eat. Traveling with a friend also means having someone to share the high and low points of the trip with, and you can rotate responsibilities and logistical chores.

An organized tour is another option. If the convenience and security of having prearranged hotel, transportation, and logistical plans sound appealing, a group tour is definitely for

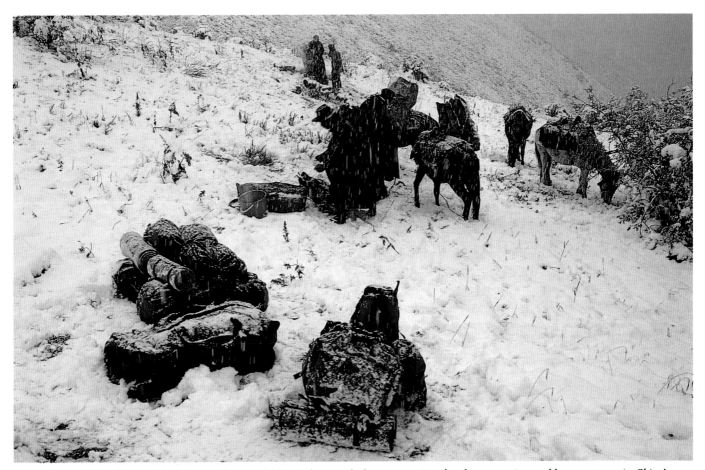

Protecting my Nikon F3 and 24mm lens with an umbrella, I photographed my companions breaking camp in a sudden snowstorm in China's Sichuan Province.

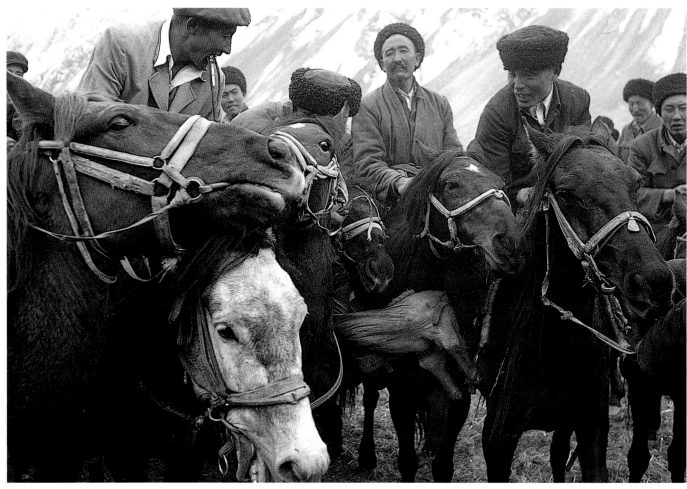

While I was staying in a Kirghiz village in China's Pamir Mountains, I was beckoned to join a group of villagers who were heading off on horseback in their best clothes. Even though we didn't speak the same language, it was clear that they wanted me to bring my cameras and that we were going someplace special. I was thrilled when we arrived at a game of bozkashi, a Turkish variation of polo played on horseback with the skinned body of a goat. At the end of the game, I walked up to the players and captured this moment with my Nikon F3 and a 24mm wide-angle lens. The exposure was 1/125 sec. at f/8 on Kodachrome 200.

you. Group tours enable you to meet new friends with shared interests and to benefit from the savings that come with traveling in numbers. There is a plethora of adventure-travel companies that run every trip imaginable in practically every crevasse and corner of the world. As a photographer, you have the choice of going on an organized adventure tour for laypersons or experienced travelers, or on a tour designed specifically for photographers.

If you're traveling on an organized tour, you may not have much control over your time, so be sure to select one with a relaxed pace, not one that tries to cover as much ground as possible. Talk to the tour leaders ahead of time and explain why you are there and that you need a certain amount of time on your own; doing this will help them understand when you

rush off from the group to photograph. Go out of your way to be polite and considerate. Try to do most of your work on your own. You aren't, of course, obliged to join the group for events that don't interest you. Be prepared to have your breakfasts and dinners late in order to free yourself up during the perfect light. Inevitably anytime you combine traveling with a group and photography, you'll have to make compromises. The challenge is to minimize them.

Unlike most conventional tours, the numerous photography tours are designed around photographic opportunities rather than around mealtimes. Planned with photography in mind, the tour schedules usually include special events or colorful festivals. In addition, you have the advantage of being with a group of people with a similar aim and focus.

It is important for you to check the qualifications of your tour guide. Ideally the guide will be a photographer who knows how to impart his or her knowledge to others. Many photographers are brilliant in the darkroom, but not in the classroom. Does the guide have a column in a photography magazine or regularly teach workshops? If that is true, get references from former workshop participants.

HOW TO SELECT AN ADVENTURE-TRAVEL COMPANY

Before you send your money to a tour operator you need to ask a number of questions. First, is the company reliable, with a proven record of successful tour operations? How long has

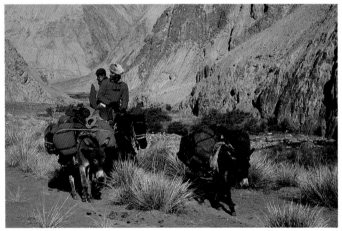

Here, a friend and I are on the final leg of a journey in the Pamir Mountains in Xinjiang Province in China.

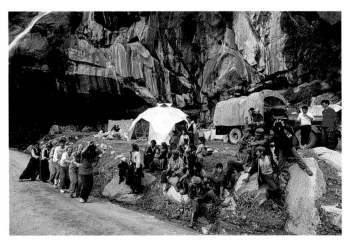

I photographed my bicycle-tour members and Tibetans doing the "Bunny Hop" outside Maerkam Town in Sichuan Province in China.

the company been in business? Does the company actually run the trip itself, or does it subcontract local outfitters? (With so many destinations, most companies subcontract some of their trips to other outfitters abroad that they've established a reliable working relationship with.) Quality control is a key factor, so it is always a good idea to get references from people who've already gone on a trip.

Next, you should carefully explore the package. What's included in the cost of the trip? Are there hidden costs, such as meals or local air fares? What equipment is provided? What is the level of physical activity? What is the guide-to-client ratio? What class of accommodations are offered? (In many remote areas, standard tourist facilities don't exist.) Is there a guaranteed departure? (Some companies cancel trips at the last minute if there is insufficient sign-on.) Is there tiered pricing? (Some companies vary the cost of a trip according to the number of participants.)

Finally, be aware that the tour leader or guide can make or break a trip. It is essential that the guide has been to the destination before and, preferably, is an expert in the area. In remote areas, it is helpful to have a Western guide, or at least one who understands Western predilections, as well as a local guide.

BEFORE YOU GO

Read everything you can put your hands on about the area where you'll be traveling, and pore through picture books and travel guides. For example, find out what is unique about the place, which tribes live there, and what their customs are. Do your homework before you go; know, as best you can, what is permissible legally and culturally. If you're planning an international trip, obtaining a passport should be one of your first steps. There is an additional fee if you need to apply in person in order to have the passport rush-processed. Your passport is valid for 10 years. Always keep it in a secure place, such as in a pouch under your shirt or a hotel or tour operator's safe. If you are unfortunate enough to lose your passport, contact the nearest United States Consulate or Embassy as soon as possible. Either one will have you fill out a "lost passport" report and issue you a replacement. For emergency assistance, call the Overseas Citizens' Emergency Center.

A visa is official permission from a foreign government to travel in that particular country. The visa is usually stamped into your passport, although some countries issue you a separate document. Each country has different visa requirements. Some countries require that you obtain a visa before your arrival, while others issue visas at an official border station. Requirements for obtaining a visa continually change. It is best to get them from the consulate of the nation you want to visit. (You can find the addresses and telephone numbers of these agencies through any knowledgeable travel agent or from a guidebook.)

Carry most of your money in the form of United States traveler's checks. Internationally recognized brands are accepted more readily than lesser-known traveler's checks. A combination of small and large denominations is best. When I fly into a new city or country, I usually exchange a small amount of money at the airport. In town I ask or look around to see where the best place is to change money. Sometimes it makes a big difference. For example, in Hong Kong you can lose a great deal of money at the street exchangers. For the intrepid, sometimes there is a black market. In some countries you can get a much better rate for your dollar, but, remember, the black market is illegal and can be dangerous.

You can also get money from an American Express office by writing a personal check on your home bank account. For a long trip this is a safer way to obtain funds instead of carrying a large wad of bills. But this works only when you travel through major cities. I always bring some United States dollars in small denominations. Some countries, such as Vietnam, prefer cash. Make sure that you do some research on how to bring your money for each country before you leave.

Major credit cards are accepted in most places around the world. The exchange rate that applies to a credit-card purchase is the one prevailing on the date of the bank notification. This can work for or against you since the charge often takes up to three months to show up on your bill.

Depending on your foreign destination, you might need proof of vaccination before crossing a border. Consult your County Public Health Service, your personal physician, or the Center for Disease Control (CDC). CDC has a very useful

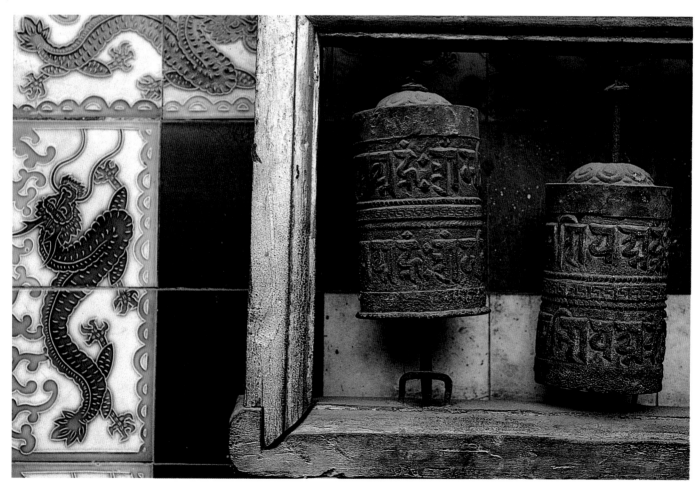

I shot these prayer wheels in a small shrine in Patal, Nepal. Handholding my Nikon N8008 and 50mm macro lens, I exposed Kodachrome 64 for 1/30 sec. at f/5.6.

automated hotline that gives travelers current information on disease prevention anywhere in the world. So does the State Department's Citizens Emergency Center.

HOW TO TRAVEL LIGHT

I have a large repertoire of cameras to fit a variety of occasions. I rarely take all of my equipment with me on my travels. I tailor my photo gear to each situation, and I ask myself the crucial question, "Who's going to carry this stuff?" Sometimes I have porters, vehicles, horses, or camels with me, but more often than not the answer is, "Me." Lamentably, I've never been accused of traveling light. I certainly don't recommend that you emulate the amount of equipment I use. I envy travelers who carry only a small, lightweight backpack. If I weren't making my living from photography, I'd bring one or maybe two camera bodies, a 24-50mm lens, an 80-200mm ƒ/2.8 lens, a 20mm lens, and a strobe. This equipment would cover almost every shooting situation.

The actual weight of the equipment I carry varies between 15 and 50 pounds, depending on the lenses and film I take along for a particular trip. For day hikes or excursions I rarely carry more than 15 pounds of gear, including my daypack or duffel bag. On an overnight trip I try to keep the weight under 25 pounds. If I'm going on a long trip, I carry quite a bit of equipment, weighing between 25 and 50 pounds. However, I don't carry all that on my person every day; this amount includes film, backup equipment, accessories, and more lens options than are usually necessary. I keep most of the equipment in my duffel, suitcase, or pack during the day and switch gear to my daypack as needed. During a long trek, I have access to everything at camp in the morning and evening when the light is best. While on the trail I keep various lenses in my photo vest and carry one camera. I don't carry extensive lighting equipment or large-format cameras. The photographers who do, usually bring assistants with them.

CAMERAS

There have been some outstanding advances in cameras in the last decade, particularly in the field of autofocus. I used to be a true purist and worked with only manual cameras, feeling smug that I was a real photographer. But during the last few years I've altered my thinking. For certain subjects and shooting situations, such as horseback riding, kayaking, mercuric sports, and low light levels, there are definite advantages to using an autofocus camera.

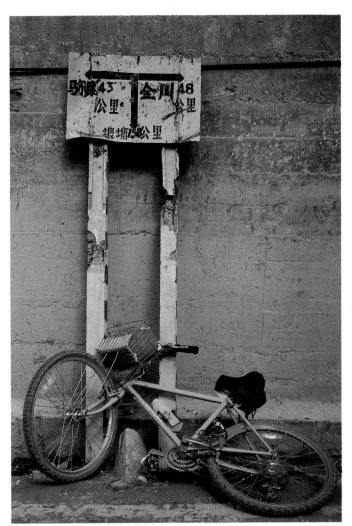

On one of my trips through China's Sichuan Province, I dropped my bike at the foot of a road sign and took this photograph. I liked the combination of colors and casualness. Shooting with my Nikon F3 and a 35mm lens, I exposed for 1/60 sec. at ƒ/8 on Kodachrome 64.

I have one Nikon F4 camera, two Nikon F3 cameras with motor drives, and one Nikon N8008 camera. The N8008 is becoming a favorite because of its lightweight construction and superb metering capabilities. I'm not abandoning my F3s; they are workhorses, and I like being able to remove the motor drive.

I'm convinced that complex professional cameras, such as the Nikon F4, require more expertise to operate than manual ones do. The marketing premise that automatic cameras are easier to use than manual cameras holds true only for simple cameras and artless expectations. After mastering the complex controls of the F4, I discovered that the camera's features enabled me to explore a new level of photography. But there is one drawback: I find the camera too large for most women's hand grips.

LENSES

Always buy the best lenses you can afford. Obscure "bargain" lenses are no bargain when it comes to shooting sharp pictures. In most cases, you are better off purchasing the same brand of lens as your camera. However, many lenses that are made by independent lens manufacturers do produce very sharp photographs if used properly, such as Tokina and Tamron. But you do get what you pay for.

I use a wide range of Nikon lenses, from 16mm to 400mm. I favor wide-angle lenses over telephoto lenses. Telephoto lenses are great but they are heavy, bulky, and expensive, so they are usually the first to be left behind. My armory of lenses includes: a 16mm $f/2.8$ lens, a 20mm $f/2.8$ lens, a 24mm $f/2.8$ lens, a 28mm $f/2.8$ perspective-control (PC) lens for correcting parallax in buildings or trees, a 35mm $f/1.4$ lens, a 35-70mm $f/2.8$ AF lens for autofocus and autoflash capability, a 55mm $f/2.8$ Micro-Nikkor closeup lens that works well as a standard lens, an 85mm $f/1.8$ lens (my favorite low-light portrait lens), a 180mm $f/2.8$ ED IF lens (Nikon's "ED IF" designation indicates that the lens is made with extra-low-dispersion glass that allows better registration and greater sharpness of primary and secondary colors on the film plane), an 80-200mm $f/2.8$ AF lens, a 300mm $f/4$ ED IF AF lens, and a 400mm $f/5.6$ ED IF lens. I also have a TC-14A teleconverter, which is a 1.4X teleconverter for lenses up to 300mm long, and a TC-14B teleconverter, which is a 1.4X teleconverter for lenses 300mm or more in length.

Until recently I shied away from zoom lenses, complaining that they weren't fast enough and that the optics were mediocre. However, they've improved dramatically in the past decade, thanks to the advancement of computer-assisted optical development and optical-glass manufacture. The ranges of both available speeds and focal lengths have expanded considerably. I now include zoom lenses in my camera bag, and I find them on my cameras more often than my old favorite single-focal-length lenses. Zoom lenses are perfect for travel photography; you can't beat the size and convenience. You can bring fewer lenses and have more flexibility because they let you use odd millimeters for cropping your compositions when you can't change your shooting position. The ability to frame precisely and quickly without changing lenses allows you to concentrate more fully on the subject.

FILTERS

Some photographers never use a filter on their lenses because it can degrade image sharpness. This is fine for studio work, but when I'm on the Mongolian Plateau with the wind hurling sand at my lenses or I'm working fast and changing lenses throwing them in my camera bag without their lens caps, I want a filter on my lenses. Filters are much cheaper to replace than lenses are. Use filters only as needed, one at a time, and only those of superb optical quality. At low altitudes, I keep a Nikon skylight filter on each of my lenses; at high altitudes, I use ultraviolet (UV) filters. These filters remove some of the blue haze and ultraviolet haze, respectively, that are found in most outdoor scenics.

Polarizers cut through high-altitude glare to strengthen the subtle color of rock and to improve the separation between the white of clouds or snowcaps and the blue of the sky. These

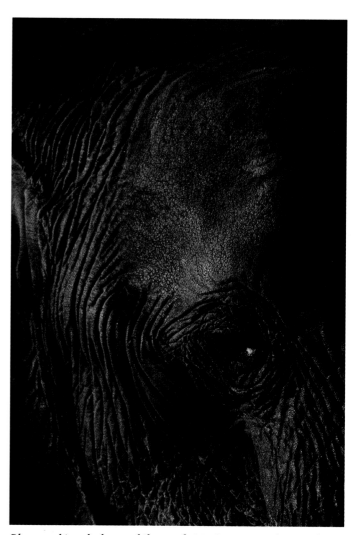

Photographing elephants while on safari in Botswana, Africa, I often focused on a detail of an animal. For this closeup, I used a 300mm telephoto lens on my Nikon F3 to frame the thick, tough folds of skin around the elephant's eye. The exposure was 1/250 sec. at f/4 on Kodachrome 64.

filters also reduce glare on water, increase visibility by cutting through haze, and cut down on reflections caused by moisture in and on plants (especially in humid countries). A polarizer won't have much of an effect on an image unless the camera's pointed approximately 90 degrees away from the sun. You lose 1 to 1 1/2 stops with a polarizer in place. Use a circular polarizer (as opposed to a linear polarizer) with an autofocus camera. With a wide-angle lens 20mm and lower, you tend to see the gradation shifts of the polarizer, going from dark blue in the center of the sky to a lighter blue at the edges.

To subtly enhance a warm feeling in an image I'm shooting in the late-afternoon sun or at sunset, I use an 81A, 81B, or 81C warming filter; these filters warm the tone of the reflected light in degrees of increasing intensity. I also keep an assortment of Cokin and Tiffen graduated and ungraduated color filters, including gray, sepia, yellow, sunset, mauve, and blue filters. No one likes to admit to using colored filters. I use them once in awhile to enhance a subtle color, to give a kick to a scene, or to try and salvage a seemingly hopeless situation.

LIGHTING EQUIPMENT

Unless you're doing a large commercial shot and you need to lug large, expensive studio strobes with you, you should avoid bringing any flash other than the one built into your camera or a shoe-mount unit. I use a Nikon SB-24 flash. Frankly, this flash is a miracle worker, offering a variety of settings, particularly for fill flash. The biggest disadvantage of an electronic flash is the inability to previsualize its effect. Even though the latest cameras do a remarkable job of automating fill flash, for optimal results your exposures need to be thought out carefully. Run tests of your flash before you set out on any trip.

Reflectors can be made of anything that reflects light. Usually they are made out of fabric or some sort of hard board. While traveling you can use bedsheets or aluminum foil, or you can bring a collapsible lightweight reflector. I sometimes bring a Flexfill 38-inch gold/white reflector for bouncing sunlight into shadows. Using a reflector usually requires an assistant. During my travels I find it easy to enlist the services of a bystander or a friend to help me.

Attach a bouncer to your flash to help diffuse and soften harsh shadows. I use both the LumiQuest Ultrasoft and the LumiQuest 80/20, which has holes to send 80 percent of the light to the ceiling and a flat area to direct the rest of the light forward, filling in shadows under people's eyes. The reflectors attach to your flash with Velcro and fold up compactly for storage in your camera bag.

TRIPODS

Although bringing a tripod with me means carrying extra weight, I always do. When it comes to choosing a tripod, the goal is to bring the lightest but sturdiest one possible for your purposes. A tripod that is too heavy to carry with you is useless. A tripod that weighs between 1 and 2 pounds is fine for small, lightweight cameras, but I find that this weight is too light for either a Nikon F3 or F4. I have a 4-pound Gitzo 226 Reporter Mode Performance tripod, which I keep in a custom-made zippered Cordura case with a shoulder strap. When I need to travel lighter, I bring a 3-pound Gitzo 106 Total Luxe tripod with me.

Of course, for the sharpest photographs you'll need your sturdiest tripod. Don't use the center post to increase the height of the camera; extend the legs fully instead. Elevating the center post turns the tripod into a unipod, which destabilizes the whole system. To help stabilize a tripod you can hang your camera bag, a heavy "stuff" sack, or a plastic bag filled with rocks, sand, or water from the center of the tripod. Hang a heavy towel over the barrel of a long lens for extra stability. Remember to recheck your image for possible focus shift. A cable release separates the camera from your body motion, preventing the transfer motion during the exposure. Whenever I use a tripod, I ordinarily use a cable release on my camera; the only exceptions are when I'm following motion or shooting with a flash.

Always lock up the mirror before each exposure, and use a cable release. Many SLR cameras have vibration problems from 1/30 sec. to 1/2 sec., particularly with lenses that are 200mm or longer. Unfortunately, many of the new cameras, such as the Nikon N8008, lack a mirror-lockup button. I'm forced to use one of my Nikon F3 or F4 bodies instead of my N8008 when I use a tripod; furthermore, the N8008 doesn't have a cable-release outlet. If your camera doesn't have a mirror-lockup button, you can use the self-timer button and put a motor drive on the camera body to absorb vibrations. Another option is to avoid shutter speeds between 1/15 sec. and 1/4 sec. by using either a faster shutter speed and a larger f-stop, or a slower shutter speed and a smaller f-stop. I've found that 1/15 sec. is especially bad on most cameras. When you use either wide-angle or standard lenses, you don't have to be overly concerned about mirror vibration. But you should still use a tripod whenever possible.

If you're working without a tripod, roll up a garment—the bulkier the better—into a ball, or jam it inside a stuff sack. Then prop it up on a window, a rock, or against a tree or building and push the camera deep into the garment. You can also brace yourself and, if possible, the camera firmly against a tree, building, or some other solid object. Take a breath, and then exhale before pressing the shutter-release button. Since most shutter-release buttons depress two-thirds of the way before they click, remember to depress the button slowly and gently to avoid camera movement.

I prefer a ball head over a two-axis tilt head. A good ball head facilitates panning on a moving person or animal, and you can quickly position the camera to focus on a stationary subject. Landscape photography benefits from the ease of correcting horizons and changing from a vertical to a horizontal format. For closeup work the ball head allows quicker and easier positioning of the camera, especially in awkward positions low to the ground. Choosing the best ball head differs from photographer to photographer. I use both the Gitzo Ball 2 Head and the Arca Swiss Monoball B1. Slick and Bogen also make a range of excellent ball heads.

The Kenyon Gyro Stabilizer KS 4 is a portable stabilizing system that you can use for shooting from boats, cars, kayaks, and helicopters, and even for handholding cameras with long lenses at very slow shutter speeds. The KS 4 is a small pod that fits beneath a camera or lens and resists any quick movements transmitted to the assembly. The pod weighs 2 pounds, 2 ounces and is attached to a battery pack that weighs 5 1/2 pounds. This advanced technology isn't cheap—it sells for close to $2,000—but it solves problems that aren't easy to resolve any other way.

ACCESSORIES

Lens shades and caps are the items usually left behind when you pack for a trip, so you should double-check to make sure that you have yours before you leave. Lens shades block glare on the front elements of your lens and are the often overlooked cause of flat colors in a final photograph. You can also use your hand to shade the lens, but this is awkward. It isn't always effective either because the photographer's hand often ends up in the corner of the picture.
I'm continually ferreting lens caps out of my pockets and camera bag after a frenetic spat of shooting. One solution is the CapKeeper. This disc-on-the-end-of-a-cord adheres to the lens cap, and the other end of the cord, both of which are elastic, hooks to the camera or around the lens.

Batteries fit into two broad categories, rechargeable and nonchargeable. You can reuse rechargeable batteries many times, which is convenient for travel photography, but only if you'll be near an electrical socket and you have an electrical 110/220 converter. I prefer bringing extra AA batteries with me

since I am usually far from electrical outlets for long periods of time, even though the practice is more expensive and translates into more weight in my bag.

When carrying a light bag is a primary factor, I depend solely on the light meter in my camera. At other times, I bring an incident meter. These meters are very helpful in difficult shooting situations when the light's rapidly changing. Handheld incident meters have a white diffusion dome and measure the brightness of the light falling on them. When using an incident meter, stand next to your subject and point the white sphere toward the main light source. This will be more or less in the direction you'll be photographing. You want to know the brightness of the light source, such as whether it is from the sun or the sky (as in backlit situations).

Split-image focusing devices and microprisms, which are usually found on most standard focusing screens, are intended to help you focus sharply. However, they always seem to obscure my view of the subject and hinder focusing. So I replace them with a grid screen that's commonly used for shooting architecture. The vertical and horizontal lines help me keep horizons level and compose. However, you should experiment with one before you invest in it. Some people find them more difficult to focus than split-image screens, especially in low-light conditions. You can also replace your standard screen with a Beattie Intenscreen. This is at least one stop brighter than most camera screens, and is also available in a grid.

Years ago cameras had thin, nylon straps that dug grooves into your shoulder. Today you can buy thick straps that help absorb the weight of the camera. I have Optech Straps on all my cameras. As a result of the shock-absorbing qualities of the thick-neoprene strap, I can easily carry two or three Nikon F3 or F4 cameras without serious stress. Domke also makes a good strap, the Gripper Strap; it has rubber tracks woven into its entire length, so it grips your shoulder and the swiveling hooks keep the camera flat against your body.

I always carry the camera and flash manuals in my accessory bag. No matter how well I know my cameras, the manuals save me from a lot of aggravation and fiddling when I try a technique I haven't used in a long time.

CAMERA BAGS

Most travel and outdoor photographers know that the proper transportation, protection, and maintenance of equipment are critical. Photographic equipment is fragile and expensive, and if you want it to remain in good working condition, you'll need to find a suitable means of protecting it during transportation or storage. I have two systems for choosing and packing my camera bag. One is designed for efficient traveling, and the other for responsive shooting. The first, which stresses protection and compactness, I use while en route to somewhere. I use the second when I arrive at my destination and convert my bag to shooting mode.

When I'm carrying a full array of photographic gear, I use the enormous Tamrac 614 Super Pro bag, which measures 18 inches wide, 10 inches deep, and 9 inches high. I also pack one or two smaller camera bags in my checked luggage for later use. The Super Pro holds my two motor-driven Nikon F3 or F4 bodies and one Nikon N8008, as well as eight lenses. The bag also has voluminous pockets for meters, filters, and film. A giant pocket underneath the bag holds my 3-pound Gitzo tripod or a 300mm or 400mm telephoto lens. As you can imagine the bag is monstrous, and I usually transport it around airports on a wheeled cart. As an alternative, I use an Eagle Creek Overland Carry-On bag. I pack it full with a Tamrac 610 bag, which is 15 inches wide, 6 inches deep, and 9 inches high, or a 709 Pro Convertible, which is 13 1/2 inches wide, 6 inches deep, and 9 inches high, as well as with my other carry-on items. The Tamrac 709 bag satisfies Federal Aviation Agency (AAA) carry-on regulations and has a backpack harness that I can zip inside a custom pocket for storage. I either keep any big lenses that don't fit into my camera bag in separate cases or wrap them in Domke Protective Wraps.

If necessary you can check your gear as luggage in a hard camera case, such as a Haliburton, but make sure that it's locked and isn't obviously a camera case. Then put the case inside a scruffy duffel bag for extra security. Hard cases work best for shooting in places where you need to protect your gear from water and dust, such as on river trips and safaris. Remember, though, they are much more awkward and harder to carry for long periods of time.

Packing your carry-on camera bag means getting the most equipment in the least amount of space, while paying special attention to protecting your equipment. Figuring out how to pack everything you need into a 9 × 14 × 22-inch space beneath your airline seat is a puzzle. Sometimes you can get away with an extra bag on a flight, but most international airlines are becoming very strict about having more than one or two carry-on bags. You don't want to get stuck arguing with the airline attendant and risk having your cameras put through as checked baggage.

You must pack carefully as you decide on the type and amount of equipment you'll bring, and how much film and which accessories you'll need. Place fragile items deep inside the bag, far away from its vulnerable periphery. Put hard

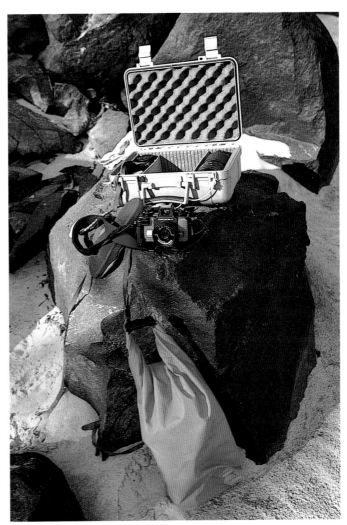

On Africa's Zambezi River I carried my non-waterproof Nikon gear in a Tundra SeaKing waterproof case and an REI waterproof bag. During the trip I kept my Nikonos V strapped around my neck and clipped to my life jacket.

objects against soft ones or against the padding of the camera bag itself to cushion them. Don't pack heavy items on top of lighter, more fragile ones. You'll probably find that you can get more in your bag if you pack the camera without a lens attached. When transporting your camera without a lens, make sure that you use a body cap.

When I reach my destination, I rearrange my gear to make it readily accessible when I'm actually shooting. For most situations, a good medium-size shoulder bag is my favorite choice. These bags have been improved remarkably during the last decade, and there is now one for all photographic needs. The hallmarks of a good shoulder bag are a well-padded shoulder strap, adjustable interiors, a dustproof lid closure system, a large film pocket, and a rigid, padded interior with a low-fashion Cordura exterior with Fastex buckles (Cordura is a rough-textured nylon material). Using the camera cradle or bridge is an intelligent way to keep a long lens in place for ready use and the camera well protected.

Avoid all stylish designer bags that scream, "Expensive cameras here!"; the uglier and older the bag, the better. Tan and gray are probably the best colors because light colors reflect heat, and bags have an unfortunate habit of standing out in bright sun more often than they should. Ballistic nylon on the backside of the camera bag helps protect your clothing from the abrasive rubbing of Cordura.

Lowe, Tamrac, Domke, and Tenba are all good brands. However, Tamrac has the best lid system, with an amply sized, Velcro-edged rain flap on its fully zippered and Fastex-buckled lid. I ordinarily use the Tamrac 709 Pro Convertible. It holds two cameras and six or seven lenses, and has a hip belt that I can tuck away in a rear pocket. I like built-in waist straps and shoulder harnesses because they make carrying equipment for long periods of time much easier—and less stressful for your body. I hope manufacturers continue to incorporate these two features into future bag designs, particularly in the larger bags that require extra carrying support.

The backpack convertible is a hybrid design that offers some of the best features of both hard cases and soft shoulder bags. The LowePro Photo Trekker is the largest of these cases and is a true backpack, offering a superb harness system for long hours of comfortable carrying. It just fits under an airplane seat and looks more like a backpack than a valuable-camera bag, especially if you take the labels off. This is a great case for backpacking and landscape photography, when you have time to set up shots and can safely put your gear on the ground while you work. However, the best backpack for outdoor photography often is a regular backpack with one or two fannypacks inside.

When I'm photographing I don't like to have my cameras on my back; I like them within easy reach without having to undo straps. Tamrac's PhotoPack has a unique design that successfully combines the qualities of a shoulder bag and a small backpack, complete with removable side pockets and a greater degree of flexibility. I like the concept but my Nikon F3 cameras with motor drives don't fit comfortably in the bag, and I get lost going through all the different pockets trying to find a particular lens. (I hope that Tamrac will continue to experiment with this design.)

When I take minimal gear with me, I like to use the Tamrac 636 Photo Traveler One. It is slim and unobtrusive and holds a surprisingly large amount of gear. The bag can also double as a briefcase or a purse. For short outdoor trips a fanny pack is a handy camera bag. It rides out of the way on your back, and then swings to the front for lens, filter, and film changes. I use one when I'm skiing, bicycling, or hiking.

Once you've arrived at your shoot, repack only the items you'll need for the specific subject you're shooting that day. Decide on your priorities in advance. Your shooting bag should be full, but not overflowing, and lighter. Try to have just a single layer of equipment. If that isn't possible, place your most-used items on top and keep your most-used lens mounted on the camera body. Support the lens with a lens cradle or similar device, especially if it is large. Distribute the weight evenly in order to balance the bag, and have it sit flat on the ground.

Be consistent and pack predictably, so you'll always know where everything is. Compartmentalize your bag; you want to be able to work by touch, whether you're removing or replacing equipment. Theoretically, you should be able to locate any item within your camera bag instantly without removing your eyes from your subject.

There are numerous other bags and excellent brands that might work better for you. Every photographer has his or her favorite system. Spend a couple of hours at your local camera store exploring the possibilities before you buy one.

FILM

Ten years ago deciding which transparency film to shoot was easy: the only real choice was Kodachrome. Now that Fuji has challenged the photographic giant, the choice is less clear and more controversial. But this has led to a dramatic rise in both the quality and the variety of film. I still primarily use Kodachrome 64 because it gives me the best balance I've found in terms of sharpness, speed, and archival properties. I usually rate it at ISO 80 for more saturated colors.

But I'm also beginning to use more Fuji Velvia. It has picked up huge accolades since its recent introduction. Some photographers consider it to be the finest landscape film available on the market. Its granularity equals that of Kodachrome 25, and its color saturation and separation of tones exceed those of Kodachrome 64 (although some people prefer Kodachrome's relatively muted colors). Fuji Velvia yields some of the most vivid colors I've seen while not picking up heightened contrast. It is, however, excellent at picking up details in shadows. Kodachrome 64's rendition of greens in shadow under a blue sky is poor, and the film turns most shadow detail to black in high-contrast situations.

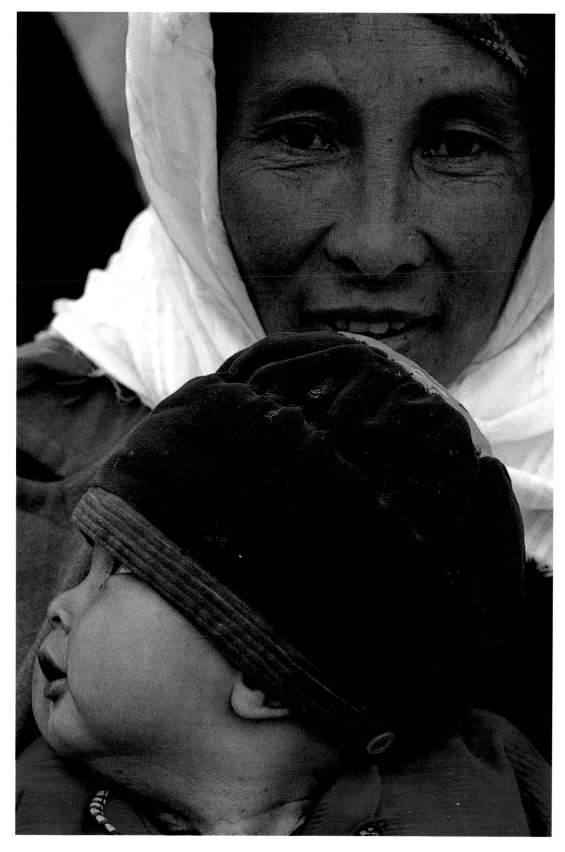

Traveling with friends through the Pamir Mountains in China's Xinjiang Province, I saw a group of people on horseback approaching me. When they stopped to make our acquaintance, I noticed this Kirghiz woman and her son. After she dismounted, I walked up to her and quickly photographed a series of shots while maintaining eye contact with her; the baby stared at his father. I like the combination of a full face and a profile, as well as the red and green framing the subjects in this image. Working with my Nikon F3 and an 85mm lens, I exposed for 1/60 sec. at f/8 on Kodachrome 64.

Velvia isn't recommended for people photography because the skin tones shift to red; Kodachrome and Ektachrome 64X (EPX) are better choices here.

Ektachrome 64X has a warmer tone and improved color saturation than regular Ektachrome 64 (EPR). EPX has both a color palette and saturation similar to those of Fuji 100, but EPX has a larger contrast range and warmer shadows. It is an excellent choice for people photography. Fuji 50 and 100 aren't as sharp as Kodachrome, and since they require E-6 processing they aren't as archivally stable. All E-6 films start to degrade after six years under realistic storage conditions. Fuji Velvia claims a 25-year life span, like Kodachrome, but there isn't any evidence to back this up. When tested, however, Fuji 50 and 100 were found to be more stable than Kodachrome for extended use with a projector or a lightbox. In rain and dim light, I like the romantic grain and muted colors of Kodachrome 200; this film can also be pushed to 400 with good results.

As to the question of whether professional film is better than amateur film, the answer varies from one photographer to the next. It depends on your preferences, the eventual use of your images, and the various circumstances you'll be working under. Professional film, which includes Fuji Velvia, isn't shipped until its optimal point: when its color rendition meets standards considered ideal by its manufacturer. It's delivered in refrigerated vans to the retailer, who keeps it in cold storage to prevent heat from accelerating the aging process. Since Kodachrome is notorious for its color shifts, I always use color-tested professional film from the same batch number (which I order from Fishkin Bros. in New York).

Professional film is perfect for people who work in studio conditions where they can keep the film refrigerated at temperatures below 55°F before and after use. But it isn't quite so perfect if you're traveling to the farthest reaches of the world. In that case, nonprofessional film is a better option because it

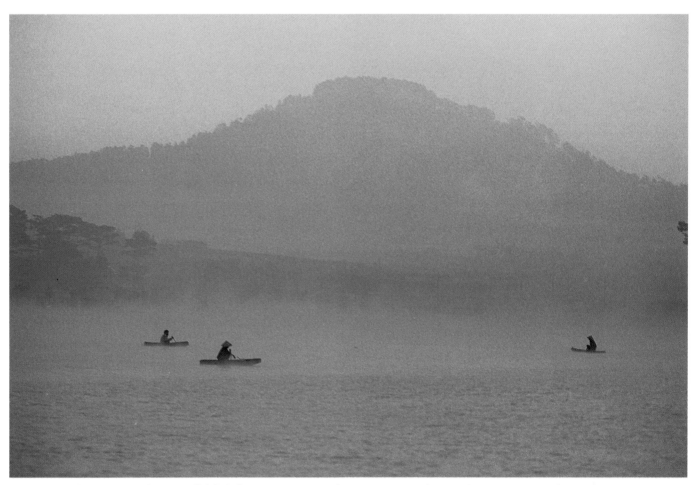

I rose very early to photograph two small fishing boats at sunrise over the Xuan Huong Lake in Dalat, Vietnam. I used my Nikon F4, a 180mm lens, and a tripod.

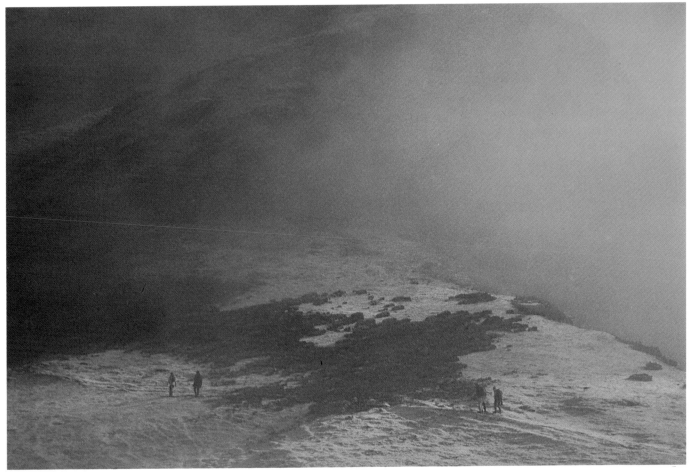

Returning to Chengdu, China, as the sun rose, I noticed these Tibetan sheepherders in the morning mist. With my Nikon F3 and a 35mm lens, I exposed for 1/60 sec. at f/4 on Kodachrome 64.

was actually designed to continue maturing to its peak performance level. The point when this film reaches its optimal color balance is typically one year before its expiration date.

Experiment with Fuji and Kodachrome, and choose the film that suits your specific needs and personal taste. Each has its own strength and weakness. There is an advantage to getting familiar with one film and using it as much as you can. The best exposures often result from long familiarity with the characteristics of a film.

I have yet to use print film for my work. For publication most magazine and book publishers prefer color-transparency film. However, if I were shooting only for myself, my family, and my friends, I'd readily make the switch. Unless you're dedicated to slide shows, transparency film usually ends up on the top shelf of your closet in cobwebs. With color-print film you can make photo albums that can be enjoyed over and over again. The past year has seen quantum leaps in the

technology and improvement of color-negative film. Kodacolor Gold, Kodak Ektar, and Fuji Reala are the films of choice in this category.

The pro-series Extapress Gold 100, 400, and 1600, excellent color-negative films for traveling photographers, are designed for storage at room temperature. Extapress Gold 1600 is specifically intended for push-processing. Even pushed to its limit of ISO 6400, it still performs remarkably well. For available-light photography in remote locations where flash isn't feasible or permitted, a few rolls of Ektapress Gold 1600 are indispensable.

A rule of thumb is to bring between 5 and 10 rolls of film per day for serious shooting. (You can certainly shoot less or more, especially if you're shooting for an assignment or stock.) I continually remind myself that film and processing are relatively inexpensive compared to my investment of time and effort.

WHILE YOU TRAVEL

There is more to photographing and traveling than being in an exotic location. You have to deal with the tedium of travel: finding a hotel, waiting for planes, and dealing with officials and permits. You have to meticulously take care of your gear from the moment you leave home. Inclement weather and unexpected dilemmas can foul up your travel plans and photographic equipment. Camera-repair technicians usually aren't available in remote locations. To avert disasters you have to anticipate possible problems before they occur. But if they do, you need the know-how and the tools to solve them.

AT THE AIRPORT

Following a few simple guidelines will make getting through the airport easier. For international flights arrive at the airport at least two hours before your flight's departure time. Never check your luggage at the curb; take it to the inside counter, and make sure that the luggage is tagged with the proper destination code. After I check in at the ticket counter, I immediately go to the security and X-ray inspection area. Although I rarely have bad experiences, I always give myself ample time in case the security guards insist on examining all my photographic equipment.

I prepare for this encounter before I arrive at the airport. At home I take all my film out of the boxes and out of the canisters. I put 50 to 60 rolls in one zip-lock, heavy-duty, gallon-size freezer bag, squeeze the air out, and seal it. Then I put it inside two or three more bags in the same manner, so it is well protected, minimizing the chance of puncturing the inner bag. I keep the film in my carry-on bag and put the film canisters inside my checked luggage. If I'm taking a large quantity of film, I take only about half of the canisters and recycle them.

When I get to the X-ray security check, I take the zip-lock bags of film out of my carry-on bag and put the cameras (I remove all film beforehand), lenses, and other items through the scanner. Without comment I hand the film to the security staff member for inspection. I try not to argue because I've found that it is more effective to use strong body language, looking firm and single-minded. If the inspector says the expected, "The X-ray is film-safe," I don't say a word. I just shake my head and hand over my film bags. I find this is usually enough encouragement, and the inspector then hand-checks my film readily.

I've never had any trouble with this method in the United States (inspectors are required to hand-check bags if asked to) and Asia, but at some foreign checkpoints, particularly in Europe, inspectors resolutely insist on X-raying your film if it isn't high-speed film. When this happens, I reluctantly let my film go through. Actually, despite all the dialogue on this issue, I know of very few situations where film has been damaged by an airport X-ray machine.

Evaluations show that after 150 cumulative exposures through a HI-CAT machine, no perceptible damage occurs to films up to ISO 400, color-slide films have less damage potential than color-negative films, and higher-speed films are more susceptible but still don't incur any visible damage after minimal exposure to HI-CAT scanners. I used to put my film in lead bags, such as a FilmShield bag, but they are heavy and bulky. I prefer the zip-lock-bag method. Also, since the machines can't see through the lead bags, in some countries inspectors crank up the power to see inside the bag, which nullifies the effectiveness of the FilmShield bag. Currently there are no foolproof measures that you can use to protect your film from being X-rayed, but never let your film go through as checked baggage. The dosage level of X-rays used on checked baggage might be 5 to 20 times higher than the carry-on-baggage screening level.

When I get to my destination I put the film back into the canisters for everyday use. Then when I've used a substantial amount of film, I remove the exposed film from the canisters and package them again in zip-lock bags so I am ready for my return flight. I then reuse the canisters for my next batch of film or discard them; of course, I recycle them if possible. Although this might sound like a lot of work—which it is—it is worth it.

CUSTOMS REGULATIONS AND PAPERWORK

Before leaving the United States you should register the camera gear you're taking with the United States Customs Service at a major international airport. This provides proof of your ownership, so you won't have to pay import duty upon your return. (For more information write for the free pamphlet entitled, "Know Before You Go," from United States Customs, P.O. Box 7407, Washington, DC 20044.)

Entering foreign countries is usually very simple and trouble-free. Most of the time I'm waved quickly through customs. You're allowed to bring in, without duty, all of your personal effects. This includes clothing, sports and travel equipment, personal appliances, camera gear, and film.

However, in some countries if you have a computer, video camera, or some other electronic item, it's recorded in your passport and you have to show the item upon departure to ensure that it wasn't left in the country duty-free.

When you return to the United States, you'll need to declare all items bought by or given to you. The first $400 of value is duty-free, and on the next $1,000 you must pay a 10-percent duty. Beyond this limit, the excess value of your goods is charged at full duty rate, which can range from 1 to 2 percent depending upon the merchandise.

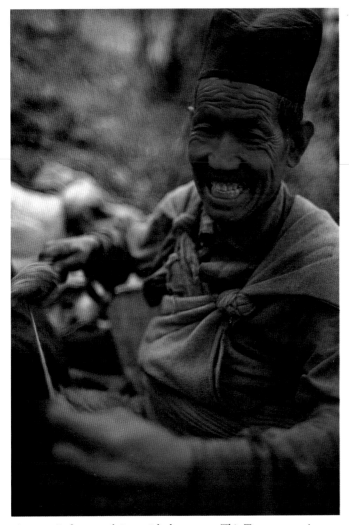

At camp I often spend time with the porters. This Tamang man is spinning hemp to make a new head strap for his doko, a basket used to carry loads. Since we were sitting under thick foliage, I shot at a low shutter speed, 1/15 sec., to ensure a workable exposure and to suggest the motion of his hands. With my Nikon F3 and a 35mm lens, I exposed for 1/15 sec. at f/2.8 on Kodachrome 64.

KEEPING JOURNALS AND CAPTION NOTES

Since I often take hundreds of rolls of film with two or three different cameras on a trip, I have to take meticulous field notes each day. I have a system that works well for me: I keep a daily chronological list of names, places, and other important caption information in a notebook. After I finish a roll of film, I label it with the date and the number of roll. For example, on July 18th when I finish my fifth roll of the day, I mark the film canister with a permanent marking pen, "7/18 #5."

Sometimes I use a microcassette tape recorder tucked in a photo-vest pocket or my camera bag, especially when I need to keep involved notes and I don't have time to write them down. I identify the roll and exposure number and speak into the recorder. You can record a lot more information more quickly onto tape than you can in a journal; usually two tapes are more than sufficient for one trip. Sometimes I transcribe the information from the tape at night into my notebook, or I wait until I get my processed film back at home. Then I play the tape back as I study the images on my light table, and transfer the information to the caption on the slide mount or on a separate piece of paper kept in my trip film journal.

OBTAINING MODEL RELEASES

In America many lawsuits against photographers arise because of a failure to have a model release when one is necessary. A model release is a document that basically says the person being photographed has given his or her consent not only to the taking of the photograph, but also to its use. The American Society of Magazine Photographers (ASMP) has sample release forms in its publication, *Professional Business Practices in Photography.* I use the forms included in that book as guidelines, and bring copies of my adult release and property release when I travel.

Whenever you include Westerners, particularly Americans, in a photograph that might be published, always get signed model releases at the time you take their picture. I usually show them the release and explain its need before I take the picture, but wait until after I've taken the photograph before I give it to them to sign. This way they know basically how they'll be portrayed in the photograph. If they refuse to sign the release, then I don't have much choice except to disregard that photograph.

If you plan to use your photograph for publication or stock, I think it is wise to have signed model releases from any people you photograph in a foreign city, no matter what their nationality or what the shooting situation is. (Even though lawsuits aren't currently common in the rest of the world, this might change.) Translate your release forms into the language of the country you'll be traveling and photographing in. In more remote regions it is a bit trickier to get signed model releases, and not always appropriate. People may be suspicious, confused, or frightened if they're asked to sign a piece of paper. Use your common sense.

PROTECTING YOUR EQUIPMENT FROM THE ELEMENTS

It is important to keep your film out of the sun and heat. When I travel to hot climates, I bring a cooler that holds all my film. I either carry the cooler on the airplane as one of my carry-ons or put it in my checked luggage inside a large duffel. Bring two ice packs, and keep a frozen one in the cooler at all times. If bringing a cooler is impossible, keep your film in the coolest place available, such as inside your sleeping bag, the hotel refrigerator, or a shady closet.

You must be constantly vigilant about keeping very fine sand and dust away from lenses and camera mechanisms. This is a particular concern in desert regions and high-altitude plateaus, such as Tibet, Ladakh, and the Middle East. Make sure all your film and lenses are protected from sand and grit. If necessary, keep your lenses in individual zip-lock bags. Pay special attention to preventing dust and sand from entering the back of your camera, or you'll find long scratches across your developed film. Getting dust into tripod works is almost unavoidable. Try to chose a tripod whose legs and locks tend not to trap sand, or that work in spite of this. I've had excellent luck with Gitzo tripods because they can be easily taken apart and cleaned.

In climates with inclement weather, I always carry a large assortment of plastic bags, trash bags, and zip-lock bags. They are the best and cheapest insurance against everyday encounters with water. You can drape one bag over your

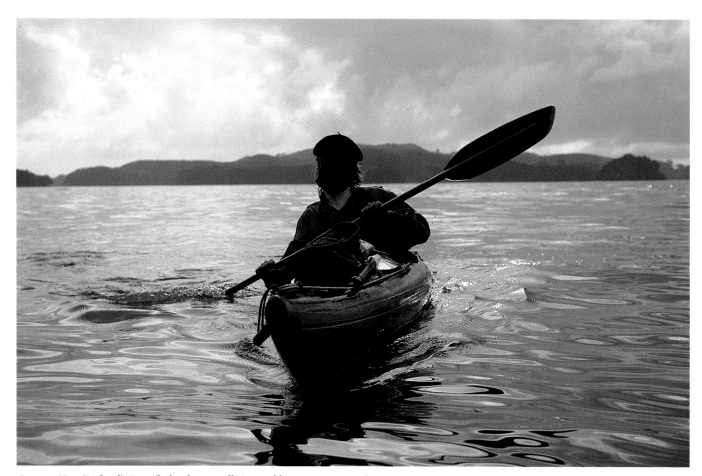

Because New Zealand's Bay of Islands was still, I was able to remove my Nikon N8008 and 80-200mm zoom lens from the case strapped on the front deck to get this shot.

camera bag for rain protection, and punch some armholes in a large trash bag for yourself. To make a temporary snow- and rain-resistant housing, slip your camera into a bag, make a small hole where you want the lens, stretch the plastic around the front of the lens protector, screw on a lens hood, and use a little duct tape to seal the edges. If you don't like sticking your head inside the plastic bag while shooting, remove the eyecup on the eyepiece, and repeat the procedure.

If too many raindrops get on the lens, tape an extension made out of cardboard or some other available material on the lens hood. Duct tape is always useful for customizing and repairing plastic bags, as well as making impromptu inventions. I usually find all sorts of situations where plastic bags and duct tape are indispensable.

Hard cases with shiny white or light-colored exteriors tend to reflect heat, which keeps the equipment (and film) inside cooler than black or dark ones do. Shoulder bags made out of Cordura or canvas should also be tan or gray. No matter what kind of bag you have, keep it and your camera out of the sun so that they don't become too hot and cook your film. Intense sun heats cameras quickly. I've touched black camera bodies that are too hot to pick up after just an hour in the sun. If there isn't any shade, place something reflective over the camera to minimize the heat.

Beware of leaving your cameras and film in a closed car. Temperatures inside will quickly soar past the safety point even in winter. I carry a small cooler complete with silicone desiccant and ice packs in my car to safeguard film. I also put my film inside zip-lock bags to protect it from moisture inside the cooler. Damp conditions also require paying special attention to film and equipment. Humidity softens the emulsion so that film becomes sticky, and condensation on a camera can seep into delicate mechanisms.

Adhering to some guidelines can also protect your equipment and film. First, keep rolls of film in their airtight containers until loading, and then try not to leave film in the camera for too long. To prevent mold and fungus from forming on your cameras or lenses, store your film and cameras in plastic bags (after you squeeze as much air from the bag as you can) with silica-gel packets. Silica gel is a crystalline compound that soaks up moisture, and changes color when fully saturated. It is usually available at a chemist's shop. Make sure you dry out the gel regularly, in the sun or in an oven. To avoid condensation when leaving air-conditioned areas, keep equipment wrapped in plastic bags until it warms to the ambient temperature. Finally, process film promptly.

Despite all of the precautions I take, I always carry an extensive repair kit with me. It is an indispensable part of my photography gear and contains: a set of jeweler's screwdrivers, needlenose pliers, a small wrench, a small pocketknife or a razor blade, lens-cleaning fluid and tissue, soft lint-free cloth, a pencil eraser for cleaning electrical contacts, a tool for extracting film leaders (this can be found in camera stores), cotton swabs for cleaning hard-to-reach places, super glue, garbage bags, tape, safety pins, rubber bands, twist ties, wire, string, and duct tape. Duct tape is the most well-used item in my repair kit. I keep some on my tripod legs, extra pens, and cable release.

CLEANING YOUR GEAR

When I am in the field I regularly clean my equipment, particularly in very dusty environments. I carry plenty of lens tissue, lens cleaner, compressed air (use the environmentally kind ones without Freon), and cotton swabs. Hold the camera and lens upside down while dusting, so dust falls away from them, not back on them. Use separate brushes for cleaning your lenses and camera bodies.

Most modern amateur cameras can go two to four years between professional servicing for normal use, but I usually end up abusing my cameras as much as I use them. As soon as I return from an extended trip or if I've been in an exceptionally harsh climate, I take my camera to a reputable camera-repair professional for a thorough internal cleaning and have its diaphragm, shutter, and exposure system checked. Older, all-mechanical cameras need professional cleaning, lubrication, and adjustment more often than modern, electronically controlled ones do. At home, I check each lens to make sure the screws are tight and the filters aren't scratched. Then I clean the lenses thoroughly.

If you aren't going to use your camera for a few weeks, remove the batteries and store them separately. This prevents the slight battery drainage that can occur if batteries are left in place, as well as removes the danger of battery-terminal corrosion.

SAFEGUARDING YOUR EQUIPMENT

From the moment you leave home until you return, you must be alert to the possibility of theft and take the necessary precautions to avoid making yourself an easy target. Not all areas of the world have the same risk factors. The highest-risk areas are in Latin America and India, and the lowest-risk countries are China, Japan, and the Muslim countries of Asia. However, don't let down your guard in so-called low-risk areas. Trouble always strikes when you least expect it to.

Your packing goals are to minimize your equipment and keep a low profile. A well-worn, somewhat-scuffed camera bag (remove the logos) isn't as noticeable as a pristine, polished leather case with an embossed "Hasselblad" or "Nikon" logo on the front.

If possible, don't put any of your valuable gear through as checked baggage at the airport. Unscrupulous airline employees have learned to recognize bright metal camera cases, such as Haliburton cases, as high-ticket items that bring a good price on the stolen-goods market. I know photographers who've shipped their large telephoto lenses in these cases without any trouble, but I wouldn't take the risk. If you must put some gear through as checked baggage, put the case inside a cardboard box or an old duffel. Most airlines won't cover the loss of camera equipment, even though anything else lost will be covered up to $1,000 or $1,200. Most airlines won't even sell you additional insurance coverage for cameras. However, some credit-card companies provide insurance if the airline ticket was purchased with the card.

Never reveal the contents of your bag to anyone (except when you go through customs or an airline security inspection). Keep your film in a separate compartment, so you won't have to show your cameras when you ask to have your film hand-checked. While you're waiting for the plane, don't leave your equipment unattended even for a moment. Keep it close to you, and wrap the bag strap around your wrist or ankle. Never ask a stranger to watch your bag while you go buy a cup of coffee.

An alternative is to send your equipment by air freight. In case of loss or damage, your gear is then insured. To collect, you must be able to show proof of the original purchase and have receipts for replacement equipment. Federal Express and Next Day Air service by the United Parcel Service (UPS) are also possibilities for shipping, but are expensive.

As you enter a hotel lobby don't advertise that you have expensive cameras with you. Keep your equipment in its bag. Leaving film and equipment in your hotel room can be as risky as taking it with you everywhere you go. This is a personal choice. So if you feel more comfortable having your equipment within sight and it is a manageable amount to carry, it is probably better to carry it with you. You can also put your camera in the hotel safe; just make sure that you get a receipt.

If you're traveling on a small budget and staying at the least-expensive hotels, then you have to be perpetually on your guard. Often the locals aren't a threat, but other travelers are. Don't advertise the fact that you have expensive cameras

by indiscriminately telling locals or fellow travelers that you are a photographer. When you leave your hotel room in dubious-security situations, lock your cameras in your suitcase or duffel. Then, for added protection, hide the bag in the closet under your dirty clothes or in the shower with the curtain drawn. If you are in an extremely high-risk area, chain your suitcase or hard camera case to a pipe or a secure post with a bicycle lock and chain. If you're staying in a higher-priced hotel, you should have more security. Still I make a habit of keeping my photographic equipment out of sight.

On the street or trail, I wear the shoulder strap of my camera bag diagonally over one shoulder and walk away from the curb so that no one can grab the bag off my body. I find the waist strap of the Tamrac Pro Convertible shoulder bag invaluable, not only for weight distribution, but also for security. I carefully fasten the belt around my waist and drape an arm around the case, holding the bottom. This helps to keep the weight off my shoulder and ensures that no thief can possibly yank the bag away from me. Wear inconspicuous, inexpensive clothing, and be aware of the people around you.

Most of the time I try to keep the zippers closed and buckles fastened on my shoulder bag. However, when I'm working at a fast pace and changing lenses often, I leave the top unzipped—but I always keep the Fastex buckles closed. When I put the camera bag down, I try to keep it close to me with a hand on the strap or around my shoulder or foot. Even when you feel confident, your gear might not be safe. Loose equipment on a table top or chair is an open invitation to theft.

Probably the most important precaution you can take is to insure your equipment adequately. While a standard homeowner's policy covers most of your possessions while traveling, there are often strict limitations when it comes to photographic equipment. Study your policy carefully to see how well you're covered. Many insurance companies sell floater policies for more expensive equipment. But keep in mind that these policies usually apply only to amateur photographers. If you use your photo equipment to earn money, you might need to take out a separate commercial policy, and these premiums can be quite high. Often photographic trade organizations offer lower group-rate insurance to their members.

PROTECTING YOURSELF

A trip can be delayed, curtailed, or terminated if you lose your money and passport. It is absolutely essential to keep them secure. I split my money into two or three different Eagle

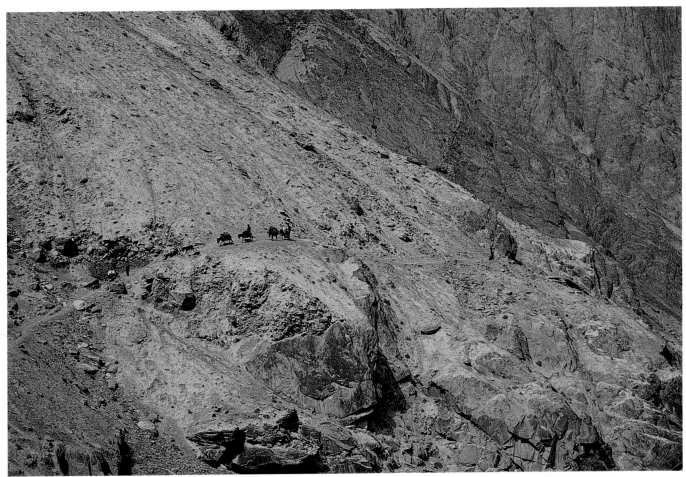

My companions and I traversed the foothills of at the Qaratash Gorge in the Pamir Mountains in China's Xinjiang Province to reach a few isolated villages. Because I was ahead of the pack horses and mules, I turned around to photograph this scene. I used a 50mm standard lens on my Nikon F3 in order to minimize the caravan in proportion to the landscape. The exposure was 1/250 sec. at f/8 on Kodachrome 64.

Creek "undercover" pouches: a waist pouch, a neck pouch, and for truly crime-ridden areas, a leg pouch. Nevertheless I've been pickpocketed a couple of times in China and South America. But since I never have more than small bills in my most accessible wallet, I've never experienced a true disaster. I have one friend who sews inside pockets into all her traveling clothes. She has never lost a dime; thieves would have to rip her apart to find any money. Keep a separate record of all your credit-card numbers and other important information. Bring photocopies of the first two pages of your passport and of any important visas. And I always have a few extra passport-size photographs with me.

I also bring a few of my favorite teas, soups, granola bars, and chocolates for those moments when sea slugs and chicken feet are the only items on the menu. Patience is a virtue, but being comfortable while being patient is even

better. In my daypack I carry a collapsible chair called "The Chair." It triples as the internal frame for my daypack, a pad for my camera gear, or best of all, a chair for me to sit on during those long hours outside waiting for the alpenglow. If you're limited in terms of weight and space, you might want to bring a ½-inch-thick ensolite pad that fits inside your camera bag instead.

Dress warmly. The weather changes quickly in the mountains; you can be pelted by hail one minute and overheated by intense radiation the next. The right clothes let you stay out in the elements in comfort. Make liberal use of modern fabrics and fills, such as Gore-Tex, Capilene, Thinsulate, and Bunting. Dressing in layers provides the warmest protection. Fingertip-less gloves or extra-thin liner gloves are helpful when you're working with cold metals and you still need to manipulate intricate camera features.

WHEN YOU RETURN

There is a bittersweetness to coming home after a long trip. I am always anxious to see my friends and a good movie, and to develop my film. But it isn't always easy to make the abrupt transition from walking in the Himalayas or riding across the plains of Mongolia to living my comparatively mundane existence in the United States. Suddenly the cinemascopic events are reduced to memories and pieces of celluloid. This change can be unnerving.

To me, coming home means hard work at my desk, indoors; it certainly isn't romantic. Being out on the road meeting people and coming across unusual situations and events is fun, but the real work associated with adventure-travel photography takes place in your office. It isn't simply a matter of selling travel photographs. The business of photography is 20 percent taking pictures and 80 percent marketing them. Magazines and publishers rarely come to you; you have to court them.

Whether you're interested in selling your photographs or just plan on producing a photo album or slide show, you'll find that both require thought, careful editing, and a pinch of tenacity.

I shot this spectacular view of Kangchenjunga Peak at sunset from a high viewpoint in Darjeeling, India. I'd been looking for a spot above the telephone wires and finally, at last light, I found a hill above town that provided this perspective. Shooting with my Nikon F3 and a 180mm lens steadied on a tree, I exposed for 1/125 sec. at f/4 on Kodachrome 64.

I made this portrait of a Tibetan woman at the Gonga Shan monastery in China's Sichuan Province. She'd just finished making some bread, and I coaxed her outside to take her portrait. I shot with my Nikon F3 and an 85mm lens, and exposed for 1/60 sec. at f/5.6 on Kodachrome 64.

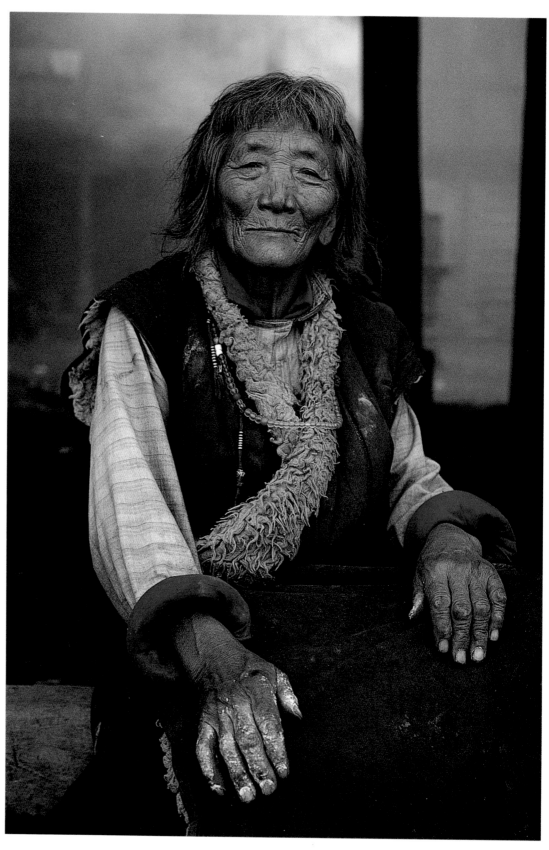

EDITING YOUR PHOTOGRAPHS

Editing and captioning slides are my least favorite aspects of photography. However, I've disciplined myself to begin the task as soon as the slides come back from the processing lab. Although I keep daily notes about my slides during my trip (sometimes written, sometimes taped), there is always some information that isn't recorded. The longer you wait to caption your slides, the greater the chance of valuable caption information being lost in your fading memory.

When the boxes of processed film arrive, first I count them to make sure I've received them all. If not, I locate the missing film-receipt stub from the mailer and contact Kodalux or the lab. Then I arrange the boxes chronologically according to the dates written on the name label. Next, I begin my preliminary edit. I spread the contents of each box on a 2 × 6-foot color-corrected Acculite lightbox, and examine each slide with a 4X Schneider loupe. (A loupe is a magnifying eyepiece used to examine slides on a lightbox.) I quickly sort through each box and toss out the obvious "no-goods." Since I sometimes use two or three camera bodies as well as different films in one day, I also have to rearrange the similar slides so that they're all grouped together.

After this first cursory edit, I start over and begin the process of fine-editing, captioning, and sorting my slides. I use a computer and caption-writing software to label my slides as I edit them. I separate them into various piles: one for assigned magazine articles, one for my stock agency, one for my personal files, and one for my portfolio. I also keep a slide projector set up so if I'm having trouble deciding on certain slides, I can run them through the slide projector and get a bigger and better viewpoint.

Throwing out slides is very cathartic. I used to hold on to every exposure and angle, afraid that I'd misjudge a slide and

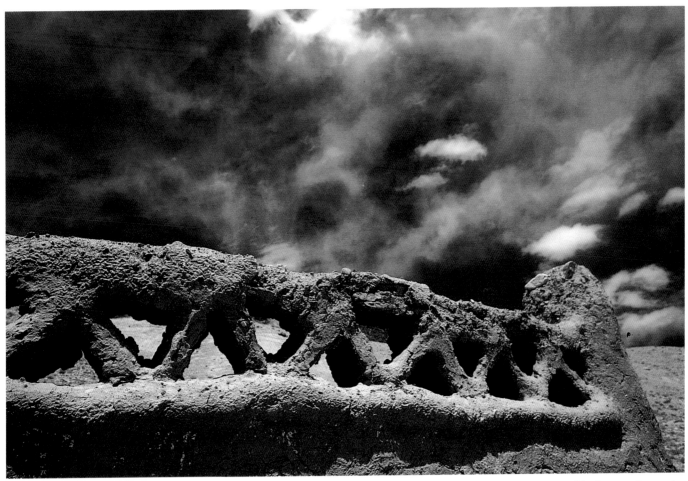

Shooting with my Nikon F3 and a 24mm lens in Tajikistan, I focused on the top section of an ancient mud tomb. I wanted both to emphasize the design and to punctuate the vast expanse of the sky. The exposure was 1/125 sec. at f/11 on Kodachrome 64.

throw out an undiscovered masterpiece. I've since learned to trust my judgement. Now I enjoy throwing the rejects into the trash basket. But before I toss them away, I study each slide to know why it is a reject. I ask myself if I could've prevented its failure, and how. I'm not completely ruthless about discarding slides. Some slides might not be aesthetic award winners, but they might have important historical, personal, or behavioral value.

I keep only slides that are tack-sharp. Spare your friends and editors fuzzy slide presentations. For wildlife and people shots, check the eyes first; if they are sharp, the slide is still a contender for the files. If only part of a slide is in focus, it means the shutter speed was adequate but that the focus or depth of field was off. If nothing is sharp, generally there was camera or subject motion because of, for example, a too-slow shutter speed. A slide doesn't have to be sharp from edge to edge; sometimes the most interesting image is partially blurred. But this is an aesthetic choice, not a technical one. Keep only your best slides. Although it is tempting to keep less-than-perfect pictures, eventually they become liabilities by cluttering your files. Your final selections should be sharp, exposed properly, and interesting.

EDITING EQUIPMENT

There are two types of light sources for editing slides: light tables and slide sorters. Light tables are usually flat, with some capability for an upward tilt, and contain one or more fluorescent lamps depending on their size. The better light tables are color-corrected but expensive. Slide sorters are ribbed to hold rows of between 40 and 80 slides at about a 45-degree angle. They're illuminated by household light bulbs, so they aren't color-corrected.

The main consideration for sorting slides is the intensity of illumination, whether it is from a light table or a slide sorter. Check the intensity of your light source with a light meter. It should read 1/125 sec. at f/5.6-8 at ISO 100. The optimal color temperature should be 5000K and have a color rating index (CRI) of 90 or more. Besides a quality light table, you need a good-quality loupe that covers the entire image, such as the Schneider 4X loupe. It is essential for editing slides. Hoya recently introduced an excellent, and considerably cheaper, 4X loupe.

After I finish editing my slides, I caption them. A computer slide-labeling program is indispensable. I use the Cradoc CaptionWriter. Essentially it works like this: you type the information you want on each slide into the computer and give the print command. The information is then transferred to the slide labels in your printer. This is neater, quicker, and more professional than writing information on the slide by hand. There are many different slide-labeling programs on the market.

Some are very basic and only create labels for slides. Others are sophisticated systems for pros who need to catalog and retrieve slides, as well as keep track of billing and accounting.

STORING YOUR PHOTOGRAPHS

When color films are processed, exposed silver is exchanged for the color dyes that make up the image. Some of these dyes are less stable than others. When a dye fades or bleaches away, the remaining colors dominate. Some color films are more archivally stable than others. Although Kodachrome has the best long-term archival-storage properties, Ektachrome and Fujichrome have better light-storage longevity than Kodachrome. If I'm going to frequently project an image in slide shows, I make E-6 dupes. And, naturally, a print hung on the wall in the light has a considerably shorter life span than one stored in the dark.

The conditions under which you store your photographs are very important. Heat and humidity have a profound effect on photographic stability. Store your prints and slides at room temperature, 68°F at about 40-percent relative humidity. If you live in a humid climate, storing your photographs in an air-conditioned room is best. If this isn't possible, do the best you can by investing in a dehumidifier for the hotter months and avoiding storage in areas subject to severe temperature swings.

The dyes in color materials are also adversely affected by storage in certain albums, sheets, boxes, and cabinets. I avoid storing my slides in polyvinyl-chloride (PVC) slide sheets. Instead I use ones made of polypropylene or Mylar, usually labeled as "archival." If you've stored your slides or negatives in the older PVC or glassine storage pages, replace them now.

I store my slides in metal file cabinets, using secretarial hanging folders and archival file folders. I make sure that I don't stuff each drawer too full; I don't want my slides pressed tightly against each other. Be sure to avoid certain wooden cabinets whose varnishes and formaldehyde can ruin emulsions, print albums with sticky adhesives, and cardboard storage boxes that aren't archival. There is a vast number of archival-storage products on the market. It is worth spending a few more dollars today to protect your photographs for future enjoyment.

PRODUCING A SLIDE SHOW

A slide show can be a great ending to any trip, but creating an interesting presentation requires thought and a lot of editing. Narrow your choices to the most informative, best-exposed, in-focus, and stunning slides. A short production, one or two trays, is enough for the average attention span of an audience. Some people make a complete audiovisual production, with music and sounds accompanying the slides.

PRODUCING AN ALBUM

Even though you might shoot transparency film, you can still have prints made from slides at a local photography store or by a less-expensive mail-order company. This process costs a bit more than making prints from negatives, but the advantage is that you can pre-select your images. Another possibility is to bring along a pocket-size point-and-shoot camera in addition to your better cameras for "album possibilities." Just be sure to edit, edit, edit. Keep your selection minimal, informative, humorous, and dazzling. Many of my friends keep an album

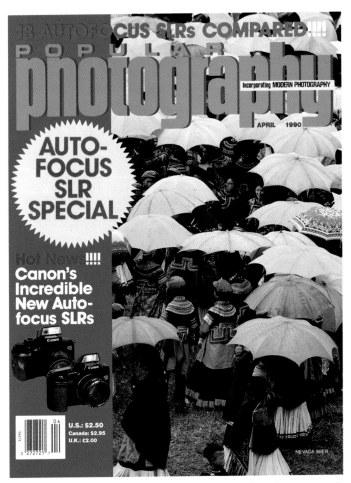

My photograph of participants at the Yi Torch Festival in China appeared on the cover of the April 1990 issue of Popular Photography magazine.

for each trip in a bookcase. These albums are well thumbed and appreciated by all curious arm-chair travelers.

However, you can also venture beyond the standard photo album into an uncharted creative domain. I have one friend who makes an extraordinary picture album/scrapbook/journal for each journey; they are masterpieces of travel reportage. She uses a small, unruled bound book with high-quality paper. She writes as she travels, jotting down conversation and observations, pasting in mementos (ticket stubs, menus, newspaper articles, napkins, and business cards), and reserves space for the photographs she inserts after she gets home. Journals and photographs can be combined in countless creative ways.

SELLING YOUR PHOTOGRAPHY

Making photography your primary source of income calls for good business sense, marketing skills, tenacity, and, finally, photographic skills. Take a serious, critical look at the quality of your photographs, and count the number of excellent images you see. Then scrutinize your commitment to devote time to pursuing more of the same. If you honestly feel that you'd like to pursue photography professionally, be aware that you have an exciting but long road ahead of you.

Begin pursuing your dream in your spare time. Get a copy of the latest edition of *The Photographer's Market*, and look up magazines and stock houses that specialize in the type of photography you actually produce—not what you want to produce. Contact these firms by mail, and ask for submission guidelines. You'll probably receive an impersonal form letter. If the intended marketplace is receptive to new work, it might ask you to submit a number of images for consideration. These should be examples of your very best work that you think fit the needs of the specific magazine or stock house. If asked to send your portfolio, select only the highest-quality originals; they should be sharp, perfectly exposed, and thoughtfully composed. Send your portfolio by certified mail or an express-mail service. Some clients might request duplicate slides instead of originals; make sure that they, too, are top quality.

All of this takes time. Art directors and picture editors have very full days and must interrupt their schedules to look at your portfolio. Don't start telephoning before a reasonable length of time has elapsed. And don't be depressed if your work's rejected. That is the nature of the business. Your "tenacity quotient" counts. If being a travel photographer is what you really want and you can cope with an erratic life and income, welcome to the world of adventure, exploration, and travel.

The opening spread for an article I wrote for the July 1988 issue of Discovery magazine is shown on the left. The other three spreads reprinted here show images that capture the lives of the Tibetan cowboys.

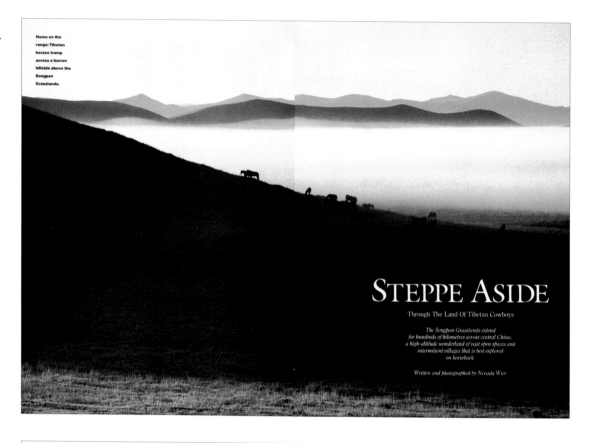

Home on the range: Tibetan horses tramp across a barren hillside above the Songpan Grasslands.

STEPPE ASIDE

Through The Land Of Tibetan Cowboys

The Songpan Grasslands extend for hundreds of kilometres across central China, a high-altitude wonderland of vast open spaces and intermittent villages that is best explored on horseback.

Written and photographed by Nevada Wier

WE ARRIVED IN ZOIGE IN OCTOBER. IT WAS an odd Chinese town. People gathered around pool tables on the main street instead of lounging in the usual tea shops. Swarthy Tibetans in thick yak coats rimmed with fake leopard fur, sent pool balls slamming wildly across the old warped tables. Their horses stood placidly beside them, reins tucked securely into the players' leather belts. An intense, high-altitude sun pierced the cool air and the streets smelled of horses, yak butter and incense. Characterless and rather ugly concrete houses flanked the streets, in stark contrast to the colourful excitement of bargaining, gossiping, pool playing and eating that was taking place around them. Outside the town the grasslands stretched off in the distance, a golden undulating sea.

Politically speaking, we were in the Sichuan province, but geographically we were on the eastern edge of the immense Tibetan Plateau, home for several Chinese cultural groups, but mainly populated by Tibetans. At 3,660 metres, Zoige is the gateway to the Songpan Grasslands, a carpet of short grass that extends for hundreds of kilometres. Only a few foreigners have visited this dusty town. It's difficult to find on a map, and even if you found it you'd need special permission to stay there.

Michael and I had been travelling companions on several expeditions in China. While in Chengdu we became intrigued by the possibility of exploring the northwest frontier of Sichuan on horseback, a region not visited by Westerners for over 30 years. Spurred on by fantasies of riding with Tibetan cowboys, we pitted ourselves against the Kafkaesque Chinese bureaucracy.

"Nothing is easy in China," a valuable motto I've come to swear by. Using every gram of *guanxi* — otherwise known as "connections" — we had acquired in our four years of travelling and guiding in China, we were able to procure this precious travel permit. Immediately we stuffed a van with tents, camping equipment, food and Double Happiness beer, then drove two days from Chengdu to Zoige in the company of a Chinese driver and two liaison officers, Mr Li and Mr Lin. Now all we needed was a guide and a few horses, and Mr Lin assured us they would be easy to find.

Unfortunately, horses and guides were not available; we had arrived a week too late. All the Tibetans were cutting hay and fattening their horses for the long winter that was beginning to sweep down from the north. As I said, nothing is easy in China. By the same token, I had also learned that nothing is impossible either. After a friendly dinner with Zoige's minis-

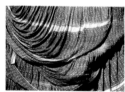

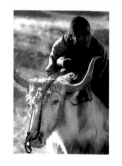

Above: A youthful Yellow River twists and turns through Songpan. **Above left:** Pattern of faded Buddhist prayer clothes in Hongyuan. **Left:** The Tibetans routinely utilize their yaks for transportation.

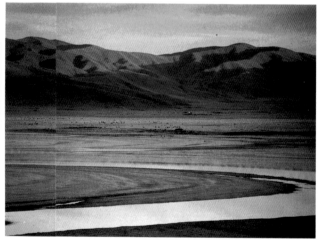

ter of foreign affairs, many toasts to cooperation and exclamations of infinite friendship, we heard that the Chinese army might be persuaded to lend us horses. And, as Michael could speak passable Chinese, it was decided that a local guide would suffice.

Next morning we were introduced to Lau Ma, a sullen-looking fellow, our guide. The day before he'd been a truck driver for the People's Liberation Army; today he was a horsepacker stuck with two foreigners for a week. And he was dazed with disbelief.

We were on our way at last — almost. We had permission, we had a guide and horses, now we needed a route. Our plan was to spend a week riding north to Lamusur on the Gansu border and then

back. Lamusur was the epicentre of tantalizing rumours about traditional Tibetan culture and huge Buddhist monasteries, but it wasn't on either of our maps. One was a photocopy of an army map, in Chinese characters. The second was a copy of a copy of a Sichuan map from an unremembered source. Our Chinese friends sketched a circle on one of our maps in a blank spot that seemed to represent the grasslands, wrote in "Zoige" and "Lamusur," then proudly announced our route. As things transpired, Lamusur was Lau Ma's hometown; he'd know how to get there.

A few hours later the horses arrived in the courtyard of our green cement guesthouse. They seemed high spirited and nervous, at least to my concerned

eyes. The truth of the matter was that neither Michael nor I were good riders. Actually, the real truth was that Michael had been on a horse once and I only a few more times than that. The Chinese didn't know this, and we certainly weren't going to tell them at this point. We both subscribe to the "learn-by-doing" philosophy.

We mounted our wary horses, assuming an outward countenance of confidence and skill. The entire population of Zoige — lamas, merchants, pool players, yaks, bundled babies and dogs — gaped at our undignified departure. Michael's knees were up to his ears, as there had been no time to adjust the stirrups. My reins were too short. Our baggage horse looked increasingly unhappy. Suddenly the awkward load shifted and slid side-

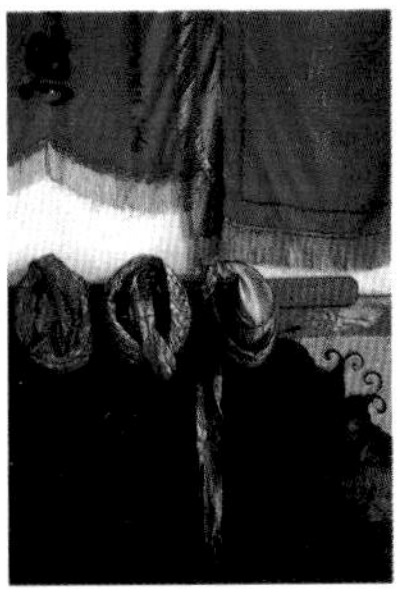 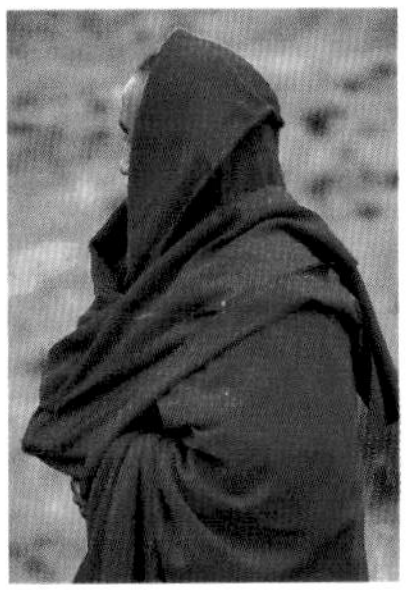

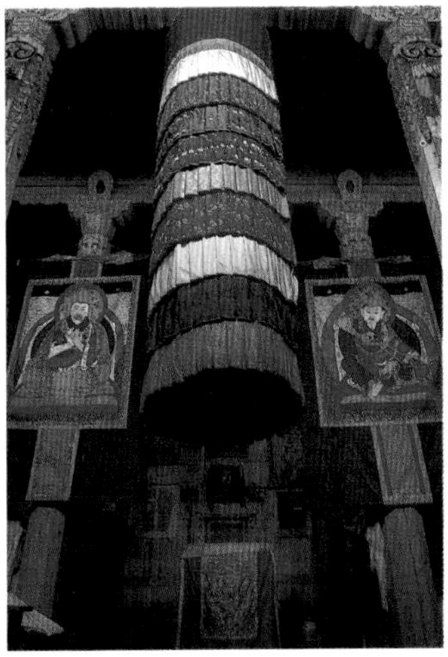

ways, strewing our belongings along the road. The amused onlookers covered their white teeth with weathered hands and laughed. Lau Ma soothed the frightened horse and bound up the load a little tighter. We waved and rode out of town.

*

Our route followed a meandering stream across a broad valley with swamps and uneven mounds of grass, sabotaging our attempts to take a direct track. We wove to the right, away from the swamps, then left, away from the yak herders' camps guarded by fierce mastiff dogs. Michael and I grinned at each other. We had done it: we were riding in the Sichuan grasslands.

We ambled through a Tibetan village festooned with long white prayer flags and encountered the wildest looking Tibetans we'd ever seen. Matted black hair was twisted in braids around their heads, fastened with turquoise rings, and silver-cased knives swung easily from their waists. They bore themselves with a bold insouciance and flashed wide smiles at us. They were real horsemen. They knew how to ride — horses or yaks, saddle or no saddle, it didn't matter.

The following day it took a long time to make that indispensable cup of morning tea. The wind, wild and energetic, blew out our camp stove every five minutes. You soon get the impression that this wind feels the plateau is its personal playground and anything that dares to cross is fair game. Relentless, it can drive men mad, and also horses I suppose, considering our current predicament: three of our four horses had run away. They had bolted from their stakes and were desperately heading for the solace of home. The fourth, our exhausted baggage horse, was not in the mood for running. He had merely trotted in the opposite direction in pursuit of fresher grass. Lau Ma frantically snatched the horse's reins and flew off, bareback, into the grasslands. There was nothing we could do, so we decided to have some more tea.

A few minutes later two Tibetans rode nonchalantly into our dismantled camp. Word was already passing from village to village that we were here. Having never seen a foreigner before they were compelled to visit. After initial greetings, the two sunbaked Tibetans sat down among our partially packed gear and accepted some tea. Their yak coats enveloped them like big warm houses. First their eyes and then their hands began to roam over our possessions with eager interest — plastic buckles, bright yellow nylon, cameras . . . zippers! They reminded me of children playing with treasured toys.

One of the Tibetans picked up a novel lying on Michael's pack and stared at the back cover photo of a white-bearded man with an amused smile. He pointed at the portrait and looked quizzically at Michael. "Hemingway," said Michael. "Hem-ming-way," the Tibetan repeated perfectly, staring at the photo. The two Tibetans glanced at each other and laughed, nodded and grunted their approval. One of the Tibetans held the book and stared at the photograph gravely. He continued to stare at the book, muttering "Hem-ming-way," then solemnly raised the book to his forehead in a reverent salute.

Before Michael could explain the true nature of the photograph he was interrupted. In the distance, a horseman with three riderless horses approached us at an easy lope. Lau Ma was back and he looked tired. The horses had gone most of the way back to Zoige; he had been chasing the renegades for three hours. It was already afternoon, but with the help of our Tibetan friends we packed the sweaty horses and rode off towards a distant row of dim blue mountains.

Far left: Traditional Muslim-style hats on the wall of a Lamusur mosque. _Left:_ Tibetan monk wrapped in the robes of his order. _Above:_ Inner sanctum of a monastery in Lamusur, once the fulcrum of Tibetan Buddhism in the Songpan region.

The two Tibetans stayed with us until their camp of yak-hide tents came into view. With sweeping gestures they insisted it was late and we should spend the night in their camp. It was tempting: we would probably sit around a warm fire and drink Tibetan yak-butter tea and laugh. But we decided that it was imperative to make up for lost time. The sun was sinking low between dark clouds, spreading honey-yellow light across the valley. We glanced back at the two Tibetans trotting towards their camp — each held a picture of their god-king outstretched before them.

By morning our world was an opaque white. Peering out from our dome tent, we could just see four shadowy figures in white felt coats, on white horses. The riders, all of them women, bent low, belly to belly with their wet horses, to peer into our tent. Seeing two blond, blue-eyed Westerners wrapped in red-and-purple nylon, they immediately began to laugh — Tibetans always laugh. Actually, Tibetans are the most amiable souls on this planet (with the meanest, snarliest dogs as balance). They live over three kilometres above sea level in a windy, barren, bitterly cold environment and I suspect that laughing keeps them warm and sane.

After pacing around our camp for a few minutes inspecting our gear and breakfast of leftover rice, the Tibetan women disappeared as silently and mysteriously as they had come.

*

For four days we rode — six to eight hours a day, often at a slow walk as the terrain was uneven and marshy. Our recalcitrant horses resigned themselves to the journey. My knees ached from being constantly bent and Michael resorted to sitting on a foam pad to relieve the hardness and deformity of the Chinese cavalry saddle. Aside from these minor unpleasantries, we were content and grateful that we were on tolerant horses. And we felt extremely cavalier in this aloof, romantic country.

The grasslands rolled out around us in a series of shallow yellow valleys and low green hills. We rode over trackless ground, occasionally crossing a narrow dirt road. The air was crisp and crystalline; winter was coming. We passed a few small villages, yak camps and families moving their belongings to winter pasture. There's a lot of space on the Tibetan Plateau, which is about the size of Western Europe but populated by only six million people and countless yaks.

Lau Ma had resigned himself to the journey. He was a Muslim from the Hui minority group in China, but his true allegiance was to trucks. "I drive big trucks," he often told us. He thought it was ridiculous to be riding to Lamusur when one could drive there faster.

Besides wondering why we wanted to travel to what he considered as the far side of the planet, riding between poor forgotten villages, he was concerned about our choice of food. According to Lau Ma, our mode of travel demanded two kinds of food in voluminous quantities: rice and *tsampa*, the Tibetan mainstay, a paste made from ground barley. Tibetans thrive on it, shovelling it into their mouths with great gusto. Our dinners of Chinese noodles with tomato sauce convinced him that all the stories about disgusting Western eating habits were true.

On the fourth morning we met a composed Tibetan boy on a black horse. We were almost to Lamusur. Once over a pass in the jagged hills confronting us, the northernmost point of the blank spot on our map was only an hour away. The boy conferred at length with Lau Ma, describing the route in detail, and escorted us up the narrow valley. As we began to ascend the hills, the boy stopped to water his horse in a small creek. We kept moving and as the distance between us lengthened, he suddenly sang out in a loud and sonorous voice. His thin arm was raised high, wishing us luck and a good journey. The sweet, melancholy song reverberated through the canyon, gradually fading as we moved up the gravel slope.

"We'll be in Lamusur soon," said Lau Ma offering a cigarette to Michael. Practically all the men smoke, and it's considered very polite to offer a cigarette to someone you've just met and to keep proffering them throughout the conversation. Michael doesn't normally smoke, but he took one and lit it.

Lau Ma smiled and pointed straight ahead, "Lamusur."

"What's Lamusur like?" Michael asked.

Lau Ma shrugged, "Dusty."

From a distance Lamusur looked unremarkable. It appeared to consist of post-Cultural Revolution architecture, sombre and boxy, typically clashing with the local minority culture. At closer inspection, however, it gave the impression of a place immensely intriguing.

We trotted into town, aware of the silent scrutiny cast in our direction from windows and doors. One wizened old man squinted his eyes at me, broke into a toothless grin and waved. As we moved through the narrow, muddy streets, we passed stones carved with the Tibetan Buddhist symbols for *Om Mani Padme Hum* (a mantra meaning "Hail to the jewel in the heart of the lotus"), and strewn with prayer flags, tattered and grey from years of blowing prayers to the unyielding wind. Row after row of shiny new golden prayer wheels lined the sides of the streets. On the hillsides all around the town, mammoth Tibetan monasteries were being constructed. In their various stages of development they looked like giant cocoons about to hatch. A tall green minaret loomed over the centre of town. This was Lau Ma's hometown. Half Hui, half Tibetan; half Muslim, half Buddhist; half in Sichuan province, half in Gansu province.

*

Lamusur was once the centre of Tibetan Buddhism for Sichuan, Qinghai and Gansu provinces. Then, in 1966, Mao Zedong launched the Cultural Revolution. For ten years the country plunged into madness attempting to purge itself of "bourgeois" elements. The minority areas were particularly hard hit. In Lamusur, all the monasteries were plundered and destroyed. Some relics were hidden and saved, but most went up in flames.

The rebuilding of Lamusur began in 1978 when the Chinese Government eased their policy of cultural hegemony and began allowing more religious freedom throughout China. Over ten monasteries are now in the process of being reconstructed. Everything is being built by hand. Even the lumber is being painstakingly shaped with hand tools from crude logs. We were impressed by the scope of the project and the complete devotion it required.

A coterie of lamas in long red robes accompanied us onto the construction site of one of the larger monasteries. We estimated that over a thousand people would fit comfortably in the main room. The smell of freshly sawed timber mingled with incense burning from small black pots. An enormous Buddha sat in a hieratic attitude on a wooden altar, a huge gilded figure looming out of the dimness. The oldest and most treasured relics rested at its base, some encased in glass, and photos of previous reincarnates hung on the front wall. It wasn't the largeness and ornateness that impressed me — there are much bigger, more opulent monasteries in other Tibetan towns — it was the overwhelming effect of seeing so many of them being diligently built at the same time so close together.

Later that day we followed the lamas to a forested canyon on the west end of town. Through it flows the White Dragon River, the head waters of one of the nine major tributaries to the Chinese mother river, the Yangtze. "The mouth of the canyon is holy," said the eldest lama. "A dragon once lived in one of the caves, a lion in another. Centuries ago the lion rode the dragon across the canyon. Here, where the lion landed, you can see the marks made by his claws." The lamas gently pressed a palm or a forehead to the series of gouges in the limestone cliff, expressing a silent devotion.

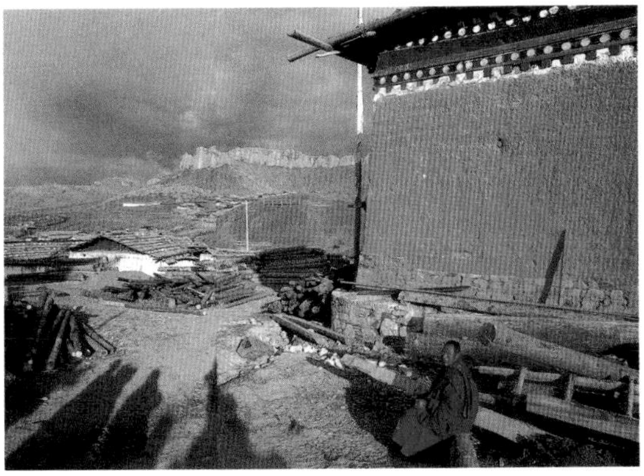

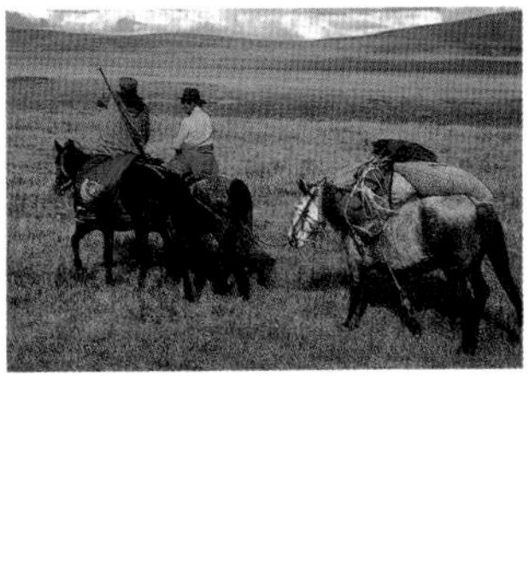

Above: At least ten Buddhist monasteries are being refurbished in Lamusur. _Right:_ Lau Ma leads the horse-trekking party across the grasslands.

Inside the cave, squatting in the darkness, was a large bulbous stalagmite, declared to be the only female Buddha in Tibet. The lamas walked deftly up to the base and rubbed the slippery rock. Outside the cave we were shown other important markings, such as a boulder that bore the signs of Buddha's feet. "This is where he hitched his horse," said a lama pointing to a natural rock handle in the canyon wall. "If you throw a rock in this hole you will have good luck," said the youngest lama, gesturing at a baseball-sized hole in the wall above us.

A day later, we ambled through the streets of Lamusur, buying turquoise-hued plastic hats, black felt boots and Himalayan snuff in the small shops that lined the main street. A black-veiled woman in sturdy shoes strolled past us, dragging her child which was mesmerized by our presence. A bent, grey-haired Tibetan woman waddled in the opposite direction, gumming devotions as she methodically rubbed her prayer beads. Around the corner were the ubiquitous ratty pool tables and Tibetan pool sharks.

That afternoon we rejoined Lau Ma, who had taken the horses to the outskirts of town to graze. We drank jasmine tea and ate preserved vegetables while plotting the route back to Zoige. I was looking forward to getting back on my horse, eager to feel again the slow rhythm of riding, back to meeting people in a leisurely manner, on their own terms. Lamusur had become another stop along the trail, another moment and place to be savoured. Every day had been perfect in its own way, and I knew the journey back to Zoige wouldn't be any different.

An American adventure holiday firm offers horseback tours of the Songpan Grasslands for those who have neither the time nor inclination to make their own arrangements. For more information contact Boojum Expeditions, 2625 Garnet Avenue, San Diego, California, USA 92109; tel: (619) 581-3301.

Cathay Pacific has seven flights a week between Hong Kong and the cities of Shanghai and Beijing, from where there are connections to Sichuan province.

Nevada Wier *is a freelance writer and photographer based in Santa Fe, New Mexico, who has spent much of the last four years exploring little-known parts of China.*

RESOURCES

ADVENTURE - TRAVEL COMPANIES *

Afro Ventures
P. O. Box 2239
Randburg 2125
Republic of South Africa
011-27-11-789-1078
011-27-11-866-1524
Fax: 011-27-11-886-2349
*Canoeing on the lower
Zambezi River, Zambia, and
other African safaris*

Boojum Expeditions
14543 Kelly Canyon Rd.
Bozeman, MT 59715
406-587-0125
*Horseback-riding expeditions
to the Tibetan Grasslands,
Mongolia, and Central Asia*

Innerasia Expeditions
2627 Lombard St.
San Francisco, CA 94123
800-777-8183
415-922-0448
*Travel to Central Asia,
Mongolia, Patagonia, and
other exotic destinations*

Intertreck
P. O. Box 126205
San Diego, CA 92112
800-346-4567
619-259-1552
Fax: 619-259-1552
*Trekking in the Pamir
Mountains in Tajikistan*

Mountain Travel/Sobek
6420 Fairmount Ave.
El Cerrito, CA 94530
800-227-2384
415-527-8100
Fax: 415-525-7710
*Rafting the Zambezi River,
going on safari in Africa,
trekking in Nepal or Vietnam,
and traveling almost
anyplace else on the globe*

New Zealand Adventures
11701 Meridian Ave. N.
Seattle, WA 98133
(206) 364-0160
Sea kayaking in New Zealand

Sourdough Outfitters
P. O. Box 90
Bettles, AL 99726
907-692-5252
*Dog-sledding trips in the
Brooks Range in Alaska*

* *For a more complete listing
of adventure-travel outfitters,
consult the "The Active
Traveler" directory in the back
of* Outside *magazine. For a
listing of adventure-travel-
photography workshops consult
the "Travel and Workshops"
directory in the back of*
Outdoor Photographer
magazine.

OUTDOOR GEAR

Eagle Creek
1665 S. Rancho Santa Fe Rd.
San Marcos, CA 92069
619-471-7600
800-874-9925

Lowe Alpine Systems
P. O. Box 1449
620 Comptorn
Broomfield, CO 80020
303-465-3706

Marmot Mountain Works
827 Bellevue N.E.
Bellevue, WA 98004
206-453-1515

Roy McClenahan
P. O. Box 313
Eldorado Springs, CO 80025
303-494-1408
*(Custom-made frontal
packs for hiking and skiing
photographers)*

The North Face
999 Harrison St.
Berkeley, CA 94710
510-548-1371

Patagonia
1609 W. Babcock St.
P. O. Box 8900
Bozeman, MT 59715
800-638-6464

REI
P. O. Box 88126
Seattle, WA 98138
800-828-5533

INDEX